Hospice and Palliative Care for Companion Animals

Hospice and Palliative Care for Companion Animals

Principles and Practice

Second Edition

Edited by

Amir Shanan, DVM
Founder, International Association for Animal Hospice and Palliative Care
Compassionate Veterinary Hospice, Chicago, IL, USA

Jessica Pierce, BA, MTS, PhD.
Center for Bioethics and Humanities, University of Colorado, Anschutz Medical Campus
Denver, CO, USA

Tamara Shearer, MS, DVM, CCRP, CVPP, CVA, MSTCVM
Western Carolina Animal Pain Clinic
Sylva NC, USA
Shearer Pet Health Hospital, USA

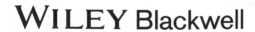

Library of Congress Cataloging-in-Publication Data
Names: Shanan, Amir, editor. | Pierce, Jessica, 1965– editor. | Shearer,
    Tamara S., editor.
Title: Hospice and palliative care for companion animals : principles and
    practice / edited by Amir Shanan, Jessica Pierce, Tamara Shearer.
Description: Second edition. | Hoboken, NJ : Wiley-Blackwell, 2023. |
    Includes bibliographical references and index.
Identifiers: LCCN 2022037174 (print) | LCCN 2022037175 (ebook) | ISBN
    9781119808787 (paperback) | ISBN 9781119808794 (adobe pdf) | ISBN
    9781119808800 (epub)
Subjects: MESH: Pets | Animal Diseases | Hospice Care | Palliative Care |
    Human-Animal Bond | Veterinary Medicine
Classification: LCC SF981 (print) | LCC SF981 (ebook) | NLM SF 981 | DDC
    636.089/6029–dc23/eng/20220826
LC record available at https://lccn.loc.gov/2022037174
LC ebook record available at https://lccn.loc.gov/2022037175

Cover image: © Anna Kraynova/Shutterstock, Lenar Nigmatullin/Shutterstock
Cover design by Wiley

Set in 9.5/12.5pt STIXTwoText by Straive, Pondicherry, India

Printed and bound by CPI Group (UK) Ltd, Croydon, CR0 4YY
C004935_100323

Contents

List of Contributors

Kristina August, DVM, GDVWHM, CHPV
Harmony Housecalls
Ames, IA, USA

Cheryl Braswell, DVM, DACVECC, CHPV, CHT-V, CVPP
Regional Institute for Veterinary
Emergencies & Referrals
Chattanooga, TN, USA

Mark D. Carlson, DVM
Stow Kent Animal Hospital
Kent, OH, USA

Nathaniel Cook, DVM, CVA, CVFT, CTPEP
Chicago Veterinary Geriatrics
Chicago, IL, USA

Kathleen Cooney, DVM, CHPV, DACAW
Companion Animal Euthanasia Training
Academy (CAETA)
Loveland, CO, USA
Caring Pathways
Windsor, CO, USA
Colorado State University
Fort Collins, CO, USA

Christle Cornelius, DVM, CHPV
Fair Winds Pet Hospice
Galveston, Texas, USA

Shea Cox, DVM, CHPV, CVPP
Founder, Medical Director, BluePearl
Pet Hospice
Temecula, California

Coleen A. Ellis, CT, CPLP
Founder, Two Hearts Pet Loss Center
Certified in Pet Loss and Grief
Companioning
Southlake, TX, USA

Mary Ellen Goldberg, CVT, LVT, SRA-retired, CCRVN, CVPP, VTS-lab animal-retired, VTS-Physical Rehabilitation-retired, VTS-anesthesia/analgesia-Honorary
Independent Contractor, Canine
Rehabilitation Institute
Boynton Beach, FL, USA

Emma K. Grigg, PhD, CAAB
Lecturer and Staff Research Associate,
University of California, Davis
Davis, CA, USA

Betsy Hershey, DVM, DACVIM (Oncology), CVA
Integrative Veterinary Oncology
Phoenix, AZ, USA

Suzanne Hetts, PhD, CAAB
Animal Behavior Associates, Inc.
Sun City, AZ, USA

Laurel Lagoni, MS
Co-founder, Argus Institute
Colorado State University Veterinary Teaching
Hospital
Co-owner, World by the Tail, Inc.
Fort Collins, CO, USA

Beth Marchitelli, DVM, MS
4 Paws Farewell Mobile Pet Hospice, Palliative
Care and Home Euthanasia
Asheville, NC, USA

Jessica Pierce, BA, MTS, PhD
Center for Bioethics and Humanities
University of Colorado Anschutz
Medical Campus
Denver, CO, USA

Gail Pope
President, Founder, and Educator,
BrightHaven Center for Animal Rescue,
Hospice and Holistic Education
Founding Partner, Instructor, and Mentor,
Animal Hospice Group
Palm Desert, CA, USA

Carol Rowehl, LVT, MAR, STM
Adjunct Chaplain, Hospital of the University
of Pennsylvania
Philadelphia, PA, USA

Amir Shanan, DVM
Founder, International Association for Animal
Hospice and Palliative Care Compassionate
Veterinary Hospice
Chicago, IL, USA

**Tamara Shearer, MS, DVM, CCRP, CVPP,
CVA, MSTCVM**
Smoky Mountain Integrative Veterinary Clinic
Sylva, NC, USA

Chi Institute Faculty
Reddick, FL, USA

Western Carolina Animal Pain Clinic
Sylva NC, USA

Shearer Pet Health Hospital, USA

Mary Beth Spitznagel, PhD
Department of Psychological Sciences
Kent State University
Kent, OH, USA

Alice Villalobos, DVM, FNAP
Pawspice and Animal Oncology
Consultation Service
Hermosa Beach, CA, and Woodland
Beach CA, USA

Tammy Wynn, MHA, LISW, RVT, CHPT
Founder and Owner, Angel's Paws, LLC
Cincinnati, OH, USA

Acknowledgments

Amir Shanan

To my parents, who taught me creativity and resilience, and whose lifelong struggle with grief and post-traumatic stress prepared me for my life's calling.

To my wife, the love of my life, thank you for half a century of friendship, love, support, and sacrifice.

To the books that taught me so much about emotions in human and non-human animals – *The Human–Animal Bond and Grief, Mental Health and Well-being in Animals*, and *The Emotional Lives of Animals* –and to (books' authors), the pioneering scholars and authors who eloquently articulated the concepts underlying the mission of Animal Hospice and Palliative Care (AHPC).

To Tina Ellenbogen, Kathryn Marocchino, Coleen Ellis, and Kathy Cooney who helped me lay the foundation of AHPC as an important new field in veterinary medicine and companion animal care.

And to my Co-editors and professional soul mates, Tami Shearer, and Jessica Pierce – thank you for your friendship, support, and guidance throughout the years.

Jessica Pierce

To Ody and Maya, who each in their own way helped me better appreciate the profound challenge and gift of taking that last walk with someone you love.

To Bella, who demonstrates adaptability and optimism in the face of life-altering disability.

To my mother, who showed me how the dying can dwell in possibility.

To my father, who was the most devoted and generous caregiver I can imagine.

To my husband and daughter, who are everything.

To my colleagues and friends in the world of animal hospice – your work on behalf of animals and their people inspires me every day.

To the many caregivers of animals who have shared their stories of pain, struggle, small triumphs, and beauty, and who understand the sacredness of human–animal friendships and the profound importance of a good and meaningful death.

To Amir and Tami, the best collaborators one could ever hope for. It has been an honor working with you both.

Tami Shearer

The support of many family members, friends, and colleagues set the stage for my contributions to this textbook.

To my parents, sister, and brother who were always there when I needed them.

To my late husband, for his tolerance and patience of being married to a veterinarian and his acceptance of the many animals that shared our home throughout the years and were instrumental in my pursuit of hospice and palliative care.

I would like to thank my past and present staff and clients who have inspired me to work hard on their behalf to find solutions to preserve the human–animal bond and prevent distress.

Professional thanks to my special mentors Drs. Don Van Vlerah, Azaria Akashi, Alice Villalobos, and Huisheng Xie who shaped my philosophy of care and improved my ability to treat my patients.

A personal thanks to Amir Shanan and Jessica Pierce who without their dedication and support this publication would not be possible.

From all of us:

We would like to thank Merryl Le Roux, Susan Engelken, Erica Judish, and the rest of the team at Wiley for their hard work on behalf of this project. We are grateful for your dedication to this book.

1

Introduction

Jessica Pierce, BA, MTS, PhD

A paradigm shift is under way in how we understand and relate to companion animals. Although neglect and poor treatment are still endemic to pet keeping, a growing number of guardians seek to provide their animals with everything they need to be healthy and happy, including good, quality food; proper socialization; ample physical and mental stimulation; and thoughtful veterinary care during all life stages. As people integrate animals into their families, they are paying more attention to the physical needs of their companions. They are also increasingly attentive to their companion's emotional and behavioral well-being.

At least some of the changes in how people view and relate to companion animals are a result of evolving ideas not just about the human–animal bond, but about animals themselves. Over the past several decades, a tremendous surge in research into animal cognition and emotions has altered our understanding of who animals are, which has led to a much greater appreciation of their intelligence, emotional sensitivity, and sociality. We now understand, for instance, that a whole range of animals, including fish and birds, feel pain in much the same way as humans. We also understand that all mammals – and perhaps other taxa as well – have the same repertoire of basic emotions as humans and many of the same patterns of social attachment. This scientific knowledge is gradually translating into a greater sense of responsibility for animals and an appreciation of all the good care that this involves for an animal. An example of this translation is the fact that nearly all discussions of well-being now pay attention not only to physical comfort, but also to the emotional and social needs of companion animals.

An outgrowth of this changing paradigm of animals and human–animal relations is that pet guardians and veterinarians are giving greater attention to the final stages of life. When animals are highly valued members of a family, it is only natural that people would strive to provide loving care even as an animal becomes elderly, sick, or otherwise near the end of life. Caregivers and veterinarians are challenging what they see as unnecessarily stark choices: allow an animal to suffer or euthanize; provide aggressive curative treatment; or do nothing. Hospice veterinarians are broadening the possibilities for providing care and helping pet caregivers take a proactive role in making sure animals are eased more gently through their final months, weeks, days, and hours. Furthermore, veterinary teams increasingly recognize that the death of a companion animal can be a source of both meaning and profound suffering for people, and as a result, they are looking for ways to make the dying process less painful not only for the animals, but also for their human families. The provision of home-based care allows animals and families a greater measure of privacy and comfort. Finally, hospice veterinary teams are paying attention to the details of death itself, whether it occurs over time and is supported by palliation, or whether euthanasia is the ultimate end point, and are helping caregivers honor their animals through ceremonies, memorials, and aftercare.

In human medicine, end-of-life care has undergone a metamorphosis. After decades of misunderstanding and fear, hospice has been firmly embraced by the public and by health professionals as a sensible and compassionate alternative to intensive, cure-oriented, hospital-based care. Palliative care, which focuses on pain and management of symptoms both in the context of curative treatments and hospice care, finally became a board certified subspecialty of internal medicine in 2006. A similar transition is now occurring within the veterinary realm: more and more veterinarians are interested in offering clients a broad range of end-of-life options, and many are specializing in hospice care and in the treatment of pain.

Hospice care and palliative care represent two separate though overlapping modes of care within human medicine; within veterinary medicine, they are comfortably paired – at least for now – and will likely develop as a single intertwined entity. Although there is currently no certification or advanced training in animal hospice and palliative care, it is our hope that this possibility will eventually be realized in the veterinary field. This book represents a step in this process, by officially introducing the field of Animal Hospice and Palliative Care (AHPC) and providing what we hope will be an indispensable text for hospice and palliative care practitioners.

Four core philosophical concepts lie at the heart of human hospice philosophy, as developed by Cicely Saunders, one of the leading voices of the early hospice movement. These concepts stand at the core of animal hospice, too. And building from these core concepts, the field can work to develop consensus over how these values can best be served.

1) Dying is a meaningful experience. The experiential process of dying involves all aspects of personhood (emotional, physical, spiritual, and social) and can be deeply meaningful, for the dying and for their loved ones.
2) Dying takes place within a system of interrelationships and a network of shared meanings. Care should support relational structures, not disrupt them.
3) Hospice takes an expansive and holistic view of the nature and relief of suffering. Saunders used the phrase "total pain" to reflect that suffering is not just physical, but also psychological and relational. When it is not possible to eliminate the physical causes of pain, the goal becomes to keep suffering below the level of phenomena experienced by the patient.
4) Care should seek to protect the integrity of the patient and allow the patient to live in ways that honor what they find most valuable and meaningful in their lives (Kirk 2014, p. 43).

Animal hospice and palliative care is an inherently moral practice, embodying in its philosophy and practice this basic set of values. It is also an area of heightened ethical complexity: the potential for prolonged life must often be delicately balanced against the potential for suffering, and decisions often have life or death consequences for an animal. As Kirk and Jennings note, ethics is more than just discussing or settling disagreements about right and wrong; it is also about "creating moments of stillness and introspection, allowing teams to identify and explore resonances and dissonances...." and finding "ways of bringing the values, hopes, and fears of team members from the background to the foreground so they can be discussed, explored, addressed" (Kirk and Jennings 2014, p. 4).

As ethicist Courtney Campbell points out (in the context of human hospice), the language we use embodies – either consciously or not – a set of values. Which phrase is chosen makes a big difference (e.g. physician-assisted suicide, physician-assisted death, aid-in-dying, or death with dignity). "One important task for hospice ethics," says Campbell, "is conceptual clarification and movement toward consensus on terminology" (Campbell 2014, p. 231). The development of an increasingly nuanced vocabulary for animal hospice and palliative care is also vitally important. The term "euthanasia" is a very blunt instrument. It carries negative connotations in human medicine; likewise, in the context of animals, the term has a huge variety of applications, not all of them salutary. Furthermore, "euthanasia" doesn't allow moral distinctions between, for example, killing a healthy animal and offering a very sick animal relief from intractable and prolonged suffering. AHPC practitioners sometimes use, instead, "veterinarian-assisted death" or "veterinary aid-in-dying" (VAD) to describe the process of humanely taking the life of a suffering animal. The phrase "natural death" similarly lacks precision and carries unwanted associations. "Hospice-assisted natural death" is a great improvement. The thoughtful choices made by the authors of the chapters in this volume contribute to the evolution of a useful and morally precise vocabulary for the field of AHPC.

The philosophical core of AHPC needs to coalesce, but the ways in which AHPC is practiced need to spread and grow, like seeds of change being carried by the winds. Many different models of care need to be developed and refined, and as practitioners innovate they need to share what they learn. There are practical and financial challenges to building a multidisciplinary care team, just as there are unique difficulties in providing mobile, home-based services. Even medically, there is a great deal of work to be done in understanding how to help animals die comfortably. Because it is so rare for companion animals to die a natural death, we don't know as much as we could about the dying process or care of the terminally ill. AHPC promises, over the next decade, to become one of the most vibrant, exciting, and important areas of veterinary medicine.

References

Campbell, C. (2014) Moral meanings of physician-assisted death for hospice ethics. In: Hospice Ethics: Policy and Practice in Palliative Care (eds T.W. Kirk and B. Jennings). Oxford University Press: New York, pp. 223–249.

Kirk, T.W. (2014) Hospice care as a moral practice: exploring the philosophy and ethics of hospice care. In: Hospice Ethics: Policy and Practice in Palliative Care. (eds T.W. Kirk and B. Jennings). Oxford University Press: New York, pp. 35–58.

Kirk, T.W. and Jennings, B. (2014) Hospice Ethics: Policy and Practice in Palliative Care. Oxford University Press: New York.

Further Reading

Quill, T. and Miller, F.G. (2014) Palliative Care and Ethics. Oxford University Press: New York.

2

What Is Animal Hospice and Palliative Care?

Amir Shanan, DVM and Tamara Shearer, MS, DVM, CCRP, CVPP, CVA, MSTCVM

Abstract Animal Hospice and Palliative Care (AHPC) is a rapidly evolving field of animal health care. It has its roots in human hospice care philosophy, striving to keep seriously ill animals as comfortable as possible and to minimize their suffering as they approach the end of life. AHPC also addresses the emotional, social, and spiritual needs of the human caregivers in preparation for the death of the animal and the subsequent grief.

A small group of innovative professionals began to educate veterinarians in the mid to late 1990s about the concept of hospice for animals. Founded in 1997, the Nikki Pet Hospice Foundation (NPHF) was the first organization in the United States dedicated exclusively to promoting the benefits of animal hospice. Veterinarian Dr. Tamara Shearer opened the first veterinary establishment solely dedicated to hospice care, Pet Hospice and Education Center in Columbus OH, in 2003. In 2008 the first International Veterinary Hospice Symposium, sponsored by NPHF, convened in Davis, CA. In 2009 Dr. Amir Shanan founded the International Association for Animal Hospice and Palliative Care (IAAHPC). The IAAHPC published the *Guidelines for Recommended Practices in Animal Hospice and Palliative Care* (IAAHPC 2013) in 2013 and launched the first post-graduate training program for veterinarians and veterinary nurses/technicians in 2016.

Human and animal hospice differ in that animal patients cannot express their preferences verbally and therefore depend on a human caregiver to serve as the patient's proxy decision maker. Human and animal hospice also markedly differ in their position on euthanasia. Lastly, third party payors are the norm in human hospice, allowing the provision of more, and more diversified, services than currently available in animal hospice.

AHPC is an emerging field, in need of continued constructive debate about underlying ethical principles, and in need of development of evidence-based best practices for the benefit of animal patients and their human caregivers.

Keywords: Animal Hospice and Palliative Care, AHPC, emerging field, human hospice, hospice philosophy, Nikki Pet Hospice Foundation, International Association for Animal Hospice and Palliative Care, IAAHPC, third party payers.

Introduction

Animal hospice and palliative care are rapidly evolving fields of animal health care. They have their roots in human hospice care philosophy on the one hand, and in the increasing recognition of the human–animal bond on the other. The terms "hospice" and "palliative care" are distinct but interrelated. Palliative care seeks to increase comfort and minimize the suffering of patients at any stage of disease, to give the patient and family a voice in prioritizing the goals of medical care, and to address the patient and family's social, emotional, and spiritual needs in addition to treating the patient's physical discomfort. Hospice is a system of delivering palliative care to terminally ill patients. Its mission is to minimize the patient's suffering in living and dying, and to support patients and their families through a peaceful and meaningful dying process. Within veterinary medicine, the two forms of care are intimately linked, and for philosophical and practical reasons, this newly emerging field is often referred to as "animal hospice and palliative care." For definitions of some of the key terminology see Box 2.1. For a more complete

---

Box 2.1 Definitions of selected animal hospice and palliative care terms.

Animal hospice: A philosophy and/or a program of care that addresses the physical, emotional, and social needs of animals in the advanced stages of progressive, life-limiting illness, or disability. Animal hospice care is provided to the patient from the time of a terminal diagnosis through the death of the animal, inclusive of death by euthanasia or by hospice-supported natural death. Animal hospice also addresses mental health – the psychological, emotional, social, and spiritual needs of the human caregivers in preparation for the death of the animal, and subsequent grief. Animal hospice care is provided by an interdisciplinary healthcare team under the supervision of a licensed veterinarian.

Animal hospice team: An interdisciplinary team of providers working together to support animal patients and their caregivers through the animals' dying process and after death. In addition to a licensed veterinarian acting as its medical director, the team may include veterinary nurses, technicians and assistants, veterinary and non-veterinary providers of physical, rehabilitation, complementary and alternative therapies, as well as mental health professionals, pet sitters, pharmacists, chaplains and spiritual guidance counselors, community volunteers, and others as required for individual cases.

Animal palliative care: Like human palliative care, animal palliative care guides caregivers (the animals' human family members or owners) in making plans for living well based on the animals' needs and concerns and on the caregivers' goals for care. It also provides caregivers with emotional and spiritual support and guidance. Palliative care is of special significance in the context of terminal illness and end-of-life care; when cure has been determined to be unachievable and relief of suffering takes center stage in caring for the patient. It is a constant and foundational component of the animal hospice philosophy.

Caregiver: The caregiver is the animal's owner, and any others involved directly in the animal's daily care and in decision-making surrounding the animal and his or her health care. The term "Caregiving Family" may be used to designate multiple people assuming responsibilities of ownership and care.

Hospice-supported natural death: Hospice-supported natural death is natural death that is supported with palliative care measures, including the treatment of pain and other signs of discomfort.

Natural death: Natural death proceeds in its own time without euthanasia, accident, or an act of violence.

Source: International Association of Animal Hospice and Palliative Care.

glossary of animal hospice and palliative care terminology see the Glossary section at the end of the International Association for Animal Hospice and Palliative Care's *Guidelines for Recommended Practices in Animal Hospice and Palliative Care* (IAAHPC 2013).

Animal hospice and palliative care seeks to keep seriously ill animals as comfortable as possible and to minimize their suffering as they approach the end of life. As such, it is perfectly aligned with the veterinary oath. Care is provided to the patient from the time of a terminal diagnosis until the peaceful and meaningful death experience of the animal, by euthanasia or by hospice-supported natural death. Animal hospice also addresses the emotional, social, and spiritual needs of the human caregivers in preparation for the death of the animal and the subsequent grief. Unresolved and complicated grief, including grief over the loss of a beloved animal, is a common human mental health problem associated with significant and prolonged suffering. Animal hospice care minimizes the risk of unresolved grief resulting from pet loss. As such, it makes an important contribution to human public health, again in line with the veterinary oath.

Hospice and palliative care provide a practical alternative to premature euthanasia. They also provide an alternative to prolonged animal suffering, either in the isolation of intensive care, under the crushing burden of futile attempts to cure what cannot be cured, or at home with inadequate treatment. The provision of care by an interdisciplinary team is a central tenet in delivering both palliative care and hospice care. Supervision by veterinarians with expertise in palliative and end-of-life care is paramount to ensure that the most effective, humane, and ethical medical treatments are provided to animals receiving hospice care. Goals of care are defined by the animal's caregivers in collaboration with the attending veterinarian. Participation of expert non-veterinary animal

hospice team members is also vital to adequately serve the complex needs of animal hospice patients and their caregivers.

This chapter will give a brief description of the development of animal hospice as a defined field of animal care and a future specialty in veterinary medicine and will briefly compare and contrast human and animal hospice and palliative care.

History of Animal Hospice

Scientific and Philosophical Roots

Animal hospice and palliative care evolved as a philosophy of care and a system for delivery of services for seriously ill and dying patients, lagging behind but strongly influenced by the remarkable success of human hospice and palliative care. This is similar to other fields within veterinary medicine that, over the past 50 years, have used new technologies and advanced, specialized training to bring many of human medicine's innovations into veterinary practice.

Offering companion animals "human grade" medical care has been driven by the human–animal bond – the increasing recognition among humans during the last several decades that the relationships they form with nonhuman animals can be emotionally profound and mutually beneficial. The term "human–animal bond" was articulated in the 1970s by ethologist and Nobel laureate Konrad Lorenz and psychologist Boris Levinson (Hines 2003). It was brought into the veterinary world by Leo Bustad. With this recognition, increasing numbers of humans have been willing to invest significant resources (e.g. time and money) to preserve the bond by maintaining their animals' well-being to the best of their abilities. The intimate relationship with companion animals also facilitates recognition of animals' identities as individuals, with unique reactions to and interactions with the world around them.

The human hospice movement developed in response to concerns about the poor quality of care for terminally ill and dying patients in human healthcare systems during the mid to late twentieth century. By that time, an astounding procession of scientific discoveries and technological innovations had significantly changed both daily life and human life expectancy in western societies. To provide access to the new disease-fighting technologies, hospitals replaced the family doctor as the basic institution providing care. Care for the dying moved from the home into the hospital. The psychological, social, and spiritual needs of patients and families were largely ignored, and discourse or information about death and dying were often avoided. The hospice movement emerged to advocate respect for the needs of dying patients and their families, recognizing the importance of their emotional, social, and spiritual needs, and providing patients with relief from their physical, mental, and spiritual pain. Kubler-Ross' book *On Death and Dying* (1969) brought professional and public attention to grief as a normal and significant emotional reaction to loss, spawning the development of social services to support individuals experiencing grief and bereavement.

The animal hospice and palliative care movement has roots in this same social movement to acknowledge that aggressive curative treatments were not the "solution" to death, and that what the dying and their families really need is *care*. This care needs to be holistic, attending to the physical, psychological, and spiritual needs of the dying, and broadening the notion of who is the object of care to include the patient's family. Parallel to the human hospice movement, animal hospice brought attention to pet owner grief and bereavement as a normal and significant part of the death of an animal.

Animal hospice and palliative care also has roots in ethology, particularly in the study of animal cognition and emotion. During the 1960s and 1970s, new knowledge and ideas were gradually changing scientific and societal attitudes toward animals. For example, researchers recognized individual differences between animals of the same species, opening the door to understanding each animal as a unique "person" with unique preferences and needs. Research into animal cognition, affective neuroscience, and comparative psychology gradually established a significant body of data on animal emotions. The evolving animal welfare movement acknowledged that animals have feelings and psychological needs that deserve to be respected with the publication of the list of "five freedoms" in 1979 by the UK Farm Animal Welfare Council. These scientific disciplines have helped shed light on how to care for ill and dying animals by helping practitioners and caregivers understand behavior as a reflection of an animal's internal experiences, which might otherwise remain inaccessible or hard to interpret accurately.

Early Beginnings

By the mid to late 1990s, a number of factors aligned to set the foundation for an animal hospice care philosophy and to give it initial momentum. New medical knowledge, innovative practitioners, lectures at conferences, and articles in veterinary journals all combined with the growing public recognition of animals' individual identities, discernable psychological needs, capacity for suffering, and the profound emotional bond they form with their human families. All of these supported the notion that hospice and palliative care at the end of animals' lives would offer benefits for both the animal patients and their human caregivers.

Emerging veterinary disciplines and better medicine increased the number of options and tools available to improve quality of life at the end of life. Recognition that animal pain management is both medically beneficial and a moral imperative began in the mid-1990s and profoundly influenced the development of animal hospice and palliative care. Veterinary rehabilitation provided new tools to manage mobility and pain. In response to the aging of the pet population, a growing number of research studies were conducted that helped to manage chronic conditions. For example, published reports elucidating the benefits of using calcitriol to control serum phosphorous in chronic kidney disease (Nagode et al. 1996) and ways to better manage gastrointestinal complications of uremia (Krawiec 1996) made it easier to treat the undesirable side effects of end-stage disease.

A small group of innovative professionals began to lecture in the mid to late 1990s to educate veterinarians about the formal nature of veterinary hospice care. In 1995, veterinarians Dr. Guy Hancock and Dr. James Harris with mental health professional Bonnie Mader gave a lecture at the Delta Society's 10th Annual Conference on the "Hospice Concept for Animals." Other veterinarians were also lecturing about hospice care. For example, in 1998, Dr. Eric Clough presented a lecture at the American Veterinary Medical Association (AVMA) Conference titled "Helping Clients Say Good-bye: Hospice care for pets," and in 2000, Dr. Alice Villalobos introduced her Pawspice concept (Marocchino 2011).

Publications and scientific articles contributed to the evolution of animal hospice care. The earliest scientific article on the subject cited on PubMed, "Pawspice: An Option for Pets Facing the End" was published in 2000 in the *Journal of the American Veterinary Medical Association* (JAVMA) (Monti 2000). The trade journal *Veterinary Economics* published articles in 1997 and 1998 featuring the animal hospice efforts of Dr. Eric Clough. In 2004, *Bark Magazine* interviewed Dr. Tami Shearer and ran an article entitled "Pet Hospice Providing Alternative to End-of-Life Care" (Edwards 2004). The same year, writer Mary Biattiata of the *Washington Post* shadowed Shearer at the Pet Hospice and Education Center and ran a feature on medical options for pets that included hospice care

(Battiata 2004). In August 2006, *JAVMA* published the article "More Veterinarians Offer Hospice Care for Pets," featuring the work of Villalobos, Shearer, and the Argus Institute at the Colorado State University College of Veterinary Medicine (Rezendes 2006).

Not until the late 1990s and early 2000 did the topic of veterinary hospice start to appear in books, including *Preparing for the Loss of Your Pet* by Myrna Milani (Milani 1998), *Pets Living with Cancer* by Robin Downing (Downing 2000), and *The Essential Book for Dogs over Five* (Shearer 2002). These books include discussion of hospice care, treatment options, nursing care, euthanasia, and decision making.

Organization and Recognition

As time progressed, more groups organized, and academia began to acknowledge the importance of hospice care. The Nikki Pet Hospice Foundation, founded in 1997 by Kathryn Marocchino, was the first organization in the United States dedicated exclusively to promoting the benefits of animal hospice. This organization developed the first set of hospice guidelines in 1999 followed by the AVMA in 2001. The Pet Hospice and Education Center was founded in 2003 by Tami Shearer to provide hospice care support to pet owners, veterinarians, and local veterinary students. The center hosted lectures for pet owners and offered an in-house daycare service for working pet owners of chronically ill pets who could not be left alone during the day. Also in 2003, the Argus Institute for Families and Veterinary Medicine in association with the Colorado State University College of Veterinary Medicine started the CSU Pet Hospice program with student volunteers, becoming the first veterinary teaching institution to acknowledge the need for exposing veterinarians in training to hospice care for dying pets. The program is still active today, with students visiting homes of terminally ill pets and acting as a liaison between the family and their veterinarian. The program supports pet owners for a more positive end-of life experience (Bishop et al. 2008).

Animal hospice began to appear in veterinary texts in 2007 with *Canine and Feline Geriatric Oncology* by Villalobos, which advocates the benefits of a hospice and palliative care philosophy and contains a chapter on "Palliative care: End of Life 'Pawspice' Care." *The Handbook of Veterinary Pain Management* by James Gaynor and William Muir (second edition) contains a chapter on Hospice and Palliative Care by Shearer, introducing a "Five-step Protocol for Comprehensive Hospice and Palliative Care" and discusses techniques for improving animal hospice patients' quality of life, including the use of rehabilitation modalities (Shearer 2009). In May 2011, the *Veterinary Clinics of North America* published its issue dedicated to palliative medicine and hospice care, which, until the publication of this volume, provided the most comprehensive compilation of printed hospice and palliative care information for veterinarians.

From 2008 to the present, animal hospice and palliative care has undergone a monumental evolution. Hospice care lectures have increased in frequency, both at veterinary schools and at conferences, and have been recognized as an integral part of continuing education. Dr. Villalobos continues to present her Pawspice concept throughout the country at various meetings. Dr. Ella Bittel has been teaching seminars through her organization, Spirits in Transition. In 2008, the first International Animal Hospice Symposium sponsored by the Nikki Hospice Foundation and Assisi International Animal Institute was held at the University California, Davis, School of Veterinary Medicine. Later that year the Central Veterinary Conference in San Diego offered a full day of hospice lectures featuring Dr. Tami Shearer. Two years later in 2010, at the AVMA Conference in Atlanta, the American Association of Human–Animal Bond Veterinarians (AAH–ABV) sponsored

another full day of lectures focusing on hospice and palliative care.

In 2009, Dr. Amir Shanan founded the International Association for Animal Hospice and Palliative Care (IAAHPC) to promote animal end-of-life care education, research, and public and professional discourse. The IAAHPCs mission is to promote knowledge of, and develop guidelines for, comfort-oriented care to companion animals as they approach the end of their lives. Profoundly influenced by the Veterinary Hospice Symposium at UC Davis in 2008, Shanan saw the need for a broad professional community, inclusive in its philosophy and committed to representing different professional disciplines and diverse viewpoints.

The IAAHPC has served as the catalyst that has propelled animal hospice toward accelerated growth and recognition. The IAAHPC has offered continuing education at its annual conferences since 2011 and offers monthly webinars. Under Shanan's leadership, the IAAHPC published in 2013 its *Guidelines for Recommended Practices in Animal Hospice and Palliative Care* (IAAHPC 2013). The document, available on the IAAHPC website (www.iaahpc.org) aims to help hospice providers and caregivers implement "best practices." The guidelines are updated periodically to include the most recent medical and ethical information and discourse. In 2016, Shanan led the IAAHPC's development and launch of its Animal Hospice and Palliative Care Certification Program to standardize and define the skills and knowledge required of individuals and/or organizations offering animal hospice and palliative care. The program offers structured, competency-based training programs for veterinarians and registered veterinary technicians/nurses. Also in 2016, the American Animal Hospital Association (AAHA) in collaboration with the IAAHPC published the *AAHA/IAAHPC End of Life Care Guidelines* authored by a panel of experts chaired by Shanan (AAHA/IAAHPC 2016).

Interest in veterinary hospice and palliative care has grown over the past two decades, and the concept has gained acceptance to become an integral part of veterinary practice. Progressive and proactive general practitioners, specialists, other professionals, and faculty in veterinary teaching institutions have embraced integrating hospice and palliative care services to better care for dying pets.

Animal Hospice and Human Hospice

Throughout the preceding discussion, many references have been made to characteristics shared by human and animal hospice. Those include compassionate care for patients facing a life-limiting illness or injury; a team-oriented approach to expert medical care; pain management; emotional support expressly tailored to the patient's needs and wishes; support provided to the patient's loved ones; the belief that each patient has the right to die pain-free and with dignity; focus on caring, not curing; preference for care to be provided in the patient's home; and a family member serving as the hospice patient's primary caregiver, helping to make decisions for the patient when appropriate. These similarities are easily understood since animal hospice care has its origins in human hospice care philosophy. However, significant differences also exist.

Ethical and Legal Differences

Patient Autonomy A central tenet in human hospice philosophy, articulated by the National Hospice and Palliative Care Organization (NHPCO, at www.nhpco.org), is that "expert medical care, pain management, and emotional and spiritual support [are] expressly tailored to the patient's needs and wishes." In animal hospice, it is assumed that patients have needs and preferences;

however, they cannot communicate these in human language, depriving animal hospice teams the benefit of verbal guidance from the patient. Animals' individual needs and preferences, therefore, must be represented in clinical decision-making by a human advocate. In animal hospice, the ideal patient advocate is a team consisting of the animal's primary caregiver and an attending veterinarian. Chapters 4 and 7 in this book provide in-depth discussions of the critical importance of animals' individual preferences, the rapidly accumulating knowledge and understanding of animal emotions and cognition, and the implications for ethical decision making for animal hospice and palliative care patients.

Right to Die and Euthanasia In veterinary medicine within the United States, euthanasia is a widely accepted and legal method for ending animals' immediate suffering. Prophylactic euthanasia is also recommended by many veterinarians to protect animals from future suffering. Many veterinarians also appear to believe that allowing an animal to die without the benefit of euthanasia is a disservice to the animal. No evidence supporting these beliefs and recommendations has been published.

Euthanasia for humans is illegal in the United States but legal in some countries. Human hospice philosophy is opposed to euthanasia. Dame Cecily Saunders, considered the founder of modern hospice, stated that the objective of hospice is "to achieve care of the dying that is so effective that no-one should reach that desperate place where he could only ask for his life to be taken." Dame Cecily was motivated not only by the inadequacy of services for terminally ill patients, but also by the rising popularity of the Voluntary Euthanasia Society (for humans) in the United Kingdom in the 1950s. Saunders realized that "hospice and euthanasia have a shared vendetta against pointless pain and impersonal indignity"; she saw the need or desire for euthanasia (of humans) as a direct reflection of society's failure to provide adequate "total care" to dying persons (James 1996, pp. 102–108).

Physician assisted suicide (PAS), in which a physician prescribes medication that the (human) patient intends to take to end his or her life, is legal in some states in the United States. There is no recognized veterinary equivalent to PAS in the United States.

Animal hospice pioneers were bitterly divided on the question whether euthanasia, or death without euthanasia, best serves animal hospice patients' needs and wishes. In the May 2011 issue of *Veterinary Clinics of North America*, which was dedicated to palliative medicine and hospice care, Kathryn Marocchino wrote that "hospice seeks to allow hospice-assisted natural death" and that "euthanasia is a 'last resort' option that should always be available for extreme cases" (Marocchino 2011, p. 491). In the same issue, Dr. Alice Villalobos wrote that "the ideal outcome is for the pet to die at home in a painless and peaceful state, using veterinary supervision that includes proper pain control and home euthanasia services," and that "natural death amounts to caring for an emaciated, dehydrated, depressed, terminal patient that must endure further deterioration, pointless pain, and suffering until liberated by death" (Villalobos 2011, p. 525).

Realizing that this bitter controversy was impeding the development of end-of-life care for animals, Dr. Amir Shanan founded the IAAHPC in 2009 as an inclusive organization committed to representing diverse viewpoints of animal hospice, palliative care, end of life, and death and dying. The IAAHPC advocates that the emphasis of animal hospice is on the care provided to the patient and family before, during, and after death, "inclusive of death by euthanasia or by hospice-supported natural death." The choice between death by euthanasia or by hospice-supported natural death is best made by the patient-advocate team, consisting of the animal's primary caregiver and attending veterinarian.

Economic Differences

Spending on human hospice in the United States is currently over $25 billion annually. In 2019, more than 1.6 million Medicare beneficiaries (including more than half of decedents) received hospice services (up from 1.38 million in 2015), and Medicare hospice expenditures totaled $20.9 billion, (Medicare Payment Advisory Commission 2021) representing about 85% of all hospice services (Fay 2021). The average cost of hospice services for one patient is between $10 000 and $15 000. No comparable figures are available for animal hospice services.

The current level of funding for human hospice care allows for a much broader spectrum and higher frequency of services than is currently feasible in animal hospice. Human hospice staff members make regular visits to assess the patient and provide additional care or other services. Hospice staff is on call 24 hours a day, 7 days a week. The hospice team usually includes the patient's personal physician; a hospice physician (or medical director); nurses; home health aides; social workers; clergy or other counselors; and trained volunteers. There is no public funding for animal hospice services, and the percentage of pet owners who have pet insurance is low. It is also unclear, at this point, precisely what kinds of palliative and hospice services are covered by pet insurance. There is considerable variability from one insurance company to another, and there are no government or even professional standards for what end-of-life services might be considered "essential." Animal hospice, at this point, must be entirely funded by the pet's family, which limits access to hospice services to those with sufficient financial resources. Although animal hospice aims to provide services by an interdisciplinary team very much like human hospice, progress toward this goal has been slow, in part due to funding limitations.

Summary

Veterinarians and other professional animal care providers are seeking ways to provide end-of-life care in an ethical and humane manner and to serve the needs of animal patients as well as their human caregivers. Animal hospice care has its origins in human hospice care philosophy, and there are many similarities as well as significant differences. Animal hospice and palliative care is an emerging field, and definitions are still being refined and debated. Continued constructive debate about underlying ethical principles will expedite the development of evidence-based best practices for the benefit of animal patients and their human caregivers.

References

American Animal Hosptial Associate (AAHA)/ International Association of Animal Hospic and Palliative Care (IAAHPC) (2016) End-of-life care guidelines, *J. Am. Anim. Hosp. Assoc.*, 2 (6):341–356.

Battiata, M. (2004) Whose life is it anyway? *The Washington Post*, Aug 29, at W16 (Magazine).

Bishop, G. Long, C., Carlsten, K., Kennedy, K., Shaw, J. (2008) The Colorado State University pet hospice program: end-of-life care for pets and their families. *J. Vet. Med. Educ.*, 35: pp. 525–31.

Downing, R. (2000) Pets Living with Cancer: A Pet Owner's Resource?. Lakewood, CO: AAHA Press, pp. 81–103.

Edwards, K. (2004) Hospice care. Exploring an alternative way to provide comfort care. *Bark Magazine* 27.

Fay, M. (2021). Hospice costs and end-of-life options. Debt.org. Available at: https://www. debt.org/medical/hospice-costs/ (Accessed on 29 October, 2022).

Hines, L.M. (2003) Historical perspectives on the human-animal bond. *Am. Behav. Sci.*, 47 (1): pp. 7–15.

IAAHPC (2013) *Animal hospic and palliative care guidelines*. Available at: https://iaahpc. org/wp-content/uploads/2020/10/IAAHPC-AHPC-GUIDELINESpdf.pdf. (Accessed 29 October, 2022).

James, N. (1996) From vision to system: the maturing of the hospice movement. In:. Death rites: law and ethic at the end of life (ed. D. Morgan and R. Lee), 102–108. London: Routledge.

Krawiec, D. (1996) Managing gastrointestinal complications of uremia. *Vet. Clin. North Am. Small Anim. Pract.* 26: pp. 1287–1292.

Marocchino, K. (2011) In the shadow of the rainbow: the history of animal hospice. *Vet. Clin. North Am. Small Anim. Pract.* 41: pp. 477–498.

Medicare Payment Advisory Commission. (2021) Report to the Congress: Medicare payment policy. Washington, DC: MedPAC, pp. 309–349. Available at: https://www. medpac.gov/wp-content/uploads/2021/10/ mar21_medpac_report_ch11_sec.pdf (Accessed on 29 October, 2022).

Milani, M. (1998) Preparing for the Loss of your Pet. New York: Crown Publishing Group.

Monti, D.J. (2000) JAVMA news: pawspice an option for pets facing the end. *J. Am. Vet. Med. Assoc.* 217: pp. 969.

Nagode, L. Chew, D., Podell, M, (1996) Benefits of calcitriol therapy and serum phosphorous control in dogs and cats with chronic renal failure. Both are essential to prevent and suppress toxic hyperparathyroidism. *Vet. Clin. North Am. Small Anim. Pract.* 26: pp. 1293–1333.

Rezendes, A. (2006) JAVMA news: more veterinarians offer hospice. *J. Am. Vet. Med. Assoc.* 229, pp. 484–485.

Shearer, T. (2002) The Essential Book for Dogs over Five. Columbus: Ohio Distinctive Publishing, pp. 216–31.

Shearer, T. (2009) Hospice and palliative care. In: Handbook of Veterinary Pain Management (eds J. Gaynor and W. Muir), 2 edn. St. Louis: Mosby, pp. 588–600.

Villalobos, A. (2011) Quality-of-life assessment techniques for veterinarians. *Vet. Clin. North Am. Small Anim. Pract.* 41: pp. 519–530.

3

The Interdisciplinary Team

Tammy Wynn, MHA, LISW, RVT, CHPT and Amir Shanan, DVM

Given the tremendous success of hospice in human healthcare (patient participation in the United States increased from about 25 000 in 1984 to over 1.5 million in 2018), it is reasonable for animal healthcare providers to review the core concepts of hospice philosophy for possible valuable lessons. One of these core concepts is the use of an interdisciplinary team of professionals in planning and sharing the care of the patient and family. The team-care aspect of hospice philosophy is as foreign to mainstream animal medical care today as it was to human medical care just one generation ago. This chapter will first briefly outline the established roles of the interdisciplinary team in human hospice and palliative care, and will then present concepts that may be practical for incorporating animal medical care.

Interdisciplinary Teams in Human Hospice and Palliative Care

The goal of hospice and palliative care is to address all the physical, psychosocial, spiritual, and practical burdens placed by serious illness on the patient and family. No single health care discipline is viewed as capable of effectively addressing all of these at once. It takes a team, or a group of people with complementary skills working together to solve a problem or perform a job. An "interdisciplinary team" implies an integrated approach in which team members actively coordinate care and services across disciplines.

The interdisciplinary team (IDT) approach encourages patients, family members, and professional caregivers to exchange knowledge, greatly facilitating communication about treatment preferences. Typically, a physician, a nurse, and a social worker function as a "core team" and act in the capacity of care managers for the patient and family throughout the patient's stay in hospice care. This core team is responsible for coordinating and managing care across all settings and providing assessment, evaluation, planning, care delivery, follow-up, monitoring, and continuous reassessment of care.

The IDT approach improves outcomes for patients and families by proactively anticipating problems, seeking them out, and addressing them, rather than waiting for consequences to manifest. Randomized clinical trials provided evidence for improvement in patient mood and quality of life (QOL) after administration of palliative care interventions focused on educational or IDT approaches.

To appreciate the importance of the IDT for hospice and palliative care's successful outcomes requires an understanding of how different it is from a traditional healthcare team. In the traditional team, the physician primarily directs care of the patient, and family needs may or may not be considered. Multiple medical specialties or healthcare disciplines may be involved in assessments and in the delivery of care, but efforts are frequently uncoordinated and independent. The primary mode of communication between disciplines is the medical chart. Frequently, the result is incomplete communication between the professions, lack of accountability, and a tendency of each discipline to develop its own list of goals and plan of care. In contrast, in the IDT model communication and decision making is collaborative, with leadership shared and based on the patient and family needs and goals. Team identity supersedes personal identities and agendas. The concept of "the whole is greater than the sum of its parts" is valued and respected. The interdisciplinary model encourages team members to directly interact with the patient and family, share information between team members, provide consultation to one another, and work together interdependently to achieve patient and family goals (Krammer et al. 2010).

According to the National Consensus Project on Clinical Guidelines for Quality Palliative Care (Dahlin 2013), palliative care is defined as medical care provided by an interdisciplinary team, and is focused on the relief of suffering and the support for the best possible quality of life for patients and their families. The document lists the interdisciplinary team as a core element in the provision of palliative care. Professionals from medicine, nursing, and social work are the core of the IDT, which may also include a combination of community volunteers, bereavement coordinators, chaplains, psychologists, pharmacists, nursing assistants and home attendants, case managers and others.

In recognition of the IDT's key role in the delivery of hospice, the US Government Medicare Hospice Conditions of Participation require that an interdisciplinary group provide or supervise the care and services offered by all hospice programs. (US Health Care Financing Administration 1983)

Interdisciplinary Teams (IDT) in Animal Hospice and Palliative Care

Over the past generation, profound changes have taken place in how human–animal relationships are perceived in the United States and other countries. Many companion animal owners/guardians now consider their animals "family members" (Burns 2018) and are willing to carry emotional, financial, and/or physical burdens in providing care for them.

The need for support services for animals' human families is increasingly recognized within the veterinary community. As one example, Malinda Larkin reported that the Center for Veterinary Specialty and Emergency Care in Lewisville, Texas hired a full-time social worker. As the social worker explained, "Every ... [caregiver] has a unique set of circumstances and bond to their animal which influence their treatment decisions. Social workers are trained to know how to take all these factors into account when working with clients." The practice owner elaborated: "The veterinarian's responsibility is to diagnose the animal's problem, communicate the diagnosis to the caregiver, go over the options, and allow the caregiver time to absorb the information and make a decision, [demonstrating support] of the client's feelings and emotions. As the caregiver is coming to grips and making a decision, that's where the social worker can come in and help. The veterinarian then follows up with a conversation about the prognosis and treatment plan" (Larkin 2016).

Several significant obstacles, however, stand in the way of IDT availability in animal healthcare systems:

1) Trained, licensed providers are not as available in veterinary nursing and social work as they are in human nursing and social work.

2) Many veterinarians are reluctant to accept the challenge of building a team that can provide support services for their human clients. Their reluctance stems from fear of increased malpractice litigation risk for the veterinary practice, lack of the necessary skills for building such teams, and/or from lack of motivation.

3) Most animal healthcare establishments are small businesses that may not be financially able to afford the addition of new employees such as social workers or even the addition of new responsibilities to current employees such as veterinary nurses. Networking with and referring to independent licensed human service professionals in one's community has been used successfully to overcome this hurdle.

4) Finally, government and other third-party payers have played a key role in carrying the financial burden of hospice and palliative care (HPC) services for humans; in comparison, third-party payers' role in financing animal healthcare is still very limited.

Despite these challenges, the effort to develop an IDT to serve animal hospice and palliative care (AHPC) patients and their families is well worthy of consideration. IDT teams serve important needs, and their benefits will be increasingly sought after.

Operating a Successful Interdisciplinary Team

Operating a successful IDT relies on several key factors:

1) Common mission and vision
2) Clarification of roles and responsibilities, and
3) Effective communication and collaboration

Common Mission and Vision

The saying "hospice isn't a job, it's a calling," says a lot about the makeup of the animal hospice IDT. Recruiting and keeping team members who are passionate about making the end-of-life experience for a pet and his or her family special is critical to the success of an animal hospice program.

As mentioned above, one definition of a team is a group of people with complementary skills who work together to solve a problem or perform a job. In the case of AHPC, the team's mission is to deliver care that attends to the pain and symptoms of a chronically or terminally ill or very aged animal patient, while also attending to the emotional and spiritual needs of the animal and his or her human caregivers.

Clarifying the team's mission and vision is an important first step in making sure that all team members are on the same page. AHPC are patient- and family-centered and comfort-oriented. This is very different from the traditional mainstream healthcare disease-focused and cure-oriented medical care, which focuses on identifying the patient's disease and then fighting the disease to achieve a patient cure. The ultimate goal for veterinary team members trained in this traditional mainstream mindset is to restore life to a disease-free or symptom-free state. When such efforts fail or are recognized as not achievable, euthanasia is often recommended. In much of mainstream veterinary care, human caregivers' goals are treated with suspicion when they are not aligned with the veterinary providers' personal values and views. Under such circumstances, caregivers' goals are often considered to contradict the animal's best interests and are presumed to be motivated by caregivers' selfishness or ignorance. In addition, the existence of animal patients' individual preferences and will to live are not recognized as relevant to the patient's care.

In contrast, AHPC occupies a middle ground between aggressive medical treatment and "doing nothing" or premature euthanasia. Medical intervention still plays a key role, but it is focused on palliating symptoms and maximizing quality of life. Treatment goes beyond the patient's disease and is now aimed at the entire family system as the "unit of care."

The needs of a family system are very different from the needs of an individual with a disease process. Helping the family system come to terms with a difficult diagnosis or unfavorable prognosis may call for mental health and spiritual interventions requiring a very different skill set than "disease fighting." Recognition that part of the unit of care will survive the patient's death is an important component of hospice care. Helping that component of the "unit of care" come through the loss experience and return to a healthy and fully functioning state is a central goal in AHPC. Nonmedical team members such as a social worker or chaplain may be best suited to provide the education, support, and aftercare that can help the family cope before, during, and after their loss. Veterinarians and veterinary nurses on the AHPC team need to have skills beyond their traditional medical training in their practice toolbox to let an animal's life end with dignity and respect and to support caregivers and loved ones.

Medical decision-making is team-based in AHPC and focused on the patient's and family's goals. This can only be accomplished through information sharing and supportive communication, empowering the family to understand the realities of the options available. See Chapter 8 in this volume for additional information about end-of-life communication principles and techniques.

Careful selection, training, and orientation of new team members are crucial to AHPC success. In human hospice care, no matter how well qualified and experienced in palliative care, new staff members go through a period of training before they start working. It is common practice for a new team member to go through a three-to-five-week preservice training period before seeing his/her first patient (Doyle 2021). The topics covered in human HPC preservice staff training can serve as an example of what AHPC staff training might entail and are listed in Box 3.1.

> **Box 3.1 Topics covered in hospice and palliative care preservice staff training.**
>
> - The principles of palliative care
> - The philosophy of the service
> - The management structure of the service
> - How the service operates
> - Communications within the service
> - Legal aspects of work in the service
> - Day-to-day routines, paperwork, etc.
> - Staff support mechanisms in the service
> - Health and safety regulations and routines
> - Security matters
> - Relationship with other health professions
>
> *Source:* Doyle 2021

The preservice staff training functions as a "reprogramming" period to help clinicians who are moving to HPC from cure-oriented care comprehend and internalize the HPC team's mission: to alleviate burdens placed by serious illness on the "patient and family" unit of care. HPC team members must remain dedicated to this mission, which is best served by the diverse set of complementary skills offered by interdisciplinary teams.

Team members, Their Roles, and Responsibilities

As in human HPC, the "unit of care" in AHPC is the patient and family system, not just the animal patient. AHPC team members providing medical care for the seriously ill animal include the veterinarian, veterinary nurse (called a registered veterinary technician in the United States), veterinary assistants and other animal care providers, as well as the animal's primary caregiver/s (usually his or her human family). Care for the animal's human caregivers may include any of the above, and in addition may include mental health professionals, spiritual advisors, respite care providers, extended family, friends, and community volunteers. Finally, the patient and family themselves are important participants in the HPC team, contributing to medical decision making and providing care and support. Brief descriptions of the roles and responsibilities of each core IDT member are presented below.

Veterinarians. Hospice veterinarians act as medical experts as well as educators and support persons. In fulfilling these roles, veterinarians play an important leadership role in the AHPC IDT. Veterinarians must have a thorough understanding of the relationship between hospice care and the human–animal bond and possess competency in team-based medical decision-making (See Chapter 7 in this volume) and in end-of-life communication (See Chapter 8 in this volume). To help owners make the best decisions, the veterinarian must offer a balanced presentation of all options available. The veterinarian must respond to owners' emotional bonds with their pets in terms of the way the owners see them, meeting owners at their "model of the world" (Lagoni et al. 1994).

Every AHPC patient must have a licensed veterinarian in the role of the medical director for the case. In this role the veterinarian is responsible for diagnosing and prescribing treatments for the pet that are in line with goals of palliation and maintaining and hopefully also improving quality of life. The veterinarian also offers insights and guidance to the family about the expected course of the animal's illness and the associated prognosis. It is the veterinarian's responsibility to assemble the list of parameters to be used to determine the treatment's success and to recommend the frequency with which those parameters should be assessed.

Veterinary nurses and technicians. Veterinary nursing for the AHPC family unit of care is a complex, challenging, yet extremely rewarding undertaking. A licensed veterinary nurse has the most suitable educational background and training to coordinate the wide range of responsibilities and skills required. Veterinary assistants can be trained to perform specific tasks under the supervision of the licensed veterinarian and/or veterinary nurse.

Laws governing the activities that can be assigned to veterinary technicians in the United States vary from state to state.

Serving the needs of the animal/caregiver unit in AHPC requires collecting information regarding the family's needs, beliefs, and goals for the animal (Shearer 2011). A veterinary nurse can be assigned to conduct an intake interview, in person or by phone, to collect this information. In addition to collecting information, the intake interview is an opportunity for the veterinary nurse to offer prospective hospice caregivers information about AHPC's goals of care, what resources might be needed, and what the AHPC team has to offer.

As the "eyes and ears for the veterinarian," veterinary nurses monitor the animal's response to the prescribed treatment plan. The monitoring includes recording progress reports from all caregivers, veterinary nurse recheck examinations, and when applicable, collection of laboratory specimens. Veterinary nurses are the foremost experts in a wide variety of animal care activities, including administering medications and performing treatments; maintaining animals' hygiene, comfort, and safety; the use of assistive devices; and practical aspects of animal behavior and handling. They can provide caregivers with information on a wide range of topics including techniques for medicating animals, observation of animal behavior, activities of daily living, symptom recognition, and death and dying.

Ensuring that AHPC patients live in a comfortable environment and are protected from injury is a primary responsibility of the veterinary nurse and requires effective communication with caregivers. It is a task requiring knowledge, understanding, and sensitivity. Empathy must be demonstrated for both the animal and caregiver. Actively listening to caregivers when sharing their stories and their concerns may be the most valuable gift hospice providers can offer caregivers (Shanan 2015). Last but not least, veterinary nurses must be accessible when they are most needed and be emotionally present whenever interacting with caregivers.

Social workers and mental health professionals. Social workers and mental health professionals are charged with monitoring and supporting the human component of the AHPC unit of care, assessing the history and current mental state of the human caregiver, and matching resources to meet identified needs. A coordinated effort with other team members is essential. For example, a social worker may recognize that the caregiver needs more education about the pet's disease to make informed decisions. The social worker can then facilitate an appointment with the veterinarian or nurse to provide that information. The additional support will help the caregivers feel positive about their conduct after the loss.

Active listening is another important responsibility of the AHPC social worker. Caregivers' interactions with their animal's medical providers, including learning of a beloved companion's unfavorable prognosis, place a heavy burden on caregivers' emotional resources, resulting in significant stress and anxiety and possibly leaving them in an impaired state at the exact moment they are facing life and death decisions for their beloved animal. Active listening by trained social workers and mental health professionals ensures that caregivers are encouraged to express emotions and are offered acknowledgement, validation, and normalization of their feelings. This process replenishes caregivers' emotional resources, relieves some of their stress, and supports their coping and decision-making capacity.

Other important responsibilities of the AHPC social workers include assessing caregivers' needs for a more intensive mental health support or intervention; assisting caregivers in financial planning for the level of care they have chosen for the patient and in making mindful decisions about what they can afford; and helping them access supportive resources that may be available to help. Services that may be offered by social workers as part of AHPC teams are listed in Box 3.2.

Box 3.2 Possible services offered by social workers as part of animal hospice and palliative care teams.

- Supportive counseling, grief support, and counseling
- Help with end-of-life decision-making and follow-up
- Advocacy and brokering of resources
- Reading materials and educational packets
- Crisis intervention
- Assessment of suicidal tendencies and mental health issues
- Facilitation of a pet loss support group
- Consultation about clients and follow-up
- Referral for outside mental health services for staff
- Debriefing sessions for staff
- Presentations to staff
- Recommendations to administrators

Source: Larkin 2016

Other animal care professionals. Many caregivers who have abandoned aggressive treatment seek the additional comfort for animals that may be provided by complementary and alternative medicine (CAM) modalities of care. Acupuncture, tui-na, healing touch, reiki, and other CAM treatments are often performed in the home and can deliver unique improvement in quality of life. Professional pet-sitters offer caregivers much needed temporary relief from their caregiving responsibilities, so they can replenish their energies and continue to provide their caregiving as a labor of love.

Volunteers. Volunteers play an important role in hospice. Volunteers can be recruited from among previous beneficiaries of the hospice experience, some of whom experience a strong desire to "give back." They may also see service to an AHPC organization as a way to honor a pet they had lost.

To make the best use of volunteers when they are available, the AHPC organization must have a system to match the time, skills, and talent the volunteers have to offer with the needs of the organization and/or families currently in hospice care. When living with a special needs or terminally ill pet, caregivers find their time and energy tapped in ways they did not expect. A volunteer can provide respite that allows the caregiver time to catch up on essentials for daily living, such as running to the grocery or simply getting some rest. Volunteers can also help the organization when they are trained or skilled in performing necessary tasks, freeing up paid staff to do other necessary tasks. Finally, volunteers can serve as effective public relations ambassadors for the AHPC organization in the community, by telling their friends about their experience, delivering brochures to area pet services (groomers, pet stores, etc.), or having meaningful conversations with their primary care veterinarian/s.

The patient and family. The patient and his or her caregivers are also considered members of the AHPC IDT. This is a diverse group made up of the animal with the disease, the human family, human nonfamily caregivers (e.g. pet-sitters), and "sibling" animals. Every family unit is unique, and its voice must be heard for the AHPC treatment plan to reflect its unique values, preferences, and needs. Caregivers participate actively in the planning of care, reporting observations to the medical team, and making treatment decisions. In addition, the patient and caregivers actively interact with each other in daily activities such as administration of medications, maintaining the patient's hygiene, and providing invaluable social and emotional support to each other.

Effective Communication and Collaboration

With multiple professional entities interacting with AHPC patients and caregivers, coordination of care is key to successful outcomes. The quality of the continuity of care across team members is directly dependent on the quality of the communication between team members.

Documentation is the foundation of health-care team communication and is important in AHPC for the same reasons that it is important in traditional medicine. The patient's chart is the central location for the deposition of information about that patient and its dissemination to all team members. Paper documentation has its drawbacks in clinic settings, and those are amplified and multiplied in the AHPC practice offering in-home services. Fortunately, recent technological advancements have made it possible to use electronic medical records and programs that allow real-time data entry and updates from any service location. Ensuring that team members document every task or interaction performed with or for the patient is critical and nonnegotiable.

Patient charts, however, aren't sufficient for effectively delivering comprehensive and well-coordinated service to fulfill the AHPC unit of care's complex needs. In human HPC, IDT meetings have been found to be so essential that in the Unites States they are mandated by law of all hospice organizations. (US Health Care Financing Administration 1983) There are many ways to format effective IDT meetings, and they can be customized to fit the particular organization, team, and patient population. Regardless of format, essential elements of all IDT meetings include debriefing about the deaths that have occurred since the last meeting, introduction of new admissions, and discussion of the needs and goals of the current patient census. Effective team meetings should last no longer than 1.5 hours and occur weekly or bi-weekly depending on the number of patients on census. IDT meetings require a significant amount of valuable staff time and need to be structured so they are optimally effective and efficient. The presence of a trained facilitator can be extremely valuable in helping a team unleash their potential for the benefit of their patients and caregivers. Among other roles, the facilitator can provide the agenda for the meeting as well as ensure adherence to it.

The purpose of the IDT meeting is to develop an individualized, interdisciplinary plan of care that meets the evolving needs and goals expressed by the patient and family. An interdisciplinary plan of care is unique to AHPC and is a foreign concept in cure-oriented medical care. Patient plan of care in cure-oriented healthcare teams is typically limited to listing the patient's medical problems and interventions directed at resolving those problems. To create the most effective plan of care for the animal and human caregivers, however, the IDT members provide different types of information that must then be absorbed and discussed by the entire team. In addition to the patient's most current medical information, provided by the team's medical professionals, information is provided by the social worker, chaplain, and others about psychosocial issues. Those may include the makeup of the family, the number of children, their history with loss, their caregiving abilities and time availability, their financial situation, the home environment of the pet, the pet's role in the family, the caregivers' spiritual beliefs and expectations, their interest in CAM treatment modalities, their views regarding euthanasia, and their goals for body care after death. Presenting the nonmedical case information first helps to focus the meeting on treating the unit of care (the pet AND the family) as a whole, as opposed to treating only the patient's illness. Once each respective discipline has had an opportunity to present their information, all disciplines collaborate in designing the care plan that will most effectively help the family achieve their goals.

The above format may be difficult to implement in smaller animal hospice teams who, due to time or financial constraints, "outsource" to mental health professionals and animal care providers in the community. Communication with such team members may be limited to phone consults that often last about 10–15 minutes, scheduled on an as needed basis. Still, smaller practices have much to gain from bi-weekly or weekly meetings dedicated to reviewing plans of care for all active AHPC patients. Such meetings offer opportunities to assess the team's handling of its caseload in its entirety, to acknowledge the team's accomplishments and concerns, and to discuss some cases in greater depth. This level of team communication is not frequently achieved during the daily rounds in which the veterinarian and the veterinary nurse discuss the AHPC case/s of the day. Input received between such meetings from other professionals involved with AHPC cases can be reviewed and discussed at that time.

Interdisciplinary collaboration maximizes the expertise that each discipline can offer and is critical to IDTs working effectively. Laura Bronstein developed a theoretical model of interdisciplinary collaboration and suggests that collaboration is most successful when team members behave in ways that support interdependence, flexibility, collective ownership of goals, and reflection on the collaborative process (Bronstein 2003).

Interdependence refers to each professional on the team relying on interaction with other professionals to accomplish their goals.

Flexibility is facilitated through purposeful "role blurring" within a team setting (see "Professional roles" below).

A **collective ownership of goals** is produced as team members share responsibility for the goal-achieving process.

Finally, **reflection** is the team's ability to evaluate itself. Thinking back on the process of working together allows future improvement through learning from past experiences specific to the group.

According to Bronstein's model, professional roles, personal characteristics, and the organization's structural characteristics are key factors influencing collaboration within an interdisciplinary team.

Professional roles influencing team collaboration include the values and ethics of each team member's discipline (e.g. chaplaincy, social work, nursing), an allegiance to the agency setting and profession, respect for professional colleagues, and a similar or complementary perspective of other team members.

Each profession socializes its members differently with regard to role, values, and practice. The differences among the professions are compounded by the high value placed on professional autonomy – the professional's ability to be "self-directed." Understanding the sense of professional autonomy, professional identity, and role expectations of each profession are prerequisites for a group of professionals from different disciplines to collaborate effectively.

Team members must be viewed as equal and each valued for her or his contribution. They must balance respect for their own professional role with respect for their role as a team member for effective collaboration to happen. Freedom to contribute is critical for the benefits of interdisciplinary collaboration to be maximized, manifesting as interdependence, collective ownership of goals, creative problem solving, and out-of-the-box thinking. If, on the other hand, the dynamic is hierarchal or if team members' freedom to contribute is limited for any reason, the creative synergy of true collaboration is lost. When the freedom to contribute is stilted (e.g., one person is dominating or talking down to other team members), some disciplines will be represented at the meeting in physical presence, yet not be able to make the unique contribution they are professionally skilled to make. As a result, the plan of care is missing valuable input, and the patient and family suffer.

Personal characteristics relevant to interdisciplinary collaboration include the ways collaborators view each other as people, outside their professional role. Trust is a critical base for collaboration, as well as respect, understanding, and informal communication between collaborators. These qualities must be given considerable weight when recruiting and in selecting the members for the team that will be comfortable and effective in collaborating with others.

Organizational characteristics influencing team collaboration include a supportive collaborative culture, systems designed for efficient case flow, a caseload that is manageable, time and space conducive to collaboration, adequate team training, and administrative support. The ways in which the organization allocates resources and assigns work can either inhibit or advance collaboration. Clear communication from the organization's leadership in words and in action that collaboration is valued and expected is essential for team success.

One such action is investing in the development of a clear, consensus-based process for efficient case flow from admission through discharge. Discussing case flow in a team setting can be challenging because of the many potential distractions from the case's substantive issues. The distractions, however, are predictable and can be dealt with systemically upfront. Organizational systems that are specifically and deliberately created to enhance case flow enable the team to move efficiently toward its goals on a superhighway rather than setting out to get through the woods with an ax in hand. The investment in creating a customized system for the organization will pay off downstream with benefits for years to come.

An organizational culture that encourages interdisciplinary collaboration requires that time and space for collaboration be allowed and rewarded. Team members must be assigned caseloads that allow them time to "think" about their cases and collaborate with other team members. When new clients present, short-term business considerations as well as humane considerations create pressure on the organization to enroll them. The organization's leadership, however, must exercise discipline and avoid taking on new cases at the expense of what the team can do to serve current patients and caregivers. Case overload will hurt team morale and sabotage its mission.

Collaborative teamwork is not achieved by knowing that collaboration is needed, but by educating the team members on how each must behave for the team to function successfully. Ensuring that team members value what each team member brings to the group should be incorporated into the new team member orientation process and then reinforced in team building activities.

All team members need to be adequately trained in the case flow process, so they are thoroughly familiar with their own roles in that process as well as others' roles. Basic team training is also extremely helpful to get all team members off on the right foot. Communication and time management techniques, such as starting and ending on time, minimizing distractions of coming and going during the meeting, and being nonjudgmental, can be explained and practiced prior to the first team meeting and are essential for the success of a meeting. Establishing these basics upfront sets up the team to emerge from the meeting feeling their time and energy were used in a meaningful and productive way.

Last but not least, the interdisciplinary team needs administrative support to manage the added level of complexity and coordination necessary to keep it working efficiently. When team members themselves are required to manage administrative tasks, they are not making the most efficient use of their professional skills. If the organization cannot provide administrative support dedicated to facilitating team meetings, administrative responsibilities can be shared evenly between team members to communicate the equal value of each discipline represented on the team.

Summary

The interdisciplinary team provides an opportunity for professionals to come together for the collective good of a patient and collaborate to achieve an outcome greater than possible with any single discipline. The reward in helping the patient die with dignity, respect, and peace is powerful. The reward in helping the surviving family members emerge from the journey optimally prepared to grieve the loss is priceless.

References

Bronstein, L.R. (2003) A model for interdisciplinary collaboration. *Soc. Work.* 48 (3): pp. 297–306.

Burns, K. (2018) *U.S. Pet Ownership & Demographics Sourcebook*, 2017–8. American Veterinary Medical Association (AVMA). Available at: https://www.avma.org/javma-news/2019-01-15/pet-ownership-stable-veterinary-care-variable (Accessed April 17, 2022).

Dahlin, C. (2013) *Clinical Practice Guidelines for Quality Palliative Care*. 3 edn. Richmond, VA: The National Consensus Project for Quality Palliative Care.

Doyle, D. (2021) Getting started: professional-education-and-training. In: Guidelines and Suggestions for those Starting a Hospice / Palliative Care Service. 3 edn., Houston: IAHPC Press.

Krammer, L.M., Martinez, J., Ring-Hurn, E.A., and Williams, M.B. (2010) Chapter 5: the nurse's role in ID and PC. In: Palliative Care Nursing: Quality Care to the End of Life (eds M. LaPorte Matzo and D. Witt Sherman), 3edn. New York: Springer Publishing.

Lagoni L, Butler C, and Hetts S. (1994) The Human-Animal Bond and Grief. Philadelphia PA: W.B. Saunders Company.

Larkin, M. (2016) For human needs, some veterinary clinics are turning to a professional. *J. Amer. Vet. Assoc.* 248 (1); pp. 8–12

Shanan, A. (2015) Pain management for end of life care. In: Pain Management for Veterinary Technicians and Nurses (eds M.E. Goldberg and N. Shaffran). Ames, IA:Wiley.

Shearer T. (2011) *Pet hospice and palliative care protocols. Vet. Clin. North Am. Small Anim. Pract.*, 41: 507–518.

US Health Care Financing Administration. (1983) Medicare program hospice care. Final Rule (A.M.P.H.C.F.R.), Agency for Health Policy Research. *Federal Register*, 48: pp. 50008–50036.

4

Quality of Life Assessments

Jessica Pierce, BA, MTS, PhD and Amir Shanan, DVM

Hospice and palliative care seek to provide animal patients of advanced age or those with life-limiting serious illness a course of treatment that allows them to enjoy their remaining life to the fullest, and that avoids prolonging life if not in the animal's best interest. A fine balancing act is often required to manage symptoms and keep pain at bay, while striving to keep an animal happy and maximize positive experiences. Effective tools to interpret and track animals' quality of life (QOL) can help veterinarians, animal hospice and palliative care (AHPC) teams, and family caregivers achieve this delicate balance.

What are Quality of Life Assessments and Why are they Important in End-of-Life Care?

The concept of health-related QOL has been in use in human medicine since the 1970s and has been developed as a measure of how much an illness or a disability affects an individual's overall physical and emotional well-being. The impetus behind developing the QOL construct was to represent the patient's interests and experiences in decisions made about health care, reflecting the growing respect among healthcare professionals for patient autonomy

and self-determination in medical decision making. What exactly health-related QOL is, how to measure it, and even whether you can measure it, has been – and still is – the subject of considerable debate.

Over the past two decades, and thanks in part to increased attention to animal end-of-life care, QOL assessments are becoming an integral part of veterinary medicine, too. As in the human realm, the conceptualization and measurement of QOL in animals has been contentious and a broad range of approaches and methods are still being explored. Deeper understanding of animal QOL and further development of assessment tools is vital to the future of the field.

Definitions of Quality of Life

Effective tools to interpret and track animals' QOL are important so their caregivers, veterinarians, and AHPC teams can make decisions that best serve animals' interests. To develop such tools and use them wisely we must first understand what "quality of life" means.

The World Health Organization defines QOL as the perception of an individual's position in life in the context of the culture and value systems in which they live and in relation to their goals, expectations, standards, and concerns (Weisman-Orr et al. 2006).

The International Association of Animal Hospice and Palliative Care defines QOL as "how well or poorly an animal is doing, considering the totality of an animal's feelings, experiences, and preferences, as demonstrated by the animal" (IAAHPC 2013).

Reid and colleagues define QOL in animals as the affective (emotional) response of an individual animal to his or her circumstances, and the extent to which the circumstances meet his or her expectations. Animal QOL is, they say, "a multidimensional construct that is subjectively experienced by and is uniquely personal to the individual animal" (Reid et al. 2015, p. 98).

Similarly, Wojciechowska and colleagues define animal QOL as "the subjective and dynamic evaluation by the individual of its circumstances (internal and external) and the extent to which these meet its expectations (that may be innate or learned and that may or may not include anticipation of future events), which results in, or includes, an affective (emotional) response to those circumstances (the evaluation may be a conscious or an unconscious process, with a complexity appropriate to the cognitive capacity of the individual)." In other words, QOL is "the subjective evaluation of circumstances that include an altered health state and related interventions" (Wojciechowska et al. 2005).

McMillan defines QOL as "the affective and cognitive ... assessment that an animal makes of its life overall, how its life is faring, experienced on a continuum of good to bad" (McMillan 2005b, p. 193).

Some terms recur within definitions of animal QOL: affect, emotion, cognition, feeling, sensation, subjective experience, well-being, and welfare. These terms overlap and sorting them out is challenging even for experts trained in the nuances of psychological and ethological terminology. A detailed analysis of all the terms used in various definitions of QOL is beyond the scope of this article.

The common thread connecting the definitions of animal QOL listed above is that it is a subjective evaluation by an animal of what he or she is experiencing under their life's circumstances. It is an internal process engaging the animal's emotions and cognition – an assessment of life overall. Subjective phenomena can be hard to evaluate from the outside (by anyone other than the individual experiencing them) and can be difficult to measure quantitatively. There is no "gold standard" for QOL that an individual animal's experience can be measured against and there are no objective units of measurement. Despite the challenging nature of the task, QOL assessments are a useful tool for documenting an AHPC patient's condition before treatment, in developing individualized treatment plans, and as a meaningful measure of treatment effectiveness over time.

Quality of Life and Well-being

In our discussion we'll use the following working definition: in the context of AHPC, "animal quality of life is a construct reflecting how an individual animal's physical, emotional, and social well-being is affected by disease, disability, or changes related to advanced age." We take QOL to be synonymous with "overall well-being" (see Sandöe 1999).

In their article "Philosophical Debate on the Nature of Well-Being: Implications for Animal Welfare," Sandöe and Appleby (2002) follow philosopher Shelly Kagan's (1992) distinction of three basic theories of well-being. One theory asserts that well-being is "objective": that certain conditions are good for an animal, whether the animal realizes it, and whether he or she desires those conditions. Such conditions might include pleasure, companionship, good health and normal physical functioning, or the expression of the animals' nature (*telos*). The list of conditions that are "objectively good for the animal" is a matter of dispute.

The other two theories of well-being assert that an individual's well-being is subjective, determined solely by the individual's feelings. One theory, often labeled Hedonism, claims that well-being depends on the experience of pleasure. The other claims that fulfillment of desires or preferences is most important to being "well-off."

Whether animal well-being should be defined in terms of feelings or functioning has been (Broom 1996; Duncan 1996) and still is an ongoing philosophical debate, as it is in discussion of human well-being. While many treat well-being as wholly subjective, others postulate "the possibility that certain changes in the body might affect well-being even though they involve no changes in one's mental states" (Kagan 1992, p. 187).

Quality of Life Assessments and Euthanasia Decisions

The Importance of Context in Quality of Life Assessment

The philosophical "feelings vs. functioning" debate takes on dramatic importance when QOL assessments are used as the basis for considering whether to end the animal's life by euthanasia. The prevailing paradigm in veterinary practice is founded on several assumptions that are widely held but rarely discussed or questioned: that animal QOL can be determined objectively; that it can be determined more reliably by humans than by the animals themselves, and more reliably by veterinarians than other humans; that a numerical scoring system for animal QOL can be developed – one that be applied to all animals of a certain type – that can help caregivers and veterinarians decide if an individual animal's QOL is acceptable; and that animal caregivers who aren't ready to euthanize their animals when the animals' QOL falls below some objective "cut-off score" are "wrong," "selfish," or even "cruel." These assumptions are reflected in educational tools designed for professionals and pet owners by leading academic institutions and practice organizations. The tools generate the QOL scores to be used to make "objective"

euthanasia decisions, based on a list of "objective criteria" for animal QOL – each tool offering a different list of criteria:

- The University of Tennessee Veterinary Social Work Department offers an "End-of-Life Values and Goals" worksheet (vetsocialwork. utk.edu/wp-content/uploads/2016/03/ EndoLifeValues-Goals.pdf) consisting of 10 questions of the format: "Would it be the appropriate time for euthanasia if my pet (is feeling pain – yes or no?/has stopped eating – yes or no?/etc.)." Of the 10 questions, only one ("no longer feels like him/herself") refers to the animal's emotional well-being.
- The Ohio State University (OSU) Veterinary Medical Center includes information on QOL assessment under its website's "How Do I Know When it's Time?" page (vet.osu. edu/vmc), which draws on Dr. Alice Villalobos' HHHHHMM QOL Scale (HHHHHMM stands for Hurt, Hunger, Hydration, Hygiene, Happiness, Mobility, More good days than bad) as a primary source.
- The HHHHHMM Scale (Villalobos 2011) is geared to generate a numerical score (out of a BEST QOL score of 70 points), stating that "a total score of >35 points is acceptable quality of life for pets."
- Lap of Love Veterinary Hospice and In-Home Euthanasia, a corporate national veterinary practice limited to end-of-life care, offers a pet Quality-of-Life questionnaire (www.lapoflove.com/quality-of-life-assessment) and a web page entitled "How Will I Know It Is Time to Say Goodbye" (www.lapoflove.com/how-will-i-know-it-is-time) with links to the Lap of Love Quality of Life Scale and Quality of Life Daily Assessment. The scale and assessment lists 16 components of QOL as questionnaire items for caregivers to score on a 0–2 scale, with 7 of those items describing aspects of the animal's behavior that in part reflect the animal's emotional well-being. The page states that (out of a WORST QOL score of 32 points), a score of "17–32 [*means that*

your pet's] QOL is a definite concern... . Veterinary guidance will help you ... make a more informed decision of whether to continue hospice care or elect peaceful euthanasia."

Can an animal's welfare be diminished by an illness that doesn't (yet) affect his or her feelings? When death is the potential outcome, the significance of understanding the underlying assumptions, merits, and limitations of animal QOL assessments cannot be overstated.

The authors of this chapter hold that QOL assessments in the context of deciding whether and when to *end* an animal's life require a qualitatively different approach from QOL assessments in the context of seeking to *improve* an animal's life. Functioning may deserve greater weight when exploring ways to improve QOL: When seeking to improve QOL, any improvement is welcome – in overall health status, physical functioning, and opportunities to experience pleasure and to fulfill individual preferences. The animal directly benefits from all of these.

In contrast, attention to feelings takes on special importance when considering whether to hasten death for a companion animal. In that context, the overriding consideration must be: *"Is this animal's life meaningful to the animal?!"* Only an assessment of the animal's mental state will answer this question. We propose that three specific aspects of an animal's mental state are most relevant to answering the question: The first is the animal's capacity and motivation to be *engaged* with their environment. The second is the animal's capacity to feel *connected* (a sense of belonging to a loving/supportive social unit). The third is a sense of *control* sufficient to protect the animal from sinking into a state of helplessness and hopelessness.

In the presence of reasonable degrees of engagement, connectedness, and a sense of hope, animals can be amazingly resilient and tenacious in their desire for life to go on. We hold that humans have an ethical obligation to consider the *will to live* animals express when deciding whether euthanasia is in the animal's best interest *as they see it*. Indeed, most caregivers facing end-of-life care decisions for their animals say their wish is to make decisions based on "what the animal wants" or "what the animal would have asked them to do." What they wish to provide their animals is patient-centered care.

Quality of Life and Patient-Centered Care

Patient-centered care is defined by the Institute of Medicine (for humans) as care that is "respectful of and responsive to individual patient preferences, needs, and values." Patient-centered care establishes a partnership among practitioners, patients, and their families to ensure that medical decisions respect patients' wants, needs, and preferences (Institute of Medicine 2001, p. 2). Over the past quarter century, patient-centered care has become one of the overarching goals of health advocacy: supporting and promoting the rights of the patient (Earp et al. 2008). To accomplish the objective of patient-centered care – making decisions that respect patients' wants, needs, and preferences – QOL assessments are used to elicit the patient's own experiences before, during, and after treatment.

This is the goal in the animal healthcare realm as much as it is in human healthcare: QOL assessments must focus as much as possible on how the animal is doing *from the animal's point of view* – how the animal perceives its own physical, emotional, and social well-being. The notion that animals have an internal mental world and therefore the capacity to have a "view of life as a whole" was met with skepticism and outright ridicule by scientists half a century ago. Unfortunately, that notion is still occasionally met with skepticism, despite the exponentially expanding evidence supporting it. It is not acceptable in the third decade of the twenty-first century to deny animals' capacities to experience rich, complex emotions, and to learn, form memories, plan for the future, and engage in other complex cognitive processes (see, for example, Panksepp 2005; De Waal 2020; Bekoff 2008).

Although animals cannot verbally tell us how they feel or what they want, we can gather a great deal of information by carefully observing their behavioral and physiological expressions of affect (Shanan 2011; see Chapter 5 "Recognizing Distress" in this volume). Interpreting observations of an animal must be based on thorough familiarity with the animal's individual preferences integrated with knowledge of that animal's species-specific behaviors.

In addition, human experience can serve as a tool to enhance understanding of the subjective experiences of nonhuman animals. When interpreting animal observations, we can refer to how a certain experience might make a person feel and assume that animals might feel similarly; this approach has limitations that must be recognized and acknowledged.

Physical Discomfort, Emotional Distress, Pain, and Suffering

Pain. Suffering. These are words we hear repeatedly in the care of animals at the end of life. Caregivers will say, "I just don't want my animal to be in pain. I won't let her suffer." This is a desire that we all share; we want to protect our animals from suffering.

Although pain and other types of physical discomfort frequently cause suffering, caregivers, veterinarians, and other animal hospice team members should bear in mind that individual animal patients have different responses to pain and other unpleasant physical sensations (e.g. extreme heat, cold, or pressure). Stimulating sensory receptors in nerve endings may cause an intense emotional reaction in one animal yet cause only a minimal or even no reaction in another. In humans, pain responses have been documented to vary considerably from one individual to the next,

and can differ according to gender, age, priming, and past experiences (Fillingim 2017). Our experience suggests that pain responses are equally individualized in nonhuman animals, and that individual animals cope differently with similar painful stimuli, as discussed below.

Pain and suffering are increasingly recognized as intimately related but distinct phenomena. Some medical fields like palliative care, pain medicine, oncology, and psychiatry address suffering more than others. But modern medicine has traditionally focused most of its attention on the treatment of physical pain, leading hospice care pioneer Dame Cicely Saunders to create the concept of "total pain" (also referred to as "total suffering"), which encompasses the complex array of physical discomfort, emotional distress and cognitive perceptions that a patient may experience (Clark 1999, 2007).

But what are pain and suffering? To assess, measure, and monitor animal patients' conditions we need first to understand what we intend to monitor.

PAIN is defined by the International Association for the Study of Pain (IASP) as "an unpleasant sensory and emotional experience in reaction to stimuli, often accompanied by physiological and behavioral arousal." A recent revision to the IASP definition (IASP 2020) emphasized that "pain is always a personal experience that is influenced to varying degrees by biological, psychological, and social factors" and that "pain and nociception are different phenomena." Pain, they note, "cannot be inferred solely from activity in sensory neurons." The experience of "physical pain" originates in unpleasant physical sensations (e.g. stimulation of nociceptive receptors) that lead to unpleasant emotional experiences (distress). Emotional distress can also be experienced as a result of unpleasant emotional experiences that involve no unpleasant physical sensations (e.g. psychological trauma). This is often described as "emotional pain." To further complicate matters, the experience of emotional distress can then trigger physiological changes and physical sensations – a physical experience caused by emotional distress – to be differentiated from physical sensations that may cause emotional distress.

STRESS is the physiological or psychological response of an animal to stressors, which include any disturbance, or a threat of disturbance to the animal's homeostasis.

DISTRESS is an unpleasant emotional reaction, triggered when an animal is unable to adapt quickly or completely to a stressor, and impacting the animal's level of functioning.

Both stress and distress are designed to bring about a desirable result: motivating the regulatory processes of coping and adaptation that help the animal regain the homeostasis that is essential for continued survival.

SUFFERING is experienced when coping and adaptation fail. The animal then feels helpless, and/or hopeless, perceiving the destruction of her or his sense of self as unavoidable. Suffering is a mental process, triggered by an emotion (distress), which in turn is triggered by stress (psychological or physiological), which is a response to exposure to a stressor (often, multiple stressors). Such stressors may include physical sensations like pain and breathlessness, and/or emotions such as frustration and loneliness. Suffering is ultimately followed by exhaustion of all psychological, psychosocial, and personal resources (Henry 2017). Box 4.1 summarizes Henry's definitions of stressor, stress, distress and suffering.

Because animals cannot verbally communicate their emotional experiences to us, we must rely on observations of their behavioral and physiological expressions of affect. But overt behaviors do not always provide an accurate measure of an animal's inner state. A grave concern for many caregivers and veterinarians is that under some circumstances animals "hide" their feelings, including pain. "Endurance of pain or hardship without the display of feelings and without complaint" is the definition of stoicism. The degree of

---

Box 4.1   Stress, distress, and suffering.

STRESSOR/S
Any disturbance to homeostasis – actual or potential,
in the animal's external or internal environment

↓

STRESS
A physiological or psychological response to stressors

↓

DISTRESS
Unpleasant emotion: motivates coping and adaptation to help the animal regain homeostasis

↓

SUFFERING
Mental process: perception that coping and adaptation failed and therefore – "destruction of the animal's sense of self is unavoidable"

AND/OR

Exhaustion of all psychological resources: helplessness, hopelessness

---

stoicism displayed varies widely among animals of the same species, indicating that it reflects an individual animal's personality, coping style, and degree of background stress (Fillingim 2017). In addition, human observers may believe that animals are hiding their feelings when they don't know what to look for. Behaviors expressing pain differ between animals and humans, from one animal species to another, and between different types of pain (e.g. acute vs. chronic pain) in the same species. Panting, for example, is a common expression of pain or anxiety in dogs but not in humans. As more studies focus on species-specific and disease-specific pain behaviors, the ability to recognize and treat pain in animals is improving (Mich and Hellyer 2015).

Suffering and pleasure are, respectively, the negative and positive affects that psychologists often identify as basic to sentient beings' emotional lives (Colombetti 2005). Physical discomfort and emotional distress both have an evolutionary role through natural selection: they warn of threats and motivate coping behaviors. The distinction between the terms "physical discomfort" and "emotional distress" should not be taken too literally: physical and emotional pain are intimately linked in mammalian brains, supporting the notion of their similar evolutionary roles.

Suffering comes in all degrees of intensity, from mild to intolerable. The duration of suffering and its frequency of occurrence significantly influence the sufferer's experience, further compounding any attempt to measure suffering on any type of scale. Attitudes toward suffering vary widely, in the sufferer and in those interacting with her or him. Attitudes toward suffering are influenced by how much it is regarded as avoidable or unavoidable, useful or useless, and numerous other factors.

The term "suffering" carries a potent emotional charge. It is often used to justify decisions to euthanize animals, and therefore one must be very cautious using it in AHPC; at the same time, avoiding use of the word "suffering" altogether leaves caregivers with one of their greatest fears unacknowledged.

"Unbearable suffering" in the animal hospice context suggests a state of suffering that is prolonged, unrelenting, intense, intractable, and unlikely to abate. It is at this point that euthanasia must be urgently considered as an ethical and compassionate option.

Coping and Adaptation

We mentioned that coping and adaptation are regulatory protective mechanisms that safeguard homeostasis, which is essential for animals' continued survival.

Coping, within the literature on animal welfare, refers to an animal's ability to reduce the physiological activation caused by stressors, by performing behaviors that either remove the stressor or reduce the emotional valence of the experience (Turner and Bateson 2014, pp. 193–194). Coping that attempts to remove the source of threat to homeostasis – pain, distress, or suffering – is called "problem-focused" coping. Coping designed to control the emotional reaction to the threat is called "emotion-focused" coping. Coping can also positively reappraise the threat's significance ("meaning-based" coping). An example of a problem-focused coping strategy is an animal displaying threatening postures to scare away an intruder. The stress induced by the intruder's presence dissipates when the intruder leaves in response to the posturing. An example of emotion-focused coping is a dog seeking reassuring social contact by snuggling close to his human companion during a thunderstorm, reducing the emotional reaction to a stressor by transferring attention away from it. Lastly, an animal who must walk to get her food may use meaning-based coping and reappraise her aversion to the osteoarthritis pain elicited by walking, so she can reach food to satisfy her hunger. Emotion-focused and meaning-based coping strategies are well suited for stressors that are difficult to eliminate and frequently encountered when living with the serious or chronic illness conditions affecting most AHPC patients.

Further complicating attempts to evaluate suffering is the process of psychological adaptation, a mechanism that stabilizes sentient beings' level of happiness throughout their lives despite events that occur in their environment (Brickman and Campbell 1971; Kuhn et al. 2008). Adaptation is the process of adjusting to both experienced and expected change. Adaptation involves both conscious and unconscious processes, is more continuous and longer in duration than coping, and is more likely to produce sustainable results. Adaptation involves cognitive changes, such as shifting values, goals, attention, and interpretation of a situation. Adaptation may reflect neurochemical processes that desensitize overstimulated hedonic pathways in the brain, preventing intense levels of joy and misery from persisting for a long time.

Psychological adaptation is highly relevant to assessing QOL in patients with life-limiting conditions. Human hospice providers report that patients' perceptions of the line separating tolerable from intolerable suffering sometimes shifts as the patients and their families spend additional time living with serious illness. Animals, too, can adapt to challenging conditions. They can, for instance, enjoy good QOL despite being blind or deaf, or having lost a limb, or needing dialysis. In one author's (Shanan) clinical experience, animals with gradually decreasing respiratory capacity due to heart failure or neoplasia may manifest an unchanged mood despite the increasing effort required for them to breathe.

Nevertheless, when psychological distress in response to either physical discomfort or unpleasant events and perceptions is prolonged, unrelenting, intense, and noxious, an animal may reach a point at which the adaptive capacities of the stress response system are overwhelmed. When the system reaches this point of overload, animals cannot adapt and will develop behavioral pathologies – often called stereotypies. Stereotypic behavior is the term used to describe animal behavior that is invariant and repetitive and serves no obvious function. Stereotypies are thought to be caused by brain dysfunction brought on by stress-induced damage to the central nervous system. Stereotypies can include locomotor behavior (e.g. pacing), self-directed behavior (e.g. compulsive grooming), and oral behaviors (e.g. air snapping). Stereotypies are a sign of very poor welfare and cause for serious concern. When such a state of poor welfare is intractable, hastening death may be the only way to relieve suffering.

Measuring Quality of Life in Animal Patients

QOL reflects how an animal's physical, emotional, and social well-being is affected by disease, disability, or changes related to advanced age. Assessing QOL involves tracking the balance between negative and positive emotional states experienced by the patient. Some of the factors that negatively impact animal's QOL include pain, nausea, inappetence, respiratory distress, loss of mobility, incontinence, dehydration, confinement, social isolation, confusion, agitation, boredom, frustration, anxiety, fear, depression, and the inability to engage in meaningful and enjoyable activities. In assessing unpleasant feelings, one must consider that some factors – notably respiratory distress and severe pain – weigh more heavily than others, such as incontinence. Some of the factors that positively impact an animal's QOL include tactile and other sensory stimulation, mental stimulation, companionship, good food, comfortable bedding, play, and a sense of control over self and environment.

In humans, it has been asserted (Kahneman et al. 1999) that "QOL cannot be reduced to a balance of pleasure and pain" due to the influence of factors such as purpose and/or meaning in life, which do not always correlate with the person's reported affect on a pain-to-pleasure scale. A hypothesis that "purpose and/or meaning in life" are important to nonhuman animals' well-being, while difficult to prove using human scientific methods currently available, is congruent with the view of fulfillment of desires or preferences as the most important to being "well-off." It is also congruent with observations of animals demonstrating a "will to live" under extremely stressful and challenging circumstances.

Our clinical experience suggests that animals' capacities and motivation to be *engaged, express preferences,* and demonstrate that they are *connected* to a loving/supportive social unit are useful indicators of animals' "purpose and/or meaning in life." While difficult to quantify, the behaviors reflecting these capacities in AHPC patients can be intuitively grasped and respected by attentive humans, and monitoring them is critically important in assessing QOL, especially when considering decisions to end an animal's life. When capable and motivated to be engaged and connected, animals can be amazingly resilient.

Unfortunately, many animals are euthanized prematurely because caregivers see only a bleak set of options: escalating but futile attempts to cure the animal, inaction and continued suffering, or immediate euthanasia. Euthanasia is elected because of a perception or fear of "suffering," and lack of ability to see the full range of capacities that animals have for adapting and coping with distress. The ideal QOL assessment tool for animal end-of-life decision-making will be one that can shift the caregiver's focus from pain and suffering to the broader concept of animal QOL acknowledging suffering as well as the animal's sources of enjoyment, fulfillment of preferences, capacity to cope and adapt, and the desire or will to live. "Suffering" then begins to shrink down to its proper place in the decision-making process. The expanse of possibilities comes into view.

A Variety of Approaches to QOL

A vast amount of research has been done and volumes published about QOL assessment in human patients. Yet, despite decades of research supported by significant budgets and driven by public interest, there is no universally accepted and uniformly applied assessment tool for human QOL. This is worth remembering as veterinarians and other animal scientists work to develop similar tools for use in animal care. There is no single best approach, and we have a lot of work still ahead of us. As veterinarians strive to develop more and better tools, they can look to research done in the sciences of animal welfare, ethology, neuroscience, psychology, and other interrelated fields, and they can draw on the ample information available from human health care.

The science and art of assessing seriously ill animals' QOL is still in its infancy, and a relatively small number of QOL assessment tools have been developed for veterinary use, which we'll review very briefly here. Measuring behavior is tricky, and so having statistically reliable and validated assessment tools is vitally important, albeit quite challenging. Reliability is the extent to which the measurements are repeatable and consistent and free from errors; validity is the extent to which a measurement tool measures what it is supposed to and gives us information relevant to the questions being asked (Martin and Bateson 2007, pp. 72–85). A validated measurement instrument helps practitioners make clinical decisions about what treatments or interventions are working or not working, based upon relatively objective information rather than on a given caregiver's hunch. And because the QOL assessment often serves (for better for worse) as a fulcrum for decision-making about euthanasia, it is clearly in the animal's best interest that the measurement tool used accurately reflects the animal's view of how he or she is feeling.

Within the context of hospice and palliative care, what's most important is that QOL assessment tools provide an accurate and comprehensive picture of the individual animal's well-being, help weigh benefits and burdens of disease and treatments, and offer a platform for discussion and shared decision-making. Generalized assessment tools for animal QOL have some use (for example, McMillan's Affect Balance Model discussed here), but it is also important to have assessment tools that are customized to the particulars of the animal at hand: different species will likely benefit from species-specific tools, and tools crafted with specific medical diagnoses in mind may also be quite useful.

Mich and Hellyer suggest that QOL assessments should address three primary factors: the physical, the psychological, and the social. Physical factors include an animal's ability to perform daily living activities including but not limited to locomotion, appetite, and sleep. Psychological factors include level of consciousness, sense of well-being, and cognitive functioning. Social factors include both quantitative and qualitative considerations of owner-animal interactions, social relationships with other pets, and societal integration into a family (Mich and Hellyer 2015).

Yeates and Main suggest that the real importance of QOL assessment is the process of assessment itself, which may lead to changes in the assessor's behavior and thereby to improvements in the animal's QOL. QOL assessment becomes, then, "both a measurement and an intervention" (Yeates and Main 2009, p. 276).

Below, we offer a brief review of several assessment tools. First, though, we would like to introduce Frank McMillan's Affect Balance Model. McMillan offers a framework (and a very good one) for understanding what information a QOL assessment tool should seek to elicit and why. According to McMillan, QOL conversations should focus, above all, on how an animal feels, as opposed to focusing on the animal's physical symptoms.

McMillan's Affect Balance Model

As the name suggests, McMillan's Affect Balance Model focuses on animal emotions (and not, for example, on physiological markers like heart rate and cortisol). He suggests that assessing an animal's QOL involves tracking negative and positive emotional states, assigning each of them relative weight based on evolutionary function and on the individual animal's preferences and then calculating the "balance." McMillan's model is discursive, involving a chapter-length discussion of the evolutionary origin and significance of affective states in animals. As such, it is extremely valuable as a learning aid for veterinarians and their team members. It would only appeal to a narrow range of veterinary clients.

McMillan argues that the QOL assessment begins with determining what factors in an animal's life affect QOL and distinguishing these from things that don't really matter to the animal. So, how do we know what matters?

Box 4.2 Examples of negative and positive affect expressed by companion animals.

Negative affect	Positive affect
sad/melancholy	peaceful
listless/dull	calm
confused	relaxed
sluggish/tired	content
clingy	connected
reluctant to engage	cuddly/affectionate
tense	stretching
subdued/resigned	inquisitive
withdrawn	attentive
disengaged	eager to engage
restless	playful
anxious	enthusiastic
complaining/groaning	energetic
crying/whining	lively
fearful	joyful
defensive	
panicky	
agitated	
screaming	
rageful/out of control	

The things that matter to animals, he says, are those things that elicit an affective response. Things that might produce positive feelings in animals include social interactions and companionship, good food, mental stimulation, play, a feeling of safety, and a sense of control. Things that might produce negative feelings include pain, hunger, a full bladder, nausea, itchiness, social isolation, frustration, boredom, and anxiety.

Examples of negative and positive affect are listed in Box 4.2.

McMillan suggests four steps (which don't really occur stepwise but are more organic and overlapping): (i) an inventory of an animal's feelings, good and bad; (ii) weighting the feelings' relevance to survival; (iii) an individualization of the weighting, because some experiences will matter more to a particular animal than others; and (iv) a scale that can quantify the weight of the individualized and importance-adjusted experiences. As he notes, "at this time this step (iv) lacks any precision," leaving "best guesses" as our only option.

Weighing Positive and Negative Affect at the End of Life

Affective responses vary not only in valence (positive or negative) but also in intensity. McMillan theorizes that "feelings that are evolutionarily associated with the most serious and immediate threats to survival" such as hypercapnia (associated with a feeling of air-hunger), pain, and fear should weigh more heavily in QOL assessments than things that produce weaker negative feelings and more heavily than things that produce positive feelings (McMillan 2005b, p. 195).

How important positive feelings are in the life of patients in advanced stages of illness and/or disability depends on what view of subjective well-being is emphasized. Pleasure is not frequently experienced by seriously ill patients. Expressing and fulfilling their individual preferences, on the other hand, remain important to experiencing life as meaningful as the end of life nears. Expressing and fulfilling their individual preferences, therefore, deserves prominent representation in assessing QOL of hospice and palliative care animal patients– no less so than the frequency and intensity of negative affect.

Quality of Life Assessment Tools

As promised, here is a brief review of several assessment tools published in the veterinary literature:

VetMetrica. Derived from GUVQuest (the Glasgow University Veterinary School Questionnaire) and developed to measure the impact of chronic pain on health-related quality of life (HRQL) in dogs (Wiseman-Orr et al. 2004), VetMetrica is a statistically validated and reliable web-based measurement instrument. It was developed by a multidisciplinary team at the University of Glasgow, using psychometric methodology well-established for the development of scientifically robust instruments (Reid et al. 2013). Unlike any of the other QOL instruments discussed below, Vetmetrica focuses on measuring QOL from the animal's perspective and in that regard is novel in veterinary medicine. As the instrument is used and more data accumulates, researchers can refine and update the instrument. A shortened version of VetMetrica (Reid et al. 2018) is a structured questionnaire in which the owner rates his or her dog's behavior using 22 easily understood terms, both positive and negative (e.g. lethargic, calm, sore, happy, tired, stiff). Instantaneous computation of scores by a computer algorithm generates a score in each of the four domains of QOL: energetic/enthusiastic, happy/content, active/comfortable, and calm/relaxed. Results are made available instantaneously and automatically to the dog's veterinarian who interprets them by comparison with age-matched norms and by the level of change relative to the minimal important difference (MID) calculated for each domain.

VetMetrica is a generic tool for use in dogs, measuring the impact of a variety of conditions and their treatment on QOL. In addition to performing well in a variety of circumstances, generic instruments such as VetMetrica are the only option when an animal suffers from more than one condition. Disease-specific instruments, however, may be more sensitive to intervention-related change.

Yazbeck and Fantoni. This instrument is designed for dogs with pain secondary to cancer (Yazbek and Fantoni 2005). In line with many instruments used in human medicine, Yazbeck and Fantoni incorporate into their QOL questionnaire items directed at assessing three broad domains: physical, psychological, and social functioning.

Hartmann and Kuffer's Karnofsky's Score Modified for Cats. Hartmann and Kuffer have borrowed the so-called Karnofsky Performance Status Scale, a tool designed for use in humans, which rates functional impairment on a scale from 0% to 100% (Hartmann and Kuffer 1998). The modified Karnofsky scale breaks down a cat's behavior into six categories. Of these categories, three address the physical functioning domain, and two address the psychological functioning domain using language referring only to positive affect. The remaining category addresses the cat's social functioning.

FETCH *(Functional Evaluation of Cardiac Health)* assesses QOL in dogs with cardiac disease (Freeman et al. 2005).

Iliopoulou et al. designed a 15-question survey instrument to assess health-related QOL in small animal patients with disseminated cancers being treated with chemotherapy (Illiopoulou et al. 2013). This instrument is for use by clients.

Wojciechowska et al. developed a 38-item discriminative questionnaire for veterinarians to use with clients, designed to assess nonphysical aspects of QOL in dogs (Wojciechowska et al. 2005; see also Wojciechowska and Hewson 2005a,b).

Lavan's CHQLS (canine health-related quality of life survey) measures 15 items grouped into 4 domains (happiness, physical functioning, hygiene, and mental status) and adds three general health and QOL questions (Lavan 2013). This instrument is unique in being designed for healthy dogs and could be valuable in offering a baseline measurement.

The main components of a good assessment tool are summarized in Box 4.3.

Box 4.3   Desirable qualities of a quality of life assessment tool.

- Guide clients to observe and monitor their animal's subjective experiences, especially the expression and fulfillment of what she sees as her individual preferences at that moment
- Take into account both positive and negative experiences
- Balance usability (for clients and hospice team) with rigor and comprehensiveness
- Allow certain experiences greater weight than others (e.g. respiratory distress and severe pain should "count" more than incontinence), based on species-specific physiology as well as the patient's individual preferences/personality/lifestyle and stage of illness
- Provide a "dynamic assessment." QOL is fluid, and assessments need to be frequent and on-going (daily, or weekly, or maybe hourly, depending on the patient's condition)

- Be based on accurate and frequent observations, recorded and aimed at recognizing trends
- Help practitioners see what we can be doing better to keep an animal comfortable and happy
- Expose gaps in caregiving
- Serve as a platform that facilitates discussion between professional providers and caregivers, working to reach a consensus on the patient's QOL
- Provide an opportunity for providers to educate caregivers about what animals need and how to look for signs of pain or discomfort, etc. (e.g. a simple ethogram of species-specific pain behaviors)
- Give attention to the influence of the human–animal bond on QOL assessments

Quality of Life Assessment Over Time

QOL, as all subjective experience, is dynamic in nature – it changes with time, and following trends is as important as specific momentary "scores." Tracking QOL over time is therefore extremely important and needs to be incorporated into all QOL assessment tools, especially those designed for use by clients. Of the tools discussed above, Iliopoulou's QOL tool and the VetMetrica module are the only ones explicitly stipulating that QOL assessments need to be repeated at regular time intervals throughout the course of the patient's illness or aging process.

Whichever system a practitioner decides to use, QOL assessments need to be frequent and ongoing (daily, or weekly, or maybe hourly, depending on the patient's condition). There are two steps to the process, summarized as follows:

Step 1. Assess the Animal's Current QOL

Assess how the animal is doing overall at the time of assessment, with attention to all three domains of QOL (physical, emotional, social).

1) Negative affect: examples are listed in the Negative affect column of Box 4.2. Negative affect can be a response to unpleasant physical sensations (pain, nausea, extreme cold, etc.) and can also be a response to unpleasant events and perceptions (anxiety, confusion, frustration, etc.).

2) Positive affect: examples are listed in the Positive affect column of Box 4.2. Positive affect can be a response to pleasant physical sensations (touch, sights, smells, etc.) and can also be a response to pleasant events and perceptions (connection to primary attachment figure/s, sense of control, enriched environment, play, etc.).

3) Expression of individual preferences or will includes responses to both desired and undesired events and/or circumstances.

4) Physical functioning (digestion, respiration, mobility, level of consciousness, etc.).

Step 2. Assess Trends in How an Animal's QOL Changes Over Time

To detect trends in QOL, repeat "Step 1" (assess of the animal's current QOL) at regular time intervals. The ideal frequency for repeating "Step 1" can be hourly, daily, weekly, or monthly, depending on how rapidly the animal's condition is changing (e.g. stable patients need to be assessed less frequently than those who are decompensating). A record needs to be kept of the repeated assessments of the animal's QOL. From this record, the magnitude of change (e.g. rate of decline) from day to day and/or week to week can be tracked and graphed as the individual patient's illness trajectory (see examples in Figure 4.1a–d).

Monitoring the impact of chronic/terminal illness progression on animals' QOL is an important component in making end-of-life care decisions for them. As has been demonstrated in the realm of human end-of-life care, there several common trajectories of decline, characteristic of major types of disease or disability (see, for instance, Lynn and Adamson 2003). Having an idea of which trajectory an animal is likely to follow can help when setting priorities for care. For example, cancers often follow a trajectory of a long period of stable QOL followed by a short period of evident and rapid decline. During the rapid-decline period, palliation of the symptoms and around-the-clock hospice care would likely be indicated. Frailty and cognitive dysfunction associated with advanced age might, in contrast, follow a trajectory of prolonged and gradual diminishment of QOL. In this case, adaptations to the home environment, enrichments that help foster social engagement, and other supportive care will be of primary importance.

Ultimately, an individual patient's disease progression is never predictable. Graphing individual patient's illness trajectories doesn't generate "answers" to end-of-life decision-making questions. It does, however, provide meaningful insights that can serve as a basis

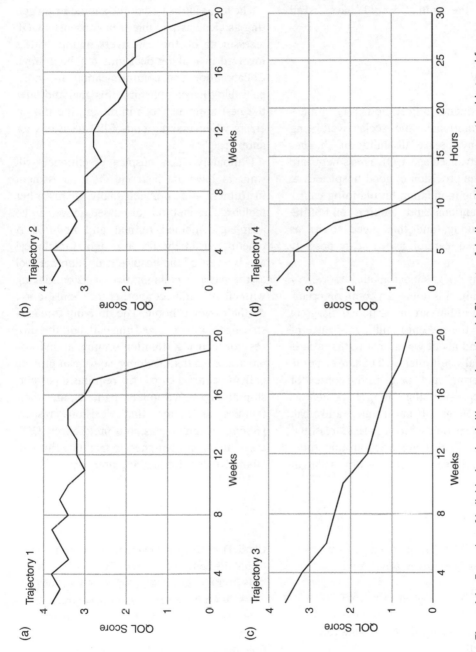

Figure 4.1 Examples of individual patient's illness trajectories. (a) Slow rate of decline, stable course: noticeable trend from month to month, with noticeable fluctuations down and up from day to day and/or week to week. (b) Moderate rate of decline, stable course: noticeable trend from week to week, but not from day to day. (c) Moderate rate of decline, volatile course: noticeable trend from week to week, with noticeable fluctuations down and up from day to day. (d) Rapid decline: noticeable trend from day to day.

for contemplation and discussion of what the animal may be experiencing from the animal's point of view, adding a rational component to the health care proxy's speculation regarding "what the animal would have asked them to do."

Summary

QOL assessments reflect how an animal's physical, emotional, and social well-being is affected by disease, disability, or changes related to advanced age. QOL assessments are crucial to the provision of good hospice care: they form the foundation for planning palliative interventions and guiding end-of-life decision-making, and thus need to be as thorough and careful as we can possibly make them.

Significant disagreement about how well or poorly an animal is doing is a common occurrence in end-of-life care, in particular disagreement about the presence and significance of suffering, and about when or if euthanasia is in the animal's best interest. The power of the terms "suffering" and "pain" in the context of end-of-life care planning is in their vagueness, invoking feelings of uncertainty and fear. Caregivers' experience becomes less stressful if one can put some boundaries around these concepts and place them within a larger

context. A thorough, methodical QOL assessment can provide that context.

The main components of a good assessment tool are summarized in Table 4.2.

The focus at the end of life should be on getting as close as possible to a consensus QOL assessment by the caregivers and providers involved in making decisions for the animal. Collaboration and communication are indispensable to accomplishing this goal and offer the best approach to minimizing the risk of errors when making end-of-life decisions for animals.

Ultimately, each hospice practitioner will want to have at least one QOL assessment instrument – and probably many – in his or her toolbox. The methods discussed above can be adapted, combined, refined, and modified. A practitioner might use one tool for clinical assessments by the hospice team, another tool as the basis of collaborative decision-making with clients, and yet another for clients to use on their own at home. The unifying thread is striving for an organized and collaborative process for focusing attention on how an individual animal patient is doing, so we can provide patient-centered care. This requires a partnership among practitioners, patients, and their families to ensure that decisions respect patients' wants, needs, and preferences. QOL assessments are designed to facilitate this collaborative decision-making process.

References

Bekoff, Marc (2008) The Emotional Lives of Animals. Novato, CA: New World Library.

Brickman, P. and Campbell, D.T. (1971) Hedonic Relativism and Planning the Good Society. Academic Press: New York, pp. 287–302.

Broom, D.M. (1996) Animal welfare defined in terms of attempts to cope with the environment, *Acta Agric. Scand. A – Anim. Sci. Suppl.*, 27: pp. 22–28.

Clark, D. (1999) Total pain, disciplinary power and the body in the work of Cicely Saunders, 1958–1967. *Social Sci. Med.*, 49: 727–736.

Clark, D. (2007) From margins to centre: a review of the history of palliative care in cancer. *Lancet Oncol.*, 8: 430–438.

Colombetti, G. (2005) Appraising valence, *J. Conscious. Stud.*, 12: 106–129.

DeWaal, F. (2020) Mama's Last Hug: Animal Emotions and What They Tell Us About Ourselves. New York: WW Norton & Co.

Duncan, I.J.H. (1996) Animal welfare defined in terms of feelings, *Acta Agric. Scand. A – Anim. Sci. Suppl.*, 27: 29–35.

Earp, J.L., French, E.A., and Gilkey, M.B. (2008) Patient Advocacy for Health Care Quality. Burlington, MA: Jones and Bartlett Learning.

Fillingim, R.B. (2017) Individual differences in pain: understanding the mosaic that makes pain personal. *Pain*, 158 (Suppl 1): S11–S18.

Freeman, L.M., Rush, J.E., Farabaugh, A.E., and Must, A. (2005) Development and evaluation of a questionnaire for assessing health-related quality of life in dogs with cardiac disease. *J. Am. Vet. Med. Assoc.*, 226: 1864–1868.

Hartmann, K. and Kuffer, M. (1998) Karnofsky's score modified for cats. *Eur. J. Med. Res.*, 3: 95–98.

Henry, B. (2017) The ethics of suffering in the era of assisted dying. *Ann. Palliat. Med.*, 6: 173–177.

Iliopoulou, M.A., Kitchell, B.E., and Yuzbasiyan-Gurkan, V. (2013) Development of a survey instrument to assess health-related quality of life in small animal cancer patients treated with chemotherapy. *J. Am. Vet. Med. Assoc.*, 242: 1679–1687.

Institute of Medicine. (2001) *Crossing the Quality Chasm: A New Health System for the 21st Century*. Washington, DC: The National Academies Press. Available at: http://nationalacademies.org/hmd/reports/2001/crossing-the-quality-chasm-a-new-health-system-for-the-21st-century.aspx (Accessed: Sept. 2016).

International Association for Animal Hospice and Palliative Care (IAAHPC) *(2013) Animal hospice and palliative care guidelines. Available at:* https://iaahpc.org/wp-content/uploads/2020/10/IAAHPC-AИГC-GUIDELINESpdf.pdf. (Accessed May 2022).

International Association for the Study of Pain (IASP) (2020) *IASP anounces revised definition of pain.* Available at: https://www.iasp-pain.org/publications/iasp-news/iasp-announces-revised-definition-of-pain (Accessed: May 2022).

Kagan, S. (1992) The limits of well-being. In: The Good Life and the Human Good (eds E.F. Paul, F.D. Miller, and J. Paul). Cambridge, UK: Cambridge University Press, 169–189.

Kahneman, D., Diener, E., and Schwartz, N. (eds) (1999) Well-Being: The Foundations of Hedonic Psychology. Russell Sage: New York.

Kuhn, P.J., Kooreman, P., Soetevent, A., and Kapteyn, A. (2008) The Own and Social Effects of an Unexpected Income Shock: Evidence from the Dutch Postcode Lottery. Santa Barbara, CA: Department of Economics, University of California, Santa Barbara.

Lavan, R.P. (2013) Development and validation of a survey for quality of life assessment by owners of healthy dogs. *Vet. J.*, 197: 578–582.

Lynn, J. and Adamson, D.M. (2003) Living Well at the End of Life: Adapting Health Care to Serious Chronic Illness in Old Age. Santa Monica, CA: RAND.

Martin, P. and Bateson, P. (2007) Measuring Behavior: An Introductory Guide. New York: Cambridge University Press.

McMillan, F.D. (2005a) Stress, distress, and emotion: distinctions and implications for mental well-being. In: Mental Health and Well-Being in Animals (ed. F. McMillan). Ames, IA: Wiley-Blackwell, 93–111.

McMillan, F.D. (ed.) (2005b) Mental Health and Well-Being in Animals. Ames, IA: Wiley-Blackwell.

Mich, P.M. and Hellyer, P.W. (2015) Objective, categoric methods for assessing pain and analgesia. In: Handbook of Veterinary Pain Management, 3edn. (eds J.S. Gaynor and W.W. Muir). St. Louis, MO: Mosby Elsevier, 78–112.

Panksepp, J. (2005) Affective-social neuroscience approaches to understanding core emotional feelings in animals. In: Mental Health and Well-Being in Animals (ed F. McMillan). Wiley-Blackwell: Ames, IA, 57–75.

Reid, J., Wiseman-Orr, M.L., Scott, E.M., and Nolan, A.M. (2013) Development, validation and reliability of a web-based questionnaire to measure health-related quality of life in dogs. *J. Small Anim. Pract.*, 54: 227–233.

Reid, J., Wiseman-Orr, M.L., Scott, E.M., and Nolan, A.M. (2015) Health related quality of life measurement. In: Handbook of Veterinary Pain Management, 3 (ed. J. Gaynor and W. Muir). St. Louis, MO: Mosby Elsevier, 98–110.

Reid, J., Wiseman-Orr, L., and Scott, E.M. (2018) Shortening of an existing generic online health-related quality of life instrument for dogs. *J. Small Anim. Pract.*, 59: 334–342.

Sandöe P. (1999) Quality of life: three competing views. *Ethical Theory Moral Pract.* 2: pp. 11–23.

Sandöe P., Appleby M.C. (2002) "Philosophical debate on the nature of well-being: implications for animal welfare" *Anim. Welfare*, 11: 283–294.

Shanan, A. (2011) A veterinarian's role in helping pet owners with decision making, *Vet. Clin. Small Anim.*, 41: 635–646.

Turner, D.C. and Bateson, P. (eds) (2014) The Domestic Cat: The Biology of its Behaviour, 3 edn. New York: Cambridge University Press.

Villalobos AE. (2011) End of life care, *NAVC Clin. Brief,* 2008: 21–23.

Wiseman-Orr, M.L., Nolan, A.M., Reid, J., et al. (2004) Development of a questionnaire to measure the effects of chronic pain on health-related quality of life in dogs. *Am. J. Vet. Res.*, 65: 1077–1084.

Wiseman-Orr, M.L., Scott, E.M., Reid, J. et al. (2006) Validation of a structured questionnaire as an instrument to measure chronic pain in dogs on the basis of effects on health-related quality of life. *Am. J. Vet. Res.*, 67(11): 1826–1836.

Wojciechowska, J.I. and Hewson, C.J. (2005a) Quality-of-life assessment in pet dogs. *J. Am. Vet. Med. Assoc.*, 226: 722–728.

Wojciechowska, J.I., and Hewson, C.J. (2005b) Development of a discriminative questionnaire to assess nonphysical aspects of quality of life of dogs. *Am. J. Vet. Res.*, 66: 1453–1460.

Wojciechowska, J.I., Hewson, C.J., Stryhn, H., et al. (2005) Evaluation of a questionnaire regarding nonphysical aspects of quality of life in sick and healthy dogs. *Am. J. Vet. Res.*, 66: 1461–1467.

Yazbek, K.V. and Fantoni, D.T. (2005) Validity of a health-related quality-of-life scale for dogs with signs of pain secondary to cancer. *J. Am. Vet. Med. Assoc.*, 226: 1354–1358.

Yeates, J. and Main, D. (2009) Assessment of companion animal quality of life in veterinary practice and research. *J. Small Anim. Pract.*, 50: 274–281.

Further Reading

American Animal Hospice Association/American Association of Feline Practitioners (2007) Pain management guidelines for dogs and cats. *J. Am. Anim. Hosp. Assoc.*, 43: 235–248.

Bekoff, M. (2005) The Emotional Lives of Animals. Novato, CA: New World Library.

Berlinger, N., Jennings, B., and Wolf, S. (2013) The Hastings Center Guidelines for Decisions on Life-Sustaining Treatment and Care near the End of Life. New York: Oxford University Press.

Boissy, A., Manteuffel, G., Jensen, M.B., et al. (2007) Assessment of positive emotions in animals to improve their welfare. *Physiol. Behav.*, 92: 375–397.

Bonica, J.J. (1979) The need of a taxonomy. *Pain*, 6: 247–248.

Cabanac, M. (2005) The experience of pleasure in animals. In: Mental Health and Well-being in Animals (ed. F. McMillan). Ames, IA: Blackwell, 29–55.

Fox, S.M. (2010) Chronic Pain in Small Animal Medicine. Manson Publishing: London.

German, A.J., Holden, S.L., Wiseman-Orr, M.L. et al. (2012) Quality of life is reduced in obese dogs but improves after successful weight loss. *Vet. J.*, 192: 428–434.

Gregory, N. (2004) Physiology and Behavior of Animal Suffering. Oxford: Blackwell.

Hewson, C.J., Hilby, E.F., and Bradshaw, J.W.S. (2007) Assessing quality of life in kenneled dogs: a critical review, *Anim. Welfare*, 16(Suppl): pp. 89–95.

Knesl, O., Hart, B.L., Cooper, L., Patterson-Kane, E., Houlihan, K.E., and Anthony, R. (2017) Veterinarians and human endings: when is the right time to euthanize a companion animal? *Front. Vet. Sci.*, 4: 45.

Lynch, S., Savary-Bataille, K., Leuw, B., and Argyle, D.J. (2010) Development of a questionnaire assessing health-related quality-of-life in dogs and cats with cancer. *Vet. Comp. Oncol.*, 9: 172–182.

Markowitz, H. and Eckert, K. (2005) Giving power to animals. In: Mental Health and Wellbeing in Animals (ed. F. McMillan). Ames, IA: Blackwell, pp. 201–209.

Mwacalimba, K.K., Contadini, F.M., Spofford, N., Lopez, K. et al. (2020) Owner and veterinarian perceptions about use of a canine quality of life survey in primary care settings. *Front. Vet. Sci.*, 7: 89.

Noli, C., Minafo, G., and Galzerano, M. (2011) Quality of life of dogs with skin diseases and their owners. Part 1: development and validation of a questionnaire. *Vet. Dermatol.*, 22: 335–343.

Panksepp, J. (1982) Toward a general psychobiological theory of emotions. *Behav. Brain Sci.*, 5: 407–422.

Panksepp, J. (1998) Affective Neuroscience: The Foundation of Human and Animal Emotions. New York: Oxford University Press.

Pierce, J. (2012) The Last Walk: Reflections on our Pets at the End of their Lives. Chicago: University of Chicago Press.

Sepucha, K., Uzogarra, B., and O'Connor, M. (2008) Developing instruments to measure the quality of decisions: early results for a set of symptom-driven decisions. *Patient Educ. Couns.*, 73: 504–510.

Strang, P., Strang, S., Hultborn, R., and Arner, S. (2004) Existential pain – an entity, a provocation, or a challenge? *J. Pain Symptom Manage.*, 27: 241–250.

Wemelsfelder, F. (2007) How animals communicate quality of life: the qualitative assessment of behaviour. *Anim. Welfare*, 16(Suppl. 1): 25–31.

Wemelsfelder, F. (2005) Animal boredom: understanding the tedium of confined lives. In Mental Health and Well-Being in Animals (ed. F. McMillan). Blackwell: Ames, IA, pp. 79–91.

Yeates, J.W., Mullan, S., Stone, M., and Main, D.C. (2011) Promoting discussions and decisions about dogs' quality-of-life. *J. Small Anim. Pract.* 52: 459–463.

Yeates, J. (2013) Animal Welfare in Veterinary Practice. Oxford: Universities Federation for Animal Welfare.

5

Recognizing Distress

Emma K. Grigg, PhD, CAAB, Suzanne Hetts, PhD, CAAB, and Amir Shanan, DVM

Stress, Distress, Emotions, and Suffering

Behavior scientists have struggled to come to general agreements about the definitions of stress, distress, and suffering, and how to recognize these states. These terms, used very loosely in everyday speech, need more precise definitions and understanding when used as the basis for making decisions about what's best for an animal.

It is not the purpose of this chapter to delve deeply into the nature of stress. The core of our discussion is dedicated to recognizing signs of distress, and it is therefore important for our discussion to consider the animal's experience of distress, its causes, and how distress is different from stress. The primary topic for this chapter, and indeed this entire book, is how we can help alleviate and/or prevent animal distress. To alleviate or prevent distress, we must be able to recognize it; this chapter will reference currently available methods for assessing emotional state in nonhuman animals.

The Stress Response

The term "stress" is often used in everyday speech to refer to both a physiological and/or behavioral stress response, as well as the stimuli that elicit it. There seems to be no single, generally accepted definition of stress, and the term is often used without any specifications as to how it is defined in that context. Drawing from several definitions of "stress" in the scientific literature, the terms we chose to use in this chapter are "stressor" for the condition causing stress, and "stress response" for the effects on the animal.

Simply defined, the stress response is a biological reaction to environmental events or conditions (stressors) that caused an upset of the animal's balance or homeostasis. The stress response has physiological (including metabolic, endocrine, and immunological), behavioral, and emotional components. The stress response may or may not have a detrimental effect on the animal's welfare or well-being, depending in part on whether the stress is acute or chronic. All animals – including humans – are exposed to stressors regularly, and the stress response is a normal reaction to stressors that does not necessarily produce long term harmful effects. An animal's response to a particular stressor can be quite specific; for example, the stress response to extreme cold will be different from that to extreme heat. In addition, a variety of environmental and internal factors, including individual resilience, will influence how an animal will respond to potential stressors.

McMillan (2005) notes that the terms "stress," "anxiety," and "fear" are often used

Hospice and Palliative Care for Companion Animals: Principles and Practice, Second Edition.
Edited by Amir Shanan, Jessica Pierce, and Tamara Shearer.
© 2023 John Wiley & Sons, Inc. Published 2023 by John Wiley & Sons, Inc.
Companion website: www.wiley.com/go/shanan/palliative

interchangeably in the literature, and provides numerous examples to support his contention. While writing this chapter, one of the authors (Hetts) attended a conference where a number of service dogs, search and rescue dogs, and therapy dogs were present. A number of these dogs exhibited behaviors generally considered to be manifestations of canine "stress," such as panting, avoidance of certain people and other dogs, ears back, eyes widened, and even a few defensive threats (growling and teeth baring). Hetts found herself remarking to a colleague that the dogs at the conference appeared "stressed," but realized she could just as easily have said they appeared anxious or fearful. Additional examples of this linkage between stress responses, fear and anxiety are seen in the promotion of "low stress handling" (Yin 2009) techniques and the "fear free veterinary visits" (e.g. the Fear Free® initiative, fearfreepets.com) promotions designed to minimize the disruptive effects of the stress response on the clinical veterinary exam. This ubiquitous overlap in terminology reflects the fact that emotions and stress responses are inextricably linked.

To further complicate matters, release of glucocorticoids such as cortisol, a measurable physiological hallmark of the stress response, also occurs in association with pleasant emotional states. Glucocorticoid release has been shown to occur in horses during exercise, restraint, and sexual stimulation (Colborn et al. 1991). Although we know of no similar research in dogs and cats, it is not difficult to imagine a release of glucocorticoids occurring when a dog is running an agility course, or a cat stalking or capturing a bird. While it could be said the animals in these circumstances are "stressed," they are also likely enjoying themselves. For this reason, studies using cortisol measurements to evaluate stress responses are strengthened by inclusion of behavioral observations, to distinguish between positive and negative affect in the study subjects.

In our attempts to understand what animals feel when stressed (e.g. positive or negative affect), we are limited to relying on our observations and interpretation of their body language and behavior, integrating any additional insights we can gain from the environmental context in which the behavior occurs.

What Is Distress?

Like "stress," the term "distress" is often not clearly defined. The experience of distress is associated with unpleasant emotional states (DeGrazia 1996). McMillan (2005) defines distress as "an unpleasant affective state . . . resulting from an inability to control or otherwise cope with or adapt to the unpleasant affect generated by altered or threatened homeostasis" (p. 105). Similarly, the National Research Council's Committee on Recognition and Alleviation of Pain in Laboratory Animals (2009) defined distress as "an aversive state in which an animal is unable to adapt completely to stressors and the resulting stress, and (as a result) shows maladaptive behaviors" (p. 23). Ward et al. (2008) describe distress as a state in which an animal, unable to adapt to one or more stressors, is no longer successfully coping with its environment and as a result its well-being is compromised. Pain, particularly chronic pain, is often a contributing factor to distress; and distress is more likely to result when multiple stressors persist for longer durations. Distress is what animals experience when no options are readily available to successfully pursue what they want, or to avoid an aversive condition such as pain or isolation. Suffering is a broader term, and encompasses a wide range of unpleasant emotional and physical states, such as pain, fear, boredom, and hunger (Dawkins 1990). Distress contrasts with eustress (Selye 1976), a positive stress response resulting from challenging but enjoyable stressors, such as attainable or worthwhile tasks (e.g. the dog running the agility course, or the cat stalking a bird).

While definitions of distress vary, the most important components in virtually all of them are the animal's inability to control, predict, cope with, or adapt to aversive conditions or events, and the experience of the associated unpleasant affective states, all of which can result in a decrease in the animal's ability to function normally. McMillan and others point out it is the animal's *perceived* degree of control over its situation that is important (McMillan 2005; Ward et al. 2008). This is borne out by various studies of human patients, who report more effective pain relief when given the ability to self-administer pain medication than those on continuous infusion, even when the actual amount of medication used was the same (Walder et al. 2001).

Preference tests have been used by behavior scientists for years as a means for animals to tell us, through their behaviors, what they want and what they prefer. Preference tests clearly demonstrate that animals can learn to choose food that relieves their pain. Broiler chickens, who gain weight quickly in order to decrease their time to slaughter, often experience lameness and joint problems. Chickens with a lameness score of three or more (on a validated one to five scale), learned to choose red or blue colored food, depending on whether it contained the pain-relieving drug carprofen. Birds with a lameness score of zero showed no such preference (Danbury et al. 2000). The fact that the birds learned an arbitrary association and then chose a response that allowed them to escape their painful state is evidence that they experienced pain and wanted to escape it (Dawkins 2005).

If a requirement is added to preference tests such that the animal must experience some degree of unpleasantness to obtain access to something it wants, investigators may be able to gain insight into just how important a particular item or experience is to the animal. Iguanas, for example, will venture into a cold section of their cages (when regular food chow and water is available in the warm part of their habitat) for a more palatable food (lettuce), until the degree of cold offsets the pleasantness of the lettuce (Balasko and Carbanac 1998). Such studies demonstrate that animals actively pursue their preferences when they can, even if it requires "paying a price" for getting what they want.

While strictly-controlled preference tests aren't practical for animals in hospice care, this perspective (i.e. acknowledging and respecting the individual animal's preferences) can guide the choices we offer them daily, and provide ongoing information about current comfort level of animals in our care. For example, Hetts' Irish Setter Blaze loved to play ball. As Blaze aged, her ability to run after the ball declined. If at some point, Hetts threw the ball but Blaze declined to go fetch it, one interpretation would be that the cost of fetching the ball had become greater from Blaze's perspective than her enjoyment of doing so.

Behavioral Needs of Dogs and Cats

An important goal of animal hospice and palliative care (AHPC) is meeting patients' behavioral needs. Therefore, it is important for caregivers to be aware of those needs. While there is general agreement regarding animals' physiologic needs, there is less agreement in the ethological or animal welfare literature regarding behavioral needs for different species or individual animals (Curtis 1987). The Five Freedoms (Brambell 1965, Farm Animal Welfare Council 2009) provided an early framework for assessing the minimum requirements for Quality of Life (QOL) in nonhuman animals:

1) Freedom from hunger and thirst (by providing ready access to fresh water and diet to maintain health and vigor)
2) Freedom from discomfort (by providing an appropriate environment including shelter and a comfortable resting area)
3) Freedom from pain, injury, or disease (by prevention or rapid diagnosis and treatment of medical issues)
4) Freedom to express normal behavior (by providing sufficient space, proper facilities, and the company of the animal's own kind)
5) Freedom from fear and distress (by ensuring conditions and treatment that avoid mental suffering)

The Five Freedoms clarified that welfare of nonhuman animals is not just accomplished by the provision of food, shelter, and basic veterinary care (e.g. Freedoms one to three), but also requires attention to the animal's behavioral needs and mental state (Freedoms four and five). An update to the Five Freedoms can be found in the work of David Mellor and colleagues (e.g. Mellor 2016), which shifts the focus from the prevention of negative experiences to the provision of positive experiences. The Five Domains model acknowledges the mental experiences of nonhuman animals, the influence of situational/environmental factors on their mental state, and the fact that QOL encompasses the perception of one's situation. This model also acknowledges that some negative experiences are unavoidable, even necessary for survival (for example, feelings of hunger or thirst may not be pleasant per se, but drive us to consume food or water necessary for survival). Thus, the Five Domains model (Mellor 2016) stresses the need for caregivers to provide opportunities for animals to behave in the ways that the animals themselves find rewarding, in addition to minimizing negative experiences to the greatest extent possible. Rault et al. (2020a) recommend that animal welfare researchers clearly define what they mean by positive welfare, and consider how various positive welfare interventions effect each facet of animal welfare (e.g. greater sense of agency, and frequency and duration of expression of natural behaviors, and so on).

This framework has been adopted by many practitioners and welfare advocates to promote welfare of owned companion animals. For example, Hetts et al. (2004) proposed a list of behavioral needs in dogs and cats that they have used to promote behavior wellness. This list includes:

- Freedom from, or the ability to escape from, unnecessary pain, fear, threats, and discomfort
- Ability to control some aspects of the environment

- Opportunities to express a range of species typical behaviors including but not limited to chewing, scratching, and elimination
- Opportunities for appropriate exercise and play
- Opportunities for mental stimulation
- Opportunities for pleasant social contact with other members of the species, and with familiar people
- Provision of a safe, comfortable place to rest and sleep

This list of behavioral needs assumes the basic needs for adequate food, water, shelter, and health care have already been met (Hetts et al. 2004).

Assessing Quality of Life in Nonhuman Animals

QOL can be defined generally as "the degree to which an individual is healthy, comfortable, and able to participate in or enjoy life events" (Brittanica.com), and reflects how an animal's physical, emotional, and social well-being is affected by disease, disability, or changes related to advanced age. There is no consensus on the definition of QOL as it pertains to animals. Yeates (2020) advises us to think of animal QOL in terms of what gives animals' lives value (*from their perspective*), and to describe it operationally as what animals would (most likely) want for themselves.

As animals age or as illness progresses, attempts to figure out what they would want for themselves are complicated by the processes of coping and psychological adaptation – mechanisms that stabilize sentient beings and modulate their responses to adverse situations, and that move humans and animals toward a balance in their mental, social, and emotional states of being. As a result of coping and/or adaptation, a life with disability, chronic or terminal illness can be a life worth living for most human and animal patients. It is important, therefore, to not equate QOL with that particular animal's reality during his/her prime; when faced with adverse reality, they go through an adaptation phase to a "new normal." It may be that family members and medical teams view the patient's "new normal" more negatively than the patient, as reported in studies with human patients (Sprangers and Aaronson 1992). Relying too heavily on "activities enjoyed before illness/aging" as a baseline for QOL assessment cheats patients out of the benefits to their QOL gained thru coping and adaptation. This is highly relevant to assessing QOL in animals with life-limiting conditions, who often adapt well to changing circumstances. Animals can still enjoy life despite being blind or deaf, having lost a limb, experiencing chronic pain, or facing many other physical and emotional challenges.

QOL in nonhuman animals is evaluated in one of two ways. In research settings, QOL may be measured by quantitative measures of observable behavior, such as frequency of stress-related behaviors, sometimes augmented by measures of physiological stress responses. For companion animals, however, QOL is usually measured by proxy (e.g. the animal's caregiver answers a series of questions about the animal's recent behavior, activities, etc.). The proxy approach, while useful when the reporter is very familiar with the animal, may be limited by the reporter's attitudes, perception of what constitutes normal behavior in that species, or even ability to interpret the body language and behavior of distress in their animal. See Chapter 4 in this volume for an in-depth discussion of animal QOL.

Relevance to Animal Hospice and Palliative Care (AHPC)

Attached caregivers involved in making end-of-life care decisions for their animals frequently say their wish is to make decisions based on what they think the animal wants, or what the animal would have asked them to do. What they wish to provide their animals is a good QOL. To provide a good QOL for animals, we must understand their wants, needs, and preferences. To do this, and to assess whether the interventions provided are effective, it is important to be able to recognize expressions of emotion in their animals (see "Are Humans Adept at Recognizing Emotional States in Animals?" in this chapter). This understanding must then be followed by caregivers' careful, well-informed observations of patients' behavior over time, leading to the QOL assessments that are so important when making animal end-of-life care decisions.

Caregivers can be encouraged to keep logs or journals documenting their observations of their animals' behavior patterns and frequencies, because behavioral patterns are practical and useful measures of animals' QOL (see "Changes in Behavioral Patterns as Indicators of Pain and Distress" in this chapter). Common activities of daily living and enjoyable behaviors that are important to track in AHPC patients include willingness to eat, drink, walk, climb stairs, engage in play, and interact with familiar humans or conspecifics. Watching for changes in animals' body language (see "Body Language of Fear, Anxiety and Pain" in this chapter) and tracking the changes noticed provides invaluable information for assessing their emotional state. As all animals are individuals, it is most meaningful to compare an animal's current behavior and body language with the typical behavior and body language of that animal in the past, e.g. a week ago, six months ago, one year ago, etc.

For these reasons, behavioral logs, photos, and videos can be powerful tools to monitor and evaluate animals' experience of declining health, and promote effective communication between the caregiver and the veterinary team. Templates for simple, easy-to-use daily or weekly QOL logs are available online. These logs or diaries are most useful when customized for an individual animal or household. For more in-depth information, weekly or monthly completion of a health-related QOL survey designed to work with both healthy and declining dogs, such as found in Mwacalimba et al. 2020, can be beneficial. For animals experiencing cognitive decline, logs should include questions based on the DISHAA framework (Salvin et al. 2010) and be designed to track changes in cognitive function over time. Senior pet checklists, such as that found in Seibert (2021), can be used by caregivers for this purpose.

Are Humans Adept at Recognizing Emotional States in Animals?

Knowledge of animal behavior and emotions is growing rapidly, and often reveals that animals' feelings aren't nearly as "hidden" as they were once thought to be (e.g. de Waal 2011). Although we cannot ask animals directly how they feel or what they want, we can gather a great deal of information by carefully observing their behavior, their physiological state, and their expressions of affect. Much can be learned about animals' individual preferences by interpreting such observations, integrating our growing knowledge of species-specific behavior with attunement to individual differences.

To recognize signs of pain and distress, caregivers must be skilled at observing and interpreting the body language of the animals under our care. Highly attached caregivers are often intimately familiar with their animals' normal behaviors, activities of daily living and individual preferences. Still, accurate interpretation of animal behavior may be challenging. Several studies have demonstrated that pet owners and less experienced pet professionals have difficulty recognizing behavioral expressions of fear and anxiety in dogs. For example, pet owners were less likely than professionals to report that ears, eyes, and mouth were features providing important information about dogs' emotional state (Wan et al. 2012).

Adding to these challenges, a caregiver placebo effect is well documented in veterinary medicine and may compromise an accurate assessment of a pet's QOL. Conzemius and Evans (2012) report this effect for dogs with osteoarthritis to be as much as 57% for dog owners and 40–45% for veterinarians, when treatment with an NSAID was compared with ground reaction forces measurement. These observations underscore that all animal caregivers should be proactively trained in recognizing the signs of pain and distress in their animals.

Body Language of Fear, Anxiety, and Pain

A comprehensive discussion of body postures and behavioral expressions of pain can be found in the excellent chapter titled "Assessing Pain: Pain Behaviors" (Wiese 2015) in the third edition of the *Handbook of Veterinary Pain Management* (Gaynor and Muir 2015). We would expect veterinarians, veterinary technicians, and other animal hospice team members to be highly experienced and readily familiar with signs of fear and anxiety in the species under their care. In reality, expertise may vary among veterinary team members, and may vary greatly among caregivers. We recommend AHPC team members make it a habit to ensure that pet owners can reliably recognize the body postures and behavioral signs associated with fear anxiety, stress/distress, or pain. Handouts, like the one-page Canine Chronic Pain Scale from Colorado State University (available at 360petmedical.com/wp-content/uploads/2020/03/Canine_Pain_Scale.pdf), the Canine Brief Pain Inventory (available at https://www.vet.upenn.edu/docs/default-source/VCIC/canine-bpi-user's-guide-2017-2107), or the Feline Musculoskeletal Pain Index (FMPI), (available at doi.org/10.1371/journal.pone.0131839.s001), can be helpful tools for practitioners and caregivers to assess and monitor QOL. Downloadable one-page handouts illustrating the body language of anxiety in dogs and cats can be obtained from Cattledog Publishing, Davis, CA (cattledogpublishing.com/poster-download/).

Fear- and Discomfort-Related Body Postures Commonly Observed in Dogs and Cats

Ears – Ears will be lowered, flattened to the side, or pulled back (Figure 5.1). Experienced professionals tend to rely much more on ear position for information than do less

(a)

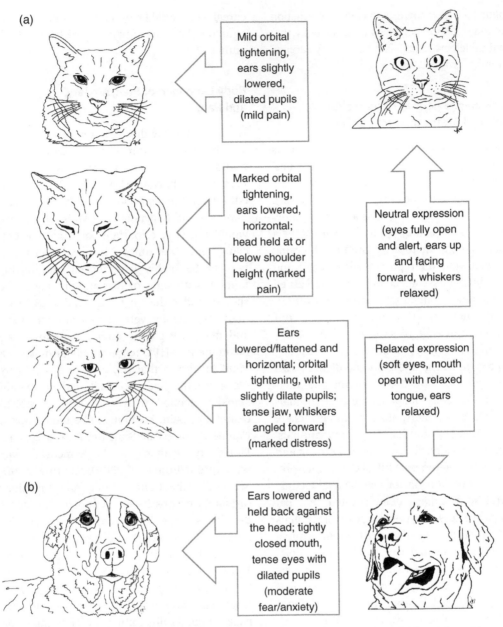

Mild orbital tightening, ears slightly lowered, dilated pupils (mild pain)

Marked orbital tightening, ears lowered, horizontal; head held at or below shoulder height (marked pain)

Neutral expression (eyes fully open and alert, ears up and facing forward, whiskers relaxed)

Ears lowered/flattened and horizontal; orbital tightening, with slightly dilate pupils; tense jaw, whiskers angled forward (marked distress)

Relaxed expression (soft eyes, mouth open with relaxed tongue, ears relaxed)

(b)

Ears lowered and held back against the head; tightly closed mouth, tense eyes with dilated pupils (moderate fear/anxiety)

Figure 5.1 Facial expressions indicating physical or emotional discomfort in cats (a) and dogs (b), contrasted with a relaxed or neutral facial expression. *Source:* Drawings: Megan Laughinghouse.

experienced observers (Wan et al. 2012). Interpretation of ear position can be complicated by differences in ear shape and coat color (e.g. floppy ears the same dark color as coat may not attract attention), and practices like ear cropping. Nonetheless, given the communicative value of ear carriage (especially in cats), it's particularly important to teach caregivers to get in the habit of watching ear position.

Tail –Tail carriage is an important indicator of emotional state. Fearful dogs and cats lower or tuck their tails, and generally do not raise them high over their backs (Figure 5.2).

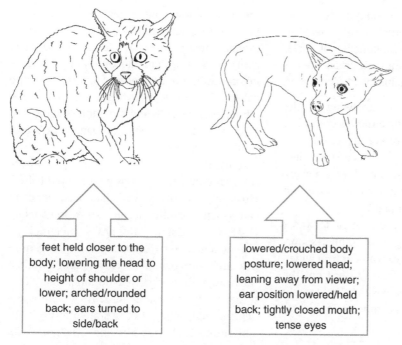

feet held closer to the
body; lowering the head to
height of shoulder or
lower; arched/rounded
back; ears turned to
side/back

lowered/crouched body
posture; lowered head;
leaning away from viewer;
ear position lowered/held
back; tightly closed mouth;
tense eyes

Figure 5.2 Body postures indicative of physical or emotional discomfort in cats and dogs. *Source:* Drawings: Megan Laughinghouse.

When lying down, fearful dogs and cats often curl their tails tightly against their bodies. Tail carriage and movement in most pets is a prominent, eye-catching aspect of their body language, and so is often used by caregivers as a primary indicator of the animal's emotional state. Professionals tend to balance the dog's tail carriage with other sources of information about the dog's intentions (Wan et al. 2012).

Body carriage – Fearful animals often duck their heads, carry their weight back on their hind legs, or assume a crouched or lowered body posture (Figure 5.2). A "roached" back (kyphosis posture) can be indicative of abdominal or hind end pain. A tense or rigid body is common, and both dogs and cats may freeze when extremely fearful. An animal in pain may be unwilling to move or change position (e.g. from standing to lying down) (Wiese 2015).

Eyes – When animals are fearful, their eyes widen and pupils dilate (Figure 5.1). Fearful dogs typically avoid eye contact or may look at you, then look away (Figure 5.2). "Whale eye" (a sideways look, eyes wide so that the sclera are clearly visible) is usually an indicator of distress or fear in dogs.

Mouth – Fearful dogs often keep their mouths firmly closed unless they are panting from fear or anxiety, or showing a submissive grin (Figures 5.1 and 5.2). The corners of a fearful dog's mouth (commissure) may be retracted backwards. Fearful cats that are not also threatening usually keep their mouths closed.

Vocalizations – Fearful dogs may be silent; or may whine, whimper or even bark. Dogs may growl when fearful and defensive. Hissing from cats occurs when the cat is also threatening/defensive, not merely fearful.

Pain-Related Facial Expressions Commonly Observed in Dogs and Cats

Intriguing new studies show how much non-human animals express their pain through facial expressions (see, for example, Cohen and

Beths 2020 for a review of mammalian pain scales used in research settings). Sotocinal et al. (2011) identified four components of facial expressions of pain in rats observed after a standardized pain-producing event. These are:

- Orbital tightening – a narrowing of the orbital area, manifesting either as (partial or complete) eye closure or eye "squeezing."
- Nose/cheek flattening – successively less bulging of the nose and cheek (see above), with eventual absence of the crease between the cheek and whisker pads.
- Ears – tend to fold, curl and angle forwards or outwards, resulting in a pointed shape. The space between the ears may appear wider.
- Whiskers – move forward (away from the face) from the baseline position and tend to bunch, giving the appearance of whiskers standing on end.

A different method (computerized measurements of differences between anatomical facial features versus analysis of video footage) has been used in an attempt to create a validated facial grimace scale in cats (Holden et al. 2014). Features that showed statistical differences between painful and pain-free cats included areas of the orbit (eyes), ears, and mouth. However, that study found that observers had difficulty recognizing these differences, with only 13% of observers able to distinguish more than 80% of painful cats. Evangelista et al. (2019) developed and validated a Feline Grimace Scale (FGS) using CatFACS, a Facial Action Coding System (FACS) similar to that used to measure facial emotional expression in humans (Ekman and Friesen 1978). Five "action units" (relevant facial features) were identified, including ear position, orbital tightening, muzzle tension, whiskers change and head position (Evangelista et al. 2019). The FGS was found to have very good inter-rater (ICC$_{single}$ = 0.89) and intra-rater (ICC$_{single}$ > 0.91) reliability, supporting its use by trained observers as a reliable tool for acute pain assessment in cats. Pain in cats was associated with, among other signs, tightening/narrowing of the eyes and lowering/flattening of the ears. An FGS training manual (Evangelista et al. 2019) is available free online (www.felinegrimacescale.com). In 2021, a Canadian animal health technology company developed a smartphone app called Tably (www.sylvester.ai/cat-owners), which uses the FGS and the phone's camera to help owners assess their companion cat's current emotional state.

At the time of writing this chapter, a grimace scale for domestic dogs has not been published. However, promising work has been done on categorizing canine facial expressions using DogFACS. Using DogFACS technology, researchers linked (for example) blinking, nose lick, and "ears flattener" (ears flattened against the head) with a negative emotional state (frustration) (Bremhorst et al. 2019). Figure 5.3 depicts facial images of a dog suffering with Chiari-like malformation and syringomyelia, before and after receiving treatment for pain (original patient images courtesy of Clare Rusbridge, DVM; University of Surrey, UK).

Relevance to Animal Hospice and Palliative Care (AHPC)

Given the existing work identifying meaningful facial expressions in dogs and cats, paying attention to the changes in an animal's facial expression and tension, as well as other aspects of body language, can help professionals and caregivers recognize when the animal feels anxious, fearful, and/or painful. Caregivers have a greater degree of familiarity with their pets, and can provide detailed information on signs of distress in their animals, including changes in "typical" or situational (e.g. when resting, or during handling) facial expression over time. This long-term monitoring is particularly important in cases of chronic pain. With the opportunity for multiple observations, caregivers can more readily recognize changes from unpainful to painful states. AHPC team members must be knowledgeable enough to educate caregivers about what facial features to look for that may suggest the

(a)   (b)

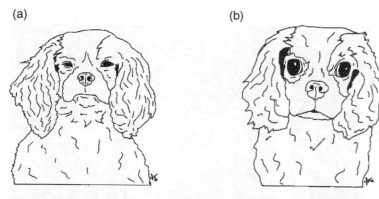

Figure 5.3 Before (a) and after (b) images of a dog treated for pain associated with Chiari-like malformation and syringomyelia; in (b) dog was receiving pregabalin and a nonsteroidal anti-inflammatory drug. *Source:* Original patient images courtesy of Clare Rusbridge, University of Surrey, UK. Drawings by Megan Laughinghouse.

animal is in pain. References cited in this chapter can be a starting point for learning to recognize pain in rats, mice, cats, horses, and rabbits (Leach et al. 2011).

Changes in Behavioral Patterns as Indicators of Pain and Distress

In addition to clues obtained through careful observation of body language, changes in the typical behavior of an individual animal can be important indicators of emotional state and the presence of physical discomfort.

Do Animals "Hide" their Pain?

Most everyone has heard the claim that animals instinctively hide their pain so as not to appear vulnerable to other animals that might hurt them or take advantage of them (e.g. Hellyer et al. 2007). This is a very difficult motivation to substantiate or refute objectively. However, the wide variation between individual animals of the same species in displaying their emotions suggest that, at least in part, the degree of "hiding pain" reflects an individual animal's personality trait or coping style (Lush and Ijichi 2018), and this may differ by breed in dogs (Hellyer et al. 2007). As Wiese (2015) notes, not all animals display pain-related behavior, and thus it is important to remember that lack of obvious pain-related behavior does

not guarantee that the animal is not experiencing pain. Signs of physical pain may be quite subtle, and may not be immediately evident to someone not familiar with the individual animal's normal state, or someone not specifically looking for these signs (Figure 5.4). Presence of stressors and environmental factors (such as being in a veterinary exam room, versus in the familiar home environment) may also alter the likelihood that an animal will display signs of pain (Wiese 2015; Reck 2012).

This situation can be further complicated when human observers do not know what to look for. A lack of activity, decreased movement, and general behavioral suppression (not doing much of anything) are all recognized as behavior changes that may occur when animals are ill or in pain (e.g. Hellyer et al. 2007; Wiese 2015). It is theorized that these behaviors' evolutionary function is to promote healing and minimize further injury (e.g. sickness behaviors; Stella et al. 2011). However, these normal but more subtle expressions of pain aren't the loud vocalizations, moans or whimpering that people expect as expressions of pain; in the absence of these vocalizations, the animals may be presumed to be "hiding" the pain. In fact, pain is almost always associated with behavioral changes, and the most common signs that an animal is in pain or mental distress are changes in

(a)

(b)

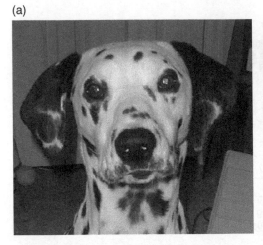
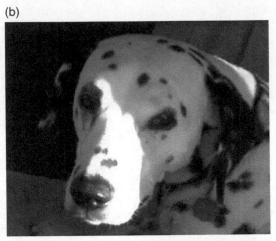

Figure 5.4 Subtle facial signs of pain in a Dalmatian dog: (a) the dog in younger years; (b) the dog on her last day prior to humane euthanasia, when she was suffering from significant physical discomfort and movement impairment, and decreased QOL. Note the orbital tightening, giving the eyes a somewhat "squinty" appearance, tightened corners of the mouth, and ears held slightly back and lowered in (b). *Source:* (Photos: S. Hetts).

behavior (Hellyer et al. 2007, Wiese 2015). Behavior changes commonly associated with pain include:

- Increased anxiety and/or fearful behavior
- Lethargy or depression
- Loss of appetite
- Reluctance to move
- Reduced interest in interactions (with familiar people or animals, for example, especially in dogs)
- Increased irritability or aggression
- Reduction in or cessation of grooming (resulting in a dull, unkempt coat, especially in cats)
- Self-mutilation
- Hiding (especially in cats)

Decreased Response to and Engagement with their Surroundings

When animals are ill, they marshal their physiological and behavioral resources to fight the disease (Hart 1988). As their physical and mental condition deteriorates, their ability and motivation to move freely and engage with their surroundings becomes more limited, and their "attentional flow" (Wemelsfelder 2005)

may decline. This may of course be complicated by sensory deficits as animals age. Varied and enjoyable behaviors may be replaced by increased lethargy, reclusiveness/hiding, inability to relax and appear comfortable, a lack of focus or ability to pay attention to any one thing for very long, and being easily startled or irritable. These behaviors are recognized as indicators of increased pain or distress, and of decreased welfare and/or enjoyment of life (e.g. Wiese 2015). Horses in pain are reported to exhibit a decrease in normal activity, lowered head carriage, fixed stare, rigid stance, and reluctance to move (Costa et al. 2014). These behaviors can be exhibited for varying amounts of time after an acute pain-producing event; for example, horses displayed decreases in exploratory behavior and alertness at eight hours after castration (Costa et al. 2014); dogs showed behavioral changes consistent with pain for up to three days (the study duration) following surgical neutering (Wagner et al. 2008). When these behavior changes persist and become more pronounced, for example in cases of chronic pain or a suboptimal environment, questions about distress, suffering, and QOL arise. Distressed animals may show little or no interest in eating or drinking, and reduce their self-grooming, further compromising physical health. Dogs and cats may become less cooperative (and more irritable) when asked to move or shift positions when they are in pain (Wiese 2015), and pets with cognitive decline may forget previously learned behaviors or cues (Salvin et al. 2010). Such animals may be mistakenly labeled as suddenly stubborn, disobedient, or "trying to be dominant" because of their unwillingness to comply with their owners' requests (Hetts, unpublished). In other cases, changes in behavior in aging dogs may be dismissed by caregivers as, "he's just getting old."

A behavior-based way to assess an animal's (continued) enjoyment of an activity is to perform a "consent test" – essentially causing the activity to stop, and then waiting and watching to see if the animal attempts to restart the activity or interaction. To optimize welfare, Rault et al. (2020b) discuss the importance of providing choice and control to the animal, particularly in the context of human interactions. More practical tips on utilizing consent as an indicator of willingness and enjoyment can be found in the progressive animal training literature, e.g. Anderson 2012, Stremming 2016, Stewart 2013.

One potentially important aspect of decreased engagement with surroundings, particularly for companion animals, would be changes to the animal's primary relationships, both with humans and with other animals. Both dogs (Topál et al. 1998, Payne et al. 2015) and cats (Vitale et al. 2019) do form attachment bonds with their human caregivers, and these bonds can be beneficial to the welfare of both the animals and their caregivers (Boissy et al. 2007; Rault et al. 2020b). For aging humans, maintaining social engagement has frequently been cited as an important predictor of quality of life during aging (e.g. Zhang et al. 2015). Distressed animals may avoid or withdraw from social interactions (Hellyer et al. 2007). Increased irritability due to pain, etc., may contribute to more threatening or aggressive behavior. When compared to younger (<7 years) dogs, older (≥7 years) dogs were reported to cope less

efficiently with distress caused by mild social challenges (Mongillo et al. 2013). Caregivers of distressed animals should be made aware of these potential changes, and accommodations made to ensure safety and minimal stress to all concerned, while still maintaining primary social relationships to the greatest degree possible. Rault et al. (2020b) define a positive human-animal relationship as evidenced by the animal showing "voluntary approach and spatial proximity (seeking) and signs of anticipation, pleasure, relaxation, or other indicators of a rewarding experience arising from interacting with humans" (p. 2). These authors recommend taking proactive steps to maintain and improve the human-animal relationship, using simple strategies such as paying attention to the animal's behavioral response to humans (Rault et al. 2020b), with approach or handling adjusted as necessary to foster a positive relationship. Low-stress (Yin 2009) or "fear free" (the Fear Free initiative, fearfreepets.com) handling approaches can provide useful tips for minimizing distress during, for example, administration of medicine or treatments. Echoing the Five Domains framework (Mellor 2016), fear of humans will preclude a positive human-animal relationship, but lack of (or low) fear is not in and of itself sufficient for individual animal welfare (Rault et al. 2020b).

Unusual Patterns of Movement or Positioning

Unusual patterns of movement may also be a sign of physical deterioration and/or increased pain. Changes in the sequence of normal locomotion are often indicators of pain and/or that characteristics of the environment are not accommodating the animal's changing needs. In one case, a dog began to go up the stairs backwards, before refusing to go up the stairs at all (Hetts, unpublished). Cattle kept on slippery floors took as long as 20 minutes to lie down; a process that would normally take much less time (Broom and Johnson 1993). Each step in the lying down sequence was prolonged. Unusual positions held while sitting, lying down or defecating have been reported in animals experiencing pain (Hellyer et al. 2007; Wiese 2015).

Suffering animals may develop abnormal repetitive behaviors or stereotypies in response to frustration, inability to cope, or central nervous system dysfunction (Overall and Dunham 2002, Mason 2006). These behaviors interfere with the normal daily function of the animal (and can be stressful for the human caregiver). These behaviors should be considered a sign of distress, and possible medical and environmental causes investigated upon recognizing stereotypies. Taking immediate measures to reduce stressors in the animal's environment, and adding appropriate enrichment (e.g. social interactions, play, mental and physical exercise, foraging opportunities in the form of food puzzle toys; with accommodations for limited mobility if necessary) may be beneficial in reducing these behaviors (Landsberg et al. 2013).

Focused Attention to One Specific Body Part

Animals who are suffering may stare at, lick, chew, or bite at a painful area, often to the point of self-trauma and acral lick dermatitis (Landsberg et al. 2013; Wiese 2015). Types of compulsive behavior like self-trauma and excessive barbering can also be exacerbated by stress, and (in addition to treating pain, skin infections, etc.) it is important to identify and remove or reduce stressors present in the animal's environment (Landsberg et al. 2013).

Displacement Behaviors

Caregivers should also watch for the expression of displacement behaviors (Leuscher and Reisner 2008) when animals show reluctance to engage in behaviors they previously enjoyed. Displacement behaviors occur when an animal experiences a conflict between two motivations, such as approach-avoidance (Breed and Moore 2015). Common displacement behaviors in dogs and cats include yawning, lip licking (dogs), scratching and self-grooming. For example, in response to an invitation to jump up next to the owner on the couch a dog (more commonly) or cat might yawn instead. The yawning is an example of a displacement behavior, shown in the context of social conflict. The animal may want to jump up, but is conflicted about doing so because the act of jumping has become painful. The internal conflict between jumping up or not produces a third, irrelevant behavior (yawning) that is displaced out of its normal context.

Can Sick Animals Suffer from Boredom?

Animals normally attend to their surroundings. When not asleep, they move their heads, eyes, ears, whiskers, and other body parts in various directions, even in the absence of specific stimuli that attract their attention (Welker 1964). This attentiveness allows an animal to obtain information and reduce uncertainty about his environment. Animals also naturally explore their surroundings, showing a variety of behaviors. Wemelsfelder (2005) argues that this "attentional flow" shows that an individual is engaged with the environment, and contributes to an animal's enjoyment of its life.

This natural ability to find meaningful things to do may be severely hindered by conditions of involuntary confinement, such as hospitalization and/or loss of mobility. In humans, serious illness often hinders patients' natural ability to find meaningful things to do, resulting in boredom and, when the illness is prolonged, in the distress associated with chronic boredom (Barbalet 1999). Boredom has been described as "difficulty in finding meaning in the activities in which one is engaged" (Gemmil and Oakley 1992, Newberry and Duncan 2001). Activities, however, are not in and of themselves meaningful. When the activities engaged in are dissociated from the individual's authentic voluntary interest, the result is often boredom – a mental state manifesting as some combination of apathy, restlessness, frustration, anxiety, hostility, and depression.

Wemelsfelder (2005) observed that "virtually all captive animals," such as those in agricultural and laboratory systems, live under conditions offering very few opportunities to express individual interests or preferences. The conditions under which companion animals live vary widely in this respect. In recent years, a growing recognition of the potential harm to animals living under conditions offering few opportunities to express individual interests or preferences has led to efforts to enrich those animals' living environments. These efforts have been found to be more successful in revitalizing animals' interest and enjoyment in some cases than in others – depending on the animals' level of genuine interest in the type of enrichment offered. Some excellent, user-friendly resources now exist for adding enrichment to the lives of companion animals: Bender and Strong's *Canine Enrichment for the Real World* (Bender and Strong 2019) and the companion workbook (Bender and Strong 2022) provide both a comprehensive overview of the theory and application of enrichment, and a diversity of practical tips; and Anderson's *Remember Me?* (Anderson 2016) offers a section on enrichment for dogs with canine cognitive dysfunction. The website *Food Puzzles for Cats* (foodpuzzlesforcats.com) has abundant information about using foraging toys with pet cats (Dantas et al. 2016).

Similarly, Nicholson and Meredith (2015) noted that ongoing disease has the potential to induce chronic stress in dogs, which may negatively impact welfare. Thus, chronically ill dogs may benefit from stress management as part of their treatment protocol and daily care. It is certainly feasible that the same would apply to other domestic species.

Relevance to Animal Hospice and Palliative Care (AHPC)

These considerations are important to include in the design of activities and environment for animals in AHPC. As an example of modifying a preferred activity to meet the animal's changing abilities, when it became too difficult for Hetts' elderly Irish Setter Blaze to run to fetch a ball, she and Blaze invented "old dog ball" as an alternative. Hetts would throw the ball so Blaze could easily catch it while lying down. Blaze would then drop the ball, and the sequence would repeat. Blaze was engaged in her surroundings, able to focus on the game for some period of time, and enjoyed it as evidenced by her interest and willingness to participate.

This modified game of fetch could be seen as giving Blaze a means to cope with her decreased function, thus relieving her distress from the inability to engage in what had been her normal play behavior. AHPC can and should include providing creative options and alternatives for dogs and cats to get their behavioral needs met when their illness has taken away their ability to enjoy past activities. When options cannot be provided, the animal patient's QOL should be closely monitored.

End-of-Life Decisions

Proficiency at recognizing and assessing an individual animal's level of distress is paramount to ongoing evaluation of QOL, as well as when making end-of-life decisions, which are emotionally laden undertakings. When human patients can no longer make decisions for themselves at the end of life, it's not uncommon to find family members in disagreement as to what course of action would be most in line with the person's wishes, despite living wills, do-not-resuscitate (DNR) directives, and other legal remedies available to take the burden off our loved ones. We should take it as a given that when a pet is in hospice care, there may be different interpretations of the animal's physical, emotional, and behavioral status, and of what the animal would or does want.

Animals cannot use human language to communicate what their wishes are regarding their end-of-life preferences as their physical and mental health declines. The best we can do is to infer what they want based on their body language and behavior. At some or many points, one or more people will have to interpret the meaning of those behaviors as best they can. The more proficiently we interpret animals' condition and experience from the animals' own point of view (e.g. by paying attention to the visible signs of the animal's affective state), the closer we can get to making decisions for them that are in line with their preferences. Advance preparation for making these decisions, including tracking QOL over time (using the methods described earlier), is essential for making good end-of-life decisions.

We must take extra caution not to confuse the animal's experience with what may be distressing to *us*. Many people are distressed, for example, when their companion animals become incontinent toward the end of their lives. How much are the animals distressed by this condition? Rather than assuming they are as distressed as we would be in their place, we should instead look for signs of distress in the animals' behavior during and immediately after an incontinent episode (or after taking a fall, after a bout of confusion, etc.).

In the context of making end-of-life decisions, it is crucial to acknowledge the limitations inherent to making decisions for someone other than ourselves, let alone someone belonging to a different species. It is not realistic, therefore, to expect certainty about making the exact same choices our companion animals would make for themselves if they had the option. We can never be certain if the animal would – or would not – prefer to continue living until the moment of "unaided" death. When it comes to choosing the moment for euthanasia for a beloved animal, we should not expect to be able to "hit the bull's eye" – to choose the exact moment the animal would say, if he or she could, "It's time, help me

pass on." A more realistic goal is to "hit the target board" – a metaphor proposed by bioethicist Jessica Pierce: we must do the best we can to construe the animal's preferences, using the best information available from knowledge of species-specific behavior and from observing the behavior of the individual animal patient. We must accept the inherent imperfection of this process. See Chapter 7 in this volume for a detailed discussion of end-of-life decision-making considerations.

Conclusion

To alleviate or prevent distress, we must be able to recognize it. The experience of distress is associated with unpleasant emotional states; it has been described as a state in which an animal, unable to adapt to one or more stressors, is no longer successfully coping with its environment, and as a result the animal's well-being is compromised (DeGrazia 1996; Ward et al. 2008). Pain, particularly chronic pain, is often a contributing factor to distress. Among the most common signs that an animal is in pain or mental distress are changes in behavior, and common body language and behavioral changes associated with pain are summarized in this chapter. New research into the facial expressions of pain is adding to our ability to detect pain and distress. Particular attention may need to be paid to maintaining the animal's primary relationship with his or her human caregiver, and to the animal's attentional flow. Scales and client handouts are available to assist AHPC team members and caregivers in reading body language and recognizing distress.

References

Anderson, E. (2012) Does your dog REALLY want to be petted? Available at: https://eileenanddogs.com/blog/2012/08/29/does-your-dog-really-want-to-be-petted (Accessed: 28 May 2021).

Anderson, E. (2016) *Remember Me? Loving and Caring for a Dog with Canine Cognitive Dysfunction*. Little Rock, AK: Bright Friends Productions, pp. 144.

Balasko, M. and Carbanac, M. (1998) Behavior of juvenile lizards (*Iguana iguana*) in a conflict between temperature regulation and palatable food. *Brain Behav. Evol.*, 52: 257–262.

Barbalet, J.M. (1999) Boredom and social meaning. *Br. J. Sociol.*, 50: pp. 631–646.

Bender, A. and Strong, E. (2019) *Canine Enrichment for the Real World: Making It Part of Your Dog's Daily Life*. Wenatchee, WA: Dogwise Publishing, pp. 230.

Bender, A. and Strong, E. (2022) *Canine Enrichment for the Real World: Workbook*. Wenatchee, WA: Dogwise Publishing, 76.

Boissy, A., Manteuffel, G., Jensen, M.B. et al. (2007) Assessment of positive emotions in animals to improve their welfare. *Physiol. Behav.*, 92: pp. 375–397.

Brambell, R. (1965) *Report of the Technical Committee to Enquire into the Welfare of Animals Kept Under Intensive Livestock Husbandry Systems*, Cmd. (Great Britain. Parliament), H.M. Stationery Office, pp. 1–84.

Breed, M.D. and Moore, J. (2015) *Animal Behavior*, 2 edn. Elsevier, Inc./Academic Press, pp. 546.

Bremhorst, A., Sutter, N.A., Wurbel, H. et al. (2019) Differences in facial expressions during positive anticipation and frustration in dogs awaiting a reward. *Sci. Rep.*, 9: pp. 19312.

Broom, D.M. and Johnson, K.G. (1993) *Stress and Animal Welfare*. Chapman and Hall Animal Behaviour Series, New York: Chapman and Hall.

Cohen, S., Beths, T. 2020. Grimace scores: Tools to support the identification of pain in mammals used in research. *Animals*, 10(10), 1726.

Colborn, D.R., Thompson, D. L., Roth, T.L. et al. (1991) Responses of cortisol and prolactin to sexual excitement and stress in stallions and geldings. *J. Anim. Sci.*, 69: pp. 2556–2562.

Conzemius, M.G. and Evans, R. B. (2012) Caregiver placebo effect for dogs with lameness from osteoarthritis. *J. Am. Vet. Med. Assoc.*, 241(10): 1314–1319.

Costa, E.D., Minero, M., Lebelt, D. et al. (2014) Development of the horse grimace scale (HGS) as a pain assessment tool in horses undergoing routine castration. *PLoS One*, 9(3): e92281.

Curtis, S.E. (1987) Animal well-being and animal care. *Vet. Clin. North Am. Food Anim. Pract.*, 3: 369–382.

Danbury, T.C., Weeks, C.A., Chambers, J.P. et al. (2000) Self-selection of the analgesic drug carprofen by lame broiler chickens. *Vet. Rec.*, 146: 307–311.

Dantas, L.M., Delgado, M.M., Johnson, I. et al. (2016) Food puzzles for cats: feeding for physical and emotional wellbeing. *J. Feline Med. Surg.*, 18(9): 723–732.

Dawkins, M.S. (1990) From an animal's point of view: motivation, fitness, and animal welfare. *Behav. Brain Sci.*, 12: 1–9.

Dawkins, M.S. (2005) The science of suffering. In *Mental Health and Well-Being in Animals*, (ed F.D. McMillan). Ames, IA: Blackwell Publishing, pp. 47–55.

DeGrazia, D. (1996) *Taking Animals Seriously*. Cambridge: Cambridge University Press.

Ekman, P. and Friesen, W. (1978) *Facial Action Coding System: A Technique for the Measurement of Facial Movement*. Consulting Psychological Press.

Evangelista, M.C., Watanabe, R., Leung, V.S.Y., et al. (2019) Facial expressions of pain in cats: the development and validation of a Feline Grimace Scale. *Sci. Rep.*, 9: pp. 19128.

Farm Animal Welfare Council (2009) *FAWC Report on Farm Animal Welfare in Great Britain: Past, Present and Future*. London: Farm Animal Welfare Council, pp. 70.

Gaynor, J.S. and Muir, W.W. (2015) *Handbook of Veterinary Pain Management*, 3 edn. St. Louis, MO: Elsevier.

Gemmill, G. and Oakley, J. (1992) The meaning of boredom in organizational life, *Group Org. Manag.*, 17: pp. 358–369.

Hart, B.L., 1988. Biological basis of the behavior of sick animals. *Neurosci. Biobehav. Rev.*, 12: 123–137.

Hellyer, P., Rodan, I., Brunt, J. et al. (2007) AAHA/AAFP pain management guidelines for dogs and cats. *J. Feline Med. Surg.*, 9: 466–480.

Hetts, S., Heinke, M.L., and D. Q. Estep (2004) Behavior wellness concepts for the general veterinary practice. *J. Am. Vet. Med. Assoc.*, 225(4): 506–513.

Holden, E., Calvo, G., Collins, M. et al. (2014) Evaluation of facial expression in acute pain in cats. *J. Small Anim. Pract.*, 55: 615–621.

Landsberg, G., Hunthausen, W. and Ackerman, L. (2013) *Behavior Problems of the Dog & Cat*, 3 edn. Saunders Elsevier, pp. 454.

Leach, M.C., Coulter, C.A., Richardson, C.A. et al. (2011) Are we looking in the wrong place? Implications for behavioural-based pain assessment in rabbits (Oryctolagus cuniculi) and beyond? *PLoS One*, 6(3): e13347.

Leuscher, A.U. and Reisner, I.R. (2008) Canine aggression towards familiar people: a new look at an old problem. *Vet. Clin. North Am. Small Anim. Pract.*, 38: 1107–1130.

Lush, J. and Ijichi, C. (2018) A preliminary investigation into personality and pain in dogs. *J. Vet. Behav.*, 24: 62–68.

Mason, G.J. (2006) Stereotypic behaviour in captive animals; fundamentals and implications for welfare and beyond. In: *Stereotypic Animal Behavior: Fundamentals and Applications to Welfare* (ed G.J. Mason), Wallingford, UK: CAB International pp. 325–356.

McMillan, F. D. (2005) Stress, distress and emotion: distinctions and implications for mental well-being. In: *Mental Health and Well-Being in Animals* (ed F.D. McMillan), Ames, Iowa: Blackwell Publishing, 93–111.

Mellor, D. (2016) Updating animal welfare thinking: moving beyond the "Five Freedoms" towards "A Life Worth Living". *Animals*, 6(2): 21.

Mongillo, P., Pitteri, E., Carnier, P. et al. (2013) Does the attachment system towards owners change in aged dogs? *Physiol. Behav.*, 120: 64–69.

Mwacalimba, K. K., Contadini, F. M., Spofford, N. et al. (2020) Owner and veterinarian perceptions about use of a canine quality of life survey in primary care settings. *Front. Vet. Sci.*, 7: 89.

National Research Council (US) Committee on Recognition and Alleviation of Pain in Laboratory Animals. (2009) *Recognition and Alleviation of Pain in Laboratory Animals*. Washington, D.C: National Academies Press.

Newberry, A.L. and Duncan, R.D. (2001) Roles of boredom and life goals in juvenile delinquency. *J. Appl. Soc. Psychol.*, 31: 527–541.

Nicholson, S.L. and Meredith, J.E. (2015) Should stress management be part of the clinical care provided to chronically ill dogs? *J. Vet. Behav.*, 10: 489–495.

Overall, K.L and Dunham, A.E. (2002) Clinical features and outcome in dogs and cats with obsessive-compulsive disorder; 126 cases (1989-2000). *J. Am. Vet. Med. Assoc.*, 221: 1445–1452.

Payne, E., Bennett, P., and McGreevy, P. (2015) Current perspectives on attachment and bonding in the dog-human dyad. *Psychol. Res. Behav. Manag.*, 8: 71–79.

Rault, J-L, Hintze, S., Camerlink, I et al. (2020a) Positive welfare and the like: distinct views and a proposed framework. *Front. Vet. Sci.*, 7: 370.

Rault, J-L, Waiblinger, S., Boivin, X., et al. (2020b) The power of a positive human-animal relationship for animal welfare. *Front. Vet. Sci.*, 7: 590867.

Reck, J. (2012) *Facing Farewell: Making the Decision to Euthanize Your Pet*. Wenatchee, WA: Dogwise Publications, pp. 70.

Salvin, H.E., McGreevy, P.D., Sachdev, P.S., et al. (2010) Under diagnosis of canine cognitive dysfunction: a cross-sectional survey of older companion dogs. *Vet. J.*, 184(3): 277–281.

Seibert, L. (2021) Management of dogs and cats with cognitive dysfunction. *Today's Veterinary Practice*. Available at: https://todaysveterinarypractice.com/management-of-dogs-and-cats-with-cognitive-dysfunction (Accessed: 29 May 2021).

Selye, H. (1976) Stress without distress. In: *Psychopathology of Human Adaptation* (ed G. Serban), Boston: Springer.

Sotocinal, S.G., Sorge, R.E, Zaloum, A. et al. (2011) The Rat Grimace Scale: a partially automated method for quantifying pain in the laboratory rat via facial expressions. *Mol. Pain*, 7: 55.

Sprangers, M.A.G., Aaronson, N.K. 1992. The role of health care providers and significant others in evaluating the quality of life of patients with chronic disease: a review. *J. Clin. Epidemiol.* 45(7): 743–760.

Stella, J., Lord, L.K., and Buffington, C.A.T. (2011) Sickness behaviors in response to unusual external events in health cats and cats with feline interstitial cystitis. *J. Am. Vet. Med. Assoc.*, 238: 67–73.

Stewart, G.(2013) Take the hint: how to use the 5-second rule for petting dogs. Available at: https://grishastewart.com/take-the-hint-how-to-use-the-5-second-rule-for-petting-dogs-2 (Accessed: 28 May 2021).

Stremming, S. (2016) Matters of consent. Available at https://thecognitivecanine.com/blog/matters-of-consent (Accessed: 28 May 2021).

Topal, J., Miklosi, A., Csanyi, V. et al. (1998) Attachment behavior in dogs (Canis familiaris): a new application of Ainsworth's (1969) strange situation test. *J. Comp. Psychol.*, 112(3): 219–229.

Vitale, K. R., Behnke, A. C., and Udell, M. A. R. (2019) Attachment bonds between domestic cats and humans. *Curr. Biol.*, 29(18): R864–R865.

de Waal, F.(2011) What is an animal emotion? *Ann. NY Acad. Sci.*, 1224: 191–206.

Wagner, A.E., Worland, G.A., Glawe, J.C. et al. (2008) Multicenter, randomized controlled trial of pain-related behaviors following routine neutering in dogs, *J. Am. Vet. Med. Assoc.*, 233(1): 109–115.

Walder, B., Schafer, M., Henzi, I. et al. (2001) Efficacy and safety of patient-controlled opiod analgesia for acute postoperative pain. A quantitative systematic review. *Acta Anaesthesiol. Scand.*, 45: 795–804.

Wan M., Bolger N., and Champagne F.A. (2012) Human perception of fear in dogs varies according to experience with dogs. *PLoS One*, 7(12): e51775.

Ward, P.A., Blanchard, R.J. and, Bolivar, V. (2008) *Recognition and Alleviation of Distress in Laboratory Animals*. Washington, D.C.: The National Academies Press.

Welker, W.I. (1964) Analysis of sniffing of the albino rat. *Behaviour*, 22: 223–244.

Wemelsfelder, F. (2005) Animal boredom: understanding the tedium of confined lives. In: *Mental Health and Well-Being in Animals* (ed F.D. McMillan), Ames, IA: Blackwell Publishing, pp. 79–91.

Wiese, A.J. (2015) Chapter 5: Assessing pain: pain behaviors. In: Gaynor JS and Muir WW (eds) *Handbook of Veterinary Pain Management* (eds J.S. Gaynor and W.W. Muir), 3 edn. St. Louis MO: Elsevier, pp. 67–97.

Yeates, J.W. (2020) Quality of live of animals in veterinary medical practice. In: McMillan, FD, *Mental Health and Well Being in Animals* (ed F.D. McMillan), 2 edn. Boston: CABI, pp. 82–95.

Yin, S. (2009) *Low Stress Handling, Restraint and Behavior Modification of Dogs & Cats: Techniques for Developing Patients Who Love Their Visits*. Davis, CA: Cattledog Publishing, pp. 469.

Zhang, W., Feng, Q., Liu, L., et al. (2015) Social engagement and health: findings from the 2013 survey of the Shanghai elderly life and opinion. *Int. J. Aging Hum. Dev.*, 80(4): 332–356.

6

Balancing Efficacy of Treatments Against Burdens of Care

Kristina August, DVM, GDVWHM, CHPV

In end-of-life care, perhaps more distinctly than care provided during any other stage of life, practitioners must consider how their actions affect the quality of life (QOL) of their patients. We should of course always consider the adverse effects of medical treatments and diagnostic testing, striving to minimize these effects by reducing stress during handling and using palliative measures when needed. In a younger or healthier animal with a comparatively long life ahead and a good prognosis for recovery, the benefits of surgery, chemotherapy, or other intensive treatments can outweigh many temporary discomforts the animal may experience. However, when time is limited and the patient is more fragile, the need to ensure that those last days and weeks are comfortable becomes critical. Futile life-saving measures may increase *quantity* of life while negatively impacting *quality* of life, a tradeoff that may not be appropriate for an animal near death. Unfortunately, a range of complicated factors can sometimes make the realistic achievement of these goals elusive.

The human hospice movement grapples with these challenges as well. As Atul Gawande writes, "Hospice has tried to offer a new ideal for how we die... But doing so represents a struggle—not only against suffering but also against the seemingly unstoppable momentum of medical treatment" (Gawande 2010).

For humans, as for animals, the tension between quantity and quality of life requires a delicate and ongoing balancing act. Research has consistently shown that, often, the choice to pursue aggressive medical interventions substantially reduces rather than improves QOL. Longer enrollment time in a hospice program has been shown to correlate with improved QOL, and sometimes even extension of life (Connor et al. 2007; Wright et al. 2008; Fadol et al. 2021).

Finding the right balance between providing curative treatment and maintaining QOL is also important for the well-being of caregivers. Surviving caregivers, who are frequently unprepared for the death of their loved one, report a significant increase in feelings of regret and major depression after the death of a loved one following aggressive curative treatments as opposed to hospice care. Studies have shown that increased communication and understanding of the disease process may help human patients and their families to accept hospice and palliative care sooner, avoiding inappropriately aggressive care near the end of life (Wright et al. 2008; Tönnies et al. 2021).

Questions about how aggressively to pursue life-saving measures factor into veterinary care as well, especially when the proximity of the end is uncertain and some families resist facing the inevitable death of their beloved companion (Quain et al. 2021). In veterinary care, we can start discussions about the end of life and begin hospice care at any time, without the six-month prognosis certification required by the US healthcare systems for human patients. Depending on the disease trajectory, there is the potential for more time to broach the subject of "advance directives" and treatment goals as the patient's condition declines. These "Serious Illness Conversations" are more commonly being broached in human and veterinary medicine today than they have in the past, and development of empathetic communication skills is thankfully gaining priority for all medical professionals (Goldberg 2019; Paladino et al. 2020; Lagrotteria et al. 2021). End-of-life discussions are initially difficult, but they contribute to improving the animal's QOL and preparing caregivers for the emotional challenges of grieving and accepting death. They can smooth the way for later decision-making when emotions are strong. In the field of animal hospice and palliative care, we endeavor to bring these conversations to the forefront.

Nonmaleficence is one of the core principles of ethical medical and veterinary practice, summarized by the phrase *do no harm*. There is something appealing in that simple phrase, and so we continue to repeat it. *If we can do nothing more, at least let us do no harm.* Trying to follow this simple guideline, however, can bring a flood of questions to mind: What is harmful? When is it acceptable to cause harm in order to cure? At what point have we done more harm than good? Who gets to decide, the veterinarian or the client? What if animals could decide for themselves? How would they like to live their last days? How do we determine if these are indeed their last days? And, ultimately, when do we stop trying to cure and decide that the best way to "do no harm" is to support the patient in their dying?

These are difficult questions, the answers to which depend on each patient's unique circumstances, including disease progression and prognosis; the physical, emotional, and financial resources of the patient's family to provide nursing care; and, not to be underestimated, the temperament and cooperation of the animal patient. In hospice and palliative care, the focus is on assessing not just the disease or medical condition, but rather on treating the whole patient and the whole family and on palliating distress even when disease can no longer be cured.

In addressing the efficacy of treatments and burdens of care, we weigh the potential risks and benefits of diagnostic and treatment options. Are they beneficial for our end-of-life patients when the primary goal is to provide comfort rather than cure? Given the burden or effort associated with this procedure, will it improve the animal's overall life experience or detract from it?

Through the establishment of hospice and palliative care goals, assessment of the efficacy and burdens of care, and consideration of potential adverse consequences of diagnostic testing and treatments, we strive to find a balance that provides the optimal QOL for our animal patients.

Establishing the Goals of Care

The efficacy of medical care is ultimately measured by its outcomes in relation to what the patient and family have hoped to achieve. Defining the goals of care involves honest and open communication between animal hospice care providers and the families and caregivers of our animal patients, starting with providing information about the disease conditions and their anticipated progression and prognosis. Armed with this knowledge, the family can then consider what it is that they hope to achieve through treatment. This may vary greatly from one family to another, based on individual preferences, previous experiences, religious or moral values, family dynamics, finances, and the practical logistics of caregiving. Goals may include minimizing discomfort for the animal, improving QOL, increasing longevity, reducing stress and fear, or reducing caregiving burdens for the family.

In addition to discussing goals for the animal's remaining time on earth, the hospice team should seek to elicit the family's goals surrounding the circumstances of death, and the team should emphasize that death does not always follow the prescribed plan. A family may prefer that their animal die at home without the stress of relocation to a clinic, or before any signs of distress are perceived, or the family may wish for death to occur naturally without the intervention of euthanasia. Some may desire to keep the animal alive and comfortable long enough for distant family members to return for a final farewell. Caregiving requirements to maintain comfort and the level of commitment needed to fulfill

these goals should be established to determine if expectations are realistic in each individual situation. Above all, goals must have a degree of flexibility as life and death are certain to be unpredictable. Frequent communication with caregivers and re-evaluation is needed as the end draws near. A document such as the "Animal End-of-life Comfort Care Plan" (see Box 6.1 a sample form for establishing goals for a comfort care plan) is useful in navigating these goal-setting conversations and defining individual interpretations of discomfort, suffering, and distress. Having a completed form nearby helps to remind families of their priorities and goals of care during stressful situations and can support communication during emergencies and visits to new care providers.

Box 6.1   Sample form for establishing goals for a comfort care plan.

Animal End-of-Life Comfort Care Plan

1) Knowing that life can take unexpected turns, do you understand the most likely disease progression and prognosis for your animal?
   - Yes
   - I need more information

   _____
   _____
   _____
   _____

2) What are your primary concerns in supporting your animal?
   - Improve/maintain Quality of Life
   - Support animal needs and desires (to the best of our understanding and ability)
   - Minimize discomfort
   - No suffering/distress
   - Control signs of discomfort: (check specific concerns for this patient)
     – Pain
     – Gastrointestinal distress (vomiting, diarrhea, nausea, pain)

   – Respiratory distress
   – Anxiety
   – Mobility
   – Skin lesions
   – Other

   _____
   _____

   - Minimize need for medications (due to difficulty administering)
   - Minimize handling or transport (due to stress/anxiety, or physical limitations)
   - Minimize need for caregiving (due to unavailability, work, other commitments)
   - Minimize expenses (due to financial limitations)
   - Other

   _____
   _____

3) Planning for death can help to alleviate feelings of regret. This can be different for everyone and there is not one "ideal" time. Some patients progress comfortably with

palliative support and others require more intensive treatment. We do not always have control over this, but if there is a choice, what do you consider to be the optimal or ideal way for your beloved animal to die?

- Quietly dying without intervention (occasionally this happens, but not likely without palliative support; please choose a second option as a backup plan)
- Euthanasia before any discomfort becomes evident
- Euthanasia when suffering or discomfort has become evident
- Euthanasia after all palliative treatments to alleviate suffering or distress have been undertaken and discomfort continues
- Euthanasia as needed, whenever and wherever it seems appropriate
- Palliative support through natural death (this may require intensive preparation, time, physical and emotional caregiving and monitoring)

4) Ideally, what is your preferred location for your animal's death?
  - Home
  - Veterinary clinic:

  _____

  - Another location:

  _____

5) What is your after-hours/emergency plan?

  _____
  _____
  _____
  _____

  Phone numbers for emergency: _____

  _____

6) How would you like to have the body prepared after death?
  - Cremation and ashes returned
  - Urn for ashes_____

- Bury ashes
- Cremation with no ashes returned
- Bury body (address special requirements here, particularly if euthanasia takes place) _____

  _____

  _____

- Other

  _____

7) What memorialization plans would help you to grieve and remember the love?

  _____
  _____
  _____
  _____

8) Do you anticipate having difficulty dealing with the grief of loss and do you have resources or counselors for help with your own personal care and that of your family members?

  _____
  _____
  _____
  _____

9) Acknowledging that my animal has entered the end stage of life, I do not wish for him/her to receive cardiopulmonary resuscitation (CPR). _____

  _____

10) Comfort Care Plan Summary of most important points and additional comments:

  _____
  _____
  _____
  _____
  _____
  _____
  _____
  _____
  _____
  _____

Assessing Efficacy and Burdens of Medical Treatment

Assessment of Treatment Efficacy

Our primary goals in providing palliative care should always be to minimize animal distress and to maximize comfort. This should begin with determining the most essential factors in an individual patient's QOL. QOL is a composite construct reflecting both physical well-being and emotional well-being. In considering animal patients' physical well-being, managing pain is a top priority. Fortunately, much progress has been made in the objective assessment and treatment of signs of animal pain by recent research and resources are available to practitioners, especially since the establishment of the International Veterinary Academy of Pain Management (ivapm.org) and the publication of recent texts (Gaynor and Muir 2015; Goldberg and Shaffran 2015), the *2022 AAHA Pain Management Guidelines for Dogs and Cats* (AAHA 2022) and the *2022 ISFM Consensus Guidelines on the Management of Acute Pain in Cats* (Steagall et al. 2022). Increased recognition of pain and discomfort through facial expression and other physical and behavioral signs has greatly improved our ability to assess treatment success (Feline Grimace Scale: www.felinegrimacescale.com; Mota-Rojas et al. 2021).

Many other factors can also affect an animal's physical and emotional comfort, including clinical signs associated with their medical condition (for example, visual impairment, decreased mobility, and urinary or fecal incontinence), nutrition, hydration, bedding quality, feelings of security, environmental stimulation, and social interactions. Various assessment tools for QOL and pain are readily available and can facilitate our evaluation of treatment efficacy (see Chapter 4 in this book for an in-depth discussion of animal QOL).

Appetite and Hydration Needs at the End of Life

A unique aspect of providing palliative care as death becomes imminent is in the provision of nutrition and hydration. QOL assessment tools can be valuable in providing a list of the most distressing signs to consider in animals, but care must be given in the interpretation of these results. Nearly every QOL assessment tool asks whether an animal has lost interest in food, and lack of interest in food is often taken to be an indicator of poor QOL and a trigger for euthanasia. Caregivers often place a heavy emotional emphasis on the appetite of their loved one, equating acceptance of food with love and happiness. Yet, human hospice patients report that there comes a time when food loses its appeal. Eating has been shown to cause discomfort when the body is no longer digesting and processing nutrients for continued use (Ross and Alexander 2001; del Rio et al. 2012; van de Vathorst 2014). Artificial nutrition through tube feeding and/or hydration through the intravenous or subcutaneous routes can be life extending and greatly improve QOL in earlier stages of terminal illness; however, in a dying patient it may cause more harm than benefit. Excess fluids may accumulate in tissues and cells causing edema, ascites, and pleural effusions (Good et al. 2014). The value of providing artificial hydration or nutrition must be determined on a case-by-case basis with frequent assessment for signs of distress such as gastrointestinal (GI) discomfort, restlessness, edema, or respiratory difficulty.

Appetite stimulants may be appropriate and beneficial in early stages of decline, but often have less effect over time and should be removed from the list of medications when they are no longer effective. An animal experiencing hunger or thirst that cannot be satisfied is different from an animal whose appetite is waning with the normal progression of dying. The experience of thirst and hunger may represent distress whereas a normal decrease in appetite and increasing dehydration at the end of life may not be distressing until well-meaning humans try to force food and water on an animal who no longer desires it. In human hospice, near the end, food is reserved for pleasure or comfort, but is not relied upon for nutrition or life-sustaining support. Water is used to moisten mucous membranes and given for comfort as desired, but concern for hydration is no longer a priority. Animals fare better when families are prepared to recognize the decreasing appetite in hospice care as simply the progression of the dying patient to the next stage. This preparation helps to reduce caregiving anxiety, though it may not reduce the grief associated with this indicator of impending, inevitable loss.

Emotional Well-Being

Reducing anxiety and stress for patients as well as caregivers is paramount to improving the animal's QOL. Assessment of emotional well-being involves the recognition of animal behaviors which are often subtle and may be specific to individuals (see Chapter 5 in this book for detailed information on Recognizing Distress). Feelings that must be supported include helplessness and the vulnerabilities associated with increased discomfort and/or decreased mobility. Animals may become cranky, anxious, fearful, and even aggressive if they feel the need to defend or protect themselves from pain or harm. Depression or boredom can result from decreased activity and social interaction. Providing supportive emotional care to these animals, along with treatment of distressing clinical signs, is vital to increase their feelings of security and comfort. Supportive care addressing emotional needs may include environmental adaptations such as creating a safe space for the animal to be near family, but also a quiet space to rest with decreased sensory input from noise, light, smells, and family activity.

Animal Individual Preferences

There are golden retrievers who are perfectly happy to visit the oncologist multiple times a week, while some cats might strenuously object to this same treatment. Though these are stereotypical examples, they serve to illustrate the many factors that must be considered when evaluating how an individual animal's burdens of care impact his or her QOL. What may be harmful or distressing to one may be a reasonable option for another. Some patients become more needy and attention-seeking, while others turn away and want to be left alone. Individual preferences can change throughout the course of illness and require close observation and adjustments in the plan of care to maintain QOL.

Individual variation in pain tolerance cannot be ignored. Recognizing and eliminating pain is an essential goal for all patients, yet, some animals will continue with their daily activities, seeming undisturbed by a level of pain that might be severely crippling to others. Especially when considering the option of euthanasia, we must study and observe our patients in the most objective and educated way possible, remembering that it is the patient's capacity for coping that determines when pain and discomfort cause distress and suffering. It is important to acknowledge and respectfully consider that spark of hope or will to carry on living, that contentment to still be present even if at a lower level of functioning and requiring more assistance. Some animals are more comfortable accepting help than others and their preferences should be respected as well.

Do-Not-Resuscitate and "Advance Directives"

People can make their own decisions about their end-of-life care and can (and should!) write them up in legal documents called "advance directives." The establishment of a hospice care relationship generally includes provisions against cardiopulmonary resuscitation (CPR). For people and animals with terminal illness, the long-term success of CPR is almost nonexistent, and when it is successful, QOL generally suffers greatly due to the trauma of bruising and potential for broken ribs and/or lung contusions (Tilley et al. 2008; Seung et al. 2016). Allow Natural Death (AND) is an alternative language to Do Not Resuscitate (DNR) orders used in some areas of human medicine. This positive reformulation removes some of the distress from providers, especially in hospital or ER settings where CPR is considered an automatic response regardless of circumstance. Animals do not have the luxury of writing advance directives, but caregivers should be encouraged to think through and even write down these proxy decisions for their animal in an end-of-life care plan (Box 6.1) before a medical crisis occurs. Having an AND or DNR order in place allows an animal that is close to death to die more peacefully, without the interference of life-saving measures that have no possibility of succeeding and only cause harm and distress.

QOL is often reflected in changes in the animal patient's preferences concerning food, resting location, noise level, interest in social interaction, and any number of other factors meaningful to the individual animal. Behaviors and indicators of contentment and discontentment can be recognized and monitored. Providers can ask caregivers to consider how their individual animal expresses happiness and comfort vs uneasiness or distress. Regular logs and journaling are also valuable in recognizing changes in physical signs such as the number of times vomited, amount, contents, and possible triggers such as food type, anxiety, or medications. Journaling can help to identify trends and avoid risk factors in the future. This would also apply to changes in appetite, stool quality (diarrhea or constipation, blood, mucous), pain, restlessness, sleep quality, respiratory events, and activity level.

Box 6.2 Assessment of efficacy of palliative care.

1) Determine elements of QOL that are especially pertinent to an individual animal under care.
2) Establish specific evaluation criteria for that individual including signs of comfort and discomfort.
3) Observe and record positive and negative influences of palliative care treatments on these QOL elements.
4) Adjust treatment plan to improve QOL using these observations.

Source: Adapted from Shanan (2011), p. 641.

When changes in any of these factors correspond to a recent change in the animal's treatment, they form the basis for evaluating the efficacy of that treatment. When efficacy is determined to be inadequate, adjustments should be made to the treatment care plan (see Box 6.2).

Assessment of Treatment Burden

As the end of life approaches, the needs of patients change. To maintain QOL, medications may need to be adjusted and prioritized. Every effort should be made to reduce the stress associated with medicating animals. This can be accomplished with food, flavored and/or compounded drugs, and positive reinforcement associated with treatments. As appetite decreases, the intake of oral medications may become more challenging, complicated, and frustrating for caregivers. We must therefore determine which medications still provide comfort and eliminate those that do not support the prioritized goals for that individual animal.

Most palliative treatments – such as those for pain, diarrhea, or vomiting – need to be given time to work. But if improvement in the patient's QOL is not seen within 12–24 hours, additional or different treatments should be considered.

Medications should be regularly evaluated, and their benefits weighed against the risk of adverse effects. The risk of decreased QOL caused by the struggle of administration must be considered. Alternate routes of administration such as injectable, transdermal, or rectal should be considered for their potential to improve patient comfort and efficacy of treatments, especially as bodily functions begin to shut down.

Assessment tools offer a starting place for evaluation and communication between providers and caregivers. Offering time to pause, discuss treatment alternatives, reevaluate goals, and to assess the burden of care can be conducive to more mindful decision-making, decreasing the risk of future regret if decisions are made during transient moments of frustration or hopelessness.

During these conversations, treatment efficacy must be weighed against the burden of providing the treatment. The key question can be asked:

Knowing that we are no longer able to cure, does this treatment support the palliative care goals established in the Comfort Care Plan?

If the answer is no, there are three choices:

1) **Reassess** the treatment goals
2) **Eliminate** the unnecessary treatment
3) **Adapt** the treatment to reduce the burden of care

Assessing Diagnostic Procedures

The same process of evaluation can be applied to diagnostic procedures such as radiography, ultrasonography, laboratory testing, or exploratory surgery. Unless the results will influence treatment decisions that can potentially increase patient comfort or even comfortable longevity, they should be approached with caution. Admittedly, diagnostic procedures may have a place in researching improved methods of palliative care and prognostication, but the broader benefits must be weighed against any distress caused to the individual patient.

Not all animals appear to be disturbed by transportation and handling, and some may even enjoy the interactions. For those patients experiencing adverse reactions, including stress and/or physical discomfort after diagnostic procedures, the balance of burdens and benefits must be frequently reevaluated, keeping the hospice and palliative care goals foremost in mind. Diagnostic monitoring for these animals should be done in the home whenever possible, to minimize the stress of transportation and handling.

Caregivers should always be apprised of any risks or potential negative outcomes involved in diagnostic or treatment procedures, especially those involving "heroic" measures. For example, an exploratory laparotomy may be needed to assess the full extent of a potentially malignant mass seen on radiographs. The hope may be that the mass can be completely resected, and the animal will recover completely from the disease. If there are doubts or concerns about metastasis, those should also be communicated, and a secondary plan should be made. Some questions to address with caregivers include: What are the chances for a full recovery? What is the best guess at life expectancy and QOL with and without surgery? Is the family prepared to euthanize the animal before awakening if the prognosis is poor, or will they wish to provide palliative care in the face of postsurgical recovery and severe disease? Are there any less invasive diagnostic tests, such as ultrasound or biopsy that could be performed first to help in making this decision? Communication in these instances is paramount so that the caregiver fully understands the full range of options and consequences. Offering time for goodbyes, even a night or a few days at home together if desired and medically advisable, can sometimes help to mitigate the shock and grief of loss.

Adverse Events: Treatment-Related Consequences

In animal end-of-life care, adverse events and treatment-related consequences can lead to euthanasia if the decision-maker concludes (accurately or not) that the animal is suffering unduly. Oftentimes, however, the adverse side-effects of treatments can be mitigated through careful attention. As an example, the diligent use of nonsteroidal anti-inflammatory drugs (NSAIDs) or steroids can dramatically improve mobility and comfort, yet long-term use of such drugs can potentially lead to various adverse effects including gastrointestinal irritation and ulcers. This may result in nausea, inappetence, and even bloody vomiting, which can be very disconcerting to caregivers and in turn may trigger a decision to euthanize. Concurrent GI protective and preventative treatments can be lifesaving for these patients, especially as they become more vulnerable and sensitive to adverse effects.

Alternatively, some consequences ordinarily thought to be significant may not be a concern when life expectancy is measured in days or months. Avoiding the potential liver and neurologic toxicity of long-term metronidazole treatment to control diarrhea in a patient with hepatic insufficiency may be a lower priority than mitigating the human and animal distress from uncontrolled diarrhea, which may prompt some caregivers to consider euthanasia. The clinician must weigh the risks and benefits. Keeping in mind that the organs are fragile at the end of life and may fail more quickly, will the dog live long enough for the medication's side-effects to be significant? Will a lower dose be safer and still be beneficial? Are there other ways to help manage ongoing diarrhea and GI discomfort?

Understanding species differences and following current research is important in assessing treatment decisions. Concern for renal damage in an already sensitive species has left many cats with osteoarthritis untreated over the years. Fortunately, studies have shown that low dose meloxicam can be safe and effective even in the face of chronic renal disease (Monteiro 2020; Steagall 2020). Awareness of potential precautions, such as the importance of hydration and the use of a multimodal approach, can enhance the comfort and longevity of these patients.

Adverse effects of, or reactions to, drugs and other treatments are always a possibility. Some happen more commonly and have a significant impact on patients' well-being, especially given the debility of patients nearing the end of life. Others may be rare or less consequential and cause more fear than beneficial precaution. The intention should be to base treatment selection on the most likely outcome and prepare caregivers to recognize potential adverse events so they can be quickly addressed, reducing the risk of decision-making based on unfounded concerns that the animal is now "suffering." Euthanasia decisions, unfortunately, are often motivated by fear of "suffering" when there are no feasible alternate choices in view.

A preventative approach to adverse side-effects involves having a plan in place for any possible adverse occurrences, which can help to alleviate caregiver concerns. To minimize the impact of adverse side-effects, the potential severity of various signs of clinical distress needs to be evaluated and prioritized (Box 6.3). Generally, pain gets high priority here, but other clinical signs can be equally distressing to animal or caregiver, such as respiratory distress or anxiety. Avoiding medications with common, clinically significant adverse effects is an important goal in palliative care, but not to the detriment of patient comfort. If the use of such medications is paramount to controlling distressing clinical signs (again, we are no longer seeking cure), then reducing their dosages may be considered to decrease the risk of adverse effects. Lower doses are often recommended for patients with reduced functioning of organ systems, especially when drug clearance time by the liver and kidneys is prolonged, and many hospice and palliative care patients

---

Box 6.3   Think preventative!

An approach to the use of medications with potentially clinically significant adverse effects:

1) **Prioritize** need for medications depending on the severity or potential for severity of signs if left untreated.
2) **Avoid** medications with potentially clinically significant adverse effects when possible, weighing the realistic risks with the potential benefits.
3) **Reduce** dosages of medications with potentially clinically significant adverse effects. This may involve combining multiple medications with complementary effects at lower doses, as is often done for pain management.
4) **Provide** additional supportive care to reduce the need for medications with potentially clinically significant adverse effects. This may include nutritional support, gentle exercise and physical therapy, acupuncture, massage, low toxicity herbs and supplements, and anxiety reduction using methods such as gentle handling, decreased environmental stimulation, and music therapy.

---

fall into this category. Be aware, though, that a higher dose of some medications may be required to achieve the desired palliative effect and titration may be in order. Using combinations or substitutions where possible and supportive care with lower potential for toxicity to decrease the need for medications with known clinically significant adverse effects can greatly benefit patients. Integrative medicine is often used in human and animal hospice to augment a multimodal approach to palliative care. Supportive care should be started early whenever possible for optimal preventative effects. See Chapters 19, 20, and 21 in this book for more details on pharmacological, physical medicine, rehabilitation, and complementary and integrative medicine supportive treatment options. A comprehensive discussion of the potential risks of individual drugs and other treatments is beyond the scope of this book.

Steroids and End-of-Life Care

Balancing the benefits of chronic steroid use with the risks of adverse effects in end-of-life care can be challenging. Used for some cancer treatments and inflammatory bowel conditions, steroids can initially keep the cancer or signs of distress at bay, maintaining comfort for a time. Eventually, higher doses may be required to achieve the same effect, and the patient may develop Cushing disease (hyperadrenocorticism, more common in dogs), diabetes (more common in cats), or other adverse effects. Caregivers should be informed of these risks, as well as the potentially severe consequences of abruptly withdrawing steroid medications, such as an Addisonian (hypoadrenocorticism) crisis. If an animal stops eating and is no longer taking medications orally, switching to an injectable steroid is recommended to avert crisis and maintain comfort near death.

Adverse Events: Indirect Consequences of Medical Care

Though they are generally the first to come to mind, the term "adverse events" does not refer exclusively to drug or treatment side-effects. Physical and stress reactions to handling for diagnostics, treatment, or travel can significantly affect an animal's QOL. For example, awkward positioning of an arthritic animal for radiographs, even if the animal is sedated, may cause soreness for days afterward (Bittel 2014). In determining the benefit or efficacy of care, we must consider the time it takes for our patients to recover and return to normal comfortable behaviors after a treatment event.

How long is too long? How can these experiences be modified to reduce adverse effects? Fortunately, strides have been taken in recent years to reduce the stress and fear experienced by animals during handling to obtain diagnostic information and provide treatment (Yin 2009; Low Stress Handling 2022; Fear Free 2022; Cat Friendly Practices 2022). In-home visits, limited contact examinations, and even video and telemedicine can provide needed ongoing care, while reducing stressful handling for some patients.

The primary approach to reducing adverse events is to think preventatively rather than reacting in crisis mode. Providers should strive to anticipate possible detrimental outcomes of treatment or disease progression and have comfort care options readily available. Offering caregivers resources and advice for the prevention, early recognition, and treatment of common concerns such as decreasing mobility, diarrhea, vomiting, nausea, restlessness, pain, and respiratory distress can greatly improve success in end-of-life care. The provision of a "comfort kit" for caregivers to have at home with medications and supplies that might be needed for emergencies may be part of this preparation.

Assessing the Burdens of Caregiving

The burdens of treatment are the "work" involved in receiving care by, as well as providing care to, end-of-life patients. This chapter focuses primarily on burdens of treatment experienced by the animal patient. However, the human burdens inherent in providing this care may strongly influence the decisions caregivers make and are therefore important for the animal patients' well-being as well. Caregiver burden, the physical and psychological load experienced by human caregivers, affects the ability to provide patient care including treatment adherence, maintaining regular hygiene, and other important aspects of care. Client communication with veterinary staff can be reduced, increased, or strained due to an array of emotions including feelings of discomfort, embarrassment, misunderstanding, anxiety, grief, or depression. (Shaevitz et al. 2020; Spitznagel et al. 2019). Different aspects of pet caregiving burden are discussed in detail in Chapters 25–29 in this book.

When caregivers become overwhelmed and no longer see viable treatment options, they are in dire need of guidance and support. This happens frequently as care for animals becomes more involved and complicated near the end of life. Clients must first be informed of the pros and cons of all the options that veterinary medicine can offer, including palliative treatments as a viable alternative to "preemptive euthanasia." The idea of considering a "Spectrum of Care" rather than limiting treatment options to a "Gold Standard," has recently been discussed as useful in veterinary practice and important enough to address in veterinary training programs. It allows the flexibility to bring treatment into grasp for some clients where either/or decisions can be emotionally straining for families and veterinary staff as well (Fingland et al. 2021; Brown et al. 2021). Euthanasia has historically been given as the only "humane" alternative when treatments are declined, potentially leaving all stakeholders with feelings of guilt and helplessness. Initially intended to address financial and "access to care" concerns, the spectrum of care approach is highly relevant in end-of-life care as well. The addition of palliative medicine, including multimodal pain management, environmental adaptations, and recognition and treatment of clinical signs of distress, expands the meaning of and allows the easier acceptance of treatment as a spectrum within humane care of animals at the end of life. With those in mind, practitioners can address financial, cultural, religious, moral, and other concerns that affect treatment decisions. Documenting discussions of treatment options and goals of care in patient records protects veterinarians and patients alike from misunderstandings and can improve case outcomes while reducing decision regret. Embracing a "Spectrum of Care" approach enhances overall client acceptance and participation in the treatment and decision-making process, allowing focus on patient-centered care. This is not a new idea in veterinary medicine, but the process of naming and acknowledging it as a legitimate, important, and necessary part of veterinary practice relieves some of the stress placed on veterinarians and clients alike. This is particularly relevant when the most expensive, most aggressive approach is not always the most appropriate for a patient nearing the end of life.

A "Spectrum of Care" approach reduces the burdens of care and enables caregivers to consistently and sustainably provide care with minimal risk of injury, undue stress, or over-exhaustion. The following statement, in a review of treatment burden for human patients with advanced heart failure, applies readily to human–animal caregiving pairings: "Considering treatment burden would force us to begin to move away from the prevalent disease centered care to more person centered models of care... There is a need to ensure care provision that prioritizes the goals of patients and caregivers, taking into account their personal context and prognosis." (Jani et al. 2013).

As medical providers, the veterinary team also carries significant burdens. These certainly include physical efforts, humane handling and restraint of patients, education of themselves, staff and clients, the effort required for empathy and listening, increased client contacts, and many others. In addition, when caregiver choices do not agree with provider views and recommendations, providers experience producing ethical conflict and moral distress (Moses et al. 2018). Clarifying goals of care helps to bring concerns from all stakeholders to the forefront, illuminating dilemmas and establishing limitations and boundaries for both caregiving families and medical providers.

Financial burdens add stress for caregivers and providers alike. This can be a difficult subject to broach, but it is important to know and understand that these limitations can have a strong influence on treatment plans and decision-making. Whether the financial limit is $100 or $100 000, it affects the ability to provide care to the patient. A few nights of hospitalization and diagnostics may clear the budget of any funding for ongoing treatment.

Conclusion

When switching our thinking from administering lifesaving, curative care to providing life-supportive, comfort care, many factors rise to the forefront that otherwise may seem insignificant. Short-term consequences take priority over long-term effects. Treatment of clinical signs becomes most important. Following disease progression through continued diagnostic testing may not lead to a more efficacious therapeutic plan, and may wind up causing unnecessary distress for the animal and their family. The goal of simplified care often takes precedence. Clinical assessment and empathic communication become the central focus of patient visits. One of the key goals of hospice and palliative care is to keep patients relatively comfortable by anticipating and preemptively treating signs that may become distressing, offering them the best possible balance between quantity and quality of life.

References

American Animal Hospital Association (AAHA) (2022) Pain management guidelines for dogs and cats. Available at: https://www.aaha.org/ aaha-guidelines/2022-aaha-pain-management-guidelines-for-dogs-and-cats/home/ (Accessed: April 2022).

Bittel, E. (2014) (How) It can be done: special needs care and complementary treatment options for animals with mobility issues. *American Holistic Veterinary Medical Association (AHVMA) Conference Proceedings.* Portland, OR (September 13–16).

Brown, C.R., Garrett, L.D., Gilles, W.K., et al. (2021) Spectrum of care: more than treatment options. *J. Am. Vet. Med. Assoc.*, 259 (7): pp. 712–717.

Cat Friendly Practices. (2022) Cat friendly practices. International Cat Care and American Association of Feline Practitioners. Available at: http://www.catvets.com/cfp/cfp (Accessed: April 2022).

Connor, S.R., Pyenson, B., Fitch, K., et al. (2007) Comparing hospice and nonhospice patient survival among patients who die within a three-year window. *J. Pain Symptom Manage.*, 33: pp. 238–246.

Fadol, A.P., Patel, A., Shelton, V., et al. (2021) Palliative care referral criteria and outcomes in cancer and heart failure: a systematic review of literature. *Cardiooncology*, 7 (1): pp. 32.

Fear Free Pets. (2022) Fear free pets. Fear Free LLC. Available at: https://fearfreepets.com (Accessed: April 2022).

Fingland, R.B., Stone, L.R., Read, E.K., et al. (2021) Preparing veterinary students for excellence in general practice: building confidence and competence by focusing on spectrum of care. *J. Am. Vet. Med. Assoc.*, 259 (5): pp. 463–470.

Gawande, A. (2010) Letting go: what should medicine do when it can't save your life? *The New Yorker* (2 August). Available at: https://www.newyorker.com/magazine/2010/08/02/letting-go-2.

Gaynor, J. and Muir, W. (2015) Handbook of Veterinary Pain Management, 3. St. Louis: Mosby.

Goldberg, K.J. (2019) Goals of care: development and use of the serious veterinary illness conversation guide. *Vet. Clin. North Am. Small Anim. Pract.*, 49 (3): pp. 399–415.

Goldberg, M. and Shaffran, N. (2015) Pain Management for Veterinary Technicians and Nurses. Ames, IA: Wiley.

Good P., Richard R., Syrmis W., *et al.* (2014) Medically assisted hydration for adult palliative care patients (review). *Cochrane Database Syst. Rev.*, (4), CD006273. https://doi.org/10.1002/14651858.CD006273.pub3

Jani, B., Blane, D., Browne, S., *et al.* (2013) Identifying treatment burden as an important concept for end of life care in those with advanced heart failure. *Curr. Opin. Support. Palliat. Care*, 7: pp. 3–7.

Lagrotteria, A, Swinton, M, Simon, J, et al. (2021) Clinicians' perspectives after implementation of the serious illness care program: a qualitative study. *JAMA Netw. Open*, 4: pp. e2121517.

Low Stress Handling. (2022) Low stress handling. Cattle Dog Publishing. Available at: https://lowstresshandling.com (Accessed: April 2022).

Monteiro, B.P. (2020) Feline chronic pain and osteoarthritis. *Vet. Clin. North Am. Small Anim. Pract.*, 50 (4): pp. 769–788.

Moses, L., Malowney, M.J., Wesley Boyd, J. (2018) Ethical conflict and moral distress in veterinary practice: a survey of north American veterinarians. *J. Vet. Intern. Med.*, 32 (6): pp. 2115–2122.

Mota-Rojas, D., Marcet-Rius, M., Ogi, A., et al. (2021) Current advances in assessment of dog's emotions, facial expressions, and their use for clinical recognition of pain. *Animals (Basel)*, 11 (11): pp. 3334.

Paladino, J., Koritsanszky, L., Nisotel, L., et al. (2020) Patient and clinician experience of a serious illness conversation guide in oncology: a descriptive analysis. *Cancer Med.*, 9 (13): pp. 4550–4560.

Quain, A., Ward, M.P., Mullan, S. (2021) Ethical challenges posed by advanced veterinary care in companion animal veterinary practice. *Animals (Basel)*, 11 (11): pp. 3010.

del Rio, M.I., Shand, B., Bonati, P., *et al.* (2012) Hydration and nutrition at the end of life: a systematic review of emotional impact, perceptions, and decision making among patients, family, and health care staff. *Psychooncology*, 21: pp. 913–921.

Ross, D. and Alexander, C. (2001) Management of common symptoms in terminally ill patients: part I. Fatigue, anorexia, cachexia, nausea and vomiting. *Am. Fam. Physician*, 64: pp. 807–814.

Seung, M., You, J., Lee, H., *et al.* (2016) Comparison of complications secondary to cardiopulmonary resuscitation between out-of-hospital cardiac arrest and in-hospital cardiac arrest. *Resuscitation*, 98: pp. 64–72.

Shaevitz, M.H., Tullius, J.A., Callahan, R.T., et al. (2020) Early caregiver burden in owners of pets with suspected cancer: owner psychosocial outcomes, communication behavior, and treatment factors. *J. Vet. Intern. Med.*, 34 (6): pp. 2636–2644.

Shanan, A. (2011) A veterinarian's role in helping pet owners with decision making. *Vet. Clin. North Am. Small Anim. Pract.*, 41: pp. 635–646.

Spitznagel, M.B., Cox, M.D., Jacobson, D.M., et al. (2019) Assessment of caregiver burden and associations with psychosocial function, veterinary service use, and factors related to treatment plan adherence among owners of dogs and cats. *J. Am. Vet. Med. Assoc.*, 254 (1): pp. 124–132.

Steagall, P.V. (2020) Analgesia: what makes cats different/challenging and what is critical for cats? *Vet. Clin. North Am. Small Anim. Pract.*, 50 (4): pp. 749–767.

Steagall, P.V., Robertson, S., Simon, B. et al. (2022). 2022 ISFM consensus guidelines on the management of acute pain in cats. *J. Feline Med. Surg.*, 24 (1): 4–30. Available at: https://journals.sagepub.com/doi/pdf/10.1177/1098612X211066268 (Accessed: April 2022).

Tilley, L., Smith, F., Oyama, M., et al. (2008) Manual of Canine and Feline Cardiology, 4 edn. St. Louis, MO: Saunders.

Tönnies, J., Hartmann, M., Jäger, D., et al. (2021) Aggressiveness of care at the end-of-life in cancer patients and its association with psychosocial functioning in bereaved caregivers. *Front. Oncol.*, 11: pp. 673147.

van de Vathorst, S. (2014) Artificial nutrition at the end of life: ethical issues. *Best Pract. Res. Clin. Gastroenterol.*, 28: pp. 247–253.

Wright, A.A., Zhang, B., Ray, A., *et al.* (2008) Associations between end-of-life discussions, patient mental health, medical care near death, and caregiver bereavement adjustment. *JAMA*, 300: pp. 1665–1673.

Yin, S. (2009) Low Stress Handling, Restraint and Behavior Modification of Dogs and Cats: Techniques for Developing Patients Who Love Their Visits. Davis, CA: CattleDog Publishing.

7

Ethical Decision-Making in Animal Hospice and Palliative Care

Jessica Pierce, BA, MTS, PhD and Amir Shanan, DVM

End-of-life care is one of the most ethically complex and challenging areas of veterinary practice and animal caregiving. Caregivers and animals are both particularly vulnerable during the final stages of an animal's life, when illness, suffering, and mortality push their way onto center stage. Clinicians and caregivers face a range of complex and emotionally charged moral issues, from the very broad (Is it ethical to allow an animal to die a natural death? Is it ethical to deliberately take the life of an animal, even one who is terminally ill?) to the very specific (How should a clinician deal with a client who is noncompliant in dispensing pain medications to her cat, who suffers from severe osteoarthritis?).

A number of factors converge to make moral decision-making in the context of animal end-of-life care extraordinarily complicated: the clinical picture is often complex and multilayered; we have a patient who cannot speak in human language but whose preferences we want to respect; we have clients with ideas (often conflicted and confused) about what they want for themselves, what they want for their animal, and what they are willing to pay. We confront a wide spectrum of beliefs and attitudes about illness, death, the hereafter, and the value of animal life; and we face different views of how the end of life is experienced by the animals themselves. This chapter addresses these real-world moral struggles that impact the daily lives and mental health of veterinarians, animal hospice team members, and millions of emotionally attached humans making life or death decisions for beloved animal companions.

Clinically and morally sound end-of-life choices matter to all stakeholders involved. They matter, above all, to the animal. If not handled well by human caregivers, the final days, weeks, or months of an animal's life can be marked by profound suffering. If the process is handled mindfully, a dying animal can feel safe, comfortable, and loved. They matter to human caregivers. Pet owners with an ill or dying animal must navigate their way through a maze of issues: understanding the physical and emotional condition of their animal, clarifying their values (e.g. what makes living worthwhile? What is the value of an animal's life? What sacrifices are they willing to make?), and taking stock of their caregiving resources (financial, emotional, practical). The decisions made at the end of an animal's life often have long-lasting effects on pet owners. Those who are uncomfortable with the choices they made – those who feel they were pressured into euthanizing too soon, or that they dragged things out too long, or that they "shortchanged" their animal by declining certain treatments – are at risk of suffering from mental health issues such as depression, unresolved grief, and post-traumatic stress, often lasting many years. They matter to veterinarians and hospice teams. Animal death can be one of the most emotionally exhausting aspects of a veterinarian's work, yet has the potential to be profoundly fulfilling, too. A nuanced approach to the ethical issues integral to end-of-life decision-making is essential to providing good end-of-life care. And how an animal's end-of-life care is handled strongly influences whether a client will continue to use a veterinary practice or not.

A Method for Moral Decision-Making

Judgments about what forms of care an animal needs are made by multiple "stakeholders": the animal, one or more human owners/caregivers (whose agendas sometimes conflict), and one or more animal healthcare providers (each of whom may offer different recommendations). These stakeholders bring to the table diverse kinds of judgment – ethical, medical, practical – which often conflict with each other.

The following discussion outlines a three-part model intended to help stakeholders think in an orderly way through decisions about care at the end of a companion animal's life, and to facilitate communication between stakeholders as they collaborate in making decisions. In the first part of the chapter, we focus on how clinicians and clients can navigate through clinical decisions with moral and emotional integrity. The second part of the chapter explores what might be called "the animal's point of view," including ethical aspects of animal quality of life (QOL), pain and suffering, individual preferences, and expressions of agency. Finally, the third part looks at human factors – psychological, financial, professional, cultural, and societal – that can influence moral decision-making in the animal hospice and palliative care (AHPC) setting.

Keep in mind that the distinctions between the three parts in this model are at times blurred, and there is a lot of interplay among them.

Part 1: Clinical Considerations and Their Moral Dimensions

Clinical considerations are those involving or relating to the direct medical treatment or testing of patients. Considerations in making medical treatment decisions for animals in hospice and palliative care are listed in Table 7.1.

Clinical considerations are dynamic, and decision-making is an ongoing process, so judgments have to evolve as an animal's condition changes. Caregivers/clients often feel that there is one right answer to how they should best care for their animal and dread getting the answer wrong. Some of the common questions that arise in end-of-life care reinforce this

Table 7.1 Clinical considerations.

- What is the diagnosis, prognosis, medical history?
- What is the animal's age?
- Are there comorbidities?
- What is the trajectory for the animal's condition?
- Is the patient's condition critical, emergent? Is it reversible? To what degree?
- What diagnostic tests/procedures are available? What are the benefits and burdens of each diagnostic option?
- What kind of information might be gained from the diagnostic process? How useful will this information be to us? Will the information change what we do?
- What are the treatment options available? What are the benefits and burdens of each option?
- Are stakeholders (patient, caregiving family, medical team, hospice team) in the clinical decision-making process "on the same page"? If not, what are the central points of disagreement/difference about diagnosis or treatment? What are the ethically acceptable options?

concern: "When is THE right time to eutha-nize?" "How much treatment is too much, and how much is not enough?" The phrasing of these questions suggests that the answers are objectively either right or wrong. This may lure clinicians and clients who prescribe to a pater-nalistic view of medical practice ("the doctor knows best") into feeling that it is the clini-cians' professional duty to provide the "right" answers; that everyone else's responsibility is to trust that "the doctor is always right." In the complex realities of animal end-of-life care, however, objectively right or wrong answers are rarely available. An alternative to the paternalistic model of medical practice is the model of "collaborative decision-making," which is used with remarkable success in human hospice and palliative care and holds equal promise for AHPC. We'll provide a sketch of this approach later in the chapter.

Being uncertain about what option is the best is not a sign that you lack competence. To the contrary, it means that you – clinician or caregiver – are aware of the complexity of the situation at hand. Acknowledging the reality of inherent uncertainty often lifts a huge and unnecessary burden off caregivers and ani-mal healthcare providers' minds. End-of-life decision-making is imperfect – we have incomplete information and an incomplete perspective.

A helpful tool the authors use in practice when making end-of-life decisions is the meta-phor of "hitting a blank target board." A realis-tic goal, practically and ethically, is to make decisions that land somewhere on the "target board." Hitting one precise point is *not* a realis-tic goal (there are no circles or "bull's eye" on the board). It is important to avoid missing the target board altogether ("morally undesirable or indefensible decisions"). This approach goes a long way to minimizing feelings of moral discomfort, regret, and guilt for all stakeholders.

It is the clinician's responsibility to acknowl-edge uncertainty and to reassure caregivers that rather than clear (perfectly right and wrong) answers there is a range of options, each one with pros and cons to be considered.

Clients need to be reminded and reassured that, other than euthanasia, treatment deci-sions aren't set in stone and changing course is frequently indicated when new information arises (for example, side effects turn out to be more severe than expected). Changing plans is not a sign of failure – it is a sign of flexibility.

In veterinary clinical contexts, other than AHPC, hospice and palliative care must be included as one of the options available to caregivers. AHPC can be best described as "comfort care," "treatments to manage pain and discomfort," or "treatments to maintain quality of life."

Part 2: Patient Considerations: How the Animal Feels and What the Animal Wants

The claim to be doing "what is in the animal's best interest" is sometimes code for doing what is in our own best interests or doing what *we* think is best for the animal. Practitioners and clients often brush off the job of figuring out what animals want, claiming that animals aren't smart enough to know what is in their best interests or, if animals do have thoughts about their own life experience, that they can-not communicate clearly enough with us to make listening worthwhile. This silencing of the animal's point of view is unethical and leads to care that satisfies only certain stake-holders. Instead of pursuing our own interests or paternalistically assuming the task of decid-ing what an animal ought to want, we should make every effort to elicit the actual experi-ences and preferences of the animal patient. Afterall, they are the center of our caring concern in AHPC.

Tools for assessing an animal's QOL strive to inject as much objectivity into this important and challenging task (see Chapter 4 in this book for a detailed discussion). It is increas-ingly accepted, however, that animals' well-being is primarily subjective in nature (Rowan et al. 2021); assessing how an animal is feeling, therefore, must rely to some extent on intuition. Clinical intuition can be difficult to articulate and explain and is not always completely trustworthy. Using an orderly process for working through tough decisions can clarify and guide intuition and can give us increased confidence about judgments and decisions. Our orderly process must start by understanding animals' emotional well-being: what determines how can we know and how well or how poorly an animal is doing.

Understanding What Animals Want

An animal's emotional well-being can be assessed from at least two different viewpoints: we can ask, "how happy or unhappy is the animal?" Well-being rests upon mental states, and the balance between mental states that are pleasurable and those that are painful or aversive. We can also ask, "are the animal's individual preferences being satisfied?" Satisfaction of preferences often contributes to happiness, but is of great significance to animals' emotional well-being even when it does not. The extent to which any particular mental state affects an individual's well-being depends on individual preferences–or *how much it matters to that individual*. A view that considers both whether animals are happy *and* whether their preferences are satisfied could be labeled, following Parfit, "preference hedonism" (*cf.* Parfit 1984, p 493). We endorse this blended account of animal well-being.

How do we know whether an animal is happy or whether this animal's particular preferences are being satisfied? We triangulate using information gathered by careful assessment and interpretation of the animal's behavior, which is monitored and documented by appropriately skilled observers. Animals are continually communicating things to us through their behavior and body language. Practicing careful, detailed observation grounded in an excellent working knowledge

of species-specific behavioral communication will help veterinarians and other hospice providers understand what animals are feeling. Caregivers (pet owners) can play an essential role in understanding how an animal feels, particularly when there is a strong human-animal bond. Caregivers will likely be attuned to their animals' individual personalities, what they like and do not like, how they are doing, and how they will fare in a given treatment regimen. Caregivers are "the experts" and should be the hospice team's primary source of insight in the patient preferences arena. We must keep in mind, however, that the ability of animal caregivers to read the behavioral signals of their dog, cat, or other animals varies widely from person to person.

We know from the human medical ethics literature that accurately predicting what another person feels and wants when making medical decisions for that other person is difficult. Making wrong assumptions is easy. For example, research shows that QOL judgments made by the parents of teens correlate poorly with judgments made by the teens themselves regarding the same scenarios. Another example is that people living with disabilities often view their own QOL very differently (generally, more positively) from how it is viewed by able-bodied people who know them. To successfully make decisions for animals based on the animals' individual preferences, our interpretations of "what animals want and need" must be cautious and open to revision.

Will to Live

A uniquely important example of individual preferences is the preference for life over death – the "will to live." Animals' will to live is a nebulous but very powerful factor to be considered in QOL assessments and in making end-of-life care decisions for them. The will to live is an important concept when attempting to understand and comprehend why individuals do what they do to stay alive, and/or find a meaning to continuing their life, when on the brink of death.

Unfortunately, there is no science exploring the will to live in nonhuman patients. But studies of human patients may offer useful insights into how both physical, psychological, and social variables may influence an individual's will to live. Chochinov et al. (1999, 2005) studied the will to live of human patients with cancer in palliative care, nearing the end of life. Patients self-reported their will to live twice daily, as part of a symptom assessment system consisting of a series of visual analogue scales measuring pain, nausea, shortness of breath, appetite, drowsiness, depression, sense of well-being, anxiety, and activity. The studies demonstrated that fluctuations in will-to-live ratings for each patient were substantial and best predicted by patient scores for depression, anxiety, shortness of breath, and sense of well-being. Satisfaction with support from family, friends, and health care providers was also highly correlated with the will to live (Chochinov et al. 2005). When a broad range of influences were considered concurrently, existential issues emerged most prominently. Those included hopelessness (the loss of a sense of meaning and purpose); being a burden to others (the loss of a sense of agency); and the loss of dignity (the loss of a sense of identity, "essence" or "personhood"). Physical variables correlated with the will to live to a lesser degree.

Respecting What Animals Want

"Respecting autonomy" is often considered the most important ethical consideration in the human medical realm, dictating that patients have the last word in decisions about their own treatment, based upon what they themselves value and want, not upon what somebody else thinks they should value and want.

The authors of this chapter advocate for using a modified principle of "respect for autonomy" in caring for animals, based on recognizing humans' ethical obligation to respect animals' unique individual preferences. We view "respecting individual preferences" as ethically analogous to "respecting autonomy." Promoting well-being in terms of animals'

preference fulfillment is therefore a sound method for "respecting autonomy" of animal patients *IF* eliciting animals' preferences are followed by giving these preferences weight in guiding our decisions about the animals' care.

Respecting the preferences of animal patients requires recognizing that each animal is an individual with his or her own personality. Research suggests that animals with different personality types respond differently to treatment protocols, to changes in their environment, and to stress (Carere and Maestripieri 2013). Animal patients' individual personalities and preferences have been all but ignored in the veterinary profession's approach to end-of-life decision-making, until recently. We are encouraged to see that this is beginning to change. Hospice teams need to assess, in each case, how well the animal patient's individual voice is being heard by the humans who are making the decisions for her. Treatment plans will be most respectful and most effective if they take into consideration the individual personality of the animal.

Suffering

In addition to a caregiver's desire to do "what my animal would want," those facing end-of-life care decisions for their animals are most preoccupied with the wish: "I do not want her to suffer!"

As is the case with QOL, assessing whether an animal is suffering often relies on an intuitive sense of what the animal is feeling. It is important to remember that in the everyday use of the word, "suffering" means many different things. Many forms and degrees of suffering – depending on how long it lasts, intensity, etc. – are very much a part of every life; a survival mechanism hardwired into all sentient living beings' nervous systems to guide them in navigating challenging life conditions.

In caring for animals who may be nearing the end of life, however, the question "is the animal suffering?!" is often asked when deciding whether or not to end the animal's life. If the answer to the question is "YES," then the animal is often, in a knee-jerk way, presumed to be "better off dead."

Suffering is subjective, difficult to define and greatly feared by animal caregivers. There is no universally accepted definition of suffering in members of our own species, the human animal, despite extensive literature and opinions articulated over millennia. No wonder it is hard to pin down exactly what suffering is in members of other species! The suffering of animals under our care is nevertheless something we have an obligation to address.

"Suffering," writes Eric Cassell, "is experienced by persons, not merely by bodies, and has its source in challenges that threaten the intactness of the person as a complex social and psychological entity" (Cassell 1982, p. 641). Drawing on Cassell's work, suffering has been defined as the distress an individual experiences when they perceive a threat to any aspect of their continued existence, whether physical, psychological, or social. Suffering is therefore determined not by the threat itself but by the individual's emotional and cognitive response to the threat. Major characteristics of suffering are () a feeling of helplessness in the face of a threat, (ii) a loss of valued relationships, and (iii) a perception that the destruction of one's sense of self is unavoidable (see, for example, Gill 2019). As mentioned above, these correspond closely to losses of the determinants of the will to live: a sense of hope, life meaning, agency, and "personhood."

While Cassell's work addresses human suffering, his reference to "the intactness of the person as a complex social and psychological entity" applies to sentient nonhuman animals as well.

Kiley-Worthington, for example, makes the argument that all mammals make choices and decisions; rationally reason and have beliefs; anticipate and predict; make judgments and develop concepts; remember and imagine; have ideas, thoughts, and dreams; have views of the past and the future based on the individual's lifetime experience; and have a subjective point of view she refers to using the term "personhood," (Kiley-Worthington 2017) supporting the notion that in respect to their capacity for suffering as defined by Cassell, nonhuman animals are "persons."

Suffering can be caused by physical symptoms of illness or aging including pain, hypoxia (lack of oxygen, difficulty breathing), nausea, and itchiness, among other things. It can also be caused by negative affective states including, but not limited to, fear, frustration, loneliness, boredom, and loss of agency (sense of control over one's choices and environment). Affective states such as anxiety, depression, confusion, and mental exhaustion can originate in processes that are either organic (e.g. central nervous system (CNS) disorders) or psychological (e.g. an emotional response to a situation or experience), or some combination of both. It is critically important to remember that not all physical discomfort, and not all emotional distress, results in suffering.

Do animals always suffer at the end of life? How do we know whether an animal is suffering? And how do we know whether an animal's suffering morally justifies relief by ending her life?

To answer these questions, caregivers and veterinarians frequently focus on the animal's physical comfort (pain and other unpleasant physical sensations) and physical function (mobility, digestion, respiration). While physical comfort and functioning are easier to measure objectively than animal emotions, this focus may overshadow the importance of the animal's emotional well-being in determining QOL. Positive affect (happiness, joy, contentment), a sense of control, and satisfaction of preferences can significantly mitigate animals' suffering.

To assess whether an animal may be suffering it is most relevant to interpret (as best we can) what affective state the animal's behavior reflects. Animals, like humans, experience long-term mood states, and not just fleeting emotions. Animals can be happy and content, overall, and they can suffer from depression and listlessness (McMillan 2005; Paul et al. 2005; Mendl et al. 2009; Paul and Mendl 2018). Recognizing suffering, therefore, requires attention not just to present-moment stressors, but to underlying long-term affective states.

Underlying long-term affective states are reflected in how animals respond to ambiguous situations: animals who are happy overall tend to interpret ambiguous signals or stimuli with curiosity and optimism, while animals in a low mood are likely to react with fear. We can therefore use animals' response to ambiguous stimuli to assess the animal's underlying long-term affective state: if an animal who has been for most of her life curious and outgoing responds to an ambiguous situation with fear or withdrawal, the animal may be suffering.

A loss of control over one's own environment – called "loss of agency" by welfare researchers – is strongly correlated with suffering in human patients and is vitally important in animal patients as well. Animals who are repeatedly unable to escape from aversive stimuli can develop learned helplessness, which is characterized by apathy, depression, and simply giving up hope. There is an enormous literature on learned helplessness in animals, much of it from animal models developed to study human depression. As in humans, a state of helplessness is associated in animals with depression and frustration (Weary 2014, p. 193) and is a strong indicator of suffering.

Serious illness and disability can create conditions in which an animal's behavior changes due to prolonged exposure to painful or aversive stimuli. For example, an animal experiencing severe pain in his hips every time he tries to stand may, eventually, stop trying to stand. This deviation from his normal behavior patterns is an important warning sign that the animal may be suffering. Especially important to watch for are reductions in an animal's normal motivated behaviors such as food seeking, social engagement, and the expression of attachment bonds (typically with the animal's primary caregiver/s). When the reduction in motivated behaviors is obvious, recurring, and/or persistent, it is likely to reflect an underlying emotional state of helplessness, hopelessness and/or suffering.

More subtle or gradual changes in animals' motivated behaviors, however, may represent adaptation rather than suffering. Animals, like humans, are capable of regaining much of their prior level of happiness after debilitating losses (e.g. loss of vision, a limb, or a loving owner). Hence, a dog who stopped chasing a ball because of painful arthritis is not necessarily suffering if the dog discovered over a period of time other activities that are pleasurable to him. Animals' capacity for adaptation therefore must be taken into consideration in the determination of animal suffering.

Concurrently facing multiple stressors increases the likelihood of suffering. So, an animal who is in pain and who also experiences frustration or loneliness is more likely to experience suffering. Hospice interventions should therefore strive to minimize factors like uncertainty and unpredictability in animals' environments and to maximize the animals' sense of security and comfort, by providing animals with familiar surroundings and caregivers, and by following a consistent routine of feeding, play, and care. In other words, hospice interventions can seek to address patients' low mood by addressing the conditions that result in low mood (e.g. pain, unpredictability in the environment, lack of social interaction, etc.). Situations that evoke negative feelings (e.g. handling by strangers, unfamiliar places) should be avoided as much as possible. Positive reinforcement techniques can help reduce the stress associated with administration of medications and other treatments. Providing animals opportunities to self-medicate with analgesics and/or anxiolytics, which would give them a measure of control, has been demonstrated by Danbury et al. (2000) Last but not least, Marty Becker's work on Fear Free veterinary care is of singular importance in the context of hospice and palliative care. Working to create interactions with veterinarians that are free of fear will likely result in greater success in improving QOL with minimal cost in creating negative feelings in animal patients. (For more information, see www.drmartybecker. com/category/fear-free).

When suffering becomes the singular focus of end-of-life discussions, caregivers and decision-makers see only a bleak set of options:

escalating but futile attempts to cure, inaction and continued suffering, or immediate euthanasia. Unfortunately, a frequent outcome in clinical practice is premature decisions to euthanize animals - decisions driven primarily by human fears. Hospice team members must exercise extreme sensitivity when using the term "suffering" in communications with caregivers, as it can be too subjective, too nebulous, too colored by preconceptions and strong negative connotations. Once the "S-word" is on the table, caregivers may get "stuck," unable to see the entire picture. The cards are then stacked very heavily in favor of euthanasia, and viable options for hospice care may be closed off.

It is critically important, therefore, to expand the discussion to include emotional well-being, the animal's preferences and will to live. The power of "suffering" then begins to shrink down to its proper place in the decision-making process. Replacing the focus on "suffering" with a focus on animals' motivated behaviors, especially those reflecting social engagement and expression of attachment bonds, is extremely helpful when caregivers, veterinarians and other AHPC team members face difficult decisions for animals at the end of life.

Whether or not, and with what degree of sensitivity, a human caregiver perceives his animal's preferences, suffering, joy, or will to live greatly depends on the nature of their bond. Research has shown that animals who are given little value (economic or emotional) are less likely to receive compassionate treatment. Supporting human-animal relationships throughout animals' lives is thus essential for promoting the best possible experience for the animals as their lives end.

Part 3: Human Factors Influencing Moral Decision-Making

The context within which decisions are being made often determines the basic spectrum of what is possible or not. Decisions for animals at the end of life are made by human stakeholders who participate in the process in different capacities – as the animal's caregiver/s, as animal service provider/s, as family, friends, and a community. The opinions expressed by different stakeholders, the interactions between them, and the decisions eventually made all take into consideration (hopefully) the animal's clinical condition, emotional well-being, individual preferences, and will to live.

Invariably, however, decisions for the animal are also influenced by considerations *other than the animal's condition*. Those considerations are referred to as the "contextual features" of the decision-making process. They include the web of relationships between the caregiver, the caregiver's family, friends and community, the medical team and the animal. They include what beliefs caregivers hold, what responsibilities they have other than caring for the sick animal, what resources they have access to for fulfilling those various responsibilities, and how they allocate those resources. And they include the values and priorities that motivate the actions of medical and other service providers participating in the decision-making process.

The contextual features of animal end-of-life decision-making are laden with possible ethical conflicts. Such conflicts, and how they are addressed, frequently impact the long-term mental health of all human stakeholders. The risk is highest for those who are most directly involved in making the decisions: the animal's primary caregiver/s and veterinarian/s.

In the next few paragraphs, we'll describe the common contextual features influencing caregivers' decisions. Then, we'll briefly elaborate on the potential mental health risks and how they can be minimized.

A primary contextual feature in the care of an animal is: who is the animal's primary caregiver, and what kind of bond does he or she have with the animal patient. Is there just one person who is clearly recognized by everyone as the decision-maker, or are there others whose opinions must be considered and respected? If more than one person, how close or far apart are these multiple decision-makers' views? What are their family and friends' opinions, and how likely those are to influence the process? How strong is the primary caregiver's emotional attachment to the animal? What value, monetary and otherwise, does the caregiver place on the animal's life? What kind of sacrifices is he or she willing to make? How tuned in is the caregiver to what the animal is going through? How good of a proxy decision-maker can he or she be for the animal?

Another contextual feature is the caregiver's beliefs about animals' cognitive and emotional capacities, the value of animal life, the meaning of illness, the nature of a good death, and the moral and religious acceptability of euthanasia. Opinions vary widely regarding the differences and similarities between what humans and animals experience close to dying, and during dying with and without euthanasia. (Selter et al. 2022) Such opinions play an important part in the decisions caregivers make. Unfortunately, empirical data relevant to answering these questions is scarce at best; Selter et al. suggest "both human and veterinary medical ethicists engage in a thorough analysis of the dissimilarities but also the similarities of their patients and their respective experiences at the end of their lives."

Stakeholders' ethnic, religious, and cultural backgrounds are also a contextual feature in animal end-of-life decision-making. Families and individuals coming from diverse backgrounds are likely to have different expectations and different values, influencing the kinds of choices they make about goals of treatment, manner of death, and timing of death. Buddhists, for example, frequently reject euthanasia because they consider deliberately taking a life to be a violation of their spiritual precepts, and because they have a unique perspective on the nature of suffering. Although the welfare of the animal patient must always stay in the forefront, respect for the values of the animal's caregiver also needs to guide the decision-making process. Conflicting values and expectations complicate decision-making and increase the risk of moral distress and future mental health burden.

Decisions are influenced by the resources that caregivers have access to for fulfilling their caregiving responsibilities to the animal. The range of reasonable treatment options for an animal whose caregiver has limited financial resources is different than for an animal whose caregiver is affluent but is never home, or one whose caregiver places low priority on the animal's well-being relative to other aspects of their life. In addition to time and money, various other resources come into play. Given the animal's body weight, is the caregiver physically capable of providing support to help the animal go up and down stairs? Do they live in a one-level home with a yard, or in a third floor walk-up apartment? Is the caregiver capable of administering medication to the animal? Is someone at home to protect the animal from anxiety and loneliness? Does the caregiver have the emotional stamina and social support needed to cope with the emotional burden of caregiving, the uncertainty, the moments of panic?

Decisions are also influenced by caregivers' responsibilities other than caring for the animal. How demanding is the job they hold? How demanding are their family and social obligations? Is there a human family member for whom the animal's caregiver needs to also provide care? Are they going through life changes such as retirement, career change, new parenting, divorce, or relocation? Are they facing recent or imminent significant losses in terms of their own health or the health of loved ones? The answers to these questions determine, based on caregivers' priorities, how much of their available time, money, and physical and emotional stamina will be dedicated to the animal's care.

And decisions are influenced by the values and priorities that motivate the actions of medical and other service providers participating in the decision-making process. Professional ethics are standards of personal and business behavior expected of a certain profession. As outlined in the American Veterinary Medical

Association's (AVMA) *Principles of Veterinary Ethics* (AVMA 2013), the veterinarian's role involves the acquisition of a body of technical knowledge and clinical reasoning skills; and the competent application of these for the benefit of patients and society. Veterinarians, like physicians, are also expected in their professional role to behave with honesty, integrity, and fairness, and to engage in open and judicious communication with clients and colleagues.

There are many situations in which two or more ethical standards of professional conduct for animal hospice team members conflict with each other. In these situations, they may experience ethical tensions in their work. A prime example is in establishing caregiving priorities, which in veterinary care is far more complex than human medicine. The Hippocratic Oath unambiguously places the patient "first in line" in physicians' ethical responsibilities. The veterinary oath and ethics guidelines of the AVMA, on the other hand, offer no such clear guidance. The needs of the animal patient are placed in tension with the preferences of the animal's caregiver. Veterinarians are in the difficult position of having to balance obligations toward the animal patient with obligations toward the human client.

In this balancing act, and in other situations where it is unclear what exactly professionalism demands, conflicts of interest and values frequently arise, resulting in ethical tension. The risk of moral distress for veterinarians and animal hospice team members is therefore high. This was documented by Springer et al., who found that veterinarians are increasingly torn between patients' interests and medical feasibility and factors related to their clients (Springer et al. 2019). To minimize the risk, animal hospice teams should proactively seek to identify values or goals that may conflict with the welfare of the animal; recognize areas of conflict (or potential conflict) between clients and the animal hospice care team; keep lines of communication open; and make timely referrals to mental health professionals as soon as they suspect moral distress.

Specifically, adherence to professional ethical standards impacts end-of-life decision-making in several important ways as outlined below.

Providing Adequate Information

A veterinarian is expected to communicate openly and honestly with his or her human clients. Yet, it is not always clear what exactly needs to be said or how best to say it. Nor is it possible to fully inform a client about their options since there is an inherent asymmetry in knowledge. The kinds of decisions a client makes about an animal will depend, to a large extent, on how much and what kind of information they are given by their veterinarian, and how this information is delivered. Sketching the pros and cons for diagnostic and treatment options must be done without disclosing one's personal preference, which is an art requiring both skill and unfailing commitment to ethical conduct. The language, terminology, and degree of information detail must be tailored to ensure caregivers are processing what they hear and to encourage them to actively engage in the decision-making process.

The question – "how much should, or must, a veterinarian disclose to the owner to have fulfilled his or her professional obligation?" – comes into sharp focus in the realm of animal hospice. Hospice care is a relatively new field, and its ethical standards of care are still evolving.

Veterinarians who fail to discuss the option of hospice care – offering only curative treatment or euthanasia – are failing to fulfill their professional obligation to provide full information, according to the International Association of Animal Hospice and Palliative Care (IAAHPC). The IAAHPC hospice guidelines argue that caregivers of animals have a right to be informed about hospice and palliative care options, and veterinarians have an obligation to be knowledgeable enough about AHPC services to advise clients how and where to find help for their animal (Shanan et al. 2017). Knowledge about what AHPC involves and how these services can benefit animals and their families would likely dispel many concerns of veterinarians suspicious that hospice is not in the best interests of animals.

The 2016 AAHA/IAAHPC *END-OF-LIFE Care Guidelines* (Bishop et al. 2016) state: "End-of-life (EOL) care and decision-making embody the critical final stage in a pet's life and are as important and meaningful as the sum of the clinical care provided for all prior life stages." Additionally, the AAHA/IAAHPC *guidelines* state that primary care veterinary practices should have a dedicated team to implement palliative and hospice care for end-of-life patients. This would ensure that quality end-of-life care is available everywhere; however, making this a reality will require a quantum leap in this critically important area of veterinary education.

An ethically difficult situation arises if a veterinarian believes that a client, eager to pursue hospice care for their animal, will be unable to provide effective pain management and comfort care to their animal. Offering AHPC in this case could result in unacceptable levels of suffering for the animal. Is it right to simply not mention hospice and palliative care as options and recommend euthanasia? In human patients, the answer is unequivocal: respect for autonomy requires that we disclose all reasonable options, even those that we feel might not be in the best interests of the patient. With animals, it is quite a bit more complicated because the animal is not the decision-maker. In ethically complex cases such as this, might it be true that some degree of paternalism may be in order? Should a veterinarian withhold information if he or she believes sharing it is likely to result in suffering for the animal?

Providing adequate information is important for minimizing the risk of decisional regret that may be experienced after making high-stakes health care decisions, further discussed later in this chapter. Therefore, taking the time to educate clients and engender their trust in the information presented by the veterinarian is a more ethical path to preventing possible animal suffering than withholding information.

Guiding Client Decision-Making: How Much Is Too Much?

In animal end-of-life decisions, caregivers are ultimately the decision-makers. Veterinarians and AHPC team members have both medical and nonmedical roles in their relationships with caregivers. Combining the two, they use their expertise to guide clients into treatment plans that are beneficial, realistic, and safe for client and patient alike. Veterinarians have years of training and experience that provide an informed perspective on the clinical situation; it is appropriate for veterinarians to encourage clients to elect a course of action that the veterinarian believes is in the best interests of the animal. Most clients are eager to know what their veterinarian would recommend.

Ethically managing end-of-life cases, however, requires veterinarians to avoid the temptation to guide clients too strongly, to use their perceived authority to guide clients toward the decision the veterinarian prefers. The values and preferences of the veterinarian are always reflected in the kinds of recommendations they offer clients, and veterinarians must carefully assess their own assumptions about their clients for the possibility that the assumptions may be inaccurate, outright wrong, and/or driven by biases. While veterinarians may be the authority on medical diagnosis, prognosis, and treatment, they are not the authority on what a client should or should not value, nor are the only experts on what an individual animal may need. Veterinarians should be careful not to abuse their power. Any attempt, overt or covert, to sway the client's decision toward the plan that is the veterinarian's preference is wrong. Presenting information and options in such a way as to nudge a client toward a particular course of action is unethical.

Some veterinarians, on the other hand, can be overcautious in their effort to avoid guiding clients too strongly, and they believe they should not offer guidance to their clients regarding end-of-life decision-making, telling the client, "Here is the information about prognosis and treatment options; you have to decide. I can offer no opinion."

AHPC patients present with complex chronic conditions, often take multiple medications, and experience a wide variety of symptoms for which explanations and treatments can be elusive. Providing good care, in these situations, requires identifying the highest priority health-related problems that emerge from the confluence of medical and nonmedical issues. Developing an optimal action plan through such a process is the objective of so-called "collaborative decision-making," making this an ideal tool for AHPC. Table 7.2 illustrates the differences between collaborative decision-making and three other clinical decision-making models.

To "collaborate" means that the parties "work together", especially in a joint intellectual effort. (O'Grady and Jadad 2010) Collaborative decision-making helps AHPC clinicians to learn from caregivers and helps caregivers learn from medical experts: clinicians have more expertise in medical issues, whereas caregivers have expertise about their animals' and their own life issues and experiences; caregivers may also have medical knowledge that should not be discounted. Collaborative decision-making uses knowledge-building principles, defined as "the social activity by which participants create new knowledge through ongoing, dynamic interaction between individuals, in which ideas are shared with others and are iteratively transformed and improved through the sharing of perspectives." (Mylopoulos and Scardamalia 2008) In collaborative decision-making, caregivers work with clinicians on a level playing field, both parties acknowledging that building a common pool of knowledge by learning from each other will lead to more balanced and satisfactory decisions.

Addressing the confluence of medical and nonmedical issues requires merging the provision of factual information with emotional support for the caregivers, working patiently through their intense emotions to enable their participation in creating new knowledge through dynamic interaction, eliciting their underlying values and beliefs, and evaluating the available treatment options in the context of those values and beliefs. This can be a tall order. Objectively, right or wrong answers are

Table 7.2 Clinical decision-making models.

Model for patient-physician interaction	Physicians' role	Patients' role	Knowledge "flow"	Objective
Paternalistic	Directive	Passive	One-way knowledge transfer (physician to patient)	Compliance of patient to physicians' directive
Autonomous	Receptive	Directive	One-way knowledge transfer (patient to physician)	Compliance of physician to patients' directive
Shared decision-making	Informative	Informative	Two-way knowledge exchange	Equity in the decision-making process
Collaborative decision-making	Supportive	Proactive	Knowledge building that goes beyond clinical issues (shared learning by exchanging information)	Optimal action plan to improve health

Source: From: O'Grady and Jadad A. (2010)

rarely available in the complexity of end-of-life realities. As eloquently described by Laurence J. Peter, "Some problems are so complex that you have to be highly intelligent and well-informed just to be undecided about them." (Peter 1982) Being uncertain about what option is the best is not a sign of lacking competence - to the contrary: it means that you – clinician and caregiver – are aware of the complexity of the situation at hand.

Guiding the Choice between Euthanasia and Continued Palliative Care

Within human medicine, there is little agreement about what constitutes good death or successful dying (for a review, see Meier et al. 2016, Selter et al. 2022). Researchers have found that some people define a good death by objective criteria, while others define it subjectively, as "the degree to which a person's preferences for dying agree with how the person actually died." Objective and subjective arguments are used by both by those in favor and those against "induced dying" (euthanasia, Physician Assisted Suicide). Veterinary literature on the concept of good death is scarce. As Persson and colleagues suggest, "the multitude of aspects shaping the ethical discourse of animal death and the morality of killing are not apprehended in veterinary medicine. Nor do veterinarians seem to be aware of the many philosophical assumptions they make in positioning themselves." (Persson et al. 2020) The following is a brief summary of Selter et al.'s discussion of concepts of a good death in human and veterinary medicine (Selter et al. 2022, pp. 74–79).

Objective arguments against euthanasia in humans generally focus on the claim that dying is an inherently meaningful and potentially transformative experience and that there is a right time for death to occur that should not be determined by either the medical team or the patient or patient's representative. Although we cannot know what goes on inside

the minds and hearts of our animals, we should be open to the possibility that they, too, might experience something profound as they die. (Pierce 2012) Other objective arguments opposing euthanasia of human as well as non-human beings consider it as a traumatic event that takes away the individual's (and maybe the caregiver's) dignity. Euthanasia is described as bewildering and a hasty transition "from pain to just being dead" (Hurn and Badman-King 2019, p. 150), and as a betrayal of the animal's trust in its caregiver.

Objective arguments offered in favor of euthanasia focus on the prevention of unnecessary suffering and are often based on an assumption that animals are not harmed by the loss of life, whether because they have no sense of the value of life, because they are incapable of mentally transcending from the present, because they do not possess individual long-term views of life as a whole, or because they do not experience mortality in the same ways as humans do. Yet these claims are little more than folk beliefs; they are not based on empirical research into the mental states or death experiences of nonhuman animals. Unfortunately, these folk beliefs are reinforced by veterinarians who vilify noninduced death, as seen, for example, in Villalobos' melodramatic description of "an emaciated, dehydrated, depressed terminal patient that must endure pointless pain and suffering until liberated by death." (Villalobos 2011).

As the IAAHPC/AAHA (Bishop et al. 2016, p. 353f) guidelines suggest, "there is limited empirical data on what animals experience during non-euthanasia-induced deaths, however the knowledge gained from human palliative medicine suggests that hospice-supported natural death does not increase suffering." A growing body of evidence-based knowledge about animal cognition starkly contradicts the assumptions that animals are incapable of possessing individual long-term views of life as a whole; Kiley-Worthington (2017), referenced earlier in this chapter, represents a miniscule fraction of that knowledge. This new understanding of what animals can experience casts a dark shadow of doubt over the claim that animals are not harmed by the loss of life.

The debate around the ethical relevance of species membership when it comes to the concept of a good death has been going on for several decades and should not be dismissed lightly. Selter et al. suggest that both human as well as veterinary medical ethicists would be well advised to engage in a thorough analysis of the dissimilarities but also similarities of their patients and their respective experiences at the end of their lives. They advise veterinarians to engage in a conversation with those palliative physicians opposing euthanasia and PAS in order to understand their reluctance and worries.

In human medicine, the growing diversity in "good death" concepts represents the plurality of preferences of the patients themselves. In veterinary medicine it seems to be based on caregivers' adaptation of concepts and procedures from human medicine. Despite good intentions, acceptance of the clients' versatile good death ideals could potentially result in damage to the animal patients' well-being if it is not scientifically based on what might be in the animal patients' best interest.

In conclusion, Selter et al. invite palliative care providers and medical ethicists to engage in the debate on whether human and animal dying actually represent two fundamentally different kinds, and if so, on what grounds.

In light of the limited empirical data available on what animals experience during death, the animal hospice team should remain open to caregivers' preferences regarding natural death and euthanasia, with the welfare of the animal always paramount. Discussing the options and making recommendations should be guided by tact and the utmost attention to the caregiver's personal beliefs. Euthanasia should never be presented as the only morally acceptable option, especially if the caregiver is unprepared or opposed for religious, spiritual, or moral reasons; neither should natural death be presented as the only morally acceptable option for an animal. Referral to a veterinarian whose philosophy is more aligned with the client's desires or needs is sometimes the most ethical course of action.

Euthanasia is currently considered by most veterinary professionals in the United States an ethically appropriate procedure. A hospice veterinarian may, nevertheless, have a principled moral objection to euthanasia and refuse to perform the procedure regardless of the circumstances. One of the primary arguments against the legalization of physician-assisted suicide is that the practice places physicians in an impossible situation. Physicians are trained to be healers and asking them to kill patients (or help patients kill themselves) threatens their core identity as medical professionals, a situation referred to as "role ambiguity." The same kind of ambiguity does not appear to plague veterinary medicine, since euthanasia of animals is a common and well-accepted social practice in many countries. Nevertheless, for those veterinarians who identify themselves primarily as healers, being asked to end the life of an animal may cause feelings of moral distress. Because euthanasia is not openly questioned, the role ambiguity is not made transparent and veterinarians are not encouraged to explore feelings of conflict and discomfort, leading to burnout and depression. Open, profession-wide discussion of the role of killing in veterinary medicine would help practitioners address feelings of moral distress.

Caregivers should be made aware of the veterinarian's position on euthanasia prior to the establishment of a therapeutic relationship with the animal and should be referred to another provider if the provider's position conflicts with the caregivers' wishes.

Veterinarians - including hospice veterinarians – are sometimes asked to euthanize animals who they judge to still have good QOL and reasonable life expectancy. A veterinarian may refuse to perform euthanasia in situations where he or she feels that the request is inappropriate and not in the best interests of the animal. In these situations, the veterinarian should clearly explain his or her reasons for refusing to perform euthanasia.

An ethically complex situation the animal hospice team may be presented with is one in which a caregiver chooses to prolong the life of an animal in profound and unrelenting pain or other forms of suffering. Caregivers can lose sight of the animal's needs or fail to recognize how poorly an animal is actually doing. A veterinarian may choose, in such a situation, to withdraw from the case and refer the client to a different veterinarian. This may not be the most effective strategy, however; educating caregivers about animal pain and suffering and human grief within the context of a hospice relationship is often in the best interest of the animal and her human caregiver.

Societal Ethics and the Role of Cultural Values

AHPC providers are influenced by social and cultural undercurrents that flow well beyond the veterinary profession. Those include moral questions about the value of animal life, the meaning and harm of death, our moral commitments to companion animals, and the attitudinal climate within which veterinary medicine and pet keeping take place. This broader attitudinal climate implicitly shapes decision-making at the professional and clinical level, and can breed feelings of confusion and ambivalence as we care for our pets at the end of life. It cannot completely escape notice, for example, that we are willing to devote tremendous care and time and money and compassion to certain individual dogs and cats, while millions of others are killed in shelters without public protest. Nor can our indifference to the suffering of animals used for food or research always sit easily next to our extreme concern for our own individual pets - who may be considered dinner staple in another part of the world. These threads of concern and indifference increasingly cut across each other as our understanding and awareness of animal cognition and emotions

increase. Awareness of these undercurrents would help us think more clearly about our moral responsibilities to animals.

From stem cell transplants to prosthetic limbs, to linear accelerators and radiotherapy cancer treatments, the range of veterinary services available to sick or disabled animals is continuously expanding. This is a good thing for animals and caregivers and veterinarians alike. Yet as we have seen in human medicine, the expansion of options is not an unalloyed good. More treatment options mean a greater need for healthcare providers to acquire strong communication skills for properly presenting them to caregivers. They also translate into more yes-or-no decisions that must be made by clients. It is much harder to decline an available treatment than not to have the treatment available in the first place. A deliberate "no" may feel like a failure, or the lack of love or caring. It is essential to remind ourselves - caregivers and healthcare providers alike - that saying no to a particular treatment is not saying no to care, and that declining a treatment is sometimes the most compassionate choice.

A greater range of treatment options - particularly those that are expensive and complex - also means that some people will be able to offer their animals a great deal, while others will not. As options expand, more and more pet owners will be forced to decline treatments that might benefit their animal.

In human medicine there is a threshold of care below which it is considered indecent to fall. Policy makers agree, for example, that basic life-saving treatments that are widely available and inexpensive such as antibiotics must ethically be provided to all patients, as must be adequate medication for pain. Currently, there is no "indecency line" for animals. Pet owners can choose to forego even antibiotics and pain pills for their ailing animals. Without broad-scale pet insurance, without some government subsidized care, and without laws enforcing basic standards of veterinary care, there is no safety net for animals. Disparities in access to care within veterinary medicine are not inherently unethical. Still, as a matter of fairness, all animals should have access to a decent minimum of care. How should a veterinarian respond when a client cannot afford to provide basic care? What does basic veterinary care mean in this context? How can the veterinarian determine what a client can or cannot afford? These are policy-level questions, but absent societal norms, each provider must make personal judgments about the limits of his or her ethical obligation to treat animals in need pro bono.

Ethical Business Practices

Hospice and palliative care should only be offered by qualified providers. The IAAHPC Certification Program for licensed veterinarians, veterinary nurses, and social workers, launched in 2016, sets the gold standard in terms of providing graduates with the most advanced skill set available to date in AHPC. Beyond IAAHPC certification, what exactly constitutes a qualified hospice provider remains somewhat ill-defined. The IAAHPC emphasizes that every animal hospice service must be medically directed by a licensed veterinarian. The veterinarian in charge should have advanced training in pain management and comfort care and well-developed euthanasia techniques. The AAHA/IAAHPC *Guidelines for End-of-Life Care* (Bishop et al. 2016) are concise, informative, and available online to any interested party at no charge.

It would be best from an ethical point of view if animal hospice providers would advertise their services clearly:

- Euthanasia services and hospice services are not equivalent, and a veterinarian who offers primarily in-home euthanasia cannot ethically advertise him or herself as a hospice care provider.
- The accessibility of services (e.g. business hours of providers, particularly if they are not available at night or on weekends) needs to be made clear before a therapeutic

relationship is formed between a veterinarian and caregiver.
- Providers also have an obligation to ensure, prior to the formation of a therapeutic relationship, that caregivers understand the financial and other resources hospice care may require and should feel reasonably confident that caregivers will be able to follow through with a plan of care.
- Veterinarians have a right to provide only those services with which they are morally and technically comfortable. They can set boundaries for clients, which must be clearly communicated to clients at the onset of veterinarian–patient–client relationships (for example, if a veterinarian or veterinary clinic adopted undestructive policies stating that no healthy animals will be killed, or if they believe that caring for animals until they die without euthanasia is unethical).

Providing these clarifications to prospective clients in writing is another way for animal hospice providers to accurately represent the specific type of AHPC services they provide.

Moral Stress, Decisional Regret, and Mental Health

Ethical struggles when making decisions at the end of an animal's life can have significant mental health consequences for the humans involved. Moral stress can be experienced both by veterinary professionals and by the human caregivers of companion animals.

Moral stress is a psychological state caused by an individual's uncertainty about his or her ability to fulfill moral obligations (Reynolds et al. 2012). Struggling with ethical dilemmas is the most common cause of poor psychological wellness in veterinary medicine, in the opinion of psychotherapist and compassion fatigue specialist Elizabeth Strand. (AVMA 2015) Preparation of veterinary teams for handling ethical dilemmas associated with caring for animals at the end of life is sorely lacking, leaving them vulnerable to moral stress and compassion fatigue.

Adrian et al. (Adrian and Stitt 2009; Adrian et al 2017) documented significant lasting psychological distress related to pet euthanasia in about 4% of the pet owners' in their study population. Multiplied by the number of pet owners in our society, these numbers represent numerous of people affected.

Much remains to be done and to be learned about the mental health impact of loss on pet owners, including the role of moral stress due to caregivers' decision-making responsibilities when caring for their animals at the end of life. How much of the grief, trauma, functional impairment, and psychological distress experienced by caregivers is rooted in moral stress, as opposed to, or complicated by the experience of loss? The evidence is yet to be collected. We hypothesize that moral distress concurrent with strong emotional bonds between caregivers and animals presents the highest risk to caregivers' mental health because it leads to decisional regret.

Decisional regret is the remorse or distress that human patients or caregivers may experience after making high-stakes health care decisions such as euthanasia. Many caregivers/pet owners report feeling tremendous guilt and anguish over the choices they made for an ill or aged animal companion. Decisional regret is exacerbated when caregivers feel that they rushed into or dragged their feet about a decision to euthanize or gave consent to futile treatment. In all these cases caregivers are left feeling that they have failed their beloved companion. These feelings can plague people for years and cause immense suffering.

To minimize the risk that caregivers will experience regret, they should be encouraged to take the time they need to make their decisions. In situations when a quick decision needs to be made, veterinarians can coach caregivers about the urgency of the decision at hand. In addition to time for reflection, veterinarians must offer caregivers options (there is *always* more than one!) and adequate information. Too little as well as too much information can lead to an increased sense of discomfort with a final decision. To minimize the risk of decisional regret, it is ideal to provide caregivers with information based on a Goldilocks approach: not too little, not too much, but just the right amount. Figuring out how much information is "just right" for each and every caregiver at a given moment in time is the challenge and art of end-of-life communication. Regret is also more likely after a decision based on partial or faulty information. "If I had known X, Y, or Z, I would not have made that decision." Given the inherent uncertainty associated with end-of-life decisions, it is no wonder decisional regret is as common after euthanasia as it is!

There are many ways in which veterinarians can ease the level of grief experienced by owners deciding to euthanize their companion animals. Soothing practices include: providing the owner both support and autonomy in the decision-making process, actively bonding over the deceased pet, validating the emotional struggle, providing support post procedure with follow-up calls, and being respectful of grieving customs (Clements et al. 2003; Davis et al. 2003; Hart et al. 1990; Shaw and Lagoni 2007). Not only does the conduct of veterinarians impact caregivers' level of grief, it can also have a direct impact on caregivers' decisional regret, which in turn, may intensify and complicate caregivers' grief.

Regret is not all bad. It is, in fact, an unavoidable part of our lives. Regret is what guides future decisions and helps us evolve into wiser people (Watson 2014). A path of least regrets is one that leaves room for learning from past experiences but avoids long-term anguish over unrealistic expectations, uncertainties, and ambiguities that were not within the decision-maker's power to resolve.

Conclusion: Finding the Path of Least Regrets

This chapter has attempted to give some structure to very nebulous material. An organized thought process allows us to put before ourselves as much information as we have, as full a picture as we can imagine of the burdens and benefits, possible outcomes, and values that are at stake. The best we can hope to achieve is a "path of least regrets." We say "*a*" path not "*the* path" because there are many permutations and possibilities in caring for animals at the end of life, and no single right answer. We say, "*least* regrets" not "*no* regrets," because the latter is simply not a realistic goal in the landscape of end-of-life decision-making.

References

Adrian, J.A. and Stitt, A. (2017) Pet loss, complicated grief, and post-traumatic stress disorder in Hawaii, *Anthrozoös*, 30: 123–133.

Adrian, J.A., Deliramich, A.N, and Frueh, B.C. (2009) Complicated grief and posttraumatic stress disorder in humans' response to the death of pets/animals. *Bulletin of the Menninger Clinic*, 73: 176–187.

American Veterinary Medical Association (AVMA) (2013) Principles of Veterinary Medical Ethics. https://www.avma.org/KB/Policies/Pages/Principles-of-Veterinary-Medical-Ethics-of-the-AVMA.aspx.

American Veterinary Medical Association (AVMA) (2015) Moral stress is a top trigger of veterinarians' compassion fatigue. Available at: https://www.avma.org/javma-news/2015-01-01/moral-stress-top-trigger-veterinarians-compassion-fatigue (Accessed March 2022).

Bishop, G., Cooney, K., Cox, S., et al. (2016) 2016 AAHA/IAAHPC end-of-life care guidelines. *J. of the Am. Anim. Hosp. Assoc.*, 52 (6): 341–356.

Carere, C. and D. Maestripieri (eds) (2013) Animal Personalities: Behavior, Physiology, and Evolution. Chicago: University of Chicago Press.

Cassell, E. (1982) The nature of suffering and the goals of medicine. *N. Engl. J. Med.*, 306: 639–645.

Chochinov, H.M., Tataryn, D., Clinch, J.J. et al. (1999) Will to live in the terminally ill. *The Lancet*, 354: 816–819.

Chochinov, H.M., Hack, T., Hassard, T. et al. (2005) Understanding the will to live in patients nearing death. *Psychosomat.*, 46: 7–10.

Clements, P.T. Benasutti, K.M., and Carmone, A. (2003) Support for bereaved owners of pets. *Perspect. Psychiat. Care*, 39: 49–54.

Coleman, P. (2006) Man['s best friend] does not live by bread alone: imposing a duty to provide veterinary care, *Ani. Law.*, 12 (7):7–37.

Danbury, T.C., Weeks, C.A., Chambers, J.P. et al. (2000) Self-selection of the analgesic drug carprofen by lame broiler chickens. *Vet. Rec.*, 146: 307–311.

Davis, H., Irwin P., Richardson, M. et al. (2003) When a pet dies: religious issues, euthanasia, and strategies for coping with bereavement. *Anthrozoös*, 16: 57–74.

Dawson, S. (2010) Compassionate communication, in Handbook of Veterinary Communication Skills (eds C. Gray and J. Moffett). Wiley-Blackwell.

Gill, M.J. (2019) The significance of suffering in organizations: understanding variation in workers' responses to multiple modes of control. *Acad. Manag. Rev.*, 44: 377–404.

Hankin, S. (2009) Making decisions about our Animals' health care: does it matter whether we are owners or guardians? *Stanford J. Anim. L. Policy*, 2: 1–51.

Harding, E., Paul, E. Mendl, M. (2004) Cognitive bias and affective state. *Nature*, 427: 312.

Hart, L.A. Hart, B.L., and Mader, B. (1990) Humane euthanasia and companion animal death: caring for the animal, the client, and the veterinarian. *J. Amer. Vet. Med. Assoc.*, 197: 1292–1299.

Hurn, S. and Badman-King, A. (2019) Care as an alternative to euthanasia? Reconceptualizing veterinary palliative and end-of-life care. *Med. Anthropol. Q.*, 33: 138–155.

Jonsen, A., Siegler, M., and Winslade, W. (2010) Clinical Ethics, 7 edn. New York: McGraw-Hill.

Kiley-Worthington, M. (2017) The mental homologies of mammals: towards an understanding of another mammals world view. *Animals (Basel)*, 7: 87.

McMillan, F. (2005) Mental Health and Well-Being in Animals. Oxford: Wiley-Blackwell.

Meier, E.A., Gallegos, J.V., Montross-Thomas, L.P. et al. (2016) Defining a good death (successful dying): literature review and a call for research and public dialogue. *Am. J. Geriatr. Psychiat.*, 24: 261–271.

Mendl, M., Burman, O.H.P., Parker R.M.A. et al. (2009) Cognitive bias as an indicator of animal emotion and welfare: emerging evidence and underlying mechanisms. *Appl. Ani. Behav. Sci.*, 118: 161–181. https://doi.org/10.1016/j.applanim.2009.02.023

Mendl, M., Burman, O.H., Paul, E.S. (2010) An integrative and functional framework for the study of animal emotion and mood *Proc. Biolog. Sci.*, 277: 2895–2904.

Mylopoulos, M. and Scardamalia, M. (2008) Doctors' perspectives on their innovations in daily practice: implications for knowledge building in health care. *Med. Educ.*, 42: 975–981.

O'Grady, L. and Jadad, A. (2010) Shifting from shared to collaborative decision making: a change in thinking and doing. *J. Participat. Med.*, 2: e13.

Parfit, D. (1984) Reasons and Persons, Oxford: Clarendon Press.

Paul, E.S. and Mendl, M.T. (2018) Animal emotion: descriptive and prescriptive definitions and their implications for a comparative perspective. *Appl. Ani. Behav. Sci.*, 205: 202–209.

Paul, E.S. et al. (2005) Measuring emotional processes in animals: the utility of a cognitive approach. *Neurosci. Biobehavior. Rev.*, 29: 469–491.

Persson, K., Selter, K., Neitzke, G. et al. (2020). Philosophy of a 'good death' in small animals and consequences for euthanasia in animal law and veterinary practice. *Animals (Basel)*, 10: 124.

Peter, L,J. (1982) Peter's Almanac, William Morrow & Co.

Pierce, J. (2012) The Last Walk: Reflections on our Pets at the Ends of their Lives. Chicago: University of Chicago Press.

Reynolds, S.J., Owens, B.P., and Rubenstein, A.L. (2012) Moral stress: considering the nature and effects of managerial moral uncertainty. *J. Bus. Ethics*, 106: 491–502.

Rowan, A.N., D'Silva, J.M., Duncan, I.J.H. et al. (2021) Animal sentience: history, science, and politics. *Animal Sent.*, 31 (1): https://www.wellbeingintlstudiesrepository.org/cgi/viewcontent.cgi?article=1697&context=animsent Available at: (Accessed October 2022).

Selter, F., Persson, K., Risse, J. et al. (2022) Dying like a dog: the convergence of concepts of a good death in human and veterinary medicine *medicine, Health. Care. Philos.*, 25: 73–86.

Shanan, A., August, K., Cooney, K. et al (2017) *Animal Hospice and Palliative Care Guidelines*. IAAHPC. Available at: https://iaahpc.org/wp-content/uploads/2020/10/IAAHPC-AHPC-GUIDELINESpdf.pdf (Accessed: May 2022).

Shaw, J.R. and Lagoni, L. (2007) End-of-life communication in veterinary medicine: delivering bad news and euthanasia decision making. *Vet. Clin. Small Anim.*, 37: 95–108.

Springer, S., Sandøe, P., Bøker Lund, T. et al. (2019) Patients' interests first, but . . . Austrian Veterinarians' attitudes to moral challenges in modern small animal practice. *Animals (Basel)*, 9: 241.

Villalobos, A.E. (2011) Quality-of-life assessment techniques for veterinarians. *Vet. Clin. Small Anim.*, 41: 519–529.

Watson, K. (2014) Reframing Regret. *J. Am. Med. Assoc.*, 311: 27–29.

Weary, D.M. (2014) What is suffering in animals? In: Dilemmas in Animal Welfare (eds. M.C. Appleby, D.M. Weary, and P. Sandøe), 188–202. Tucson, AZ: CAB International.

8

Supportive Relationships: Veterinarians and Animal Hospice Providers' Nonmedical Roles

Amir Shanan, DVM and Laurel Lagoni, MS

In the last few decades, the role of companion animals in the United States and other countries has evolved to that of a family member in most households. As animals near the end of life, families experience emotional turmoil similar in some ways to what caregivers of seriously ill or dying human patients experience. The experience of caregiving for seriously ill companion animals has been documented by recent research (See Chapters 25 and 26 in this volume for a detailed discussion of pet caregiving experience).

When their animals approach end-of-life (EOL) and when they die, caregivers expect to draw strength and look for guidance and leadership from veterinarians, and expect their feelings to be acknowledged with sincerity and respect. These expectations are separate and in addition to the expectations that veterinarians will provide competent and compassionate medical care for their animals. To fulfill these additional expectations veterinarians must invest time and energy in building supportive (also referred to as "helping") relationships with their clients.

Box 8.1 lists what is helpful and what is NOT helpful to do when helping caregivers during EOL care, loss, and grief.

There are good reasons why veterinarians and animal hospice providers should actively work to build supportive relationships with animal caregivers and be personally involved with them during EOL care, loss, and grief: doing so goes a long way to ensure caregiver satisfaction with the services provided because their needs and expectations have been more consistently and sensitively met. This is true regardless of the medical outcomes for the animal. Caregiver satisfaction, in turn, contributes to both veterinary job satisfaction and practice financial health. A classic survey of pet owners who stopped using the services of a veterinary practice showed that 68% of them did so due to the indifferent attitudes of one or more of the practice employees (Anonymous 1989).

While most veterinarians and other animal medical professionals choose their careers because they love animals and have deep concerns for animals' health and well-being, many are also compelled by caring about people and having a strong, internal need to be of service to them. This drive to serve humanity, while rarely discussed openly, is likely an important reason why caregivers' trust in veterinarians – and expectations of them – are high.

Being in a helping relationship of any kind often results in experiencing a "helper's high" – positive emotions following selfless service to others. Participants in a study

Hospice and Palliative Care for Companion Animals: Principles and Practice, Second Edition.
Edited by Amir Shanan, Jessica Pierce, and Tamara Shearer.
© 2023 John Wiley & Sons, Inc. Published 2023 by John Wiley & Sons, Inc.
Companion website: www.wiley.com/go/shanan/palliative

Box 8.1   What is Helpful and What is NOT helpful to do when Helping Caregivers.

It is NOT helpful to:

- Offer sympathy or cliches
- Compare one caregiver's struggle to another
- Shift the focus of conversation to yourself
- Attempt to divert caregivers' attention away from their struggle
- Attempt to cheer up grieving caregivers
- Discount caregivers' concerns, thoughts, and feelings
- Give advice, reinterpret, or try to change caregivers' beliefs
- Scold, lecture, give pep talks
- Encourage caregivers to medicate their emotional pain
- Encourage pet replacement

It is helpful to:

- Offer empathy and genuine feelings verbally and nonverbally
- Talk about and ask openly about the current struggles
- Encourage caregivers to talk and engage in emotional catharsis
- Encourage caregivers to slow their lives down and make time for their feelings
- Be there for caregivers, offer support, companionship and help with everyday tasks
- Acknowledge and validate caregivers' feelings
- Listen actively
- Be silent
- Help caregivers prepare and plan
- Reinforce caregivers' trust in their own problem-solving and decision-making

Source: Adapted from Lagoni et al. (1994).

---

conducted in the 1980s reported feeling better physically and emotionally when they helped other people on a regular and frequent basis. They reported increased energy levels, a reduction in symptoms of stress, a heightened sense of emotional well-being and calm, feelings of increased self-worth, and gains in such areas as happiness and optimism. Helpers also reported decreases in feelings of helplessness and depression (Luks 1993). Many animal hospice providers report deep satisfaction from their work, despite the fact that the medical outcome is almost always death. The sense of helping suffering animals and their suffering human caregivers often brings deep emotional satisfaction.

Finally, according to the Veterinarian's Oath, veterinarians are sworn to use their knowledge and skills "for the benefit of society" in several ways including "promotion of public health." Research suggests that social support is an important factor in human physical and mental health. Recognizing human emotional well-being as included in the definition of public

health makes establishing helping relationships with caregivers in need veterinarians' professional and ethical responsibility (Lagoni et al. 1994).

Lagoni et al. (1994) proposed a model that veterinarians can use to build helping relationships with clients/caregivers, that are beneficial both personally and professionally. Lagoni et al. labeled their model "Bond-Centered Practice" to describe veterinary practices that include in their mission "concurrently providing medical care for animal patients and emotional care for human clients" – an idea that also serves as a core principle of all animal hospice and palliative care (AHPC) services.

In the bond-centered model, it is the responsibility of veterinarians and animal hospice providers to learn to:

- Assess and respond to animal EOL-related human emotions
- Facilitate treatment decisions
- Prepare clients for their pets' deaths with or without euthanasia

- Normalize clients' feelings of grief
- Provide clients with short-term, direct support referrals to qualified human mental health professionals when deemed likely to be helpful

Box 8.2 lists caregivers' emotional needs related to the bond they share with their animals and ways in which these needs can be met within a "Bond-Centered Practice."

A study panel for the Pew National Veterinary Education Program wrote in a 1989 report entitled "Future Directions for Veterinary Medicine":

In the future, *the veterinarian will play an important role in bereavement* following the death of an animal companion.

Box 8.2

All veterinarians strive to be highly responsive to their patients' and clients' needs. However, due to the nature of their work, bond-centered pet hospice veterinarians are called upon more often to meet the needs of their clients.

A. Caregivers' Emotional Needs Related to the Bond

Veterinarians working in a Bond-Centered Practice support and respond to the emotional needs created by the bond. Some of these needs are for:

- trust
- personalized and focused attention
- information
- acknowledgement of the human-animal bond
- confidence in veterinary team's ability to identify and respond to sensitive issues
- validation of intuition, observations, and perceptions regarding the pet's health
- communication skills that sooth anxiety and fear
- a feeling of partnership during decision-making and treatment procedures
- direct honest communication
- access to veterinarian/Approachable and available staff
- referrals to specialists and related experts
- commitment to identify and work through differences
- skilled support during crises, pet loss, and emotionally vulnerable times
- empathy

B. Bond-Centered emotional needs are met by:

- demonstrating respect for the human-animal bond across the life span of the relationship
- working from a holistic perspective of care, viewing entire families as clients
- using interpersonal support skills to provide pro-active, preventative case management, particularly during crises and emotional situations
- creating a practice culture that is emotion-friendly
- committing to making trust and loyalty, behavior wellness, and pet loss and grief as much a priority as the delivery of high-quality medicine
- offering comprehensive patient and client care through a well-designed referral network
- implementing policies and plans that enhance self-awareness, self-esteem and client/staff well being
- committing to annual continuing education and training for key staff in interdisciplinary, nonmedical subject matter
- taking a leadership role in promoting the concept of Bond-Centered Practice
- regularly eliciting and listening to feedback from caregivers and staff; incorporating suggestions

Source: Adapted from Lagoni et al. (2001).

Veterinarians must learn to recognize and appreciate the importance of dealing effectively with client symptoms and signs of grief, anxiety, depression, and behaviors associated with the loss of a pet. They can be useful by helping a bereaved owner cope with his-[or]-her loss and identify those cases in which additional professional assistance is needed. . . The veterinarian's role in coping with bereavement plus the growing understanding of *the importance of companion animals to good mental health and wellbeing suggest that veterinarians might have a place in the structured social and mental health services of the country* (emphasis added) (Pritchard 1989, p. 35).

Defining the Nonmedical Roles of Veterinary Professionals and Other Animal Hospice Providers (except licensed mental health professionals)

In the book *The Human-Animal Bond and Grief*, the Lagoni, Butler and Hetts suggest that there are four specific roles veterinary professionals can add to their already established role of medical experts to effectively support caregivers' grief before, during, and after pet loss. These roles are:

- source of support
- educator (source of relevant information)
- facilitator
- resource and referral guide

Striving to stay within the boundaries of these roles helps to effectively teach caregivers about the normal emotions associated with pet caregiving burden and grief; assist them in their processes of decision-making; calm them during crises, and prepare them for the deaths of their companion animals. For caregivers and/or for the animal hospice and veterinary

professionals supporting them, it also minimizes the potential ethical, moral, or interpersonal concerns that come with role ambiguity. Serving in the four roles listed creates a delicate balance among supporting (primarily listening), educating (primarily talking), facilitating (primarily guiding), and referring (primarily suggesting). When this balance is achieved, caregivers are likely to feel that their emotional needs have been attended to and the bonds they share with their animals are duly respected.

The Role of Source of Support

Providing effective emotional care for distressed caregivers depends on the ability to establish trusting relationships with them that are truly caring and supportive. Supportive relationships are based on communicating respect for others and an awareness of the limits and boundaries of personal responsibility. Every person possesses the knowledge and skills needed to heal her or his own emotional wounds. Supporting others requires respecting their abilities to do so by giving them permission to express their emotions rather than making them (or yourself) feel responsible for changing them into "happier" thoughts and feelings. Trying to change or take away caregivers' feelings in order to "cheer them up" or "make them feel better" is not helpful, and it may sometimes aggravate a person's emotional pain. People have a right to their feelings, whether they seem justified or not. Lagoni et al. describe verbal as well as nonverbal communication techniques useful in supportive relationships in the book *The Human-Animal Bond and Grief* (Chapters 6 and 7, pp. 118–165). In addition, caregivers can be supported by expressions of empathy, which can be both verbal and/or nonverbal. Empathy means having an intellectual and emotional comprehension of another's condition without actually experiencing his or her feelings.

Empathy is not sympathy. Sympathy is "feeling sorry for" someone. Being the recipient of someone's pity is not helpful when dealing with strong feelings. Feeling like they are pitied by others often shames and embarrasses people and therefore counter-productive for their needs.

Many health care providers have been conditioned to feel that they aren't of much help unless they know the "right" thing to say or the "right" thing to do. However, lending support to hospice caregivers means listening to their nonmedical concerns *without* giving advice or taking action to solve their problems. It is not helpful for animal hospice providers to rush in with their personal advice and agendas regarding what caregivers should do to feel better. Caregivers need to feel, and they need to talk about their feelings in order to move forward in their loss-induced personal growth journey. Therefore, the comfort animal hospice providers can offer is most helpful when it is characterized by small gestures of support, along with an actively listening ear. Simply sitting with someone in silence may be more comforting than providing unwanted advice. Examples of nonverbal ways to offer support include holding a caregiver's hand while she talks about her pet, offering a tissue when she cries, and allowing one's own tears to fall when a patient dies. Verbal ways to offer support include acknowledging, normalizing, giving permission, asking open-ended questions, self-disclosure, and paraphrasing. Sending sympathy cards, making memorial donations in patients' names, or making keepsake paw prints when beloved pets die are also effective ways to offer caregivers emotional support.

The basic tenets of successful, supportive relationships are listed in Box 8.3.

Box 8.3   Basic Tenets of Helping Relationships.

1) Helpers realize that, in general, the person seeking help is in a less powerful position than the helper. Helpers always keep this in mind when they offer their services to others. Humility and wisdom on the part of the helper is required. Helpers approach clients democratically, with respect, dignity, and nonjudgmental attitudes.

2) Helpers and clients enter into helping relationships by mutual agreement. Helpers use the client's "model of the world" as their therapeutic context and allow clients to move at their own pace and to set their own goals and agendas.

3) Helpers abide by a code of ethics. They convey information according to ethical guidelines in honest and truthful ways. They realize that censoring or withholding information under the pretext of protecting clients is unethical and, ultimately, not helpful.

4) Helpers abide by a code of confidentiality and do not repeat the details of what clients tell them unless they have verbal or written permission from the client. With the exception of situations that involve "harm to self or others," they do not discuss their clients' names or identifying information. Confidentiality also extends to colleagues.

5) Helpers are never the focus of the experience. Helpers' roles, along with the boundaries of their helping relationships, are well-defined and clearly understood by both helpers and clients. Helpers know their limits and view their jobs as the equivalent of medical triage, where the goal is to stabilize people and refer them to the proper resources.

6) Helpers are responsible to their clients, not for their clients. Helpers ensure that they are physically, mentally, and emotionally present while they interact with clients but know how to detach themselves from their clients' case outcomes.

7) Helpers sincerely examine their own values, beliefs, attitudes, and experiences, especially those that relate to the persons with whom they are involved. Personal values, beliefs, attitudes, and experiences are reconciled, or if need be, set aside so as not to interfere with the development of effective helping relationships.

8) Helpers do not necessarily pursue credentials from formal, accredited counseling programs. They do, however, seek education and training from credentialed counseling professionals in subjects pertinent to the areas in which they plan to intervene.

9) Helpers seek feedback from qualified supervisors and knowledgeable peers regarding their helping styles and intervention skills. They also attend regularly scheduled case debriefing sessions during which they receive further guidance and stress management support.

Source: Adapted from Lagoni et al. (1994).

The Role of Educator

Educating clients about animal health in general and about specific diseases is an integral part of every practicing veterinarian's professional responsibilities. Providing information about the processes of death and dying, what to expect when one's animal is near the end of life, and about normal human emotions in the face of impending loss, on the other hand, requires an altogether different set of skills. These skills are essential to serving animal hospice clients because animal death is an inevitable part of both veterinary and animal hospice care. It is therefore imperative for animal hospice providers to educate themselves first about death and dying, the emotional burden of caregiving, and the emotions of loss and grief. They must also be knowledgeable and familiar with resources that caregivers can use to educate themselves about these sensitive topics.

Information about death and dying is not widely available in our society, and in addition, many people are not comfortable seeking that information. As a result, there are commonly held myths and misconceptions that confuse caregivers and further complicate the difficult decisions they have to make for their animals. It is widely believed that dying without euthanasia is frequently traumatic, that animals hide pain, that animals are better off euthanized before they suffer, that there is only one right time to euthanize an animal, and that euthanasia decisions can be reliably based on loss of physical functions such as food intake or mobility. None of those beliefs are based on scientific evidence or logic. Presenting information that replaces these beliefs with sound considerations during the hospice intake interview is tremendously helpful to the animals' caregivers.

There are also many informal opportunities to teach caregivers about death and dying, and about the human emotions associated with an animal's life coming to an end. During conversations, animal hospice providers can listen for caregivers to bring up the topic, or providers can be bold and ask caregivers about their thoughts and feelings on these topics. Then, when caregivers are ready and willing to receive it, offer bits of information that are timely and pertinent to their situations.

The Role of Facilitator

When their animals approach EOL, and when they die, caregivers face difficult decisions and frequently look for guidance from veterinarians and hospice team members. This is especially helpful when a caregiver feels "stuck," unable to make any progress toward making a decision, or when multiple stakeholders cannot agree with each other on what are the best next steps to undertake. When providing such guidance, veterinarians and hospice team members act as facilitators.

Facilitators ask questions, make suggestions, review pertinent medical information, attempt to gain consensus on decisions, and, in general, move interpersonal interactions along at a pace that is appropriate to the goals and time constraints of the situation. Facilitators remain neutral, nonjudgmental, and respectful of caregivers' individual wishes. Facilitators never "take charge" but provide just enough structure to prevent emotions from interfering with the tasks to be accomplished.

Veterinarians and hospice team members can go a step beyond facilitation and engage with caregivers in collaborative decision-making, in which participants create new knowledge through an ongoing, deliberative interaction of sharing information, ideas, and perspectives. In collaborative decision-making caregivers and clinicians learn from each other and recognize that a shared pool of knowledge will lead to more balanced and satisfactory decisions. With objectively right or wrong answers rarely available in the complexity of EOL realities, openness to new ideas is not a sign of lacking competence but exactly what the situation at hand demands.

The Role of Resource and Referral Guide

Resources are qualities, assets, people, or supplies that can be drawn on during times of need. The people and programs offering expertise in particular areas of loss and grief-related services certainly qualify as resources. These resources exist so that those in need can be directed or referred to them.

Guiding caregivers toward referral resources means leading or showing them the way. As a referral guide, you inform caregivers about available resources and sometimes make recommendations about resources most appropriate for them to contact. The general rule about making referrals is to give complete and thorough information about how to contact the resources recommended, but then let the caregivers do the leg work. The reasoning behind this rule is that the more invested they are, the more likely caregivers will be to engage in creating the outcome they desire.

Resources

When asked to identify the most important resource for their clients, most veterinarians say *they* are their clients' most important resource (Lagoni et al. 1994). While that answer may be true in terms of medical care, it is not true in terms of supporting caregivers' emotional struggles. When it comes to providing emotional support or guiding caregivers through the maze of decision-making and problem-solving that are part of AHPC, caregivers' most important resource is the *caregivers themselves* because after all no one else is more accessible or knows the situation better.

The next group of resources caregivers can draw on for support is family and friends. These people are the next most important and appropriate sources of help for caregivers because they are generally available night and day, during crises, and are usually personally committed to both the caregivers' and the affected animal's well-being.

A third group of resources caregivers can draw on for support consists of professionals they personally know. These might include a caregiver's therapist, doctor, or spiritual counselor. Hospice providers most often fit into this category, as well. Veterinarians have chosen a career in which they are considered a resource for resolution of any pet-related problem. They are most likely to be a trusted and useful resource when they have a preexisting relationship with caregivers, and even more so if they are available to their clients 24/7.

The final group of resources for caregivers to draw on for support is professionals and paraprofessionals, trained to establish "helping" relationships, whom they have no prior knowledge of or relationship with. Examples might include grief therapists, facilitators of pet loss support groups, crisis hotline volunteers, or suicide prevention counselors. These are usually only available during certain times.

Each category of available resources is useful during certain times and in its own way. It may be helpful to encourage caregivers to identify and use resources from each level as their needs change throughout their journey with their animals.

Extended Services

One of the hallmark characteristics of a bond-centered animal hospice team is that the care provided extends beyond the medical treatment of animals. To do this, a bond-centered animal hospice team should have a referral network in place. This referral network can be composed of professionals and paraprofessionals available locally, by phone, or virtually, and might include veterinary specialists, veterinary grief counselors, pet cemeteries and crematories, pet loss support groups, and vendors who provide pet memorial items and other pet loss-related businesses and organizations. Together, these services comprise a human–animal bond-related network and create a continuum of care for animal hospice caregivers. See Box 8.4 for extended resources to include and a sample form for organizing their contact information.

Limiting the Role of Animal Hospice Veterinary Professionals and Other Providers (except licensed mental health professionals)

When animal hospice patients near the end of their lives, both caregivers and hospice providers may feel stressed and vulnerable. Providers who genuinely care about their patients and clients can find themselves struggling to balance their own personal response to death with their professional role and identity. Caregivers can become confused about hospice providers' roles, too. When providers work hard to be supportive and to develop trust, rapport, and respect with caregivers, the boundaries of the relationships can be easily blurred.

Role ambiguity is correlated with higher levels of job tension, lower levels of job satisfaction and self-esteem, and depression (Kahn et al. 1964). In the preceding section we defined what roles animal hospice team members can play in terms of providing support for caregivers. It is equally important to clearly define what is *not* within the scope of animal hospice team members' professional roles when providing emotional support for caregivers.

Licensed mental health professionals have an important place in the AHPC team. Due to several reasons, it is not likely that every caregiver and family caring for an animal in hospice will be evaluated by a social worker or another mental health professional as part of the routine hospice intake protocol. These reasons may include the additional cost involved, social stigma ("something is really wrong with me if I'm talking to a counselor"), or simply the lack of availability of such professionals on the animal hospice team.

An evaluation of caregivers' needs, beliefs, and goals for their pet is an essential component of the intake protocol for animal hospice patients and their families. A psychosocial concern assessment is an important part of that evaluation (Shearer 2011, p. 510). For the foreseeable future, however, veterinary professionals (veterinarians and veterinary technicians) will be performing the vast majority of hospice caregivers' intake evaluations. A thorough understanding of the boundaries between veterinary professionals' nonmedical helping roles and the responsibilities of mental health professionals and spiritual counselors is critical to performing such

Box 8.4   Using a Referral Network to Create a Continuum of Care for Clients.

It's rarely possible for veterinarians to meet all their clients' emotional needs. Therefore, creating a strong client support referral network is helpful.

Ideally, referral resources are a balanced mix of local, regional, national, and online programs, services, and professionals. Referral resources should be thoroughly researched to assure they are credible, then entered onto a Referral Network form that is prominently posted in the practice, as well as easily accessed online. Annual updates should be done to keep contact information current.

A sample list of suggested resources related to pet loss and client grief follows:

Resource	Location	Contact person	Contact number
Pet loss counselor	Local		
Pet loss counselor	Online		
Support group	Local		
Support group	Online		
Memorials	Local		
Memorials	Online		
Pet cemetery	Local		
Pet crematory	Local		
Website for grief information	Online		
Grief therapist	Local		
Mental health professional	Local		
Minister	Local		
Priest	Local		
Rabbi	Local		
Spiritual counselor	Local		
Spiritual counselor	Online		
Veterinary chaplain	Local		
Veterinary chaplain	Online		
Crisis helpline	Local		
Crisis helpline	National		
Suicide prevention	Local		
Suicide prevention	National		
Police	Local		
Ambulance	Local		

evaluations effectively, and when communicating with caregivers throughout the hospice relationship.

According to the text *The Human-Animal Bond and Grief,* (Lagoni et al. 1994) while supporting caregivers' grief, the veterinarian or veterinary technician is *not* a:

- Psychiatrist, psychologist, social worker, or therapist.

    Most pet hospice veterinary professionals are compassionate people who want to help caregivers in any way possible. Due to this overwhelming desire to help and to be of service it may be tempting for them to try to "fix" or "resolve" caregivers' feelings of distress and grief. However, without advanced training in the principles of grief therapy, "fixing" often takes the form of problem-solving, advice-giving, rationalizing, or rescuing, none of which are helpful or appropriate when dealing with other peoples' emotions.

- Member of the clergy, chaplain

    Caregivers sometimes question their religious or spiritual beliefs as they face loss and grief. For example, they may feel their God or Higher Power has betrayed or abandoned them when their pets die. Others may discover or deepen a religious or spiritual belief due to their experience with death and grief. Some caregivers might even attempt to bargain with God (or with the animal hospice team!) in exchange for their pets' lives. For instance, they may promise to donate great sums of money to a veterinarian's favorite charity in return for a guarantee that their pets will recover. When pets die despite these heartfelt pleas, caregivers may be consumed with feelings of guilt, emptiness, and failure. Without their priests or ministers in attendance, they may turn to their veterinarians and animal hospice providers, asking for spiritual guidance or religious explanation.

    However, veterinary professionals are not trained to provide spiritual counseling and it is not part of their job. It is *far more supportive to refrain from religious instruction* and explanations and instead refer caregivers to their own ministers, priests, rabbis, or spiritual counselors. On the other hand, suggesting books they can read and websites they can visit for more specific information about pet loss and the afterlife of animals *is* appropriate and may be helpful (see a list of suggested resources at the end of this chapter).

- Suicide prevention counselor.

    Occasionally, caregivers hint at suicide or designate the end of their pets' lives as the end of their own. While it is very important to take these threats seriously, and to ask caregivers gently but honestly whether or not they are considering suicide, veterinary professionals' role in suicide prevention is extremely limited. Actual suicides due to pet loss are rare. However, in case of suicidal threats, it's imperative to know what to do. The animal hospice team *should know which local professionals to contact in case a potential or attempted suicide* needs to be reported or prevented. Suicide resource networks (hotlines, emergency clinics, therapists) should be diligently researched and frequently updated, with referral telephone numbers and other contact information available to the animal hospice team at all times.

Veterinary professionals should never make a pact or contract (e.g. "Promise to call me, day or night, if you think you're going to hurt yourself") with a potentially suicidal client. Professional ethics dictate keeping the boundaries between treating animals and treating humans clear. Trying to prevent a suicide attempt without the involvement of mental health professionals or police assistance indicates that this important boundary is being violated and the veterinary professional is overly involved. Veterinary professionals who provide skilled emotional support for caregivers often develop an extremely loving and loyal clientele. Once caregivers have experienced this quality of comfort and care, many of them think of their veterinary professionals as a friend and may naturally turn to them – as "friends" – for assistance with *other* problems in their lives, especially when those problems involve a personal medical issue or death. Such conversations can be intimate and emotional, and it may be difficult to set boundaries or limit the support offered.

However, it's important for veterinary professionals to take care of themselves, too! They must not lose track of the following basic client-support principle: the hospice team has a responsibility *to*, rather than *for,* caregivers (See Box 8.3). This principle helps to keep some perspective on the relationship and to recognize the boundaries of caregiver support responsibilities.

As stated earlier, veterinary professionals are not psychiatrists, psychologists, social workers, family therapists, members of the clergy, or suicide prevention counselors. These are professional roles that require years of study and experience. As members of an animal hospice team, veterinary professionals' job *is* to deal with the thoughts, feelings, behaviors, and issues associated with caring for and losing a beloved *pet* and their efforts should consistently be limited to addressing the issues that arise surrounding the *animal*.

Know Thyself, Healer

Providing supportive relationships does not begin and end with assessing *caregivers' needs* and making referrals. Animal hospice team members must also prepare *themselves* to deal with the rigors of facing loss on a daily basis. Before one can help others during grief, it can be helpful to develop an awareness of one's own loss-related issues. Personal experiences with grief can affect the way one interacts with clients. For example, discussions about death can be highly emotional and they can touch on

feelings about one's own past losses. They can also stimulate fear about one's own mortality and the potential for one's own loved ones to die. When animal hospice providers lack awareness of their own reactions to this subject matter, their efforts to help caregivers can be seriously compromised.

An awareness of one's own fears and anxieties about death, as well as an awareness of one's personal skills and strengths, can have positive effects on emotional work with caregivers. Awareness allows members of an animal hospice team to feel fear, doubt, and apprehension, but go ahead and intervene anyway. Such emotional risk-taking and the courage mustered when helping caregivers through a hard time often makes a significant difference in the experience of both the helper and the one being helped in dealing with loss and grief. When that happens, the work is often healing for both.

Conclusion

Providing clients with emotional comfort requires animal hospice providers to assume several supportive nonmedical roles. This chapter describes the basic tenets of these nonmedical roles within the context of a bond-centered hospice team's relationship with animal caregivers.

Bond-centered animal hospice teams represent an important element in the future of veterinary medicine. Their true effectiveness isn't only in their network of support-based services. Rather, it is their own daily work. Consistently offering caregivers comfort, respect and support infuses the basic principles of bond-centered care into the mainstream of the veterinary profession. In turn, the enriched quality of veterinarian-client care improves the image of veterinary medicine overall. Animal hospice veterinarians, veterinary technicians, and other team members can be sure that their willingness to care for patients, clients and for "the bond" that exists between them will have a significant impact on the future growth and development of veterinary medicine.

Grief Support Resources

This list represents a sampling of current, credible resources and continuing education programs of interest to animal hospice veterinarians and caregivers.

Memorials and Grief Support Resources

World by the Tail, Inc.
126 West Harvard Street, Suite 5
Fort Collins, CO 80525
www.veterinarywisdom.com

Up-to-date referral resources, veterinary client handouts, a Facebook pet parent group, and memorial products, like ClayPaws® paw print kits, for veterinary practice teams.

Counselors and Grief Support

Argus Institute
Colorado State University
James L. Voss Veterinary Teaching Hospital
300 West Drake, Fort Collins, Co 80 525
www.argusinstitute.colostate.edu

Clinical service providing client grief support and pet hospice program.

PetLoss.com
www.PetLoss.com

A well-known website offering grief education for pet parents, as well as a weekly candle ceremony in honor of pets who have died.

Grief Support Training

International Association of Animal Hospice and Palliative Care (IAAHPC)
www.iaahpc.org

Professional organization providing training and information for animal hospice and palliative care providers, as well as for caregivers.

Association for Pet Loss and Bereavement (APLB)
www.aplb.org

National organization providing training and "certification" for pet loss support counselors. The association's website offers information, counselor referrals, and online forums/support for pet owners. Also includes state directories for finding pet loss counselors and veterinary chaplains.

Center for Loss and Life Transition
www.centerforloss.com

Directed by bereavement expert Dr. Alan Wolfelt, the center offers a "Pet Loss Companioning" Certification Program, as well as books and information.

Institute for Healthcare Communication, Inc.
100 Great Plain RoadDanbury, CT 06811
www.healthcarecomm.org

A nationally accredited, not-for-profit organization that trains physicians and, in recent years, veterinarians throughout North America in effective communication skills. The veterinary communication training initiative is funded by a grant from Bayer Animal Health.

Association for Death Education and Counseling (ADEC)
9462 Brownsboro Road, #164
Louisville, KY 40241   USA
www.adec.org

A national membership association that provides certification and distance learning programs, as well as resources, information, and an annual conference.

Books for Caregivers

Barton, R.C. and Baron-Sorenson, J. (2007) *Pet Loss and Human Emotion: A Guide to Recovery*. New York, NY: Routledge.
Carmack, B.J. (2003) *Grieving the Death of a Pet*. Minneapolis, MN: Augsburg Fortress.

Davy, J. (2015) *Healing Circles: Grieving, Healing and Bonding with Our Animal Companions.* CreateSpace Independent Publishing.

Kowalski, G. (1991) *The Souls of Animals.* Walpole, NH: Stillpoint Publishing.

Kowalski, G. (1997) *Goodbye, Friend: Healing Wisdom for Anyone Who Has Ever Lost a Pet.* Walpole, NH: Stillpoint Publishing.

Nakaya, S.F. (2005) *Kindred Spirit, Kindred Care: Making Health Decisions on Behalf of Our Animal Companions.* Novato, CA: New World Library.

Books for Veterinarians

Cornell, K.K., Brandt, J.C., and Bonvicini, K.A. (eds.) (2007) *Veterinary clinics of North America: Effective communication in veterinary practice* (Vol. 37, No. 1). Philadelphia, PA: W.B. Saunders Co.

Durrance, D. and Lagoni, L. (2010) *Connecting with Clients: Practical Communication for 10 Common Situations.* Lakewood, CO: AAHA Press.

Lagoni, L. and Durrance, D. (2011) *Connecting with Grieving Clients: Supportive Communication for 14 Common Situations,* Lakewood, CO: AAHA Press.

Lagoni, L., Butler, C., and Hetts, S. (1994) *The Human-Animal Bond and Grief.* Philadelphia, PA: W.B. Saunders Co.

Odendaal, J. (2002) *Pets and Our Mental Health: The Why, the What, and the How.* New York, NY: Vantage Press.

References

Anonymous. (1989) Good communication keeps clients coming back. *DVM Manag. Consult. Rep.* 20: 1.

Kahn, R.L., Wolfe, D.M., Quinn, R.P. et al. (1964) Organizational Stress: Studies in Role Conflict and Ambiguity. New York, NY: Wiley.

Lagoni, L., Butler, C., and Hetts, S. (1994) The Human-Animal Bond and Grief. Philadelphia, PA: W.B. Saunders.

Lagoni, L., Morehead, D., Brannan, J. et al. (2001) Guidelines for Bond-Centered Practice. Fort Collins, CO: Argus Institute, Colorado State University.

Luks, A. (1993) The Healing Power of Doing Good. New York, NY: Ballantine Books.

Pritchard, W.R., ed., (1989) Future Directions of Veterinary Medicine. Pew National Veterinary Durham, NC: Education Program,.

Shearer, T. (2011) Pet hospice and palliative care protocols. *Vet. Clin. North Am. Small Anim. Pract.*, 41: 507–518.

9

Management and Administration: Business Models

Kathleen Cooney, DVM, CHPV, DACAW

While a blend of both philosophy and medicine, animal hospice remains a business. Businesses require products/services, management, profitability, and other components to keep them viable in the marketplace. By building a hospice service with strong foundations in profit plus compassion, and good leadership, the service has the makings to be successful and extend countless benefits to the community. There is no shortage of animal death in the world, only the lack of skill and business acumen to support it. This chapter seeks to increase awareness of animal hospice care business models and how to get started.

Guidelines for Animal Hospice and Palliative Care Practice

Providing quality hospice care, be it human or animal, is one of the most rewarding fields out there. It is complicated yet very feasible to achieve the results expected by the stakeholders: the caregiver, team, and patient. The team must be well organized and devoted to the mission of serving dying patients. Everyone must be held accountable for their work, advancing together in modern best practices. If a patient cannot be cared for in a timely manner by one, another must be called in to carry on or suffering may occur. A well-managed team has

outstanding communication among each other and caregivers. A background in human hospice is helpful for those providing animal hospice, but not necessary.

Passion for the work includes the desire to offer something special to the community, to go beyond traditional veterinary medicine into those often-sad spaces that few seek out. Being part of an animal hospice team is a calling for individuals who find fulfillment in the complete circle of life. The desire to serve can offset some of the inherent challenges with animal hospice, such as long hours, complicated cases, and the inevitable loss of life. Passion will not diminish the risk of compassion fatigue, and management will need to closely monitor for it.

Most animal hospice services are for-profit entities and as such, caregivers will need to fund the medical and emotional support their pet receives. In human hospice, the "Medicare Hospice Benefit" is designed to meet the financial needs of the dying and is closely monitored (DHHS 2020). Hospices have to keep records, perform assessments, and develop updated plans of care. In short, human hospice is managed with impressive detail, with financial resources provided for enrolled patients expected to survive up to six months. To date, animal hospice does not have an enrollment based on the projected time frame for natural death, nor does pet insurance cover every

Hospice and Palliative Care for Companion Animals: Principles and Practice, Second Edition.
Edited by Amir Shanan, Jessica Pierce, and Tamara Shearer.
© 2023 John Wiley & Sons, Inc. Published 2023 by John Wiley & Sons, Inc.
Companion website: www.wiley.com/go/shanan/palliative

conceivable medical, emotional, or respite type of care the patient may need. Care plans are very individual to the patient and caregiver and match the level of services the hospice team is set up to provide.

Patient care would no doubt improve with unlimited financial support provided by pet insurance, should that become the norm for dying animal patients. In a review of multiple pet insurance websites in 2021, all of them covered traditional medical procedures, treatments and diagnostics linked to disease in patients who hold coverage. Many reimburse for home/mobile visits and some for alternative therapies, plus euthanasia and even deceased pet aftercare. None were identified as covering respite care, social work services, dietary consulting, or grief support common in human hospice coverage (DHHS 2020). Perhaps in the future, animal hospice enrollment may be better defined and insurance available to cover all expected and unexpected care needs. In the meantime, animal hospice services must design care plans that are affordable and achievable.

The written guidelines that exist for animal hospice establish the framework for care required to minimize suffering and enhance quality of life. They appear by this author to be in line with human hospice, even though many of the strategies may not be in consistent use around the world. A large difference between the two is the use of collaborative or standing orders in human hospice (Conner 2009). These are given to nurses to facilitate ongoing hospice care without the requirement of a doctor to directly alter the plan in real time. Based on the presentation of such symptoms as diarrhea, pain, anxiety, and breathing difficulty, the nurse is authorized to adjust medications and therapies for quick comfort. This enhances patient relief, gives nurses more freedom, and reduces the pressure on doctors to respond quickly. In animal hospice, well-trained veterinary nurses should be capable of similar collaboration and trust by the veterinarians in charge of cases. The ability to see this through

will depend on state and federal veterinary practice laws, but the idea is very attractive and worth exploring in the coming years.

Service Delivery Models

To date, there are four basic animal hospice business models: veterinary-hospital based, mobile-practice based, animal hospice case manager guided, and hospice sanctuaries or rescues. The provision of care by an interdisciplinary team (IDT) is a central tenet in palliative care and hospice philosophy and therefore is necessary regardless of the model of care (see Chapter 3). Supervision by veterinarians with expertise in palliative and end-of-life care is paramount to ensure that the most effective, humane, and ethical medical treatments are provided to animals receiving hospice care. Goals can be defined by the animal caregivers in collaboration with the attending veterinarian. Participation of expert non-veterinary animal hospice team members is vital to adequately serve the complex needs of animal hospice patients and their caregivers.

Since this book's first edition in 2017, the business models listed here have become more streamlined and specialized and the animal hospice industry continues to evolve. Nevertheless, all four models still strive to maintain a bond-centered approach by keeping the caregiver–animal relationship in focus. Ethical and logistical considerations are made based on hospice and palliative care best practices. Each business model will have unique factors that may affect outcomes. For example, the veterinary-hospital model provides ample opportunities for diagnostics that can guide care. Mobile services are given a realistic view of home life that can help determine limitations to caregiving. Animal hospice sanctuaries with numerous volunteers to manage the often intense, daily physical, and emotional requirements of the dying patient may be better suited for hospice-supported natural death (HSND) than the average caregiver. For now,

---

Box 9.1   The five-step strategy for comprehensive palliative and hospice care.

1) Evaluation of the pet owner's needs, beliefs, and goals for the pet.
2) Education about the disease process.
3) Development of a personalized plan for the pet and pet owner.
4) Application of palliative or hospice care techniques.
5) Emotional support during the care process and after the death of the pet.

(Shearer 2011).

---

as animal hospice continues to take shape, we will watch and learn which models provide the most consistent, thorough support for the dying animal and which models are best suited to a caregiver and animal's individual needs. The aim is to ensure each animal is provided a comprehensive, personalized care plan following the Five-Step Strategy, developed by Dr. Tami Shearer (see Box 9.1), regardless of which model of care is used.

Model 9.1 Hospice in the Veterinary Hospital Setting

The plan of care begins when the veterinarian and caregiver feel the animal can be kept most comfortable through palliative care, and when curative efforts are no longer sought. Veterinarian and caregiver begin by discussing the animal's condition in the hospital during the initial assessment. As with any model, support may conclude after the assessment. Alternatively, the patient may be enrolled in a continuing plan of care. The caregiver is sent home with basic medications and recommendations for comfort care, plus educational resources to understand symptoms and applicable disease trajectory expectations. A communication schedule is outlined, and check-ins are often conducted through a trained staff member or veterinary nurse who relays information to the veterinarian so adjustments to

care can be made. A veterinarian can maintain all communication with the caregiver if they find it best for their patient, but the team approach is very useful.

One of the main benefits of hospital-based hospice programs are the resources they hold. They tend to maintain larger pharmacies than mobile-based services and are able to provide most if not all necessary medications with relative ease. Palliative medicines and therapies are regularly used in traditional hospitals with or without hospice departments, however those well suited to comorbidities commonly seen in hospice patients and those open to integrative medicine are likely to have more robust offerings.

Another benefit to this model is the built-in team who often work together: oncologists, surgeons, ultra-sonographers, veterinary social workers, etc., to diagnose and care for animal patients as well as the caregiver. Rechecks and diagnostics are typically done in the hospital, although if available, nurses and other support staff may travel to the home. Some hospitals provide a company vehicle, but if not, the staff commonly use their own.

As the field of animal hospice grows, so do the number of mobile services available to support patients, thus increasing the opportunity for hospitals to refer out care. If veterinary teams find themselves ill-equipped to manage any part of hospice, including euthanasia, it is advised to refer to those trained in end-of-life care. Each hospice service should have their own referral list outside of the hospital to call upon to help clients. If the euthanasia is to be conducted in the hospital, the setting is softened and prepared for the patient and caregiver (Figure 9.1).

Teamwork is essential to any animal hospice service. Those working through established animal hospitals commonly meet weekly to discuss cases and explore ways to improve palliative care services, pet loss support, and euthanasia. This intimate environment helps to reduce the sense of isolation sometimes felt by one-person mobile hospice units. In 2020,

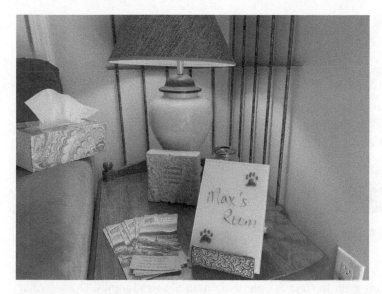

Figure 9.1   Personalized room for the patient. *Source:* Used with permission by Kathleen Cooney, DVM.

American Animal Hospital Association (AAHA) developed the world's first End-of-Life Accreditation Standards to complement their hospital accreditation program (AAHA 2020). Those gaining accreditation are called upon to improve patient monitoring, client education, palliative medicine support, communication, recordkeeping, and much more. The goal is to enhance team organization and patient care. This End-of-life Accreditation is eligible for AAHA-accredited hospitals as well as specialty mobile end-of-life services outlined in Model 9.2.

HSND rarely occurs in the hospital setting. If so, it usually occurs when an animal is brought in during a crisis event or dies unexpectedly. If an animal is expected to die within a relatively short amount of time, and the hospital team feels they can be safely transported, the caregiver and animal are usually encouraged to be at home. When this happens, hospice staff can go along for added support. In the event the animal cannot travel safely home without risk of extreme discomfort, hospitals may have designated "comfort rooms" where caregivers and animals can gather together. These spaces are designed to be a "home away from home" for patients and their families, setting a calm and

safe tone. If warranted, euthanasia can be offered either on site or at the home (home most commonly preferred).

Before or shortly after an animal dies at the hospital, the staff arranges aftercare with the local crematory or cemetery on behalf of the client (clients may choose to handle all arrangements independently). Hospice departments often work diligently to provide added respect when caring for the body. They may use body coolers instead of freezers or have the aftercare service come directly to the hospital to avoid lengthy hold times. Burial is another option when it can be achieved safely and within local, regional governing regulations. Hospitals may send home deceased animals in leak-proof containers (Figure 9.2).

Caregiver follow-up usually comes in the form of sympathy cards, phone calls, kind words when caregivers return to the hospital for ashes/memorial items if applicable, and during future visits with other pets. More and more hospital-based hospices are providing pet loss support groups and honoring ceremonies either immediately after the death of the pet or during other times of remembrance. Some caregivers develop long-standing relationships with veterinarians, nurses, social workers, and

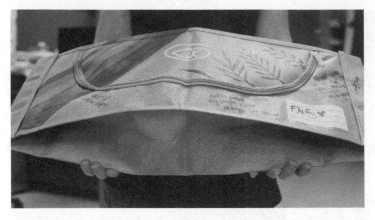

Figure 9.2 Respectful body bag for a pet traveling home for burial. *Source:* Used with permission by Kathleen Cooney, DVM.

other personnel, and wish to remain in close contact for years to come.

Model 9.2 Hospice with Specialized Mobile Veterinarians

Mobile hospice veterinarians often work alone or may have one or two support staff. To date, this is the most common type of veterinary hospice service available in most areas of the United States. Its great advantage is the low start-up cost, making it possible for any veterinarian passionate and knowledgeable about providing end-of-life services to start a business. To provide hospice services, the veterinarian working alone must build a network of relationships with veterinary nurses, grief counselors, pet care providers, specialists, and others to function as members of the hospice team. At times, however, the veterinarian must function as a "one-person IDT team" dedicating a considerable amount of time to tasks, and requiring aptitude in clinical, communication, and business skills. This model is ideal for veterinarians who find great interest in and derive satisfaction from both medical and nonmedical roles.

The initial phone call is commonly handled by the hospice veterinarian directly or by office personnel. Assessments take place only in the home setting where the patient can be seen in his or her natural surroundings. The veterinarian will go to the home for rechecks and modifications to the plan as needed throughout the hospice time frame. A mobile service robust enough to staff veterinary nurses can utilize them for many hospice-related needs. Depending on state/province/national regulations, nurses are capable of recording medical notes, demonstrating treatments, ordering prescriptions, and providing all manner of medical nursing support, with either direct or indirect supervision by a veterinarian (depending on state requirements). Ideally trained nurses are able to provide in-home care without the veterinarian being present In some cases, nurses can also perform euthanasia (AVMA 2019).

Diagnostics in the mobile setting are advancing, including the ability for radiography and mobile laboratories providing blood and other fluid analysis. Additional diagnostics are often available in the hospital but require an animal to leave the home. Many caregivers will forgo additional diagnostics to spare their animals from potential stress and discomfort associated with travel even though diagnostics give useful information to direct treatments. This means that the veterinary medical director of care needs, in such instances, to focus on managing symptoms rather than managing precise physiological/disease changes.

Because of the mobile nature of the work, it is common to carry a limited supply of drugs and medications. Mobile veterinarians often script out palliative medications to pharmacies, either local or national, or collaborate with the animal's primary veterinary care hospital to fill prescriptions. As with hospital-based hospice, the caregivers will provide almost all the care themselves including the administration of medications as needed. When beneficial, the hospice plan can direct support staff to serve up daily in-home care to reduce caregiver requirements, especially when animal patients are difficult to manage.

Mobile veterinarians are well suited to support families with both HSND and euthanasia in the home. Because natural death or a medical crisis can come at any time, many mobile hospice veterinarians offer 24/7 services or know who to call if they are unavailable. When death does come, mobile veterinarians typically transport the body to the crematory/cemetery themselves or instruct staff to pick up the deceased animal at the caregiver's home. Hospice veterinarians may offer to return the animal's ashes directly to the home or partner with the crematory to do so on their behalf. Mobile services are less suited to hold pet loss support groups but will often refer caregivers to those who can help in the community. Most other support is similar to the hospital setting.

As the field of animal hospice and palliative care grows, larger mobile services are being created to meet the demand. As of 2021, Caring Pathways, a mobile end-of-life veterinary service in Colorado (and the first AAHA End-of-life Accredited Service) has more than 40 team members composed of veterinarians, nurses, and other support staff, and the company is set to expand nationally to serve more communities. BluePearl Pet Hospice has blended both hospital and mobile models to leverage the best of both. Their comprehensive hospice services are fully integrated within BluePearl specialty hospitals, providing access to specialists, diagnostics, and often 24/7 accessibility while maintaining the majority of care in the home setting. Lap of Love Veterinary Hospice, a well-established mobile service, has many locations across the United States, with each one ranging in veterinary team size.

Model 9.3 Animal Hospice Case Managers

Case managers can be brought in to assist the primary hospice veterinarian or they are sought out by caregivers themselves. Case managers can be lay people trained in human hospice but more commonly are people with some veterinary training such as licensed veterinary technicians (nurses). The medical plan is developed by the primary veterinarian, also referred to as the medical director. The case manager may participate by facilitating communication between the veterinarian and the family. Once the hospice plan has been agreed upon by the family, the case manager is the one to maintain ongoing communication and report back to the veterinarian any changes they are seeing with the animal.

Medical care is typically carried out by the case manager if they hold veterinary medical licensure, or a veterinary nurse on the team, and includes basic nursing care, tracking of daily changes, and working closely with the caregiver to make sure everyone's needs are being met. The main challenge here is that case managers are reliant on the veterinarian to make changes to protocols when needed and are unable to prescribe medications if they do not have medical licensure to do so. This can be difficult when fast resolution to a medical issue is needed.

Case managers are ideally suited to help pets achieve HSND at home. They are already well connected with the caregiver(s) and tend to be willing to stay with them for long periods of time as the animal nears death. They tend to be very aware of the emotional and spiritual needs of everyone present. If euthanasia is elected, a veterinarian or licensed veterinary nurse will need to be called (laws on this vary state to state). Pet loss support and body care preparations are handled as in other models of care.

Model 9.4 Animal Hospice Sanctuaries/Rescues

There are a small number of free-standing animal hospice facilities around the country, all of which are self-designated because to date there are no specific state or federal legal classifications for "animal hospice facility." Ultimately, these are rescue organizations that focus their care on elderly and senior animals. Animals are typically obtained from shelters, other rescue groups, or are directly relinquished by owners who can no longer meet an animal's advanced medical needs. Financial support is obtained through donations and by direct payment from caregivers who "hire" the staff to provide a peaceful death for their pet. When managed properly, sanctuaries/rescues are operated similar to the case manager model.

Because the managers of these sanctuaries are essentially the legal guardians of the animals in their care, they are responsible for all decision making. A veterinarian, or team of veterinarians, will be called upon to establish the care plan, to make changes to the plan when necessary, and to facilitate euthanasia if needed. HSND is typically guided by trained sanctuary staff with veterinary support. Sanctuaries have staff of varying sizes to provide care, with outside hospice team members called upon to help. While the philosophy of care is entirely dependent on the hospice sanctuary operators, many appear to be oriented toward holistic and alternative medicine.

Practicalities of Starting an Animal Hospice Service

Many veterinarians and devoted support staff have taken the leap to start an animal hospice service. While the industry remains young, human hospice has provided a template to follow, and existing animal hospice guidelines/books like this one offer insight into what it takes to manage cases. Because all companion animals will someday die, there should be no shortage of patients to care for. What is unknown is how many caregivers will seek out hospice care for their pets. There are very few if any concrete death statistics on owned pets in the United States to tell us what kind of labor force is necessary to meet the demand.

Euthanasia remains the most common end-of-life procedure performed on animal hospice patients. Those wanting to start a hospice service will be expected to provide euthanasia regularly, even if they would prefer to furnish more palliative medicine and non-euthanasia-related support. This is because community awareness for what hospice offers is still lacking. It is common for caregivers to ask for euthanasia more than they do for other hospice services and do so on the day they want the procedure performed. This means it is often too late for the hospice service to implement medical support. As pet owners begin to learn about hospice, veterinary teams should have more opportunity to outline the benefits and assist with preplanning.

At present, anyone with a license to practice veterinary medicine can refer to themselves as a hospice provider, regardless of their training. Yet those who have sought advanced training in this area will be significantly better prepared to provide care to the dying. While there is still no veterinary specialty board certification in palliative medicine or hospice, there does exist a certification program through the International Association for Animal Hospice and Palliative Care (IAAHPC) designating veterinarians and technicians as trained hospice providers. In the AVMAs *End-of-Life Care Guidelines*, it recommends that where available, preference should be given to IAAHPC-certified veterinary end-of-life care services, and that referring a client for end-of-life care does not imply that excellent care is not being delivered by the referring veterinarian but provides an option for those clients specifically desiring more comprehensive end-of-life care (AVMA 2018). When starting a hospice service, it is advisable to be as knowledgeable as possible in the subject to meet the expectations of clients and to ensure ideal patient welfare.

Tips for starting an animal hospice service

- Learn the fundamentals of care, and continue learning
- Invest in equipment and business infrastructure
- Create handouts and materials for caregiver support
- Utilize cloud-based medical record systems
- Build awareness through marketing
- Find a company name that aligns with the mission
- Identify IDT members to service patients and caregivers

Regardless of the chosen business model, caregivers involved in animal hospice can be expected to have heightened emotions, evoked by the attachment and love they feel for their pets. Strong emotions can lead to periods of disconnect and difficulty focusing. Caregivers frequently absorb only parts of the information given to them by the hospice team. It is difficult to know who is fully "tuned in" to what is being said, and caregivers may forget details. Professionals should do everything in their power to give caregivers the tools they need to be successful, such as clear and concise directives and educational resources.

Every hospice and palliative care service should have proper forms and documentation to clearly define the plan of care (Box 9.2). Written protocols, policies, and educational material will help ensure caregivers have the following:

1) A good grasp of daily hospice protocols and expectations
2) An understanding of disease progression and natural decline
3) A clear outline of policies such as controlled substance management, communication requirements, and fee schedules
4) A well-defined overall plan to which the whole team can refer

Many services will use a hospice intake form to gather information pertinent to the "Five-Step Strategy for Comprehensive Palliative and

---

Box 9.2 Examples of forms to support hospice care.
1) Intake form: history, physical exam notes, caregiver goals, etc.
2) Legal consent for care form – signed
3) Zoonotic disease risk form – signed
4) Controlled substances agreement – signed
5) Information sheet on full services
6) Daily health calendar log sheet
7) Pain scales
8) Information on common medications used in hospice
9) Daily care instruction sheet – signed

Hospice Care" discussed early in at the beginning of this chapter and in Box 9.1. This plan takes into consideration caregiver psychosocial concerns, outlines medical care, lays the foundation for emotional support, and more. Outlining the team's communication plan is also a key tool and is best addressed with the caregiver during the initial assessment.

Informed consent is vitally important in hospice. Whether talking about medical care, euthanasia, or body care following the death of the animal, consent forms should clearly contain the following information:

1) Caregiver's information: name, address, phone, email
2) Animal's information: name, breed, age, weight, color
3) Reason for hospice care or euthanasia if chosen
4) After-death body care directives
5) Owner/agent signature
6) Cost of services and agreement to pay by the owner/agent
7) Date of service

Informed consent means the caregiver is informed and understands what animal hospice is, what services are being offered, and what alternative medical options exist (Box 9.3). Further detailed forms can include

Box 9.3   Example of informed consent wording for a legal contract of care.

This informed consent is for the hospice treatment of the animal listed here and for the support of the named caregivers. This caregiver(s) represents that she/he is the legal owner of said animal and is authorized to make all treatment decisions pertaining to the animal. The owner accepts sole responsibility for the payment of veterinary costs and expenses relating to treatment and care. Pursuant to the terms set forth below, and as may be added from time to time with the express consent of the owner(s), (service name) and all associated staff are authorized to provide veterinary care and treatment as described here. (Service name) is not responsible for damages or legal issues brought forth from contracted, independent pet care providers.

The owner/caregiver has been advised of the current disease processes and subsequent prognosis and has been provided with relevant information prudent to maintaining the strongest quality of life possible. It is understood that treatments are palliative in nature, not curative, and that any prescribed therapies may be modified as needed to prevent suffering by the animal. The owner acknowledges that the approximate costs, as well as the risks and benefits of each of the treatment options identified here, have been discussed. The owner also recognizes that further treatments may always be explored out of the range of care offered by (service name). Various outcomes have been discussed and options put forth for this animal and the owner is agreeing to perform said palliative care in the best interest of the animal faced with terminal or end-of-life conditions.

The owner has been advised of zoonotic disease risk, understands these risks, and by agreeing to this particular course of treatment, has hereby agreed to assume these risks. The (service name) staff is not held responsible for any injuries to the owner/caregiver, animal being treated, and other household pets resulting from the owner's rendering of medical care and treatment to the animal receiving care.

Whether treatment includes dispensation of controlled substances, all medications will be dispensed in strict accordance with the veterinarian's instructions. The (service name) staff must be consulted before disposing of any medications, especially those indicated as controlled substances. All sharps (needles, blades, etc.) should be placed in hard plastic (non-puncture) containers and turned over to a disposal service.

Owner acknowledges that because the care of the animal will be rendered at home, the (service name) staff will be limited in their ability to observe all symptoms, progress, and reactions to treatments and disease progression. The owner understands that a prompt update on the animal's condition helps to minimize suffering and a rapid decline of health. The owner does not hold (service name) responsible for any injuries arising from or relating to said treatments, including damage to private property. If necessary, (service name) staff members are authorized to provide home care for said animal in the absence of the owner/caregiver if they request.

Agent/Caregiver Signature   Date
   Agent/Caregiver Printed Name
Animal Hospice Representative   Date
   Representative Printed Name

diagnosis, prognosis, treatment options, and potential risks and benefits of those options, as well as an "assumption of risk." An assumption of risk means the caregiver has a clear description of specific warnings/risks, including what may happen if they fail to deliver adequate care.

In 2014, the US Congress passed the Veterinary Medicine Mobility Act, which allows veterinarians to carry controlled substances outside of their DEA registered address (H.R. 1528 – 113th Congress 2014). This legislation lifted the Controlled Substances Act prohibition on the transport of controlled drugs away from a registered address and was a huge victory for all mobile veterinary services, including those who focus solely on end-of-life care. Many controlled drugs are used for the management of pain, to aid in managing respiratory distress, for palliative sedation, euthanasia, and more. This change in controlled substance transport opened doors for advanced home care and will no doubt continue to help prevent and alleviate unnecessary animal suffering.

Controlled substances have been given a classification system or "schedules." Substances are placed in their respective schedules based on whether they have a currently accepted medical use in the United States, their relative abuse potential, and likelihood of causing dependence when abused (DEA 2016). The closer to zero the schedule number is, the more controlled the substance is. In 2021 for example, pure pentobarbital is a schedule II drug while lorazepam is a schedule IV. They both require tracking, but pentobarbital will require more rigorous tracking and additional paperwork because it is deemed a higher abuse risk.

Controlled Substance Handling Tips for Animal Hospice Services:

- Log drugs daily and reconcile them as often as the DEA recommends
- Reach for the least controlled drugs first, then more controlled as patient care mandates
- Keep drugs in safes and lockboxes until ready for use

- Label drugs properly at all times, sharing between other patients is not permitted
- Destroy unused drugs and record as such

Finding answers from the DEA to questions about controlled substances can be challenging. To aid practitioners, the AAHA provides tools for record keeping and information about storing and dispensing drugs. These are accessible to anyone and can be found on AAHAs website. All drugs, whether controlled or not, should be respected and the rules followed extremely closely to avoid fines and loss of licensure. As mentioned above, caregivers should be left with information about safe handling and use of all medications.

Telehealth as a Bridging Component for all Models

Telehealth is the use of telecommunication and digital technologies to deliver and enhance veterinary services, including health information, medical care, and veterinary and client education (AVMA 2021). Referred to commonly as virtual care, telehealth includes such categories as teleadvice, telemedicine, telemonitoring, and teleconsulting (Figure 9.3). Animal hospice has been utilizing components of telehealth since its inception, with necessity leading to a significant uptick in usage during the COVID-19 pandemic beginning in late 2019. The often-remote nature of animal hospice work is fertile ground for telehealth, and the ability for veterinary teams to guide caregivers via phone calls, electronic messaging, virtual appointments, and all digital communication platforms could diversify and improve animal hospice across all the models of care discussed in this chapter. Teleadvice, a category of telehealth, allows providers to offer generalized health information and guidance without an established veterinary-client-patient relationship (VCPR), which can be a huge benefit for caregivers unsure if their pet needs end-of-life assistance. A conversation opens up the door for improved care, then it can be followed

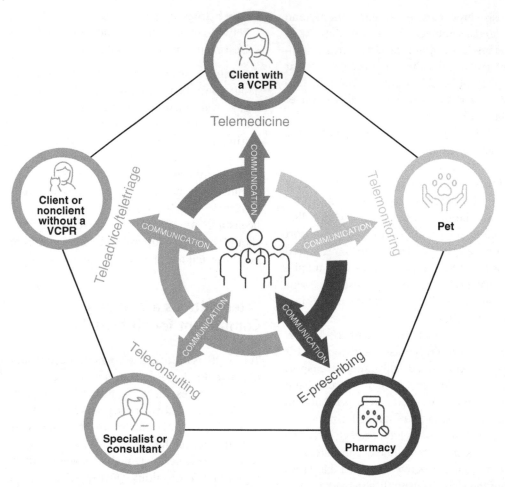

Figure 9.3 Components of telehealth in small-animal practice. *Source:* Reprinted with permission from the *2021 AAHA/AVMA Telehealth Guidelines for Small-Animal Practice.* Copyright © 2021 American Animal Hospital Association (aaha.org) and American Veterinary Medical Association (avma.org). All Rights Reserved.

by an in-person assessment to establish the VCPR, which in most states currently mandates an in-person physical exam.

Animal hospice and palliative medicine providers are able to monitor patient progress from outside the home setting, which can decrease the cost of care for clients. Telemedicine through video chat, wherein the team can visualize the patient, its environment, and treatments, increases the understanding of patient health compared to a simple phone call. Telemonitoring of patient health is now readily available thanks to wearable monitoring devices that can track physiological markers. This connectedness improves patient care and ultimately patient

welfare by avoiding suffering that may have gone undetected. Telehealth can be leveraged throughout the hospice care plan by the entire IDT. Groups such as the AVMA, AAHA, and Veterinary Virtual Care Association (VVCA) are developing guidelines for all veterinary industries to follow, and a purposeful continuation of telehealth is expected.

Conclusion

This is an important time in the animal hospice industry. Models of care continue to be developed that will provide ideal veterinary care, while maintaining career satisfaction for those delivering it. Veterinary teams are able to craft care plans that align with individual patient and caregiver needs, leveraging all available resources. Going forward, animal hospice will be well served with a broader understanding of human hospice models and business benchmarks for others to follow.

References

American Animal Hospital Association (AAHA). (2020) End-of-Life Accreditation Standards. Available at: https://www.aaha.org/accreditation--membership/specialty-accreditation/end-of-life-care-accreditation (Accessed: 18 July, 2021).

American Veterinary Medical Association (AVMA). (2018) End-of-Life Care Guidelines. Available at: https://www.avma.org/resources-tools/avma-policies/veterinary-end-life-care (Accessed: 30 August, 2021).

American Veterinary Medical Association (AVMA). (2019) Euthanasia Laws. https://www.avma.org/advocacy/state-local-issues/state-laws-governing-euthanasia (Accessed: 18 July, 2021).

AAHA/AVMA. (2021) AAHA/AVMA telehealth guidelines for small-animal practice. AAHA Guidelines. Available at: https://www.aaha.org/aaha-guidelines/telehealth-guidelines/telehealth-home (Accessed: 31 August, 2021).

Conner, S. (2009) Hospice and Palliative Care: The Essential Guide, 2 edn. New York, NY: Routledge.

Department of Health and Human Services (DHHS). (2020) Medicare Hospice Benefits. Baltimore, MA: Centers for Medicare and Medicaid Services, DHHS. Available at: https://www.medicare.gov/Pubs/pdf/02154-medicare-hospice-benefits.pdf (Accessed: 30 August, 2021).

H.R. 1528 – 113th Congress. (2014). Veterinary Mobility Practice Act of 2014. (2014, August 1). Congress.gov, Library of Congress. Available at: https://www.congress.gov/113/plaws/publ143/PLAW-113publ143.pdf (Accessed: 1 August, 2021).

Drug Enforcement Agency (DEA). (2016) Controlled Substance Schedules. Springfield, VA: Diversion Control Division, US Department of Justice. Available at: http://www.deadiversion.usdoj.gov/schedules/#define. (Accessed: 1 August, 2021).

Shearer, T.S. (2011). Pet hospice and palliative care protocols. *Vet. Clin. North Am. Small Anim. Pract.*, 41(3): 507–518. https://pubmed.ncbi.nlm.nih.gov/21601743/

Part II

Patient Care

10

Cancers in Dogs and Cats

Alice Villalobos, DVM, FNAP and Betsy Hershey, DVM, DACVIM (Oncology), CVA

Cancer is the leading cause of death in dogs and the third most common cause of death in cats. Dogs over 10 years are at 50% risk of dying from cancer. One in four dogs under age 10 years will die of cancer. Cats are at 33% risk of dying from cancer. Certain breeds are predisposed to various malignancies. Male Golden Retrievers over 90 pounds are at 67% risk while large females are at 57% risk. Boxers, Bernese Mountain Dogs, Flat Coated Retrievers and Portuguese Water Dogs are at greater risk for cancer than other breeds. Giant breed dogs are at a 60 times greater risk of developing bone cancer and Scottish Terriers are 19 times greater risk of bladder cancer than other dogs. Although hemangiosarcoma (HSA) only accounts for 7% of all canine tumors, German Shepherds, Golden Retrievers, Labrador Retrievers, Boxers, and Rottweilers are affected at 32.7%, 31.5%, 22%, 7.5%, and 6.9%, respectively (Withrow and Vail 2007; Villalobos and Kaplan 2007; Coto et al. 2013; Morrison 2002).

Cancer in companion animals is often diagnosed in its later stages and often at emergency clinics. Patients with advanced cancer are at greater risk for recurrence and metastases despite the best treatment. Cancer causes great heartbreak and sorrow for the pet's family members as their beloved pet declines toward the very end of life.

Cancer can cause illness due to paraneoplastic syndromes such as hypercalcemia of malignancy, cachexia, gastroduodenal ulceration, hemorrhage, coagulopathies, disseminated intravascular coagulopathy (DIC), hypoglycemia, and hypertrophic osteopathy (to name the most common).

Some cancer patients suffer acute issues. Unfortunately, "crisis oncology" may precipitate great emotional distress for the unprepared family if they are advised to euthanize their pet within minutes or hours of presentation for veterinary care. A typical scenario is a dog that presents at a veterinary primary care, emergency, or referral center facility after suddenly collapsing due to acute hemoabdomen secondary to HSA of the spleen or liver. The dog's family is often offered only two choices: "either operate now at great cost, despite an 89-day median survival post op, or euthanize now." This scenario represents veterinary failure to offer the third option: hospice and palliative care. If the family chooses to take their pet home for hospice care, they should be willing and required to sign an informed consent form (or medical record describing the situation) that releases the hospital from responsibility so that the patient can go home for comfort palliative care and/or hospice vigil. This option may give the family precious time to say farewell privately before they make the

Hospice and Palliative Care for Companion Animals: Principles and Practice, Second Edition.
Edited by Amir Shanan, Jessica Pierce, and Tamara Shearer.
© 2023 John Wiley & Sons, Inc. Published 2023 by John Wiley & Sons, Inc.
Companion website: www.wiley.com/go/shanan/palliative

final call for help with euthanasia, either at home or at their local veterinary hospital. Some dogs auto-resorb their red blood cells after a few days and may regain quality of life for some precious additional time with their loving family.

Approach to End-of-Life Cancer Patients

Greater expertise in palliative care cancer medicine and hospice care is urgently needed for pets enduring cancer at the end of life. It is frequently sought after by pet owners who want to safely address their pets' cancer, whether their pet is currently well but has been given a poor prognosis, is burdened with concurrent conditions, or is sick and gradually declining toward death. Animal hospice and palliative care offers a broader approach to caring for end of life cancer patients. This author (Villalobos) refers to animal hospice and palliative care as "Pawspice" (rhymes with hospice). Pawspice is not giving up. It is about embracing kinder, gentler cancer care and integrative palliative medicine when a sick pet or well pet is diagnosed with a life-limiting cancer and a poor prognosis. In "Pawspice," palliative care transitions to hospice when the pet declines toward death. The details of specific therapy for kinder and gentler palliative cancer are beyond the scope of this chapter, and readers are referred to other sources (Withrow and Vail 2007; Villalobos and Kaplan 2007; Coto et al. 2013; Morrison 2002). Cancer has many pathways that can be targeted with second-line treatment even for end-of life patients. A pathway that is common to almost all tumors is angiogenesis, which is the formation of new blood vessels that allow tumor growth. Other pathways that are being targeted for inhibition are the tyrosine kinase receptor pathway, major growth factor receptors, signaling pathways, drug resistance pathways, etc. Each of these pathways has a specific role in mitosis, angiogenesis, growth, vascular invasion, and metastases. Ideally, more than one pathway can be targeted simultaneously using combinatorial therapy. Metronomic chemotherapy (mCTx) is considered second line and is continuous low-dose chemotherapy given daily. These combinations may slow down, stabilize, reprogram, and slowly reduce cancer without causing adverse side effects (Veterinary Cancer Society Newsletter 2008).

When a cancer patient's end-of-life trajectory nears death, there is energy loss, weakness, functional failure, discomfort, pain, and finally active dying. Many veterinarians encounter cancer patients that are not yet ready to die, and they are asked to compassionately minister to these patients. Hospice care alleviates pain and helps patients escape the unnecessary ordeal of suffering to death. This chapter describes and offers tips on managing end-of-life patients with specific techniques and palliative cancer medicine that may slow down individual malignancies.

Tumors of the Skin and Soft Tissues

Mast cell tumors (MCT) are the most common fatal tumors of the skin in dogs. Release of histamine and vasoactive products from MCT may cause paraneoplastic gastroduodenal ulceration, hemorrhage, coagulopathies, and shock. Nonresectable and metastatic MCT can respond to combinations of prednisone and tyrosine kinase inhibitor drugs (toceranib, masitinib, imatinib) that can result in reduction of tumor burden and improved quality of life. A new intratumoral injectable treatment Stelfonta® (tigilanol tiglate) can achieve complete response in 75% of canine MCT with a single injection (De Ridder et al. 2021). This treatment has been effective in the definitive treatment of nonmetastatic canine MCT where surgical treatment is either not possible or would be aggressive and disfiguring (i.e. limb amputation).

Various types of sarcomas, carcinomas, and mammary tumors originate in the skin and soft tissues. The most common soft tissue sarcomas (STS) include MCT, fibrosarcomas, nerve sheath tumors, myxofibrosarcoma, liposarcomas, and malignant melanomas. The most common carcinomas include solar-induced squamous cell carcinoma (SCC) and mammary, anal, and apocrine gland adenocarcinomas.

These malignances may recur locally after initial surgery if surgical margins are not adequate. Most tend to metastasize to draining lymph nodes, especially the higher grade MCT, carcinomas, and malignant melanoma. Anal sac adenocarcinoma may cause difficult defecation and enlarged sublumbar lymph nodes, which may cause obstructions of the pelvic canal. Therefore, radiation therapy, chemotherapy, and novel therapies to control metastases are recommended.

Some STSs may grow into huge masses causing pain, ulceration, necrosis, dysfunction, and obstruction at the primary site. As the masses enlarge or metastasize, the pet's quality of life may drop precipitously. The approach for hospice doctors that would be most useful to take is to maximize pain control, provide wound care (instructing the client to put sugar on the wound and cover it with absorbent newborn baby diapers at least twice daily), control for infection, and complement the treatment plan with any other comfort care applicable. In addition, second-line palliative cancer medicine may be recommended using oral metronomic and antiangiogenesis therapies to slow down tumor growth. Those will be described later in this chapter.

Canine Lymphoma

Canine lymphosarcoma (LSA) most often appears as enlarged lymph nodes in middle-aged and older dogs; however, it may originate anywhere in the body, especially in the spleen and skin. Dogs are diagnosed via cytology and clinically staged. Most untreated LSA dogs die within three weeks to three months of diagnosis.

Prednisone palliates the lymphadenopathy but does not extend survival time.

LSA is most effectively treated with combination chemotherapy, using versions of the Modified Wisconsin Protocol, which yields an 87% remission rate and a 12–14-month survival. T-cell versus B-cell immunophenotyping using immunohistochemical stains on the cytology slides or polymerase chain reaction for antigen receptor rearrangement (PARR) testing is recommended at the time of diagnosis. Traditionally, B cell has been considered "better" and T cell as "terrible" with overall shorter survival times of 4–5.3 months. However, knowing the immunohistochemical results may improve treatment for T-cell patients, who may respond better to mitoxantrone, more alkylating agents such as melphalan, and to the mechlorethamine, vincristine, melphalan, and prednisone (MOMP) protocol. Personalized chemotherapy response prediction through Imprimed can help determine the most effective drug or drugs to treat an individual patient's lymphoma (see Precision medicine discussion below). When LSA dogs come out of remission, the induction protocol may be repeated or rescue protocols may be given (Back et al. 2015). Newer chemotherapy drugs are now available that can be beneficial in treatment of relapsed lymphoma including rabacfosadine (Tanovea®-CA1) and verdinexor (Laverdia™-CA1).

Development of effective immunotherapy for lymphoma has been challenging, and some of the products previously available such as Aratana T-cell and B-cell monoclonal antibodies (Tactress® and Blontress®) are no longer available due to lack of efficacy. Immunotherapy alone has not been effective at achieving remission or improving survival times for lymphoma but may help to improve remission and survival times when combined with chemotherapy. Autologous vaccine combined with cyclophosphamide, doxorubicin hydrochloride (hydroxydaunorubicin), vincristine (Oncovin) and prednisone (CHOP) chemotherapy has been shown to improve outcomes in B-cell lymphoma compared to chemotherapy alone (Marconato et al. 2019). The cost of immunotherapy can add significant additional expense to treatment.

Many families opt for chemotherapy, but many are not able to afford the standard best practice which may cost $7000–10000. Oncologists can recommend oral protocols that are less costly and may effectively palliate LSA dogs. A new oral twice weekly targeted chemotherapy called Laverdia-CA1 (verdinexor) has recently been conditionally approved by FDA for treatment of lymphoma in dogs. Laverdia-CA1 may be given with or without prednisone and may be used to treat both naïve and relapsed lymphoma. Overall response rate to single agent Laverdia-CA1 is 37% with T-cell lymphomas having a 71% response rate; however, duration of the response is short (18–34 days). (Sadowski et al. 2018). Laverdia-CA1 can be considered without prednisone to immediately start treatment in dogs waiting to see an oncologist without concern for inducing multidrug resistance to CHOP chemotherapy.

One of the most common challenges for oncologists is providing rescue treatments for recurrent and resistant LSA. The first remission from multicentric lymphadenopathy is generally the longest. The second remission is half the first remission and the third remission half of the second remission.

Most dogs and cats can live in hospice care with enlarged peripheral lymph nodes; however, if the tonsils or the hilar lymph nodes are greatly enlarged, then the patient has difficulty eating, exercising, breathing, and sleeping. If the sublumbar lymph nodes are greatly enlarged, then the patient has trouble defecating.

The hospice doctor may approach end-stage LSA dogs with a treatment that may give a response for a short time. The hospice doctor can administer palliative dexamethasone at $20\,mg/m^{-2}$ given intermuscular (IM) or subcutaneous (SQ) divided over two days and repeated weekly. This is a modification for the use of dexamethasone in a well-known rescue protocol used by C. Guillermo when he was at Ohio State University. The family should be instructed to give famotidine and other gastroprotectants and antibiotics at this time. Families are asked to monitor their dog's temperature and quality of life.

Head and Neck Cancer

Oropharyngeal and Neck Tumors in Dogs and Cats

In cats, oral tumors only account for 3% of all cancers, but are considered common in older cats. They are generally discovered in advanced stages. SCC is the most common feline orofacial cancer. This condition is painful, and cats should be entered into the Pawspice/hospice program at the time of diagnosis. The clinician should educate the family to consider esophageal feeding tube placement to help their cat maintain body weight and hydration and to administer palliative medication.

Selected cats with SCC and fibrosarcoma or osteosarcoma of the mandible and maxilla may be treated with surgical excision, a feeding tube and follow-up radiation therapy followed by chemotherapy. However, they remain at high risk for recurrence.

For families that decline surgery for their cat but wish to fight for more time, palliative radiation therapy may help. A combination of meloxicam with the bisphosphonate, zoledronic acid, has been reported to reduce bone invasion and inhibit tumor growth in mice (Martin et al. 2015). This author uses Fosamax at 10 mg twice weekly per os or by mouth (PO) or risedronate at one-quarter of a 150 mg tablet PO weekly along with meloxicam as a second-line treatment of feline bone invasive SCC. Great caution must be taken to instruct owners to provide at least 6–10 ml of water as a chaser so that the bisphosphonate passes through the esophagus and enters an empty stomach directly to avoid esophagitis.

In dogs, oral cancer is the fourth most common cancer overall, although it only comprises 6% of all canine cancers. It affects males 2.4

times more than females. Oral tumors in dogs generally appear in the mandible or maxilla as malignant melanoma, SCC, fibrosarcoma, osteosarcoma, acanthomatous epulides, and miscellaneous other types. Small size (<2 cm), no metastasis, and a more rostral location bodes the best prognosis. Because dogs open their mouths to pant, many of their oral tumors are discovered earlier than cats. Radiographs may show bony lysis and loosening of teeth. Magnetic resonance imaging/computed tomography (MRI/CT) allows improved treatment planning for the surgeon and radiation oncologist.

Definitive surgery with various indicated maxillectomies and mandibulectomies with adequate margins and follow-up radiation provides the most success for local control. Palliative radiation therapy may help reduce large inoperable lesions. Malignant melanoma has a high rate of recurrence after maxillectomy (48%) and mandibulectomy (22%) (Withrow and Vail 2007; Coto et al. 2013; Morrison 2002). Metastasis to regional lymph nodes and lungs occurs despite the use of the canine melanoma vaccine following definitive surgery and/or chemotherapy with only modest improvement in this author's experience (Villalobos). Toceranib phosphate (Palladia) has been effective in inducing durable partial or complete remission in dogs with oral SCC, but is not effective in cats with this oral cancer (Hershey, anecdotal experience).

Dogs with end-stage primary or recurrent oral cancer may bleed excessively. They may become anorectic and cry out when opening their mouth because invasive tumors affecting the bone can be very painful. The hospice veterinarian's approach should entail aggressive pain control, hemostasis (apply a corn starch paste on the mass and Yunnan Baiyao), nutrition, and hydration for as long as comfort can be maintained.

All pets with oropharyngeal cancer eventually develop dysphagia and weight loss from the inability to eat. Feeding tubes may help improve patients' comfort but may also cause choking and other discomfort.

Nasal Passage Cancer

Dogs with nasal tumors often have night stridor, facial deformity, pain, and epistaxis, and they may spray a bloody nasal discharge when they sneeze. Nasal tumors are often diagnosed late, after boney invasion of the turbinates and septum have occurred. Radiation therapy is recommended as the best standard therapy, but for many families and compromised dogs, it is not a feasible option due to financial and other reasons. Carboplatin administered at $300 \, \text{mg/m}^{-2}$ q21 days for six treatments has been very helpful in some cases. Toceranib phosphate (Palladia) has activity against nasal carcinoma as a primary agent and when combined with radiation therapy (Ehling et al. 2021). Toceranib has also been shown to reduce the clinical signs associated with nasal carcinoma (Merino-Gutierrez et al. 2021).

Patients experiencing pain may be palliated with nonsteroidal anti-inflammatory drugs (NSAIDS) and a protocol for using gabapentin, amantadine, and opioid. Many pets will sleep more comfortably and with less stridor if they receive evening sedation, for example butorphanol. Dogs who have trouble sleeping due to stridor and obstruction of the nasal passages by expanding tumor tissue can be taught to sleep holding a ball or bone that is big enough to keep their mouth open, which allows air to flow freely in and out of their trachea (as when awake).

Other cancer palliative treatments to be considered by the hospice veterinarian include combinatorial antiangiogenesis therapy, targeted therapy, and metronomic therapy, which may be of some benefit. Descriptions and doses are provided below.

Brain Tumors

Patients with brain tumors often experience seizures and/or tumor-related neurological deficits. The immediate standard diagnostic procedure suggested is MRI or CT scan to confirm the size, location, and operability of the mass. Neurologists have great surgical skills to offer eligible candidates, especially cats with operable meningioma. Radiation therapy, especially stereotactic radiation therapy, is considered the best adjuvant postoperatively. It is also considered the best standard treatment option to effectively treat all types of brain tumors in any location when surgery is not recommended (Winninger and Selting 2014).

Many pet owners cannot afford surgery or radiation therapy for pets who are suspected to have brain tumors. Clients may be properly advised by their local veterinarian or hospice doctor to waive the imaging if they do not have the money or the desire to follow up with definitive surgery and/or radiation therapy.

Breakthrough seizures may be controlled at home with confidence if the pet is owner is given instruction on how to administer injectable diazepam into the nasal passages via syringe or into the rectum via suppository, reducing the need for emergency visits.

If seizures cannot be controlled with oral antiseizure medications and steroids, 2–3 days with IV antiseizure drugs under the supervision of a neurologist may be successful. If the patient cannot be stabilized, then the hospice veterinarian must discuss euthanasia as the most effective way to prevent continued suffering.

High-percentage linoleic acid from safflower oil (currently available only from eSutras at www.eSutras.com) has been used by this author (Villalobos). A combinatorial protocol using steroids, metronomic lomustine at $3–4\,mg/m^{-2}$ daily, and eSutras linoleic acid at $3\,ml/kg^{-1}$ daily on three consecutive days a week along with seizure control, was shown to palliate and benefit some brain tumor patients in a clinical trial conducted by the author and colleagues (unpublished). Cats can't convert linoleic acid to linolenic acid. Cats with brain tumors may be palliated with oil of evening primrose capsules, which is linolenic acid. One 458-mg capsule twice daily along with the above combination may be of benefit for some cats, including previously operated cats with recurrent meningioma, in this author's experience (Iwamoto et al. 1992).

Cancer of the Skeletal System

Bone cancer occurs mainly in giant breed dogs, who are at 60 times greater risk than other dogs. It is rarely seen in cats. Most dogs who are treated for appendicular bone cancer are treated by amputation of the affected limb followed by four to six cycles of carboplatin chemotherapy. Without IV carboplatin chemotherapy given every 21 days for 4–6 treatments post amputation, most osteosarcoma dogs develop metastases to the lungs and other limbs within 4–6 months versus gaining 1-year survival rate of 50%. Chondrosarcoma dogs live longer. Dogs who are not amputated suffer from severe pain. Their pain can be palliated with multimodal pain control and with palliative radiation therapy. Families should be advised to purchase lifting harnesses, ramps, floor mats, and walking casts to help their three-legged dogs walk and to prevent pathological fractures in untreated dogs. The use of piroxicam at $0.3\,mg/kg^{-1}$ once daily for pain control yielded rare remissions on a sporadic basis due to its antiangiogenesis effect (Knapp 1991). Carprofen, deracoxib, meloxicam, and other NSAIDS may also be used for their role in COX-2 inhibition to help control pain and inflammation and angiogenesis, with caution about renal and hepatotoxicity, especially in debilitated dogs. The use of gabapentin and amantadine protocol with an optional opioid is very helpful in combination with an NSAID. The efficacy of tramadol and other synthetic opioids for the use in bone cancer pain control has been questioned. If used, higher doses and frequency of administration (given at least every eight hours) are recommended. The cautious use of full-strength mu-agonist opioids is more likely to alleviate severe pain. Trazadone may be helpful when anxiety is a significant concern for the osteosarcoma patient.

Abdominal Tumors

Hemangiosarcoma in Dogs

All but dermal HSA are very aggressive, infiltrative, metastatic, and fatal. One of every five Golden Retrievers dies of HSA in the United States (Glickman et al. 1999). It is prevalent in German Shepherd Dogs, Portuguese Water Dogs, and Boxers, but any breed may be affected. It is rare in cats. HAS may originate in the spleen (50%), right atrium (25%), and liver (5%) with 5% showing multiple visceral sites. Solar-induced dermal HSAs are not aggressive but should be treated with cryotherapy or laser ablation when small because some lesions may grow large and metastasize to visceral organs. Subcutaneous HSAs are not highly metastatic but may cause death due to extensive subcutaneous hemorrhage. HSA may cause thrombocytopenia, disseminated intravascular coagulopathy (DIC), and other coagulopathies.

Dogs with HSA may present in a state of collapse due to acute hemoabdomen. Some may develop arrhythmias, cardiac tamponade, and hemopericardium due to a right atrial HSA bleeding into the pericardial sac.

Palliative cancer medicine for a dog with HSA pre- and postoperatively should include Yunnan Baiyao, antiangiogenesis agents, pain management, and comfort care. Yunnan Baiyao helps control hemorrhage and has been shown to inhibit the growth of HSA cells. Some HSA dogs may be helped by an abdominal wrap that includes the hind limbs. The purpose of the wrap is to restrict abdominal distention. However, many clinicians are concerned that the wrap could slip and have a negative effect. The wrap should be carefully checked and removed after 12 hours. Most dog will die from HSAs aggressive recurrence and metastasis to the lungs. Its multifocal attacks on visceral organs may cause coagulopathies, hemorrhage, arrhythmias, and profound weakness.

Transitional Cell Carcinoma

Transitional cell carcinoma (TCC) is more common in dogs than cats. Scottish Terriers are 19–20 times more predisposed to developing TCC and even more so if they have been exposed to the commonly used weed killer 2,4-D. TCC patients may live many months to over a year on combination chemotherapy, and sometimes without treatment (Knapp 1991). Treatment with the combination of mitoxantrone with piroxicam has shown one year survival for 50% of patients. Vinblastine and metronomic chlorambucil are also effective treatment options for TCC. (Arnold et al. 2011; Schrempp et al. 2013). The efficacy of targeted chemotherapy drugs trametinib and lapatinib in combination is currently under evaluation and efficacy and duration of response appears to be similar to other protocols (Dr. Garrett Harvey, Fidocure, personal communication). Masitinib, toceranib, and metronomic therapy using Xeloda® in combination with piroxicam or meloxicam have been used by this author to sustain remissions (Villalobos).

If pollakuria and urine leakage does not regress, clients are encouraged to use diapers when the pet is in the house and to keep the pet's bed close to the doggie door. These precautions help the family to endure the house soiling problems resulting from their pet's stranguria and pollakuria.

Occasionally, hematuria can become severe enough to cause extreme blood loss. Measures to control the blood loss may include Yunnan Baiyao orally, a mix of 1% solution of formalin with a vial of the topical ear solution, Synotic® (Zoetis US, Parsippany, NJ), which contains DMSO (dimethyl sulphate), instilled into the bladder with a urinary catheter has been used, but no studies have been done to confirm efficacy. The mixture remains in the bladder for

10–15 minutes and then removed through the catheter. This may reduce the hematuria for 7–10 days, and it may be repeated as needed.

In some patients, TCC tumors at the trigone area obstruct urine outflow. These patients may benefit from a prepubic cystostomy as a palliative procedure. Pet owners are instructed to void the patient's bladder four times a day to maintain a quality of life for the pet. The skillful placement of urethral stents offers TCC patients another potentially lifesaving option. Although stents are costly and not always guaranteed to work, they may extend the patient's life with welcome satisfaction.

When bladder cancer patients decline toward death, they may develop hydronephrosis or become unable to void urine. Ureteral stenting may be considered in those patients with hydronephrosis. The metastatic component of TCC may cause abdominal and back pain, constipation, and neurological disability.

Hepatic, Pancreatic, Intestinal, Adrenal, and Renal Cancer

Most dogs and cats with abdominal tumors share a similar trajectory. Exploratory surgery may be helpful if the tumors are operable. However, the patients are at risk for recurrence. The hospice doctor can approach the patient to control ascites and to control serosal pain caused by capsule distension of the affected abdominal organs. Frequent small meals with soft food and broth are recommended so as not to distend the stomach. The hospice team members may show the family how to massage their pet and help keep up pleasurable moments during their final decline. The recent availability of targeted chemotherapy drugs such as toceranib, sorafenib, trametinib, rapamycin, lapatinib, and others has improved management of these cancers. These oral targeted drugs are well-tolerated and cost effective and can improve clinical symptoms of the cancer as well as slow cancer growth and prolong survival time.

Chest Cavity Tumors

The metastatic process frequently transports cancer cells from primary locations (tissue of origin) into the microvasculature of the pulmonary parenchyma. Lymphomas may involve the hilar and sternal lymph nodes and occasionally appear as a granular infiltrate and rarely as masses in the lungs. Symptoms such as coughing, shortness of breath or labored breathing, and pulmonary effusion may be the first clinical warning signs of a cancer that has metastasized. Primary carcinomas of the chest cavity are uncommon in dogs and cats. Tumors that originate in the thymus may be lymphoma or thymoma. Heart base tumors and HSA of the right atrium may appear in older dogs.

The hospice team approach would be to alleviate respiratory distress by draining pulmonary effusions as needed, using bronchodilators, antihistamines, and supporting oxygen intake. Oxygen support can be given at home with the use of oxygen concentrators that can be purchased or rented. A make-shift oxygen tent can be made with a plastic kennel. The animal is placed in the kennel with a sheet over the openings and oxygen flow to the patient of $4–5 \, 1 \, min^{-1}$. The temperature and humidity of the kennel should be monitored closely. The animal can be placed in the oxygen tent several times per day or in times of respiratory distress. However, if the patient is suffering significant oxygen starvation, nothing else matters as life is not worth living. The Pawspice approach would be to provide palliative cancer medicine if the patient's breathing can be restored to a comfortable level. Such was the situation for Comet Rome, who became acutely dyspneic and was diagnosed with pulmonary carcinoma after he developed pulmonary effusion. The mass occupied most of Comet's thorax (Figure 10.1). Surprisingly, Comet survived over three years from his initial acute dyspneic episode on mCTx and masitinib at 50 mg s.i.d. (Figure 10.2).

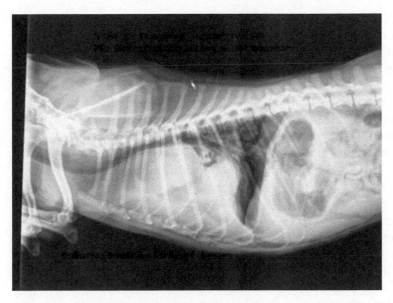

Figure 10.1 Chest X-ray 2-2-2015 after thoraocentesis. Comet Rome, a 10.6 year-old Chihuahua mix. Mass displacing trachea and heart. Despite a poor prognosis of 3–6 months, he responded to palliative care for over 22 months.

Palliative Cancer Medicine

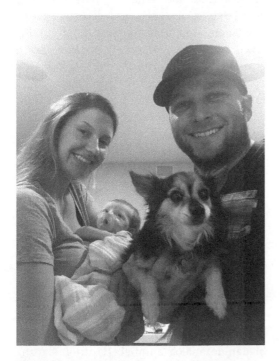

Figure 10.2 Comet Rome shown here at 22 months past diagnosis with a good quality of life. He attended his caregiver's wedding and welcomed a new baby girl into the family.

Most animal cancer patients who undergo first-line surgery or chemotherapy or radiation therapy are considered to be at moderate to great risk for recurrence of their cancers. Although they are not yet in decline, these patients are candidates for palliative "Pawspice" care that addresses the threat of recurrent cancer with kinder, gentler palliative cancer medicine. These animals qualify for Pawspice because over 50% of them experience recurrence or die from metastases of their malignant disease within less than 12 months. This sad situation is especially vivid for post-amputation osteosarcoma dogs, postsplenectomy HSA dogs, and cats following mastectomy for mammary carcinoma. Dog with untreated osteosarcoma, HSA, adenocarcinoma, and lymphoma and cats with mammary cancer, feline injection site sarcoma (FISS), and lymphoma, all face "the reality of mortality" as Atul Gawande describes in his insightful and timely book, *Being Mortal: Medicine and What*

Matters in the End (Gawande 2013). In addition, many cancer patients have comorbidities such as arthritis, degenerative myelopathy, diabetes, heart disease, and kidney disease, and up to 3% may have synchronous primary tumors (Marcello et al. 2015). It is not unusual for comorbidities to be multiple in the same cancer patients. Each comorbidity competes for attention and may result in an early death for the cancer patient.

Nutritional advice and a supplement program that supports the immune system may benefit pets who have been treated with first-line therapies, pets who are untreated, or pets who are terminally ill. Providing supplements that are proven to support the immune system addresses the cancer, and it may be professionally and sensibly supervised as palliative management. Chemoprevention is also being accepted as a palliative approach for cancer patients. An integrative approach including acupuncture, massage therapy, and many other treatment modalities creates further client confidence that the end-of-life care veterinarian is helping to address their cancer patient's pain, failing immune system, nutritional status, and organ function as much as possible.

Companion animals of any health status who are diagnosed with life-limiting cancer or are at high risk for recurrence may benefit when treated with second-line palliative therapies. These patients may experience fewer adverse events and reduced risk of infections compared to first-line standard treatment. As a result, they enjoy enhanced quality of life during palliative and hospice care and some experience improved survival time as well. Second-line palliative therapies utilize a combinatorial or multimodality approach with medications and supplements in the categories described below.

Antiangiogenesis Therapy Tyrosine kinase inhibitors such as toceranib (Palladia®) can be used at 2.5–2.75 mg every other day or Monday, Wednesday, and Friday and masitinib (Kinavet -CA1) at 12.5 mg/kg^{-1} s.i.d. Several other agents that are used for mCTx at low doses, listed below, also have antiangiogenic action. Patients on tyrosine kinase inhibitors must be monitored with bloodwork to check complete blood cell count (CBC) and serum chemistries as well as periodic urinalysis and/or urine protein creatine ratio. This author (Villalobos) uses AngioStop® (from sea cucumber) at one capsule per 60 lbs body weight b.i.d. with asparagus extract at one capsule per 60 lbs body weight b.i.d. and Revivin® at one capsule per 60 lbs body weight s.i.d. This combination has also been shown to have tyrosine kinase and telomerase inhibition and also increases apoptosis. This author (Villalobos) has been very impressed with the effectiveness of combinatorial therapy that includes the multimodality effect of these agents.

mCTx This has no intent to cure and will not induce remissions or make solid tumors shrink. Hospice team members can educate clients to appreciate the value of pursuing more achievable goals such as attaining partial remissions, stabilizing the disease, or slowing down the progression of disease (Leach et al. 2012). Typical drugs used in mCTx that are documented to have antiangiogenic mechanisms of action and immune modulation to boost antitumor activity include cyclophosphamide at 10 mg/m^2/day, chlorambucil at 4 mg/m^2/day (Leach et al. 2012), and lomustine at 4 mg/m^2/day (Mutsaers and Henry 2014). This author (Villalobos) has had success with low-dose Xeloda® (capecitabine) (Zoetis, Parsippany, NJ) (never use if for cats) at 250 mg/m^2/day for canine carcinomas. CBC, urine output, and liver enzymes should be monitored.

Chemoprevention NSAIDS such as piroxicam, meloxicam, carprofen, and others can be used for their chemopreventative actions but should be given with gastroprotectants. This author (Villalobos) uses metformin, a biguanide analog antidiabetic drug, starting at a quarter of the final dose with a gradual dose escalation to 500 mg per 60 lbs body weight b.i.d. Metformin has been shown to target cancer energetics in a subtle way. It reduces levels of hormones that can stimulate cell growth, including insulin. It also reduces the multidrug resistance genes in canine lymphoma and allows human lymphoma patients to live longer. Some patients develop gastrointestinal (GI) disturbances when receiving metformin at escalated doses; however, the drug offers potential chemoprevention benefit for those patients that can tolerate it (McDonald et al. 2014). Numerous other agents that are being studied for their chemopreventive actions such as loperamide, green tea extracts, vitamin D, bisphosphonates, chlorpromazine, pentamidine, and others. Additionally, drug repurposing, i.e. identifying new uses for approved or investigational drugs outside of the original medical indication, can offer new options for therapy. One example of this is the use of fenbendazole (Panacur), an antihelmentic that has been shown to induce apoptosis of cancer cells (Son et al. 2020).

Targeted Therapy Immunotherapy and gene therapy have been developed to target certain antigens and signaling pathways that mediate mutations, mitosis, angiogenesis, diapedesis, metastases, cytokine production, telomerase activation, and apoptosis activity. This author (Villalobos) uses T-cyte (T-cyte Therapeutic, Murrieta, CA), which stimulates T cells and related cytokine production. Cancer vaccines are being developed to target and B- and T- cell lymphoma and osteosarcoma, with more on the way. New tyrosine kinase and other major pathway inhibitors are being developed. The use of toceranib at 2.5–2.75 mg/kg^{-1} every other day or on a Monday, Wednesday, and Friday schedule and masitinib at 12.5 mg/kg^{-1} s.i.d. are considered targeted therapy as well as antiangiogenesis therapy, as described above. Another example of targeted therapy would be the use of low-dose demethylation agents that may reprogram tumor cells epigenetically to revert to a less tumorigenic state. These agents may induce fewer adverse events and may be useful in combinatorial protocols to palliate advanced cancer patients who are treatable.

Autologous Cancer Vaccines: Autologous cancer vaccines are now available through both Torigen Pharmaceuticals and Ardent Animal Health. These vaccines are derived from the patient's own cancer cells, which are obtained at the time of surgical removal of the tumor or via incisional biopsy. The tumor cells are treated in a way that makes them a target for the immune system. They are then injected into the patient where immune cells can recognize them and then potentially destroy any remaining tumor cells in the body. The vaccines can be combined with other therapy modalities and are commonly used postsurgically in combination with chemotherapy to reduce the risk of cancer recurrence and/or metastases. The vaccines are safe with minimal to no side effects and cost effective. A small pilot study of autologous cancer vaccine in canine splenic HSA showed survival times similar to standard of care chemotherapy without any observed adverse events (Lucroy et al. 2020).

Precision, Personalized or Individualize Medicine: Precision oncology is an approach to cancer therapy that tailors the treatment based on the patient's genetic tumor profile to identify mutations or alterations that can be targeted with drug therapy. Through tests offered by One Health Company (FidoCure) and Vidium Animal Health, it is now possible to obtain information on genetic changes in a canine tumor. This information can then be used to prescribe "targeted" drugs that block or turn off signals that make cancer cells grow and/or metastasize. Many of these targeted drugs are now routinely available to veterinary patients through compounding, and additional drugs are becoming available as clinical trials are completed to evaluate safety and dosing in the dog. Targeted drugs in this author's experience (Hershey) have few side effects and have been beneficial in reducing tumor burden or slowing the progression of disease and improving survival. Imprimed offers personalized medicine for canine lymphoma, analyzing Flow Cytometry, PARR analysis, and chemotherapy drug sensitivity to predict the most effective treatment for individual patients.

Immunonutrition Supplements that have known efficacy to enhance immune modulation include OncoSupport by Rx Vitamins for Pets, which contains vitamins A, E, and D, along with other vital nutrients. The Agaricus mushroom stimulates macrophage activity, which counters the immunosuppression caused by steroid therapy. Agaricus Bio (Atlas World, Pasadena, CA) is dosed at 600–1200 mg per 60 lbs body weight b.i.d. (available at www.atlasworldusa.com). Agaricus also has anticancer effects by stimulating natural killer (NK) cells and antidiabetic effects by reducing adiponectin (Borchers et al. 1999; Borchers et al. 2004). Inositol hexaphosphate (IP6) at one capsule per 15–20 lbs twice daily on an empty stomach is rapidly taken up into cells and dephosphorylated to lower inositol phosphates, further affecting signal transduction pathways resulting in cell cycle arrest. A striking anticancer action of IP6 was demonstrated in different experimental models. In addition to reducing cell proliferation, IP6 also induces differentiation of malignant cells. Enhanced immunity and antioxidant properties also contribute to tumor cell destruction (Vucenik and Shamsuddin 2006). Platinum Performance Plus (Platinum Performance, Buellton, CA) for dogs and Feline Platinum Performance for cats contain almost 40 agents that are restorative to the body. Additional information on complementary and alternative therapies for the cancer patient can be found in Chapter 11.

Advances in Noninvasive Technology for the Diagnosis of Cancer

Obtaining a definitive cancer diagnosis can be challenging in some patients. For some cancers such as intestinal lymphoma, definitive diagnosis via tissue sample requires surgical or endoscopic biopsies. Surgical and endoscopic biopsies that require general anesthesia can pose increased risk for the sick cancer patient and can be costly for the client. Not every client will have the financial means to pursue these diagnostic tests. For other cancers, such as urogenital cancers, percutaneous needle biopsy risks the seeding of tumor cells along the needle biopsy track. The recent development of noninvasive diagnostic tests for the diagnosis of cancer offers a simple, safe, and cost effective modality for diagnosis and monitoring of certain cancers.

BRAF and Braf Plus Mutation test: The majority of canine TCC harbor a mutation in the Braf Gene. The Braf and braf mutation test is performed on a free-catch urine sample for diagnosis of transitional cell and urothelial cell carcinomas (TCC/UC) in dogs and can identify 95% of these tumors. This test can be used to diagnosis patients with clinical symptoms or confirm ultrasound findings consistent with TCC/UC as well as to monitor response to treatment or relapse/progression following treatment.

VDI TK1 tests: Veterinary Diagnostic Institute offers a blood test panel for both cats and dogs that detects biomarkers in the blood that are often elevated in cancer: thymidine kinase and C-reactive protein (dogs) and thymidine kinase and haptoglobin (cats). These panels have been validated in lymphoma (dogs and cats) and HSA (dogs) and are most helpful in differentiating between lymphoma and inflammatory bowel disease in both cats and dogs. These panels can also be used to monitor response to therapy and/or relapse in patients post therapy, particularly lymphoma.

Nu.Q Cancer Screening test: This test is a blood test that measures and identifies nucleosomes, early markers of cancer, from a blood sample. This test has been shown to detect 74% of lymphomas and 89% of HSAs in dogs and is most helpful in diagnosis and monitoring of these cancers. This test is offered by Texas A&M Gastrointestinal Laboratory.

OncoK9 Liquid Biopsy: A liquid biopsy is a noninvasive alternative to surgical biopsies that tests for tumor DNA in a blood sample. All cells release DNA into the bloodstream, and

DNA released from tumor cells contains unique genomic mutations that can be detected by liquid biopsy technology. This technology has been validated in dogs and is capable of detecting 30 different cancer types with overall specificity and sensitivity similar to what has been reported in liquid biopsy technology in human cancers (OncoK9 White Paper 2021). This test is offered by PetDx.

Summary

Cancer is one of the most prevalent conditions seen in companion animal hospice practice. Standard options for treatable lower-grade and lower-stage cancers include surgery, chemotherapy, and radiation therapy, and, more recently, targeted therapy, immunotherapy and gene therapy. Adverse events associated with first-line standard cancer treatment may negatively affect quality of life for many senior and geriatric pets with comorbidities such as heart, kidney or liver disease, obesity, diabetes, and/or other primary tumors. These competing issues make it difficult for pet owners to justify aggressive first-line cancer therapy for older pets, frail pets, and pets with comorbidities. Many pet owners may be reluctant to proceed with first-line standard cancer treatments due to the increased risk of adverse events and poor outcomes for their compromised older pets. Palliative and hospice care offers second-line kinder, gentler palliative cancer medicine along with palliative supportive care and comfort care at the end of life. Most animal cancer patients endure their tumors initially, and they can be managed with effective pain control and palliative cancer medicine. Hospice teams can play an important role in improving quality of life for cancer patients and serve as steadfast pillars of support as caregivers struggle to cope with the burdens of caring for their pets in final decline.

Conflicts of Interest

This author has no financial and personal conflicts of interest that could inappropriately influence the work in this section.

References

Arnold, E.J., Childress, M.O., Fourez, L.M. et al. (2011) Clinical trial of vinblastine in dogs with transitional cell carcinoma of the urinary bladder. *J. Vet. Intern. Med.*, 25 (6):1385–1390. https://doi.org/10.1111/j.1939-1676. 2011.00796.x. Epub 2011 Sep 13. PMID: 22092632.

Back, A.R., Schleis, SE, Smrkovski, O.A. et al. (2015) Mechlorathamine, vincristine, melphalan and prednisone (MOMP), for the treatment of relapsed lymphoma in dogs. *Vet. Comp. Oncol.*, 13: 398–408.

Borchers, A.T., Stern, J.S. Hackman, R.M. *et al* (1999) Mushrooms, tumors and immunity. *Proc. Soc. Exp. Biol. Med.*, 221: 281–293.

Borchers, A.T., Keen, C.L., and Gershwin, M.E. (2004) Mushrooms, tumors and immunity: an update. *Proc. Soc. Exp. Biol. Med.*, 229: 393–406.

Coto, G., Moreno, N., and Zaragoza, S. (2013) Canine and Feline Oncology: From Theory to Practice. Spain: Servet.

De Ridder, T.R., Campbell, J.E., Burke-Schwarz, C. et al. (2021) Randomized controlled clinical study evaluating the efficacy and safety of intratumoral treatment of canine mast cell tumors with tigilanol tiglate (EBC-46). *J. Vet. Intern. Med.*, 35 (1):415–429. https://doi.org/10.1111/jvim.15806. Epub 2020 Jun 16. PMID:32542733; PMCID:PMC7848366.

Ehling, T.J., Klein, M.K., Smith, L. et al. (2021) A prospective, multi-Centre, veterinary radiation therapy oncology group study reveals potential efficacy of toceranib phosphate (Palladia) as a primary or adjuvant agent in the treatment of canine nasal carcinoma. *Vet. Comp. Oncol.* 20 https://doi.org/10.1111/vco.12776. Epub ahead of print.

Gawande, A. (2013) Being Mortal: Medicine and What Matters in the End. New York: Metropolitan Books, Henry Holt and Company.

Glickman, L., Glickman, N., and Thorpe, R. (1999) The Golden Retriever Club of America National Health Survey, 1998–1999. Available at http://www.grca.org/wp-content/uploads/2015/08/healthsurvey.pdf (Accessed: September 2016).

Iwamoto, K.S., Bennet, L.R., and Norman, A. et al. (1992) Linoleate produces remission in canine mycosis fungoides. *Cancer Lett.*, 64: 17–22.

Knapp, D. (1991) Piroxicam therapy in twenty-four dogs with transitional cell carcinoma of the bladder. *Proceedings of the Annual American college of Veterinary Internal Medicine Forum*, p. 108.

Leach, T.N., Childress, M.O., Greene S.N., et al. (2012) Prospective trial of metronomic chlorambucil chemotherapy in dogs with naturally occurring cancer. *Vet. Comp. Oncol.*, 10, 102–112.

Lucroy, M.D., Clauson R.M., Suckow, M.A. et al. (2020) Evaluation of an autologous cancer vaccine for the treatment of metastatic canine hemangiosarcoma: a preliminary study. *BMC Vet. Res.*, 16 (1):447. https://doi.org/10.1186/s12917-020-02675-y. PMID: 33208160; PMCID: PMC7672887.

MacDonald V., Gaunt, C., Arnason, T. et al. (2014) Validation of adjunct use of metformin in reversing multiple drug resistant (MDR) biomarkers in canine lymphoma. *Veterinary Cancer Society Proceedings*, October 9–11, 2014, p. 59.

Marcello, A.B., Geiger, T.L., Jimenz, D.A. et al. (2015) Detection of comorbidities and synchronous primary tumors via thoracic radiography and abdominal ultrasonography and their influence on treatment outcome in dogs with soft tissue sarcomas, primary brain tumors and intranasal tumors. *Vet. Comp. Oncol.*, 13: 433–442.

Marconato, L., Aresu, L., Stefanello, D. et al. (2019) Opportunities and challenges of active immunotherapy in with B-cell cymphoma: a 5-year experience in two veterinary oncology centers. *J. Immunother. Cancer,*: 7 (1):146.

Martin, C.K., Dirksen, W.P., Carlton, M.M. et al. (2015) Combined zoledronic acid and meloxicam reduced bone loss and tumor growth in an orthotopic mouse model of bone-invasive oral squamous cell carcinoma. *Vet. Comp. Oncol.*, 13: 203–217.

Merino-Gutierrez, V., Borrego, J.F., Puig, J. et al. (2021) Treatment of advanced-stage canine nasal carcinomas with toceranib phosphate: 23 cases (2015-2020). *J. Small Anim. Pract.*, 62(10):881–885. https://doi.org/10.1111/jsap.13387. Epub 2021 Jun 16. PMID: 34131916.

Morrison, W.B. (ed.) (2002) *Cancer in Dogs and Cats: Medical and Surgical Management*. Jackson, WY: Teton New Media.

Mutsaers, A.J. and Henry, C. (2014) Metronomic chemotherapy: theory and practice, State of the Art Presenter, Caroline Henry. *Veterinary Cancer Society Proceedings*, October 9–11, p. 56.

OncoK9 White Paper (2021). Clinical Validation of Oncok9, a blood-based multi-cancer early detection "liquid biopsy" test for dogs.

Sadowski, A.R., Garnder, H.L., Borgatti, A. et al. (2018) Phase II study of the oral selective inhibitor of nuclear export (SINE) KPT-335 (verdinexor) in dogs with lymphoma. *BMC Vet. Res.*, 14 (1):250.

Schrempp, D.R., Childress, M.O., Stewart, J.C., et al. (2013) Metronomic administration of chlorambucil for treatment of dogs with urinary bladder transitional cell carcinoma. *J. Am. Vet. Med. Assoc.*, 242 (11):1534–8. https://doi.org/10.2460/javma.242.11.1534. PMID: 23683018.

Son, D.S., Lee E.S., Adunyah S.E. (2020) The antitumor potentials of Benzimidazole Anthelmintics as repurposing drugs. *Immune*

Netw., 20(4):e29. https://doi.org/10.4110/ in.2020.20.e29. PMID: 32895616; PMCID: PMC7458798.

Villalobos, A. and Kaplan, L. (2017) Canine and Feline Geriatric Oncology: Honoring the Human–Animal Bond. *Can. Vet. J.*, Veterinary Cancer Society (2008) *Newsletter. Metronomic Chemotherapy.*

Vucenik, I. and Shamsuddin, A.M. (2006) Protection against cancer by dietary IP6 and inositol. *Nutr. Cancer*, 55: 109–125.

Winninger, F. and Selting, K.A. (2014) Brain tumors: location, location, location. *Veterinary Cancer Society Proceedings*, October 9–11, pp. 141–144.

Withrow, S.J. and Vail, D.M. (eds) (2007) *Withrow and MacEwen's Small Animal Clinical Oncology*, 4th edn. St. Louis, MS: Saunders/Elsevier.

11

Integrative Therapies for Palliative Care of the Veterinary Cancer Patient

Betsy Hershey, DVM, DACVIM (Oncology), CVA

Complementary and Alternative Medicine (CAM) refers to those therapies that are not considered to be "mainstream" or "standard of care" medical therapy such as surgery, chemotherapy, radiation therapy and immunotherapy. These therapies include acupuncture, chiropractic and other manipulative body-based practices, energy work such as Reiki and therapeutic touch, homeopathy, nutrition, and/or herbal therapies and supplements. Integrative Medicine is an approach to medical care that combines "standard of care" medicine with complementary or alternative therapies. Integrative therapy has become increasingly sought after by owners for their pets with cancer. According to a 2003 Survey by the American Animal Hospital Association, 21% of pet owners had used some form of complementary therapy for their pet compared to just 6% in the 1996 survey. Owners' interest in seeking integrative care for their pets is likely to increase. A 2019 retrospective study from the University of Florida examined patient characteristics of dogs and cats referred specifically for acupuncture and herbs. Of the patients presenting for these therapies, 14.9% sought care for oncologic conditions. Cats were more likely to be treated for oncologic complaints than dogs (Schmalberg et al. 2019).

Reasons that owners may seek integrative care for their pet with cancer include: to decrease the side effects of standard cancer therapies such as nausea, vomiting, and hyporexia; decrease symptoms of the cancer such as nausea, fatigue, and pain; take an active role in treating their pet for cancer, ease stress, and bond with their pet; and provide end-of-life comfort in the final stages of the pets' cancer. For owners that decline "standard of care therapy" due to cost or other factors, CAM can help provide a method of treatment that can benefit the pet by improving quality of life, slowing growth of the cancer, and in some cases, improve survival time. The following are examples of CAM, and how they can benefit the pet with cancer. Many of these treatment modalities require extensive training and practice. It is best to refer a client interested in these modalities to a trained, experienced practitioner. Practitioners with additional training in CAM can be found at websites for the American Holistic Veterinary Association (www.ahvma.com), Chi University (www.tcvm.com), and American Academy of Ozonotherapy (www.aaot.us).

Nutrition and Food Therapy

Nutrition is an important component of cancer therapy in veterinary patients. Too many owners associate a healthy appetite in their pet

Hospice and Palliative Care for Companion Animals: Principles and Practice, Second Edition.
Edited by Amir Shanan, Jessica Pierce, and Tamara Shearer.
© 2023 John Wiley & Sons, Inc. Published 2023 by John Wiley & Sons, Inc.
Companion website: www.wiley.com/go/shanan/palliative

with well-being and perceived good quality of life. A pet that has a diminished appetite or is losing weight is concerning for owners. With more advanced treatment options, including the ability to target specific mutations of individualized cancers, our patients are living longer, and in many patients, cancer may be managed as a chronic disease. However, malnutrition remains a concern for cancer patients. Malnutrition (cancer cachexia) in cancer patients is very common and is a consequence of the increase in inflammatory cytokines associated with cancer, metabolic alterations, and inadequate availability of nutrients. In human cancer patients, malnutrition combined with loss of muscle mass is very common and can negatively impact prognosis. Additionally, the gut associated immune lymphoid tissue (GALT) comprises the majority of the immune system. Therefore, good nutrition is important in supporting immune system function for the cancer patient.

The ideal cancer diet is one that is low in carbohydrates, but moderate in fat and protein. Cancer likes sugar as an energy source, and carbohydrates are broken down into sugar. Changes in the metabolism of sugar can occur before any clinically detectable cancer. Blood glucose can increase, favoring the growth of the cancer. Glucose intolerance is one of the earliest metabolic abnormalities found in human cancer patients. In one study, elevated fasting serum glucose levels and diabetes were independent risk factors for several major cancers, and the risk increased with increased level of serum fasting glucose levels (Ha Jee et al. 2005). Therefore, feeding a diet low in carbohydrates can "starve" the cancer. In this author's opinion, there is no one-size-fits-all for how to achieve a low carbohydrate diet. Enhancement of diet should be directed to improve the diet that the pet currently is eating. Diets should be tailored according to the pet's preferences as well as the owner's time and financial constraints. A low carbohydrate diet can be achieved through either raw, home-cooked, or low-carbohydrate kibble diets. To be considered low carbohydrate, a diet should have less than 30% carbs, with some foods having between 5 and 15% carbohydrates.

Raw diets are naturally low-carbohydrate diets and an excellent choice for many cancer patients. There are many commercial raw diets available, both frozen and dehydrated. Some raw diets are obtained via prescription and tailored for various diseases including cancer (i.e. Darwin's Pet foods). This author favors a commercial raw diet over homemade because a commercial diet is more likely to be nutritionally balanced/complete and processed to reduce bacteria and other toxins. Raw diets are easy to feed, and most dogs and cats will readily accept the diet. If prepared and stored properly, illness from eating a raw diet is unlikely. It has been this author's experience that raw diets are well tolerated in chemotherapy patients, with minimal to no increased risk of diet borne infections. Raw diets are not recommended for older, frail patients because this diet is too energetically cold for these patients. For some owners, particularly those with large breed dogs or multiple dogs, the cost of an exclusively raw diet may be cost prohibitive. In these patients, incorporation of a partial raw diet with home-cooked or low-carbohydrate kibble can be considered. Home-cooked diets are another option for the cancer patient. Exclusive home cooking can be time consuming for owners, particularly those with large breed dogs, and some owners will not have the time or capability to cook for their pets. There are multiple companies now that deliver home-cooked, personalized meals right to the owner's door. For those owners that do elect home cooking, there are many excellent books with recipes for home cooking, such as Dr. Becker's *Real Food for Healthy Dogs and Cats: Simple Homemade Food.* When home cooking, food can be "batched" in larger quantities and frozen for feeding at a later date. This author advises owners to rotate the meat protein, vegetables, and fruits per batch to help with balance. Additionally, a vitamin/mineral supplement and calcium supplement should be incorporated. A low-carbohydrate, dry food can be difficult to find. Some brands will list the carbohydrate content on the label. For those that don't, the listed ingredients may be added up, and that number subtracted from 100% will give the carbohydrate percentage. To be considered a low-carbohydrate diet, the carbohydrate percentage should be below 30%.

A ketogenic diet is a diet consisting of high fat, moderate protein, and low carbohydrates. A ketogenic diet of 4:1 high fat, low carbohydrate mimic the fasting state, forcing the body to burn fats and produce ketones for energy. Research shows that a ketogenic diet may display anticancer effects through three main mechanisms: glucose deprivation, reduction of insulin and insulin-like growth factors, and antioxidant and anti-inflammatory properties (Tan-Shalaby 2017). Since the diet deprives the body of glucose, it also deprives the cancer of its main source of fuel. The cancer cells are then forced to use a mechanism called mitochondrial oxidation to obtain energy. However, this process leads to increased oxidative stress and damage to the cancer cells and can potentially sensitize the cancer cells to the further damaging effects of radiation and chemotherapy (Weber et al. 2020). In a mouse model of systemic metastatic cancer, a ketogenic diet was noted to decrease blood glucose, slow tumor growth, and increase mean survival time. These effects increased when a ketogenic diet was combined with hyperbaric oxygen therapy (Poff et al. 2013). A case series in humans showed that feeding a ketogenic diet to patients with advanced and rapidly advancing cancers stabilized, or resulted in, partial remission (Fine et al. 2012). A ketogenic diet alone is not a cure for cancer but can be considered as a part of a multimodality treatment plan. Formulating a homemade ketogenic diet can be very time consuming for owners and not feasible for every owner. The Ketopet Sanctuary has an online calculator (https://www.ketopetsanctuary.com/pages/keto-diet-calculator) that can be used in helping clinicians guide their clients in formulating a ketogenic diet at home.

Chinese Food Therapy is the practice of using food to heal and regulate the body. It is based on Traditional Chinese Medicine (TCM) with the core belief that food shares the same origins as medicine and therefore can be used like medicine to heal the body. Use of food therapy requires knowledge of TCM patterns and energetic properties of food to select food that nourishes the body and promotes healing. These patterns of disease may seem confusing to some because they mirror the ancient description of disorders. Disease patterns can be translated to a more modern understanding with continuing education in TCM. Food has properties that can heat or cool the body (think spicy food to heat on a cold day and watermelon to cool on a hot summer day), dispel phlegm, and nourish deficiencies. Even if owners cannot feed/cook entirely based on TCM principles, supplementing the diet with food according to TCM patterns can help. Like other diseases in Chinese medicine, cancer is considered a result or manifestation of an underlying imbalance. The tumor is the uppermost branch not the "root" of the illness. Spleen Qi Deficiency is a common underlying pattern of many cancers, which can lead to dampness and phlegm and tumor formation. Feeding a diet rich in Yang (warming) tonics and foods to dispel dampness and resolve phlegm are helpful in supporting the patient (examples: shrimp, lamb, chicken, anchovy). For some cancers such as transitional cell carcinoma and osteosarcoma, clearing toxic heat can be important. Chemotherapy and radiation therapy can also create toxic heat in the patient. Food to help clear heat include melon, rabbit, mung beans, lentil, dandelion, cucumber, and apple. Both cancer and cancer treatments can result in blood deficiency manifested clinically by anemia and weakness. The feeding of blood-building foods such as sardines, liver, spinach, and chicken eggs can help improve these symptoms in patients. A good resource for food therapy is the book *Helping Ourselves: A Guide to Traditional Chinese Food Energetics* by Katheryn Trenshaw. Additional training in food therapy can be obtained at the Chi University of Traditional Chinese Veterinary Medicine.

Congee is a traditional rice porridge that can be served plain, or meat, fish, eggs, vegetables, and spices can be added to treat the underlying disease pattern. Congee is a highly digestible and palatable food and therefore suitable for the ill cancer patient. Another palatable option is bone broth, made from boiling animal bones and connective tissue. The addition of vegetables can increase the nutritional value of the broth. Bone broth can be helpful with hydrating the sick cancer patient as well as providing some nutrition including protein and trace nutrients. Bone broth is palatable, and many patients will drink it, but it can also be syringed to the sick patient.

Inappetence in the veterinary cancer patient is often multifactorial and can complicate treatment. Certain tumors can cause dysphagia or alter gastrointestinal function. Tumors can also alter nutrients, cause hypoxia, and alter the release of peripheral hormones that can alter feeding (ghrelin, peptide tyrosine). Pain can also cause decreased appetite and addressing pain in the cancer patient may improve eating. Nausea can also cause inappetence and may be a side effect of chemotherapy as well as certain cancers. Nausea does not always manifest as vomiting, but can include other symptoms such as decreased appetite and/or drooling. If nausea is suspected, treatment with antinausea medications such as maropitant (Cerenia), ondansetron, prochlorperazine or promethazine may be beneficial. Appetite stimulants may be used to improve appetite in cancer patients. Appetite stimulants to consider include mirtazapine, capromorelin (Entyce, Elura), cyproheptadine (more effective in cats than dogs), dronabinol (Marinol), megesterol acetate, and cannabidiols. Nutritional support with feeding tubes may be considered for a pet that will not eat on its own and can help facilitate administration of medications via tube. Feeding tubes can be beneficial in the short term for patients recovering from surgery or radiation therapy. For many owners, however, feeding tubes can be seen as a drastic measure to prolong a pet with a terminal diagnosis. Esophageal tubes are well tolerated in both cats and dogs, easy to place, and cost effective.

Prolonged loss of appetite can lead to weight loss and malnutrition. Cachexia is a metabolic and paraneoplastic condition in patients with advanced cancer that results in involuntary weight loss and muscle mass loss. The loss of appetite combined with cachexia is referred to as anorexia-cachexia syndrome and is associated with a poor prognosis. Although supporting or improving appetite in the veterinary cancer patient can be important, it is also important for both the owner and clinician to recognize that complete loss of desire to eat and drink are a natural and normal part of the dying process. The needs of the dying patient for food and water are very different than those of a healthy animal. As the end of life nears, the body loses its ability to process food and water normally, and minimal amounts of food and water are needed, if at all, as organs and bodily functions shut down.

Herbs and Supplements

Herbal Supplements

TCM and natural herbal remedies have been used worldwide, particularly in China, for thousands of years to treat cancer. Research has increasingly shown that Chinese medicines can have less side effects, inhibit pro-inflammatory cytokines, enhance the immune system, inhibit protein catabolism, and improve appetite and body weight (Wang 2020a). Herbal therapies can be used to improve immune system function, slow growth of the cancer, and reduce side effects of treatment, as well as reduce the symptoms of cancer (Wang 2020b). Herbal therapies may be used as an adjunct to conventional cancer therapies, although care must be taken to avoid potential interactions between herbs and conventional medications. Many owners will consider treatment with herbal therapies when conventional treatments have either failed or have been declined. Herbal medicines can be prepared as capsules, tablets, tea pills, powders, and/or tinctures. Dogs will generally accept herbal medicines in various forms, and if appetite is good and consistent, herbal therapies can be added to food for consumption. For patients with decreased appetite, tinctures can be easier to administer by direct oral route. Herbals can also be baked into other foods, such as home-made dog treats, for better palatability. Cooking can reduce the potency of the herbs by approximately 20%, so an owner may have to give an increased amount to achieve effect. Cats can be more difficult to medicate with herbals because the strong taste of many herbals can prohibit cats from consuming voluntarily in food. Glycerin-based herbal tinctures are more palatable than alcohol-based tinctures. Some cats will eat powders in wet food or pill pockets, while others will readily accept liquid tinctures. This author uses herbals commonly and has found herbal therapies to be beneficial in improving quality of life as well as extending survival time by slowing the progression of the cancer. Side effects of herbals are minimal, although it can be challenging in some patients to get them to consume the herbals. Advanced training in Traditional Chinese Veterinary Medicine (TCVM) is essential to properly diagnosis Chinese disease pattern for proper selection of herbal therapies. However, the basic principles are to treat the underlying root pattern, strengthen Qi and the immune system, dispel stasis and soften hardness, dispel damp, and stop the pain. As mentioned above, Chinese disease patterns can be translated to a more modern understanding with continuing education in TCVM. Most patients are prescribed a combination of an immune supporting herbal formula (F*u-Zheng* herbs) along with a formula to relieve stagnation and pathogens (*Qu-Xie* herbs). In some patients, additional herbal formulas may be used as a transporter to the organ affected by the cancer and/or herbal formula to address symptoms of the cancer. Courses in traditional Chinese veterinary herbal medicine for various organ systems are taught at the Chi University and the College of Integrative Veterinary Medicine. Training in Western Herbology is offered by the College of Integrative Veterinary Medicine.

An herbal called Yunnan Bai Yao deserves special mention due to its use in tumors that are prone to bleeding. Yunnan Bai Yao is a proprietary TCM used to stop bleeding and improve circulation in traumatic injuries. It has also been promoted for wound healing, anti-inflammatory, and pain-relieving properties. Its safety and efficacy have not yet been evaluated by the FDA. However, a limited number of studies in humans shows benefit in cancer patients. Topical Yunnan Bai Yao was effective in improving control of bleeding in adolescent cancer patients in combination with conventional hemostatic treatments (Ladas et al. 2012). This herbal is most commonly used in treatment of hemangiosarcoma in dogs and has been anecdotally reported to improve survival of this cancer. A recent study shows Yunnan Bai Yao causes a dose- and time-dependent cell death of hemangiosarcoma cell lines through initiation of caspase-mediated apoptosis (Wirth et al. 2016). Further research of actions and efficacy of Yunnan Bai Yao are warranted.

Yunnan is available in capsule form as well as powder, aerosol, and plaster. The oral dose of Yunnan capsule is 1 capsule per 40 lbs body weight administered twice daily for maintenance. This dose can be increased for active bleeding. A small red pill resides in the middle of the package and is used in case of "emergency" severe hemorrhage. The red pill can be given every 12–24 hours until bleeding stops or significantly reduces. The capsule can be dissolved in water and administered rectally during surgery or in patients that cannot take the herbal orally. This author frequently uses Yunnan Bai Yao in cancers that are prone to bleeding such as nasal tumors, bladder tumors, rectal tumors, and hemangiosarcoma. Yunnan Bai Yao has been effective at reducing bleeding in these cancers, although the hemorrhage that can occur with hemangiosarcoma can eventually become too frequent and severe for the herbal to remain effective.

Antioxidants

Common antioxidant vitamins used in cancer patients include beta-carotene, vitamin C, vitamin E, ubiquinone (coenzyme Q10), and selenium. Radiation therapy produces reactive oxygen species (ROS) that induce cellular damage (Ziech et al. 2010). Some chemotherapy drugs such as alkylating agents, platinum drugs, and antitumor antibiotics also exert cytotoxicity by generating free radicals. The use of antioxidants may alleviate adverse effects of radiation therapy and chemotherapy, but they may also antagonize antitumor effects of these therapies by reducing the oxidative damage. A systematic review of the use of antioxidants as an adjuvant therapy in human cancer patients indicates it is still unclear whether the use of antioxidants affects treatment outcomes or ameliorate the adverse effects of radiation and chemotherapy (Yasueda et al. 2016). Thus, this author recommends that antioxidants not be used concurrently with radiation therapy, and initiation of the use of antioxidants should be delayed for at least four weeks post completion of radiation therapy. For patients receiving chemotherapy, antioxidants should be temporarily discontinued for three days pre and post chemotherapy administration. The use of antioxidants in the palliative care setting may be beneficial in slowing disease progression.

Medicinal Mushrooms

Medicinal mushrooms have been used in Asian countries for hundreds of years for the treatment of infections, pulmonary disease, and cancer. Medicinal mushrooms have been approved as standard adjuncts to cancer therapy in China and Japan for over 30 years. There is extensive clinical research to support the safe use of mushrooms as a single agent for cancer or in combination with radiation therapy and chemotherapy (Jeitler et al. 2020). Over 100 species of mushrooms exist, the most common include: Ganoderma Lucidum (Reishi), Trametes versicolor or Coriolus versicolor (turkey tail), Lentinun edodes (shitake), and Grifola frondosa (maitake). Medicinal mushrooms have immunomodulating properties mediated through the mushroom's stimulation of innate immune cells such as monocytes, natural killer cells, and dendritic cells. The immune effects of the mushrooms are generally believed to be caused by the presence of high molecular weight polysaccharides (beta-glucans) in the mushrooms (Wasser 2017). Polysaccharopeptide (PSP), the bioactive compound in coriolus versicolor (turkey tail) mushroom, significantly delayed the development of metastasis and improved survival time in dogs with splenic hemangiosarcoma post-surgery (Brown and Reetz 2012). Medicinal mushrooms are generally well tolerated with few side effects and can be safely used in combination with conventional therapies. Medicinal mushrooms can also be considered for patients with advanced cancer, where advanced treatments may not be accessible or have been declined by the owner. Medicinal mushrooms are considered dietary supplements and as such are not approved by the FDA as a treatment for cancer or other medical conditions.

B Vitamins

Cobalamin (B12) and folate (B6) are commonly decreased in gastrointestinal cancers, particularly lymphoma, due to malabsorption. Supplementation with these vitamins can improve symptoms in these patients. It is recommended that both feline and canine patients with gastrointestinal cancers, particularly lymphoma, have baseline B12 and folate performed and supplemented accordingly. These panels are offered through both the Veterinary Diagnostic Institute Laboratory and Texas A&M Gastrointestinal Laboratory (GI Lab). Both parenteral and oral administration of B12 appear effective. The dose of B12 in cats is 250 mcg, dosing in dogs ranges from 250 to 1000 mcg, depending on the size of the dog. Parenteral administration is administered once per week for six weeks, then once monthly. Oral forms of B12 could be considered for patients that cannot be given injections. B12 levels should be rechecked after 12 weeks of administration. Folate dose is 200 mcg for cats and small dogs and 400 mcg for larger dogs once daily for four weeks.

Digestive Enzymes

Digestive enzymes are proteins made by the pancreas to help break down fats, proteins, and carbohydrates. Most digestive enzyme supplements are made from the pancreas of either cows, pigs, or lambs. Other enzymes may come from plants such as bromelain from pineapple, papain from papayas, and lactase from purified yeasts of fungi. Digestive enzymes supplementation may help reduce complications of treatment, particularly for patients with pancreatic or gastrointestinal cancers. Recent research in humans suggests a possible role for proteolytic enzymes in pathogenesis and progression of cancer, further research is warranted (Tabrez et al. 2020).

Probiotics

The gut microbiota is important in regulating host immunity. Dysbiosis and impaired systemic immunity is common with many cancers as well as cancer therapy, particularly chemotherapy. Probiotics are helpful in the treatment of side effects of cancer therapy. The use of probiotics can improve intestinal environment and enhance intestinal mucosal barrier function and reduce the incidence of diarrhea in patients receiving chemotherapy. Probiotics are also useful in reducing the painful oral mucositis that can occur with chemotherapy and reducing systemic inflammation. Probiotics have been shown in human medicine to potentially decrease the severity and frequency of diarrhea in the cancer patient and reduce the need for antidiarrheal medication (Redman et al. 2014). Increasing evidence in human oncology demonstrates the gut microbiome's influence on response to cancer treatment, with evidence suggesting that modulating the gut microbiome can positively impact response to various cancer therapies (Guven et al. 2020; Kroemer and Zitvogel 2018). Probiotics are commonly used by this author to support cancer patients, particularly those undergoing chemotherapy.

Vitamin D

Vitamin D is a liposoluble steroid hormone primarily involved in calcium and phosphorus homeostasis and in mineralization of bone. Vitamin D is available in two forms: ergocalciferol (vitamin D2) and cholecalciferol (vitamin D3). Both are inactive prohormones that need to undergo hydroxylation to become active. Low levels of vitamin D in humans have been associated with solid and non-solid cancer risk, as well as development and growth of the cancer. Supplementation with vitamin D in cancer patients has been associated with a more favorable prognosis, and evidence exists that vitamin D can increase the efficacy of chemotherapy drugs and potentially overcome the drug resistance seen with chemotherapeutic agents (Negri et al. 2020). Thus, there is increasing evidence to support the benefits of supplementation of vitamin D in veterinary cancer patients. Several laboratories, including the Veterinary Diagnostic Institute (VDI) offer vitamin D-level testing in dogs and cats. It is recommended to routinely perform vitamin D testing on veterinary cancer patients and supplement accordingly.

Omega-3 Polyunsaturated Fatty Acids (PUFAS)

Omega-3 Polyunsaturated fatty acids (PUFAS) comprise three active molecules, Alpha-linolenic acid (ALA) synthesized in plants and available in nut and seed oils such as flaxseed oil and Eicosapentaenoic acid (EPA) and docosahexaenoic acid (DPA), which are found in cold water fish and certain marine algae. ALA can be converted to EPA and DPA in dogs, but cats do not have this ability. Also, the use of flaxseed oil in cats is ineffective. Omega-3 fatty acids have anti-inflammatory effects and can preserve muscle mass. Omega-3 fatty acids may exert their anticancer actions by influencing multiple targets implicated in various stages of cancer development, including cell proliferation, cell survival, angiogenesis, inflammation, metastasis, and epigenetic abnormalities that are crucial to the onset and progression of cancer (Jing et al. 2013). In some human studies supplementation of fish oil was shown to enhance the response rate to chemotherapy (Murphy et al. 2011). However, a more recent study cautions the use of fish oil with chemotherapy due to increased levels of fatty acid 16:4, which has been shown to induce chemoresistance in mice (Daenen et al. 2015). These concerns cannot be tested in clinical trials with cancer patients due to ethical concerns. If fish oil is being given to a patient receiving chemotherapy, it is recommended to stop fish oil one day pre and one day post chemotherapy. There are also concerns regarding heavy metals in fish oils. Using fish oils (or fish) derived from smaller fish such as anchovy, herring, and sardine may be safer. Algal oil can also be used as a source of omega-3 PUFAS and may be a safer alternative for chemotherapy patients without concern for heavy metal contamination or interference with chemotherapy.

Curcumin

Curcumin is a compound extracted from *Curcuma longa* (known as turmeric). Curcumin has been shown to have both antioxidant and anti-inflammatory benefits, and these benefits have been demonstrated in multiple chronic diseases in humans including arthritis, metabolic syndrome, liver disease, obesity, and neurodegenerative diseases, as well as cancer. Curcumin affects different signaling pathways and molecular targets associated with the development of cancer and acts on cellular components such as macrophages, dendritic cells, and lymphocytes. Curcumin has shown *in vitro* activity against multiple human cancers including breast, pancreatic, lung, and hematologic. The bioavailability of curcumin is poor due to low absorption and rapid metabolism and systemic elimination. Interestingly, a clinical study in pancreatic cancer in people using curcumin as monotherapy showed two patients with clinical responses despite the low levels of curcumin measured in plasma (Dhillon et al. 2008). A recent study evaluating curcumin added to dog food fed to young Beagle dogs concluded that curcumin supplementation improved health, with emphasis on stimulation of the antioxidant system and evidence of an anti-inflammatory effect (Campigotto et al. 2020). Liposomal formulation of curcumin can enhance the antitumor effect and pharmacological activities of curcumin. Piperine, a component of black pepper, when combined with curcumin has been shown to increase the bioavailability of curcumin by 2000% in humans (Shoba et al. 1998). Curcumin is fat soluble and combining curcumin with a fatty meal can also potentially enhance absorption. Combining curcumin with black pepper and coconut or olive oil, known as "golden paste," can be a beneficial supplement for dogs and cats.

High Dose IV Vitamin C Therapy

High dose IV vitamin C has been in use with CAM practitioners both human and veterinary for decades. Administration of IV vitamin C (but not oral) can produce pharmacological plasma concentrations of the vitamin. Vitamin C in pharmacological concentrations can kill cancer cells but not normal cells *in vitro* by mechanism of hydrogen peroxide formation. In human studies, side effects of high dose IV vitamin C were minimal. This author has used IV vitamin C in dogs and cats with minimal side effects in doses ranging from 0.5 to 1 g per pound of body weight. High dose IV vitamin C has been administered twice per week for six weeks and then monthly as maintenance if deemed beneficial in controlling the patient's cancer. However, efficacy has been limited in patients with advanced malignancies that have been heavily pretreated. IV Vitamin C therapy is time consuming and laborious as the infusion must be protected from light and infused over a two hours period of time. Higher doses of vitamin C can be emetic and anti-nausea medications have been helpful in reducing emesis during infusion. Additionally, patients must be walked periodically as patients will need to urinate frequently during treatment. The challenge remains in veterinary patients in knowing whether pharmacologic and therapeutic levels are being achieved with the current doses. The levels of vitamin C in the blood dissipate quickly once the infusion has been completed and there has not been a quick and reliable way to measure vitamin C levels in the blood in veterinary patients.

Acupuncture

Acupuncture is the use of thin metallic needles to stimulate anatomical points on the body. Although acupuncture is considered a relatively "new" alternative medicine in the Western world, acupuncture is a practiced medical treatment that is over 5000 years old. Acupuncture has been practiced on both humans and animals for thousands of years in China. Acupuncture is one of the four key components of the system of TCVM. The other components include food therapy, tui-na (Chinese body work and massage) and herbal therapies. In Chinese medicine the body is seen as a delicate balance of opposing and connected forces: Yin and Yang. Among the major assumptions in Chinese medicine is that health is achieved by maintaining the body in a balanced state and that disease is due to an imbalance of Yin and Yang. Acupuncture and the other components of TCVM act to restore that balance.

Acupuncture may be beneficial in care of the veterinary cancer patient and can be used in conjunction with surgery, chemotherapy, and/ or radiation therapy. Acupuncture may be helpful in reducing cancer pain, reducing side effects from conventional therapies, including nausea and vomiting associated with chemotherapy, and enhancing immune system function. There are many publications evaluating the efficacy of acupuncture for cancer pain in humans and for alleviating side effects of conventional therapies. However, few published reports exist on the effects of acupuncture in veterinary cancer patients. A retrospective analysis of dog and cat patients referred exclusively for acupuncture indicates 14.9% presented for treatment of cancer (Schmalberg et al. 2019). A 2017 review of the literature evaluating acupuncture in companion animals (dogs, cats, and horses) found the most common indication for acupuncture's use was musculoskeletal conditions, and the most common parameters evaluated in experimental trials were pain and cardiovascular parameters (Rose et al. 2017). One case report describes using Korean Sa-Ahm Acupuncture to treat a Golden Retriever with an oral fibrosarcoma for greater than eight months (Choi and Flynn 2017).

Acupuncture points are selected based on the patient's constitution and TCVM pattern diagnosis (discussion of TCVM pattern diagnosis is beyond the scope of this chapter). Patients may receive 10–20 needles per session or as many as they will tolerate. The frequency of treatment depends on the symptoms being treated. For general immunity and overall well-being, patients may be treated every two to four weeks, or longer. For cancers such as osteosarcoma, where acupuncture is used to help with pain management, treatments may be administered every one to two weeks. Needles should not be placed in or adjacent to the tumor because needling near the tumor could potentially increase blood flow to the tumor and accelerate tumor growth and/or progression. When acupuncture is used to help alleviate side effects of chemotherapy, acupuncture may be given before or after treatment as well as the same day as treatment. This author commonly uses acupuncture concurrently on the same day the patient receives chemotherapy. An ongoing multi-institutional clinical trial is investigating the use of acupuncture and herbal therapies in dogs with lymphoma undergoing CHOP chemotherapy

In terminal patients, acupuncture can help facilitate a peaceful passing. A peaceful passing can help ease the patient's pain or fear. Acupuncture points on the liver and lung channel can allow the pet to surrender and let go and facilitate transitioning to spirit.

Manual Massage Therapies

Massage therapies include Tui-na, myofascial release, and craniosacral therapy. Myofascial release is a technique that focuses on releasing restrictions in the fascia such as trigger points, muscle tightness, and dysfunctions in soft tissue that can contribute to pain and decreased mobility. Craniosacral therapy is a technique that relieves tension in the central nervous system by using light touch to examine membranes and movement of fluids in and around the central nervous system. Craniosacral releases the body's fascia, but with focus on the central nervous system. Tui-na is a Chinese method of massage that treats the meridians and acupoints of the body through pushing, holding, lifting, and pinching techniques. Tui-na may incorporate other massage techniques such as acupressure, myofascial release, and reflexology. Sometimes techniques that are common to osteopathy and chiropractic such as stretching and joint mobilization are used. All these

systems of manual therapies function with the belief that the body is interrelated at all levels and work with the body on a deeper energy level. These manual therapies can help boost immune function and help the body to self-regulate, self-correct, and self-heal. These therapies can help with emotional and mental well-being as well as physical well-being.

Pain is a common symptom in veterinary patients with cancer. Conventional treatments do not always control cancer pain satisfactorily, and many owners turn to complementary therapies to help improve pain control in their pet. Studies in humans have shown massage therapies to significantly reduce cancer pain compared with no massage treatment or conventional care (Lee et al. 2015; Boyd et al. 2016). Massage therapies can also reduce cancer-related fatigue (Kinkead et al. 2018). Myofascial release has been shown in one study to improve overall shoulder movement and functionality as well as improved perceived pain in women after breast cancer surgery and radiotherapy (Serra-Ano et al. 2019). Pets can also benefit from the reduction of cancer-related symptoms these therapies can offer. Additionally, some of the basic techniques of these therapies can be taught to the owner by the practitioner to help the owner provide relief for the pet at home. Touch is important in the care of both humans and animals with cancer. Providing therapies the owner can give at home is important for the owner and pet bond and provides a way for the owner to be involved in their pet's cancer care. It has been well established in human medicine that caregivers can benefit from the relaxation and stress reduction that giving massage can provide (Collinge et al. 2013).

Tui-na is taught at the Chi University of Chinese Veterinary Medicine in Reddick, FL. Courses in Canine Myofascial Release Techniques are offered by EquiLearn Instititute along with Canine and Equine Body Worker Certifications. Certification in Canine Craniosacral Therapy is offered online through holisticanimalstudies.com.

Energy Therapy (Biofield Therapy)

Sound Therapy

Sound therapy is the use of rhythms, vibrations, and tones for healing. Gongs or metal bowls (Tibetan or "Himalayan" singing bowls) are most often used for sound therapy. Tibetan singing bowls are metal bowls usually consisting of a combination of metal alloys and originally used by Tibetan monks for spiritual ceremonies.

At a molecular level, every molecule in the body is moving and vibrating at all times. Energetic blockages can occur, and to relieve those blockages, another frequency or vibration, either faster or slower or at the same speed, can be introduced through sound therapy to release the blockage. Sound healing uses both audible and inaudible sounds and vibrations to achieve a therapeutic effect that shifts brainwaves into alpha (waking consciousness) or theta (relaxed consciousness) states in order to activate the body's regenerative pathways to allow for healing on a cellular level. An observational study in humans demonstrated significantly less tension, anger, fatigue, and depressed mood following Tibetan singing bowl meditation (Goldsby et al. 2017). Tibetan singing bowl therapy has also been shown to decrease blood pressure and heart rate in humans (Landry 2014).

Animals are very receptive to Tibetan singing bowl therapy. Many patients have a bowl frequency that they "prefer," which can change from each singing bowl session. Subjective observations by this author is that the use of singing bowl therapy reduces stress and anxiety of the treated patient. Singing bowl therapy is often used in conjunction with acupuncture sessions in individual patients but has also been used in the general treatment room to treat multiple patients at the same time. This author uses Tibetan singing bowl therapy as part of multimodality therapy to treat pain and reduce stress and anxiety in the veterinary cancer patient.

Reiki, Therapeutic Touch, and Healing Touch Therapies

Reiki, Therapeutic Touch (TT) and Healing Touch (HT) are all energy healing techniques where the practitioner uses their hands to allow or direct the flow of energy into the body to improve the balance and flow of energy and promote self-healing. In touch therapies, the practitioner can choose either the direct laying on of hands on the body or holding the hands over the body. The differences in these touch therapies are primarily in the philosophical intent of the discipline and the way practitioners are trained. Touch therapy is used to promote relaxation, decrease anxiety, and promote well-being and healing. In human cancer patients, therapeutic touch has been shown to decrease pain and fatigue in cancer patients undergoing chemotherapy (Aghabati et al. 2010). When compared to rest, human cancer patients receiving Reiki showed significant improvement in cancer-related fatigue, pain, and anxiety (Tsang et al. 2007). Animals are very receptive to touch therapies, and touch therapies can be used to augment other therapies in treatment of cancer-related pain, fatigue, and treatment-related side effects. Touch therapy can also be used to comfort patients at the end of life.

Ozone Therapy

Ozone therapy is becoming more popular as an adjunctive treatment in veterinary medicine for a number of conditions. Its therapeutic mechanism involves the following: Oxygen as a single atom is deficient in electrons. This makes the atom very unstable, and as a result, single oxygen atoms are not able to exist in nature. Oxygen atoms will pair together to share electrons forming the stable molecule of O_2, which is the oxygen we breath in the atmosphere. When an energetic force such as electricity (lightening) or ultraviolet light (solar exposure) acts on a molecule of O_2, the molecule will split apart into single oxygen atoms. Very quickly, these single oxygen atoms will reform into O_2 molecules; however, some will form into a trio of oxygen atoms known as ozone or O_3. Ozone is also a relatively unstable compound, and the molecules will react with each other to form the more stable compound of O_2. This breakdown of O_3 into O_2 is a process known as dismutation. Ozone generators create ozone by exposing medical grade oxygen to an electric spark inside the machine. The oxygen molecules are split apart and what emerges from the generator is a combination of oxygen and ozone. The parameters of the generator can be set to produce a given amount of concentration of the ozone in that mixture. Once ozone has been generated for a medical application, it must be used quickly rather than stored for later use.

Ozone stimulates oxygen metabolism in cells by causing an increase in the red blood cell glycolysis rate (Ciboroski et al. 2012). In contrast to normal tissues, tumors thrive in hypoxic environments. Tumor ischemia and tumor hypoxia are well-known adverse factors in cancer that can lead to treatment resistance as well as progression and metastases. It has been proposed that autohemotherapy ozone delivery can increase oxygen delivery in hypoxic tissues, may correct tumor hypoxia, lead to less aggressive tumor behavior, and may improve efficacy of radiation therapy and/or chemotherapy (Bocci et al. 2005) while reducing side effects such as nausea, vomiting, opportunistic infections, hair loss, oral ulcers, and/or fatigue. Evidence exists in human oncology patients to support the use of ozone as treatment for the side effects of cancer treatment such as osteoradionecrosis of the jaw following radiation or bisphosphonate therapy (Ripamonti 2011, 2012), persistent pelvic pain (Clavo et al. 2021), persistent radiation-induced rectal bleeding (Clavo et al. 2013), and progressive radiation induced hematuria (Clavo et al. 2005). Ozonated olive oil has been shown to significantly reduce the incidence and severity of hand-foot skin reactions in people induced by sorafenib chemotherapy (Chen et al. 2020). Ozone when delivered by autohemotransfusion was found to significantly improve fatigue in cancer patients both during cancer therapy and in palliative setting with no side effects (Tirelli et al. 2018).

There are multiple methods by which ozone may be delivered to the patient. These methods include rectal insufflation or rectal suppositories, intravesical insufflation, topical use through ozonated oils, ozonated subcutaneous fluids, ozonated drinking water, autohemotherapy transfusions, or via nasal cannula or ear buds. The method and frequency for ozone administration will depend upon the condition being treated, owners financial or time constraints, and clinician preference. As ozone generators become more cost effective, many owners are purchasing ozone generators for home use and can be taught how to administer ozone by rectal insufflation to their pet.

This author uses the methods of rectal insufflation and autohemotherapy most commonly for cancer therapy. Patients often receive ozone therapy in combination with other complementary therapies, such as herbs and acupuncture, or as an adjunct to conventional therapies. Ozone may be given directly in and around tumors at low concentrations to decrease tumor associated pain and slow tumor growth. Direct intra-tumoral injections of ozone are often combined with rectal insufflation or autohemotherapy. This author has found intravesical instillation of ozone to be superior to other methods for treatment of chemotherapy-induced sterile hemorrhagic cystitis. Most patients will have complete resolution of clinical signs of cystitis with one ozone treatment. Ozone acupuncture involves administration of small volumes of ozone (2–5 ml) into acupuncture points and has been helpful in reducing localized pain and inflammation. Topical application of ozonated olive oil can be useful in wound management of open and ulcerated masses or in treatment of chemotherapy-induced oral ulcers.

As ozone therapy gains significant momentum in veterinary medicine, training programs and equipment specific to the veterinary patient are now available. O_3VETS manufactures ozone equipment specific to the veterinary patient. O_3VETS also coordinates continuing education including onsite and regional training in ozone as well as annual meetings and summits to share experiences and techniques. Additional training and certification is offered through the American Academy of Ozonotherapists.

Hyperbaric Oxygen Therapy

Hyperbaric Oxygen Therapy (HBO) is the breathing of pure oxygen in a pressurized chamber. In a hyperbaric oxygen chamber, the air pressure is increased two to three times greater than normal air pressure. This allows oxygen to diffuse into the lungs at a higher concentration than would be possible by breathing 100% oxygen at normal air pressure. This increased oxygen is carried by the blood to other tissues in the body and can kill bacteria and stimulate growth factors and stem cells that promote healing. Hyperbaric oxygen therapy is used to treat injuries where loss of blood flow has occurred, nonhealing wounds, diabetic ulcers, radiation injury, inflammatory conditions such as ulcerative colitis, inflammatory bowel disease, and arthritis.

The role of HBO in the treatment of cancer is still being defined. Hyperbaric oxygen therapy has been beneficial in reducing pain and inflammation in cancer patients, can reduce tumor-associated edema in brain tumors, treat secondary infections, and potentially improve efficacy of other cancer treatments by overcoming tumor hypoxia. Tumor hypoxia is a common feature of many solid tumors and can be an impediment to effective cancer treatment with radiation, chemotherapy, and immunotherapy. Tumor hypoxia occurs due to inadequate oxygen delivery of the abnormal vasculature of the tumor, which cannot meet the growth and demands of the rapidly growing cancer cells. The level of oxygenation within the tumor will be highly variable from one region to another and can change over time. Chronic, profound hypoxia in tumor cells can promote changes that result in genomic instability and promote more aggressive behavior including metastases.

However, HBO as a single modality gives a limited curative effect and is best used as an adjuvant treatment along with other therapies such as radiation and chemotherapy. HBO can be used as palliative therapy to treat pain and inflammation in cancer patients. There has been some concern that HBO may enhance tumor growth; however, recent results strongly indicate that HBO does not promote tumor growth or recurrence or enhance metastases (Daruwalla and Christophi 2006). There has also been some concern that HBO when given in combination with chemotherapy can potentiate chemotherapy side effects. An in-house clinical trial performed by this author attempted to answer this question (unpublished data). Multiple canine patients with various cancers were treated with a combination of chemotherapy and HBO. Chemotherapy drugs evaluated included carboplatin, doxorubicin, vincristine, lomustine, and vinblastine. The chemotherapy drug was chosen based on the patient's cancer type. HBO was administered on the same day as chemotherapy and was administered every one to three weeks as determined by the individual patient's chemotherapy protocol. Because the veterinary chambers are monoplace and chemotherapy cannot be administered during the HBO session, chemotherapy was administered within the first 30 minutes of the patient exiting the chamber when oxygen saturation levels of tissues are highest. The study concluded that a combination of HBO and chemotherapy is safe, and the majority of patients can tolerate the full standard dose of chemotherapy in combination with HBO. No increased gastrointestinal (GI) side effects were seen with the combination. Some patients required 20–25% dose reduction of chemotherapy drug due to neutropenia, but the number of patients requiring dose reductions was not considered to be higher than what would be expected with chemotherapy alone. Efficacy of this combination was not the primary purpose of this study; however, the addition of the HBO did not seem to be detrimental to tumor control and in fact one patient with a rib osteosarcoma survived five years after combination HBO and carboplatin chemotherapy. Interestingly, a murine study investigating HBO as a chemotherapy adjuvant in the treatment of osteosarcoma showed concomitant HBO enhanced the effects of carboplatin on both tumor growth and lung metastases in osteosarcoma-bearing mice and decreased mortality (Kawasoe et al. 2009).

In humans, HBO has been used to treat and prevent osteoradionecrosis, particularly in patients receiving radiation for head and neck cancer. Radionecrosis of the bone and other tissues such as skin and muscle occurs as a consequence of radiation therapy for cancer where the tissues die and a wound develops, often exposing bone. Necrosis of the brain can also occur as a result of radiation of brain tumors. Radionecrosis can be seen in veterinary patients, and often occurs approximately six months after completion of radiation therapy. Although HBO seems to play a prominent role and is effective at treating radionecrosis in people, this author has not found HBO to be effective in the treatment of radionecrosis in veterinary patients. This author postulates that one reason may be that the frequency and duration of HBO treatments necessary to improve this condition in humans is not financially feasible for owners, particularly after the cost of cancer treatment.

The ideal treatment protocol and schedule for HBO in cancer patients has not been clearly defined. In this author's clinic, HBO is administered at 1.5 ATA for 45 minutes for non-CNS tumors and 2.0 ATA for 30 minutes for CNS tumors. When combining HBO with chemotherapy to potentially increase the efficacy of chemotherapy, the HBO is administered according to the chemotherapy protocol schedule for the cancer on the same day as chemotherapy. HBO is administered first, and chemotherapy administered within 30 minutes of completion of HBO. When using HBO for palliation of inflammation and pain, this author treats for five consecutive days, then one to two times per week for four weeks, then every two to four weeks depending on patient response.

Several hyperbaric companies and chambers exist including Hyperbaric Veterinary Medicine and Sechrist Veterinary Health. Advanced training and certification as a Hyperbaric Technologist Veterinary® (CHT-V®) is now offered through the Veterinary Hyperbaric Association®.

Cannabis and Cannabidiol (CBD) Oil

Cannabis is a generic word used to describe plants from the genus *Cannabis*, as well as the bioactive substances derived from these plants. *Cannabis sativa L* is commonly known as marijuana. These strains are more stimulating and uplifting, whereas strains of *Cannabis indica* cause more calming or relaxing effects. Cannabis plants contain more than 400 bioactive metabolites including phytocannabinoids, terpenoids, and flavonoids. Terpenoids give the plant its aroma, while flavonoids comprise the largest category of plant-based antioxidants found in plants. The two most widely studied extracts of the phytocannabinoids from *Cannabis sativa* are delta-9 tetrahydrocannabinol (THC) and cannabidiol (CBD). CBD is thought to have a greater potential value for medicinal purposes than THC due to lack of psychoactive properties. CBD has been found to temper the toxicity of THC by reducing its psychoactivity. Cannabis contains other phytocannabinoids that have their own benefits, each of which will work in concert with the other compounds to create a medical benefit. This combined interactive effect is known as the "entourage effect." This effect is why it is believed that using the whole plant works better than pharmaceutically isolating a fraction of the plant.

Two cannabinoid receptors have been identified, cannabinoid receptor type 1 (CB1) and cannabinoid receptor type 2 (CB2). These cannibinoid receptors have been identified in all areas of the human brain and peripheral nervous system (Kleckner et al. 2019). THC directly binds to CB1 and CB2. CBD does not bind to CB1 and CB2, but rather blocks the fatty-acid binding protein that transports endogenous cannabinoids (endocannabinoids) to be hydrolyzed, thereby prolonging the activation of the CB1 receptor. One of the major mechanisms by which cannabinoids can elicit a therapeutic response is via the immune response. Endocannabinoids (cannabinoids produced in the body) are produced as part of the innate immune response, and monocytes, B cells, T cells, and other immune cells all have cannabinoid receptors. In cancer, the endocannabinoid system is altered in numerous types of tumors and can relate to cancer prognosis and outcome. Cannabinoids display anticancer effects in several models by suppressing proliferation, migrations, and/or invasion of cancer cells as well as tumor antiangiogenesis. Dysregulation of the endocannabinoid system can occur in cancer and may include variation in the expression and/or function of cannabinoid receptors as well as alterations in the concentration of endocannibinoids. Terpenes and flavonoids also exhibit cytotoxicity against a variety of cancers (Tomko et al. 2020). Cancer and its treatments often lead to systemic elevated inflammation responsible for chemotherapy-induced symptoms including fatigue, neuropathy, and cognitive deficiencies. Cannabis is a promising approach to symptom management for human cancer patients. Although there still exists a dearth of research in human patients with cancer, there is an increasing body of evidence in humans to suggest that cannabis relieves chemotherapy-induced nausea and vomiting, relieves cancer-related chronic and neuropathic pain, reduces

chemotherapy-induced peripheral neuropathy and associated symptoms, and reduces chemotherapy-induced GI distress such as bloating, cramps, flatulence, and abdominal pain. Additionally, minimal drug–drug interactions have been reported, reported side effects tend to be mild (lethargy), and very preliminary research indicates that cannabinoids tend to have anticancer rather than procancer effects (Kleckner et al. 2019).

Cannabis is quickly becoming a popular treatment option for owners to consider for their pets with chronic illness, including cancer. With marijuana legalized for both medicinal and recreational use in multiple states, many pet owners are inquiring about the use of cannabis for their pet with cancer. At the time of this writing, medical marijuana is not legalized at the federal level, and the THC in marijuana is considered a class I controlled substance by the Drug Enforcement Agency. Therefore, true marijuana is not considered legal in any state for veterinarians to prescribe or dispense even if legalized for medicinal or recreational use in humans. The non-psychotropic fractions (i.e. phytocannabinoids and terpenes) of marijuana are not illegal and can be dispensed or prescribed in any state, as long as the product is derived from the legally grown industrial hemp plant. Industrial hemp has less than 0.3% THC on a dry-matter basis as determined by an analysis of the plant material at harvest. Hemp can be concentrated as an extract oil made from the 0.3% THC dry-matter plant material. This is called "hemp oil." Hemp oil is not to be confused with hemp SEED oil, which is from the seed and primarily contains omega-3 and omega-6 fatty acids and does not contain CBDs or THC in any substantial amount. For legal reasons, the scope of the remaining discussion and recommendations will be regarding these products known as CBD oil or hemp oil (Silver 2015).

Much of the research on CBD oil to date has been in humans or laboratory animal species and not domestic pet species. However, recent studies in dogs have shown positive benefits with the use of CBD oil. CBD oil when given to dogs with osteoarthritis has been shown to decrease pain and improve activity (Gamble et al. 2018; Verrichio et al. 2020). CBD oil when used in addition to conventional antiseizure medications can reduce the frequency of seizures in dogs with intractable epilepsy (McGrath et al. 2019). The effective dosage of cannabinoids in pets for specific conditions has not been well defined. Randomized, placebo-controlled studies are needed to define these dosages. Safe and effective doses as well as increased information on the biological activity of specific strains of cannabis are needed. Additionally, information regarding interactions of CBD oil with other drugs or herbs is also needed as CBD oil is rarely a stand-alone therapy. In the meantime, medication with cannabinoids is done cautiously, starting with a lower dosage and gradually working up to a higher dosage that is effective for the treated condition. In laboratory and human studies, dosages for CBDs range from 0.1 to 10 mg/kg/day. In dogs with osteoarthritis, a 2 mg/kg dose b.i.d. was found to be effective in decreasing pain (Verrichio et al. 2020), and in dogs with refractory seizures a dose of 2.5 mg/kg b.i.d. was found to decrease seizure activity (McGrath et al. 2019). A recent pharmacokinetic study in dogs shows CBD oil to be tolerated up to 62 mg/kg/day with only mild adverse events of lethargy and hypothermia, although effective doses are likely to be much lower and more cost effective (Vaughn et al. 2020).

This author uses CBD commonly as an adjunct in veterinary cancer patients to support overall well-being, treat cancer pain, reduce side effects of chemotherapy and/or radiation therapy, and for potential anticancer effects. Anecdotal evidence suggests CBD oil to be safe in combination with conventional medications and most herbs. This author has not found CBD oil to be as helpful in directly stimulating appetite. However, CBD oil can improve weight gain and food consumption indirectly in some patients by reducing pain (which can cause appetite loss) and providing a better sense of overall well-being in the patient. In the cancer patient the dose is started at 0.25–0.5 mg/kg b.i.d. and gradually increased by 25% every seven days until desired effect is achieved (pain relief, nausea/vomiting relief, improved appetite) to a total dose of 2.5 mg/kg b.i.d. or until side effects occur (generally lethargy). As there appears to be a wide safety margin for dosage of CBD oil, doses higher than 2.5 mg/kg b.i.d. can be considered, especially for cancer pain, as long as the dose is titrated gradually. Higher doses of CBD oil in larger breed dogs can be costly.

When recommending formulas or products to owners, I prefer to use liquid tinctures and extracts of hemp oil. These formulas are easy to measure dosage accurately, especially for small dogs, cats, and pocket pets. Liquid products also are ideal for starting the dose low and increasing the dose incrementally based on how the patient is responding to therapy. Dog Treats are generally a very low dose of CBD oil (2.0–5.0 mg) and a considerable number of treats may be needed to achieve higher effective doses, particularly in large breed dogs. Cats will often not eat treats or chews. Capsules can be used for cats but are hard to titrate to more effective dose slowly. Use of human edibles is discouraged as the dosing can be difficult to control and can contain products that are toxic to pets (nuts, raisins, chocolate). There are many different products on the market, many of which are not closely regulated and may contain low levels of CBD or higher than normal levels of THC or heavy metals, which can be toxic to pets. In the human cannabis market, ratios of the bioactive compounds vary between plant strains and growth conditions, and this can potentially effect therapeutic benefits and cause unpredictable side effects even with repeat purchasing of the same product. Pharmaceutical companies and medical marijuana growers produce medicinal preparations with specific THC:CBD ratios (e.g. 1:1; 1:20). This author prefers to use CBD products where veterinarians have been involved in the formulation and development of the product such as VetCBD, Rx Vitamins Hemp, Dr. Jyl's PetnPeople Hemp Spray, Shampoo, and Drops, and CompanionCBD. Third party certification is also vital to ensuring a quality product is used.

Essential Oils

Aromatherapy, or essential oil therapy, is the use of a plant's aroma-producing oils to treat disease. The essential oils are taken from a plant's leaves, flowers, bark, stalk, rind, or roots. The oils are then mixed with a base such as oil, alcohol, or lotion. The oils can be diffused and inhaled, ingested, or placed topically on the skin. Aromatherapy as practiced today originated in Europe and has been in use since the early 1900s. It is believed that the fragrance in the oils stimulates olfactory nerves in the nose that send impulses to the part of the brain involved in memory and emotion. Depending on the oil, the effect can be either calming or stimulating. The oils are also believed to interact with hormones and enzymes to cause changes in blood pressure, pulse rate, breathing and emotional responses and can stimulate production of endorphins.

Several essential oils have been shown to exert anticancer activity in *in vitro* studies of human cancer cell lines including cinnamon for head and neck squamous cell carcinoma (Yang et al. 2015), *Boswellia sacra* in breast cancer (Suhail et al. 2011), *Croton tiglium* in lung cancer (Niu et al. 2020), and *Salvia officinalis* in colon cancer (Luca et al. 2020). Essential oils have also been used to treat the side effects of cancer and cancer treatment. Topical frankincense essential oil improved cancer-related fatigue in a human patient (Reis and Throne Jones 2018). Inhaled ginger aromatherapy showed improvement in nausea score in women with breast cancer undergoing chemotherapy, although not in incidence of vomiting. However, ginger essential oil inhalation significantly improved role functioning and appetite loss from baseline (Lua et al. 2015).

Lavender oil aromatherapy improved sleep quality as well as trait anxiety values in human patients undergoing chemotherapy (Ozkaraman et al. 2018). Other benefits of essential oils to cancer patients include relief of emotional stress, pain, muscular tension, and fatigue (Fellowes et al. 2004). A systematic review of essential oils in human patients suggests a short-term benefit to reduce anxiety and depression, improve sleep, and increase overall well-being, this effect has been suggested to last up to two weeks (Boehm et al. 2012). Single oils that have been used in the cancer patient include frankincense, grapefruit, lemon, orange, palo santo, sandalwood, copaiba, and lavender. Lavender is an incredibly mild oil that is well suited for use in all species of animals. It can be used for a variety of ailments, including skin conditions, but is well known for its calming effects. Essential oils can be used in the veterinary cancer patient to help reduce pain and inflammation (marjoram, clary sage, clove, thyme, chamomile, sandalwood, lavender), support emotional well-being (frankincense, lavender, citrus oils, peppermint, clary sage, and cedarwood), and reduce side effects of chemotherapy or cancer such as appetite loss (peppermint, oregano, bergamot, ginger, tangerine), vomiting, nausea (peppermint, ginger, tarragon, lemongrass), and diarrhea (peppermint and chamomile).

When using aromatherapy for any medical condition, it is important to use 100% pure, medical grade oils. Quality essential oils should list the Latin name of the plant, information on purity (100% essential oils with no fillers), and the country in which the plant was grown. Pure essential oils are very concentrated and will break down plastic bottles over time, tainting the oil. Most companies will package essential oils in brown or blue glass bottles to preserve the quality of the oils. Fragrance or perfume oils contain chemicals and are not suitable for aromatherapy. It is important to note that many essential oils have to be diluted to avoid sensitivities or toxicity. Examples of reputable essential oils include those from

Young Living, doTerra, and animalEO, the line of essential oils for animals created by Melissa Shelton, DVM.

There are various methods of the application of essential oils for animals include diffusing (inhaled), topical through petting technique, raindrop technique, or water misting technique, and oral administration. Essential oils can be added to drinking water, mixed with food, or administrated orally via capsules, buccal route, or oral drops. Modifications to techniques may need to be considered for different species of animals and individual patients depending on need and tolerability. More detailed information on the use of essential oils can be found in the *Essential Oils Desk Reference and The Animal Desk Reference: Essential Oils for Animals* by Melissa Shelton, DVM.

Homeopathy and Homotoxicology

Homeopathy is a branch of alternative medicine that is based on the theory that "like cures like," the notion that a disease can be cured by giving small amounts of a substance that causes similar symptoms in healthy individuals. Homeopathic remedies are made from natural substances such as plants (red onion, poison ivy, arnica), minerals (sulfur, arsenic), and animals (crushed honeybees). Classical homeopathy is an exacting practice in which single remedies are selected based on careful observation of a patient's symptoms. This method of remedy selection is called "proving." The remedy selected will be the one that has the most similar symptoms to that of the patient. It takes careful observation and skill for the practitioner to be able to select the appropriate remedy. Once the appropriate remedy is selected, the degree of dilution needs to be determined, which also requires skill. Homeopathy is also based on the "law of minimum dose," which suggests that the lower the dose of the medication, the greater its effectiveness. These substances are weakened or diluted with water or alcohol. The mixture is

then shaken as part of a process called "potentization," which is believed to transfer the healing essence. Many homeopathic medications are so diluted that no molecules of the original substance remain.

Homotoxicology is a "bridge" between classical homeopathy and modern allopathic medicine. Homotoxicology uses remedies based on the syndrome or indication of the patient. Most anti-homotoxic preparations are combinations of remedies in the low to middle ranges of dilution. Each preparation carries an indication, so there is no need to determine the remedy from a variety of preparations or the potency (dilution). Homotoxins include all the substances (chemical or biochemical) and nonmaterial influences that can cause illness in a patient. These homotoxins result in regulation disorders in the patient. Every illness is due to the effects of these homotoxins. Homotoxins may be produced from the environment (exogenous) or within the body (endogenous). In homotoxicology, cancer is viewed as the body's expression of accumulated homotoxins and the damage that has been done to normally functioning systems. This represents the outcome of dedifferentiation phase disease. The homotoxicology remedies are developed to restore regulation (balance) of the body.

Homeopathy has grown in popularity in both human and veterinary medicine for treating cancer. Homeopathy, with a prevalence of 30.7%, is the most used complementary medicine in integrative oncology in Strasbourg, France, with an increase in use of 83% in a 12 year span. Fatigue, pain, nausea, anxiety, sadness, and diarrhea were improved with the use of homeopathy in 80% of patients (Bagot et al. 2021). Limited *in vitro* research has suggested that homeopathic remedies appear to cause cellular changes in some cancer cells. For example, *Lycopodium clavatum* has been shown to induce apoptosis in cancer cells *in vitro* (Samadder et al. 2013). Calcarea carbonica induces apoptosis in cancer bearing mice via by modulating the immune system of the host

(Saha et al. 2013). Homeopathic remedies were shown to significantly slow the progression of cancer and reduce cancer incidence and mortality in a rat model of prostate cancer (Jonas et al. 2006). Clinical studies of homeopathic remedies combined with conventional care have shown that homeopathic remedies improve quality of life, reduce symptoms, and possibly improve survival in patients with cancer (Frenkel 2015). Arnica was successful in reducing postoperative seroma and bleeding in women undergoing unilateral mastectomy for breast cancer (Sorrentino et al. 2017). Individualized homeopathy was successful in inducing remission in three human patients with mycosis fungoides (Nwabudike 2019). Homeopathic treatment as an add on therapy was shown to significantly improve quality of life as well as improved survival (possibly due to improved quality of life) in patients with Stage IV non-small cell lung cancer (Frass et al. 2020).

In veterinary patients, homeopathy can be used as part of a multimodality approach and is safe to use in combination with conventional therapies (surgery, radiation, chemotherapy). Homotoxicology contains many useful agents for improving general well-being in the cancer patient. As the risk for serious side effects are low with antihomotoxic therapy, clients may readily accept this form of therapy to palliate their pet with cancer. Most antihomotoxic protocols use a mixture of Galium-Heel, lymphomyosot, Hepar Compositum, Solidago compositum, Tonsilla compositum and/or Thyrodiea compositum, Coenzyme Compositum, and Ubichinon Compositum. This combination of antihomotoxic remedies is commonly referred to as the modified deep detoxification formula and assists cases in the dedifferentiation phase. This formula should be started out slowly, using twice weekly for two weeks. If the patient's symptoms improve, the formula can be continued at this level or given orally every other day. If the patient develops excessive signs of homotoxin off-loading (diarrhea, vomiting, nasal, aural, or ocular discharge or coughing), then reduce the dose or stop entirely for several days. Berberis homaccord

should be considered daily in cancer patients. Berberis homaccord helps support the adrenal glands, liver, gallbladder, renal tubules, and colon from the daily bombardment from homotoxins. Berberis homaccord contains *Viscum album* to support the dedifferentiation phase condition. This agent can be added to any cancer protocol with good effect. Symptom remedies are used to manage signs that arise during therapy. The simplest approach is to note the main symptoms and research them in the *Biotherapeutic Index* and then select the agents that assist that symptom and reevaluate the patient (excerpted in part from Goldstein et al. 2008). A Tonsilla Compositum and Ubichinon Compositum combined injection can be used to inject into subcutaneous hemangiosarcoma and osteosarcoma to good effect. Administer 0.5 cc of each into a tumor every two weeks. This protocol can cause partial or complete regression of tumors in some patients (Rick Palmquist, personal communication). For more advanced homotoxicology protocols for individual tumor types, the clinician is referred to Dr. Goldstein's book *Integrating Complementary Medicine into Veterinary Practice*. Training in *classical* homeopathy is provided by the Pitcairn Institute of Veterinary Homeopathy. Certification can then be achieved through the Academy of Veterinary Homeopathy. Training in veterinary Homotoxicology can be obtained through the College of Integrative Veterinary Therapies.

Chiropractic

Chiropractic therapy is a treatment that focuses on the musculoskeletal system and the connection to the nervous system. Treatment generally involves manual therapy from stretching and sustained pressure, specific joint manipulations, and spinal manipulations. These manipulations are done by hand and consist of a quick and gentle thrust. Manipulations are most commonly done on the spine but can be done on other parts of the body. The goal of the manipulations is to improve joint motion and function, correct misalignments, ease pain, and improve mobility and performance. In addition to spinal and joint manipulations, chiropractic care may also incorporate other treatments such as laser therapy, electrostimulation, rehabilitation and exercise, and nutritional counseling. Veterinary chiropractic has become a fast- developing field in animal alternative therapy, and certification programs exist through both the American Veterinary Chiropractic Association and the International Veterinary Chiropractic Association.

Veterinary chiropractic care is most often sought by owners for their pet with musculoskeletal symptoms. Cancer patients can have multiple comorbidities including musculoskeletal symptoms such as back pain, degenerative arthritis, and/or joint pain. Additionally, pain can be a symptom of both the cancer and treatment, and a proportion of patients may not have significant pain relief with conventional therapies. However, it is important to recognize that certain cancers such as lung cancer, myeloma, and osteosarcoma may present with musculoskeletal symptoms. Caution should be exercised in performing spinal manipulative therapy in these patients. In humans, chiropractic care is one of the leading alternatives to standard medical treatment in cancer pain management (Evans and Rosner 2005). In a survey of European chiropractors, the panel of chiropractors agreed unanimously that the role of chiropractic treatment in patients with cancer could help with pain relief, empathy, mobility, energy levels, quality of life, sleeping patterns, and function (Laoudikou and McCarthy 2020). Similar effects/benefits would be expected in veterinary cancer patients with the use of chiropractic care.

Photobiomodulation Therapy (PBM)

Photobiomodulation therapy (PBM) is a form of light therapy that utilizes nonionizing forms of light sources including lasers, LEDS (light emitting diodes), or broadband light in the visible and infrared spectrum. The nonthermal photons of light produced from the laser pass through the skin layers and subcutaneous tissues. Once the light passes through the skin and reaches the tissue, the light is absorbed and interacts with the light-sensitive components in the cell. When the cells absorb this light, it initializes a series of events in the cell that can result in normalizing damaged or injured tissue, reduce pain and inflammation, reduce edema, and reduce healing time (Martin 2003). This laser therapy is often referred to as "cold laser therapy" because the low level of light is not enough to significantly heat the tissues compared with other forms of laser therapy such as surgical lasers. Traditionally, cold laser therapy has referred to the treatment that has utilized the Class IIIB and Class IV lasers, which emit power output of 60–200 and 500 mW, respectively. The power of these lasers requires eye protection when in use. Although the Class IIIB and Class IV lasers have been beneficial in treatment of musculoskeletal injuries and pain, there is some heat produced that can be detrimental to certain fragile healing tissues. Additionally, cold laser therapy is contraindicated in the cancer patient because the vasodilation effects and potential for increased blood flow can contribute to progression or growth of the cancer.

Low-level laser therapy (LLLT) or frequency-specific low-level laser therapy (FSLLLT) refers to treatment with lasers of much lower power, with output of 5–7.5 mW, depending on the device used. These lasers are considered Class II and produce wavelengths of light in the visible light spectrum at 635 or 405 nm, depending on the device. As the light produced is in the visible light spectrum, no protective eyewear is needed. The potential advantage of LLLT is the ability to decrease pain and inflammation, increase circulation and lymphatic drainage, and generate stem cells that can aid in regeneration of nerve and other tissues. Studies in humans have shown benefit in treatment of cancer-related toxicities including breast cancer-related lymphedema, oral mucositis, radiation-induced dermatitis, and chemotherapy-related peripheral neuropathy. LLLT demonstrated significant benefits for relieving symptoms and improvement of emotional distress in breast cancer patients with lymphedema (Kilmartin et al. 2020). In the treatment of oral mucositis, there is moderate evidence that LLLT is effective in resolving oral mucositis lesions in adult patients undergoing cancer therapy and that LLLT demonstrates potential for decreasing the resolution time of such lesions by as much as 4.21 days (Anschau et al. 2019).

One of the challenges in the acceptance of LLLT use in cancer patients is whether or not there is potential for the light effects to stimulate the growth of other residual tumor cells that have evaded treatment, resulting in tumor recurrences or progression/growth of gross nonresectable tumors. A systematic review in humans evaluating the tumor safety and side effects of LLLT in management of cancer treatment toxicities found this treatment did not lead to the development of tumor safety issues and that most studies showed no side effects observed with the use of LLLT (De Pauli Paglioni et al. 2019). A case series in dogs demonstrated the use of FPLLLT as palliative care for cancer. All dogs had improvement in quality of life with reduction of cancer-related symptoms, with some having temporary

reduction in tumor burden as well (Grognet and Janes 2014).

Based on current information, this author does not advocate the use of Class IIIB and Class IV lasers in cancer patients. The use of FSLLT to treat cancer-related toxicities has shown promise in humans with demonstration of minimal to no side effects and no development of tumor safety issues. Use of FSLLT, although promising, should be used with caution in veterinary cancer patients until more information on benefit and risk is assessed.

Summary

The use of CAM for palliation of veterinary cancer patients offers many options for improving comfort and quality of life for the patient and potentially improving survival time. Many modalities of CAM can be used safely together, as well as adjunctly to conventional cancer therapies. Which modality or modalities to use can be individualized for each patient and family based on factors such as cost, treatment time and frequency, receptivity of the patient, availability of equipment/supplies, and training/experience of the practitioner.

References

Aghabati, N., Mohammadi, E., and Esmaiel, Z.P. (2010) The effect of therapeutic touch on pain and fatigue of cancer patients undergoing chemotherapy. *eCAM* 7(3): 375–381.

Anschau, F., Webster, J., Zanella Capra, M.E. et al. (2019) Efficacy of low-level laser for teatment of cancer oral mucositis: a systematic review and meta-analysis. *Lasers Med. Sci.*, 34(6): 1053–1062.

Bagot, J-L., Legrand A.,Theunissen I. (2021) Use of homeopathy in integrative oncology in Strasbourg, France: multi-center cross-sectional descriptive study of patients undergoing cancer treatment. *Homeopathy*, 110(3): 168–173.

Bocci, V., Larini, A., and Micheli, V. (2005) Restoration of normoxia by ozone therapy may control neoplastic growth: a review and a working hypothesis. *J. Altern. Complement. Med.*, 11(2): 257–265.

Boehm, K., Bussing A., Ostermann, T. (2012) Aromatherapy as an adjuvant treatment in cancer care – a descriptive systematic review. *Afr. J. Tradit. Complement. Altern. Med.*, 9(4): 503–518.

Boyd, C., Crawford, C., Paat, C.F. et al. (2016) The impact of massage therapy on function in pain populations – a systematic review and meta-analysis of randomized controlled trials: part II, cancer pain populations. *Pain Med.*, 17(8): 1553–1568.

Brown, D.C., Reetz, J. (2012) Single agent polysaccharopeptide delays metastases and improves survival in naturally occurring hemangiosarcoma. *Evid. Based Complement. Alternat. Med.*, 2012: 384301. https://doi.org/10.1155/2012/384301. Epub 2012 Sep 5. PMID: 22988473; PMCID: PMC3440946.

Campigotto, G., Alba, D.F., Sulzbach, M.M. et al. (2020) Dog food production using curcumin as antioxidant: effects of intake on animal growth, health and feed conservation. *Arch. Anim. Nutr.*, 74(5): 397–413. https://doi.org/10.1080/1745039X.2020.1769442. Epub 2020 Jun 30. PMID: 32602378.

Chen, X., Jiang, Y., Zhang, Y. et al. (2020) Effect of ozone oil for prevention and treatment of sorafenib-induced hand-foot skin reactions: a randomized controlled trial. *Nan Fang Yi Ke Da Xue Xue Bao*, 40(10): 1488–1492.

Choi, K.H. and Flynn, K. (2017) Korean sa-ahm acupuncture for treating canine oral fibrosarcoma. *J. Acupunct. Meridian Stud.*, 3: 211–215.

Ciboroski, M., Lipska, A., Godzien, J. et al. (2012) Combination of LC-MS-and GC-MS metabolomics to study the effect of ozonated autohemotherapy on human blood. *J. Proteome Res.*, 11(12): 6231–6241.

Clavo, B., Gutierrez, D., Martin, D. et al. (2005) Intravesical ozone therapy for progressive radiation-induced hematuria *J. Altern. Complement. Med.*, 11(3): 539–541.

Clavo, B., Ceballos, D., Gutierrez, D. et al. (2013) Long term control of refractory hemorrhagic radiation proctitis with ozone therapy. *J. Pain Symptom Manage.*, 46(1): 106–112.

Clavo, B., Navarro, M., Federico M., et al. (2021) Long term results with adjuvant ozone therapy in the management of chronic pelvic pain secondary to cancer treatment. *Pain Med.* (22)9: 2138–2141.

Collinge, W., Kahn, J., Walton, T. et al. (2013) Touch, caring and cancer: randomized controlled trial of a multimedia caregiver education program. *Support. Care Cancer*, 21(5): 1405–1414.

Daenen, L.G., Cirkel G.A, Houthuijzen, J.M. *et al.* (2015) Increased plasma levels of chemoresistance-inducing fatty acid 16:4(n-3) after consumption of fish and fish oil. *JAMA Oncol.*, 1(3): 350–358. https://doi.org/10.1001/jamaoncol.2015.0388. PMID: 26181186.

Daruwalla, J. and Christophi, C. (2006) The effect of hyperbaric oxygen therapy on tumour growth in a mouse model of colorectal cancer metastases. *Eur. J. Cancer*, 42(18): 3304–3311.

Dhillon, N., Aggarwal, B.B., Newman, R.A. et al. (2008) Phase II trial of curcumin in patients with advanced pancreatic cancer. *Clin. Cancer Res.*, 14(14): 4491–4499. https://doi.org/10.1158/1078-0432.CCR-08-0024. PMID: 18628464.

Evans, R.C. and Rosner, A.L. (2005) Alternatives in cancer pain treatment: the application of chiropractic care. *Semin. Oncol. Nurs.*, 21(3): 184–189.

Fellowes, D., Barnes, K., and Wilkinson, S. (2004) Aromatherapy and massage for symptom relief in patients with cancer. *Cochrane Database Syst. Rev.*, Issue 3: CD002287. https://doi.org/10.1002/14651858.CD002287.pub2.

Fine, E.J., Segal-Isaacson, C.J., Feinman, R.D. *et al.* (2012) Targeting insulin inhibition as a metabolic therapy in advanced cancer: a pilot safety and feasibility dietary trial in 10 patients. *Nutrition*, 28(10): 1028–1035.

Frass, M., Lechleitner, P., Grundling, C. et al. (2020) Homeopathic treatment as an add-on therapy may improve quality of life and prolong survival in patients with non-small cell lung cancer: a prospective, randomized, placebo-controlled, double blind, three-arm, multicenter study. *Oncologist*, 25(12): e1930–e1955.

Frenkel, M. (2015) Is there a role for homeopathy in cancer care? Questions and challenges. *Curr. Oncol. Rep.*, 17(9): 43.

Gamble, L.-J., Boesch, J.M., Frye, C.W. et al. (2018) Pharmacokinetics, safety, and clinical efficacy of cannabidiol treatment in osteoarthritic dogs. *Front. Vet. Sci.*, 5: 165. Published online 2018 Jul 23. https://doi.org/10.3389/fvets.2018.00165.

Goldsby, T.L, Goldsby, M.E., McWalters, M., et al. (2017) Effects of singing bowl sound meditation on mood, tension, and well-being:

an observational study. *J. Evid. Based Complement. Altern. Med.*, 22(3): 401–406.

Goldstein, Broadfoot, Palmquist, Johnston, Wen, Fougere and Roman. (2008) Integrating Complementary Medicine into Veterinary Practice, Wiley-Blackwell.

Grognet J. and Janes L. (2014) Palliative cancer care using frequency-specific low level laser therapy: four case reports. *JAHVMA*, 35: 28–34.

Guven, D.C., Aktas, B.Y., Simsek, C., et al. (2020) Gut microbiota and cancer immunotherapy: prognostic and therapeutic implications. *Future Oncol.*, 16(9): 497–506. https://doi.org/10.2217/fon-2019-0783. Epub 2020 Feb 26. PMID: 32100550.

Ha Jee, S., Ohrr, H., Sull, J. W. et al (2005) Fasting serum glucose level and cancer risk in Korean men and women. *JAMA*, 293(2): 194–202.

Jeitler, M., Michalsen, A., Frings, D. et al. (2020). Significance of medicinal mushrooms in integrative oncology: a narrative review. *Front. Pharmacol.*, 11: 580656. https://doi.org/10.3389/fphar.2020.580656. PMID: 33424591; PMCID: PMC7794004.

Jing, K., Wu, T., and Lim, K. (2013) Omega-3 polyunsaturated fatty acids and cancer. *Anticancer Agents Med. Chem.*, 13(8): 1162–1177. https://doi.org/10.2174/18715206113139990319. PMID: 23919748.

Jonas, W.B., Gaddipati, J.P., and Rajeshkumar, N.V. et al. (2006) Can homeopathic treatment slow prostate cancer growth? *Integr. Cancer Ther.*, 5(4): 343–349.

Kawasoe, Y., Yokouchi, M., Ueno, Y. et al. (2009) Hyperbaric oxygen therapy as a chemotherapy adjuvant in the treatment of osteosarcoma. *Oncol. Rep.*, 22(5): 1045–1050.

Kilmartin, L., Denham, T., Fu, M.R. et al. (2020) Complementary low-level laser therapy for breast cancer-related lymphedema: a pilot, double-blind, randomized, placebo-controlled study. *Lasers Med. Sci.*, 35(1): 95–106.

Kinkead, B., Schettler P.J., Larson, E.R. et al. (2018) Massage therapy decreases cancer-related fatigue: results from a randomized early phase trial. *Cancer*, 124(3): 546–554.

Kleckner, A.S., Kleckner, I.R., Kamen, C.S. et al. (2019) Opportunities for cannabis in supportive care in cancer. *Ther. Adv. Med. Oncol.*, https://doi.org/10.1177/1758835919866362.

Kroemer, G. and Zitvogel, L. (2018) Cancer immunotherapy in 2017: the breakthrough of the microbiota. *Nat. Rev. Immunol.*, 18(2): 87–88. https://doi.org/10.1038/nri.2018.4. PMID: 29379189.

Ladas, E.J., Karlick, J.B., Rooney, D. et al. (2012) Topical Yunnan Baiyao administration as an adjunctive therapy for bleeding complications in adolescents with advanced cancer. *Support Care Cancer*, 20(12): 3379–3383.

Landry, J.M. (2014). Physiological and psychological effects of a himalayan singing bowl in meditation practice: a quantitative analysis. *Am. J. Health Promot.*, 28(5): 306–309.

Laoudikou, M.T.and McCarthy, P.W. (2020) Patients with cancer. Is there a role for chiropractic? *J. Can Chiropr. Assoc.*, 64(1): 32–42.

Lee, S-H., Kim J.-Y., and Yeo S. et al. (2015) Meta-analysis of massage therapy on cancer pain. *Integr. Cancer Ther.*, 14(4): 297–304.

Lua, P.L, Salihah, N., and Mazlan, N. (2015) Effects of inhaled ginger aromatherapy on chemotherapy-induced nausea and vomiting and health-related quality of life in women with breast cancer. *Complement. Ther. Med.*, 23(3): 396–404.

Luca, T., Napoli E., Privitera G. et al. (2020) Antiproliferative effect and cell cycle alterations induced by salvia officinalis essential oil and its three main components in human colon cancer cell lines. *Chem. Biodivers.*, 17(8): e2000309. https://doi.org/10.1002/cbdv.202000309. Epub 2020 Jul27.

Martin, R. (2003) Laser- accelerated inflammation/pain reduction and healing. *Pract. Pain Manage*, 3(6): 20–25.

McGrath, S., Bartner, L.R., and Rao, S. et al. (2019) Randomized blinded controlled clinical trial to assess the effect of oral cannabidiol administration in addition to conventional antiepileptic treatment on seizure frequency in dogs with intractable idiopathic epilepsy. *JAVMA*, https://doi.org/10.2460/javma.254.11.1301.

Murphy, R.A., Mourtzakis, M., and Chu, Q.S. et al. (2011) Supplementation with fish oil increases first-line chemotherapy efficacy in patients with advanced nonsmall cell lung cancer. *Cancer*, 117(16): 3774–3780. https://doi.org/10.1002/cncr.25933. Epub 2011 Feb 15. PMID: 21328326.

Negri, M., Gentile, A., de Angelis, C. et al. (2020) Vitamin D-induced molecular mechanisms to potentiate cancer therapy and to reverse drug-resistance in cancer cells. *Nutrients*, 12(6): 1798. https://doi.org/10.3390/nu12061798. PMID: 32560347; PMCID: PMC7353389.

Niu, Q-L., Sun H., Liu C. et al. (2020) Croton tiglium essential oil compounds have anti-proliferative and pro-apoptotoic effects in A549 lung cancer cell lines. *PLoS One*,15(5): e0231437.https://doi.org/10.1371/journal.pone.0231437.

Nwabudike, L.C. (2019) Homeopathy as therapy for mycosis fungoides: case reports of 3 patients. *Homeopathy*, 108(4): 277–284.

Ozkaraman, A., Dugum O., Ozen Yilmaz H. et al. (2018) Aromatherapy: the effect of lavender on anxiety and sleep quality in patients treated with chemotherapy. *Clin. J. Oncol. Nurs.*, 22(2): 203–210.

de Pauli Paglioni, M., Damaceno Araujo, A.L., Aristizabal Arboleda, L.P. et al. (2019) Tumor safety and side effects of photobiomodulation therapy used for prevention and management of cancer treatment toxicities. A systematic review. *Oral Oncol.*, 93:21–28.

Poff, A.M., Ari, C., Seyfried, T.N. et al; (2013). The ketogenic diet and hyperbaric oxygen therapy prolong survival in mice with systemic metastatic cancer. *PLoS One*, 8(6): e65522. https://doi.org/10.1371/journal.pone.0065522.

Redman, M.G., Ward, E.J., and Phillips, R.S. (2014) The efficacy and safety of probiotics in people with cancer: a systematic review. *Ann. Oncol.*, 25(10): 1919–1929. https://doi.org/10.1093/annonc/mdu106. Epub 2014 Mar 11. PMID: 24618152.

Reis, D. and Throne Jones, T. (2018) Frankincense essential oil as a supportive therapy for cancer-related fatigue: a case study. *Holist. Nurs. Pract.*, 32(3): 140–142.

Ripamonti, C.I., Cislaghi, E., Mariani, L., Maniezzo, M. (2011) Efficacy and safety of medical ozone (O(3)) delivered in oil suspension applications for the treatment of osteonecrosis of the jaw in patients with bone metastases treated with bisphosphonates: Preliminary results of a phase I-II study. *Oral Oncol.*, 47(3):185-90. doi: 10.1016/j.oraloncology.2011.01.002. PMID: 21310650.

Ripamonti, C.I., Maniezzo, M., Boldini S., Pessi M.A., Mariani, L., Cislaghi, E. (2012) Efficacy and tolerability of medical ozone gas insufflations in patients with osteonecrosis of the jaw treated with bisphosphonates-Preliminary data: Medical ozone gas insufflation in treating ONJ lesions. *J. Bone Oncol.*, 24;1(3):81-7. doi: 10.1016/j.jbo.2012.08.001. PMID: 26909261; PMCID: PMC4723354.

Rose, W.J., Sargeant J.M., Hanna, W.J.B. et al. (2017) A scoping review of the evidence for efficacy of acupuncture in companion animals. *Anim. Health Res. Rev.*, 2: 177–185.

Saha S., Hossain, D. M.S., Mukherkee S. et al. (2013).Calcarea carbonica induces apoptosis in cancer cells in p53-dependent manner via an immuno-modulatory circuit. *BMC Complement. Altern. Med.*, 13: 230. https://doi.org/10.1186/1472-6882-13-230. PMID: 24053127; PMCID: PMC3856502.

Samadder A., Das S., Das J. et al. (2013) The potentized homeopathic drug, lycopodium clavatum (5C and 15C) has anti-cancer effect on hela cells in vitro. *J. Acupunct. Meridian Stud.*, 6(4): 180–187.42.

Schmalberg, J., Xie H., and Memon M. (2019) Canine and feline patients referred exclusively for acupuncture and herbs: a two year retrospective analysis. *J. Acupunct. Meridian Stud.*, 5: 160–165.

Serra-Ano P., Ingles M., Bou-Catala C. et al. (2019) Effectiveness of myofascial release after breast cancer surgery in women undergoing conservative surgery and radiotherapy: a randomized controlled trial. *Support. Care Cancer*, 27(7): 2633–2641.

Shelton, M. (2012) The Animal Desk Reference Essential Oils for Animals. CreateSpace Independent Publishing Platform.

Shoba, G., Joy, D., Joseph, T. et al. (1998) Influence of piperine on the pharmacokinetics of curcumin in animals and human volunteers. *Planta Med.*, 64(4): 353–356. https://doi.org/10.1055/s-2006-957450. PMID: 9619120.

Silver, R.J. (2015). Medical marijuana and your pet: the definitive guide. Lulu Publishing Services.

Sorrentino L., Piraneo S., Riggio E. et al., (2017) Is there a role for homeopathy in breast cancer surgery? A first randomized clinical trial on treatment with Arnica Montana to reduce post-operative seroma and bleeding in patients undergoing total mastectomy. *J. Intercult. Ethnopharmacol.*, 6(1): 1–8.

Suhail, M.M., Wu, W., Cao, A. et al. (2011) Boswellia sacra essential oil induces tumor cell-specific apoptosis and suppresses tumor aggressiveness in cultured human breast cancer cells. *BMC Complement. Altern. Med.*, 11: 129.

Tabrez, S., Jabir, N.R., Khan, M.I. et al. (2020) Association of autoimmunity and cancer: an emphasis on proteolytic enzymes. *Semin. Cancer Biol.*, 64: 19–28. https://doi.org/10.1016/j.semcancer.2019.05.006. Epub 2019 May 14. PMID: 31100322.

Tan-Shalaby J. (2017) Ketogenic diets and cancer: emerging evidence. *Fed. Pract.*, 34(Suppl 1): 37S–42S.

Tirelli, U., Cirrito, C., Pavanello M. et al. (2018) Oxygen-ozone therapy as support and palliative therapy in 50 cancer patients with fatigue- a short eport. *Eur. Rev. Med. Pharmacol. Sci.*, 22(22): 8030–8033.

Tomko, A.M., Whynot, E.G., Ellis, L.D. et al. (2020) Anti-cancer potential of cannabinoids, terpenes, and flavonoids present in cannabis. *Cancer*, 12(7): 1985. Published online 2020 Jul 21. https://doi.org/10.3390/cancers12071985.

Tsang K.L., Carlson L.E. and Olson K. (2007) Pilot crossover trial of reiki versus rest for treating cancer-related fatigue. *Integr. Cancer Ther.*, (6)1: 25–35.

Vaughn, D., Kulpa, J., and Paulionis, L. (2020) Preliminary investigation of the safety of escalating cannabinoid doses in healthy dogs. *Front. Vet. Sci.*, Feb 11. https://doi.org/10.3389/fvets.2020.00051.

Verrichio, C.D., Wesson, S., Konduri, V. et al. (2020) A randomized, double-blind, placebo-controlled study of daily cannabidiol for the treatment of osteoarthritis pain. *Pain*, 161(9): 2191–2202.

Wang S., Long, S., Deng, Z. et al. (2020a) Positive role of chinese herbal medicine in cancer immune regulation. *Am. J. Chin. Med.*, 48(7): 1577–1592. https://doi.org/10.1142/S0192415X20500780. Epub 2020 Nov 13. PMID: 33202152.

Wang, Y., Zhang, Q., Chen, Y. et al. (2020b) Antitumor effects of immunity-enhancing traditional Chinese medicine. *Biomed. Pharmacother.*, 121: 109570. https://doi.org/10.1016/j.biopha.2019.109570. Epub 2019 Nov 9. PMID: 31710893.

Wasser, S.P. (2017) Medicinal mushrooms in human clinical studies. Part I. anticancer, oncoimmunological, and immunomodulatory activities: a review. *Int. J. Med. Mushrooms*, 19(4): 279–317. https://doi.org/10.1615/IntJMedMushrooms.v19.i4.10. PMID: 28605319.

Weber, D.D., Aminzadeh-Gohari, S., Tulipan, J. et al. (2020) Ketogenic diet in the treatment of cancer-where do we stand? *Mol. Metab.*, 33: 102–121.

Wirth, K.A., Know, K., Salute, M.E. et al. (2016) in vitro effects of *Yunnan Baiyao* on canine hemangiosarcoma cell lines. *Vet. Comp. Oncol.*, 14 (3): 281–94.

Yang, X-Q, Zheng, H., Ye Q., et al. (2015) Essential oil of cinnamon exerts anti-cancer activity against head and neck squamous cell carcinoma via attenuating epidermal growth factor receptor-tyrosine kinase. *JBUON*, 20(6): 1518–1525.

Yasueda, A., Urushima, H., and Ito, T. (2016) Efficacy and interaction of antioxidant supplements as adjuvant therapy cancer treatment: a systematic review. *Integr. Cancer Ther.*, 15(1): 17–39.

Ziech, D., Franco, R., Georgakilas A.G. et al. (2010) The role of reactive oxygen species and oxidative stress in environmental carcinogenesis and biomarker development. *Chem. Biol. Interact.*, 188: 334–339.

12

Chronic Kidney Disease

Shea Cox, DVM, CHPV, CVPP and Christie Cornelius, DVM, CHPV

Description of Disease

Chronic kidney disease (CKD) is defined as any disease causing structural and/or functional impairment of one or both kidneys and persisting over a time period longer than three months (Polzin 2011). Chronic kidney disease is irreversible and characterized by a progressive reduction in functioning nephrons. When there is a more than 75% reduction in renal function, the urine-concentrating ability of the kidneys is impaired, leading to polyuria and polydipsia (Tilley and Smith 2011). Retention of nitrogenous waste products of protein catabolism leads to azotemia, and as renal function is further compromised, uremia results. In the later stages of disease, decreased erythropoietin and calcitriol production by the kidneys may result in anemia (common) and renal secondary hyperparathyroidism (uncommon), respectively. Because of its irreversible nature, early diagnosis of CKD affords the greatest opportunity to slow progression of disease.

The International Renal Interest Society (IRIS) recommends a dynamic staging system based on serum/plasma creatinine concentration, presence of proteinuria, and presence and degree of systemic arterial hypertension. Patients are categorized into four stages along a continuum of disease progression. Based on staging, therapeutic interventions may be undertaken, and the IRIS staging system provides a framework to guide strategies for treatment and management of CKD, which are applicable to hospice and palliative care patients.

Disease Trajectory

Dogs and cats with CKD typically progress to terminal kidney failure over months to years.

Clinical Manifestations of Disease

Clinical signs are related to the stage of CKD and the presence of complications such as proteinuria and hypertension. Common symptoms of and sequelae to CKD can include polyuria/polydipsia, declining appetite or anorexia, reduced activity or lethargy, mental depression, nausea/vomiting, ptyalism, weight loss/loss of muscle mass/cachexia, dull and unkempt haircoat, nocturia, hypertension, constipation, diarrhea, pale mucus membranes secondary to anemia, uremic stomatitis, and uremic halitosis.

Less common symptoms of and sequelae to CKD can include gastrointestinal (GI) bleeding, impaired thermoregulation, heart murmur

Hospice and Palliative Care for Companion Animals: Principles and Practice, Second Edition.
Edited by Amir Shanan, Jessica Pierce, and Tamara Shearer.
© 2023 John Wiley & Sons, Inc. Published 2023 by John Wiley & Sons, Inc.
Companion website: www.wiley.com/go/shanan/palliative

(secondary to dehydration and/or anemia), retinal detachment/acute blindness (secondary to hypertension), ventral neck flexion (secondary to hypokalemic myopathy), renal osteodystrophy, calcinosis cutis, and head or bone pain. Gait imbalance, muscle tremors, and seizures may be seen in the more advanced cases and those nearing the end of life.

In most cases, renal failure is not considered a painful process; however, some sequelae and complications such as urinary tract infections, pyelonephritis, uremic stomatitis, and uremic gastritis are often painful. Renal failure secondary to renal lymphoma can be mildly to severely painful due to stretching of the renal capsule.

Management

Specific therapies are directed at slowing the primary disease processes affecting the kidneys. Focus should be placed on targeting factors that accelerate CKD progression. Symptomatic, supportive, and palliative therapies aim to ameliorate the clinical signs of disease (e.g. inappetence, GI dysfunction, electrolyte imbalance, and weakness) as well as addressing its complications (e.g. urinary tract and oral infections).

Management of Factors that Accelerate Chronic Kidney Disease Progression

Dehydration

Minimizing prerenal azotemia by ensuring adequate hydration and renal perfusion is paramount to protecting the patient's kidneys from hypoxia, especially as CKD progresses. Whilst intravenous therapy may provide a short-term solution during periods of acute crisis, this measure is often not readily accepted by families who wish for conservative hospice measures only. For pets that struggle to maintain adequate hydration with oral intake alone, subcutaneous fluid administration or placement of an e-tube should be considered. The fluid volume to be administered should be based on the severity of dehydration as well as taking into account any comorbidities, such as heart disease.

Hydracare® is a highly palatable, liver-flavored, liquid oral product designed to improve hydration in cats. The calorie content is minimal, but it contains whey protein and potassium and may be a useful way to try to increase voluntary water intake.

Nonregenerative Anemia

Progressive decreases in packed cell volume (PCV), red blood cell (RBC) count, and hemoglobin are predictable features of progressive CKD and are proportional to the stage of disease. The use of erythrocyte-stimulating agents (ESA) should be implemented when the PCV approaches 18–20% and/or when the pet is clinically affected by the anemia.

In recent years, a modified human erythropoetin product called darbopoetin alfa (Aranesp) has become the preferred ESA due to an apparent lower prevalence of antibody production and pure red cell aplasia (PRCA), as well as the convenience of once-weekly administration.

1) **Darbopoetin alfa (Aranesp):** initial dose is $0.45–0.6\,\text{mcg/kg}^{-1}$ for larger dogs, and 2.5–5 mcg/small dog or cat, SC once weekly until PCV reaches the low end of the target range, then decreasing the frequency to q2 weeks; maintenance dosage is 2.5–5 mcg SC q2–3 weeks; if PCV exceeds the target range, discontinue until target range is achieved and then resume treatment decreasing the previous dosage by 25–50%.

PCV should be monitored weekly to semi-monthly for three months, then monthly to bimonthly as clinically indicated. Concurrent iron supplementation, preferably by intramuscular injection (iron dextran) is required, as well as blood pressure (BP) monitoring as systemic hypertension is a recognized side-effect of ESA therapy (Chalhoub et al. 2011).

Systemic Hypertension

Systemic hypertension is a persistent increase in blood pressure that generally occurs in conjunction with some underlying disease condition. Hypertension is commonly associated with CKD, and 20–65% of cats with CKD are reported to develop hypertension at some point in the disease process (Syme et al. 2002). In dogs and cats, systolic BP >140 mmHg or diastolic BP >90 mmHg is considered abnormal.

Stage I (mild hypertension) is defined as systolic BP between 140 and 159 mmHg. A BP within this range poses minimal risk for target organ damage (which includes kidneys), and treatment is generally not recommended. Stage II (moderate hypertension) is defined as systolic BP 160–179 mmHg, while stage III (severe hypertension) is defined as systolic BP >180 mmHg, which can result in acute blindness, which may be irreversible, or hemorrhagic strokes. Treatment is recommended for both stage II and III in order to limit ongoing damage to the kidneys. BP measurements of <140/90 mmHg are the treatment goal, although systolic BP <160 mmHg is reasonable and will minimize the risk of progressive renal impairment and retinal hemorrhage/detachment (Elliott et al. 2001).

1) **Amlodipine:** dogs, 0.1–0.6 mg/kg^{-1} PO q24 h; cats, 0.625–1.25 mg/cat PO q24 h. Amlodipine is more effective than angiotensin converting enzyme [ACE] inhibitors in cats with CKD-induced hypertension.
2) **Telmisartan** (Semintra®) was recently approved by the US Food and Drug Administration (FDA) for the management of moderate hypertension in cats, defined as systolic pressure <200 mmHg. The dose for this purpose is significantly higher than for proteinuria (1.5 mg/kg^{-1} q 12 h for 14 days, followed by 2 mg Telmisartan/kg PO q24 h), and creatinine must again be monitored to look for any deleterious effects

on Glomerular Filtration Rate (GRF) test (Cook 2021). The dose recommended to control proteinuria is 1 mg/kg^{-1} daily.
3) **Ace inhibitors (enalapril or benazepril):** dogs and cats, 0.5 mg/kg^{-1} PO q24 h. Benazepril use is recommended in cats with proteinuria and urine protein to creatinine (UPC) ratio > 0.4; monitor for worsening azotemia and hyperkalemia when using ACE inhibitors. In general, as solo agents, ACE inhibitors only drop systemic blood pressure by 10 mmHg, so are poor first choices for substantially hypertensive patients. If refractory to monotherapy, consider a combination of amlodipine and ACE inhibitor with frequent monitoring of blood pressure.

Proteinuria and Activation of the Renin–Angiotensin–Aldosterone System

It is thought, in humans at least, that proteins in the tubular fluid passing through a damaged glomerulus provoke an inflammatory response, which produces further renal damage. As a result, the greater the level of proteinuria, the more rapid the progression of CKD. Reducing proteinuria can be accomplished by blocking renin–angiotensin–aldosterone system (RAAS) activation with ACE inhibitors or angiotensin receptor blockers (ARB).

Although proteinuria in cats with CKD (UPC ratio > 0.2) has been shown to be a negative prognostic indicator, interventional treatment with ACE inhibitors has not yet been shown to have a survival benefit. Telmisartan is an ARB that is licensed in Europe for treatment of proteinuria and in the United States for hypertension in cats and has been found to be more effective than benazepril for treating proteinuria (Sent et al. 2015).

Renal Secondary Hyperparathyroidism

Renal secondary hyperparathyroidism is a clinical syndrome characterized by a high concentration of biologically active parathormone (PTH) secondary to CKD, due to the relative lack of calcitriol synthesis. Low calcitriol and serum ionized calcium concentrations result in increased PTH production and parathyroid gland hyperplasia. Sustained PTH production increases the low serum calcitriol and calcium concentrations, at the expense of sustained elevated PTH concentration. PTH may act as a uremic toxin and further promote nephrocalcinosis and progression of CKD.

1) **Calcitriol:** starting at $2\,ng/kg^{-1}$ PO q24 h, while monitoring effect on PTH and ionized calcium weekly for 4 weeks to avoid hypercalcemia and/or hyperphosphatemia, then monthly if the patient is stable, and then every 3–4 months; a pharmacy that specializes in reformulation of calcitriol is needed to provide these low doses.

Symptomatic, Supportive, and Palliative Therapies

Oral Ulcerations and Uremic Gastritis

Gastrin concentrations are increased in pets with CKD due to reduced renal clearance, and in dogs may result in a uremic gastritis contributing to inappetence and vomiting (Goldstein et al. 1998).

The etiology of dysrexia in CKD is typically attributed to uremic effects on the intestinal tract such as hyperacidity, uremic gastritis, and ulceration, but our understanding of this pathophysiology in cats has changed. Although cats with CKD have been shown to have elevated concentrations of gastrin that increase with the severity of kidney disease, more recent information demonstrates this is likely not related to gastric pathology or hyperacidity (Quimby 2021). In a study evaluating the type and prevalence of histopathologic lesions in the stomach of cats with CKD, gastric fibrosis and mineralization were the main changes found rather than the uremic gastropathy lesions previously described in dogs and humans (uremic gastritis, ulceration, vascular injury, edema) (McLeland et al. 2014). A recent study provided evidence that CKD cats may in fact not be hyperacidic (Tolbert et al. 2017). However, if used, studies of the effect of omeprazole on the gastric pH in normal cats indicates that it is superior to famotidine in its ability to inhibit acid production at $1\,mg/kg^{-1}$ q12 h (Parkinson et al. 2015).

Use of gastroprotectants and analgesics can be beneficial and can include omeprazole, sucralfate (Carafate), transmucosal buprenorphine, and "magic mouthwash."

Nausea/Vomiting

A multimodal use of antiemetics is often needed to control symptoms of nausea/vomiting and can include:

1) **Maropitant:** SC dogs and cats, $1\,mg/kg^{-1}$ (recommend giving in subcutaneous fluid line during administration to reduce injection discomfort) q24 h up to 5 days. PO $2\,mg/kg^{-1}$ (dogs) and $1\,mg/kg^{-1}$ (cats) PO q24 h up to 5 days. May be used long term (extra-label). A pharmacokinetic and toxicity study in cats indicated that longer-term usage appears safe (Hickman et al. 2008). A recent study assessed the efficacy of Cerenia for management of chronic vomiting and inappetence associated with feline CKD (Quimby et al. 2014). When given daily for 2 weeks at a $4\,mg/24\,h$ dose, Cerenia was demonstrated to palliate vomiting associated with chronic kidney disease; however, it did not appear to significantly improve appetite or result in weight gain in cats with stage II and III CKD within the timeframe of the study. A study in dogs revealed no adverse effects after repeated oral doses of $5\,mg/kg^{-1}$ q24 h for 93 days (Plumb 2015).
2) **Ondansetron:** dogs and cats, 0.1–0.5 mg/kg^{-1} slow IV, SC, PO q8–12 h.
3) **Metoclopramide:** dogs and cats, 0.2–0.4 mg/kg^{-1} PO or SC q8 h can be used in addition to PPIs to treat uremic vomiting.

Constipation/Obstipation

Constipation secondary to dehydration from renal failure is a common finding. Subcutaneous fluids and stool softeners, such as MiraLAX® or lactulose, should be considered for long-term administration if straining or pain with defecation is repeatedly observed, or whenever the average frequency of defecation falls significantly below once a day. If these measures are not enough to control the episodes of constipation, an intestinal motility enhancer, such as cisapride, should be considered. Enemas may also need to be considered if obstipation develops.

Loss of Appetite

Recent exploration of Mirtazapine pharmacodynamics and pharmacokinetics have provided information that has allowed for more effective use in cats. Pharmacodynamic studies have illustrated that it can be a potent appetite stimulant, but higher doses are more commonly associated with side effects (hyperexcitability, vocalization, tremors). Therefore, smaller, more frequent doses are recommended. Mirtazapine demonstrates antinausea properties in addition to its appetite stimulating properties as it acts at the 5HT3 receptor similarly to ondansetron.

Capromorelin, a ghrelin-receptor agonist that stimulates growth hormone release and causes the feeling of hunger, is FDA approved to stimulate appetite in dogs and cats. Diarrhea and polydypsia may occur with use. Vomiting and hypersalivation may also occur (Plumb 2015). A warning to pet owners about hypersalivation with the off-putting taste should be reviewed.

If pets are too nauseous or critical to consider oral feeding, or have not responded to appetite encouragement after 3–5 days, placement of an enteral feeding tube should be considered.

1) **Mirtazapine:** Typical feline dosage is 3.75 mg PO every 3 days; however, smaller, more frequent dosing appears to have less side effects while remaining effective; for cats, the author recommends using 1.875 mg every other day; the half-life is short enough that it could be administered daily in normal cats, but renal disease delays clearance in CKD patients and thus every other day administration is recommended (Quimby et al. 2011); compounded formulations can allow for ease of dosing, or one-quarter of a 7.5 mg tablet can be used. Canine dose, $0.6 \, \text{mg kg}^{-1}$ PO q24 h not to exceed $30 \, \text{mg day}^{-1}$.

2) **Mirataz®:** Transdermal mirtazapine ointment is FDA approved for the management of unintended weight loss and efficacy has been documented in pharmacokinetic and pharmodynamics studies (2 mg to inner pinna q 24 h) (Buhles et al. 2018). The appetite effect of transdermal preparations is much more subtle than oral mirtazapine due to a flatter drug concentration curve (Benson et al. 2017), a phenomenon that also results in fewer side effects.

3) **Capromorelin:** (Entyce®) for appetite stimulation in dogs: $3 \, \text{mg kg}^{-1}$ PO once daily. In cats (extra-label) $1–2 \, \text{mg kg}^{-1}$ PO once daily for up to 21 days. Elura® is FDA approved for the management of weight loss in cats with CKD; cats in the field trials gained an average of 5% of their body weight over the eight-week observation period. $2 \, \text{mg kg}^{-1}$ PO q24h.

4) **Cyproheptadine:** The typical feline dosing is 2 mg/cat SID-BID. This medication and dosing may be anecdotal due to lack of scientific evidence of efficacy in this species.

Urinary Tract Infection

Urinary tract infections are identified in approximately 16–30% of pets with CKD, with *Escherichia coli* being the identified organism in approximately 80% of the cases (Mayer-Roenne et al. 2007). Adequate length and type of antibiotic therapy is ideally based on culture and sensitivity; however, this may not be an option in a hospice setting when caregivers prefer empirical therapy only. Options for empirical therapy can include amoxicillin/cla-vulanate, amoxicillin, enrofloxacin, marbo-floxacin, and cefovecin sodium (Convenia).

Hyperphosphatemia

As renal disease progresses, dietary phosphorus restriction may no longer be enough to avoid hyperphosphatemia, and phosphate binders may be necessary. If diet modification does not address hyperphosphatemia, intestinal phosphate binders can be implemented.

1) **Aluminum hydroxide:** dogs, 30–100 mg/kg/day PO divided with meals; cats, 30–60 mg/kg/day PO divided with meals; there are both liquid and granule formulations available; a caregiver tip is to place kibble and the appropriate amount of aluminum hydroxide into a baggie and shake vigorously – each kibble will be lightly coated by the binder, and it will be more evenly distributed throughout the food.

Hypokalemia

Hypokalemia is recognized in approximately 20–30% of cats with IRIS stage II–III CKD, resulting from decreased dietary intake, increased renal loss, and activation of the RAAS (Jepson 2013). The most common clinical signs include polymyopathy resulting in generalized weakness and cervical ventroflexion. Mild hypokalemia (3.0–3.5 mEq l^{-1}) can be treated by oral potassium supplementation. To avoid over supplementation, frequent monitoring is recommended. Adding potassium chloride to fluid solutions for SC administration is also an option.

1) **Potassium gluconate (such as Tumil-K):** dogs and cats, initial dosage is one-quarter teaspoon (2 mEq) per 4.5 kg of body weight in food twice daily.
2) **Potassium chloride:** add 20 mEq to 1 l of fluid for SC administration (2 mEq per 4.0 kg of body weight if giving 100 ml to a 4 kg patient).

Seizures

Seizures can occur in end-stage renal failure and can be due to hypertension, secondary cerebrovascular accident (CVA), or worsening of underlying metabolic disturbances (such as worsening azotemia, hypocalcemia, electrolyte imbalances). Anticonvulsants can be utilized for short-term palliation, but in the author's experience, seizures generally indicate approaching death or euthanasia. Common antiseizure therapies used at home to control seizures in renal patients include phenobarbital, diazepam (rectally), and intranasal midazolam.

Dietary Considerations

A renal diet is generally recommended when a patient is in late stage II or more advanced CKD. Dietary protein restriction has been considered a cornerstone of nutritional management and helps to delay the onset of a uremic crisis and has been shown to extend survival in dogs and cats with CKD stages II–IV (Jacob et al. 2002). Important components of a renal diet include reduced protein, phosphorus, sodium, and net acid content, while supplementing omega-3 fatty acids and antioxidants. Free access to fresh water at all times is imperative.

Other Comfort Measures

Other comfort measures include:

- Supplemental heat support
- Warming subcutaneous fluids prior to administration as well as trying different needle sizes
- Warming food to stimulate appetite by increasing smell
- Rotating diet options to help prevent food aversions.

Conclusion

Chronic kidney disease affects many geriatric patients; in fact, it is the leading cause of death in geriatric felines. A good quality of life can often be maintained with appropriate care. Specific therapies are directed at slowing the primary disease process affecting the kidneys. Symptomatic, supportive, and palliative therapies ameliorate the clinical signs of disease and address its complications.

References

Benson, K.K., et al. (2017) Drug exposure and clinical effect of transdermal Mirtazapine in healthy young cats: a pilot study. *J. Feline Med. Surg.*, 21: 402–409.

Buhles, W., et al. (2018) Single and multiple dose pharmacokinetics of a novel mirtazapine transdermal ointment in cats. *J. Vet. Pharmacol. Ther.*, 41: 644–651.

Chalhoub, S., Langston, C., and Eatroff, A. (2011) Anemia of renal disease: what it is, what to do and what's new. *J. Feline Med. Surg.*, 13: 629–640.

Cook, A.K., (2021) Feline chronic kidney disease: initial assessment. *VMX (Veterinary Meeting and Expo)*, Orlando, FL. (June 5–9).

Elliott, J., Barber, P.J., Syme, H.M. et al. (2001) Feline hypertension: clinical findings and response to antihypertensive treatment in 30 cases. *J. Small Anim. Pract.*, 42: 122–129.

Goldstein, R.E., Marks, S.L., Kass, P.H., and et al. (1998) Gastrin concentrations in plasma of cats with chronic renal failure. *J. Am. Vet. Med. Assoc.*, 213: 826–828.

Hickman, M.A., Cox, S.R., Mahabir, S. et al. (2008) Safety, pharmacokinetics and use of the novel NK-1 receptor antagonist maropitant (Cerenia) for the prevention of emesis and motion sickness in cats. *J. Vet. Pharmacol. Ther.*, 31: 220–229.

Jacob, F., Polzin, D., Osborne, C. et al. (2002) Clinical evaluation of dietary modification for treatment of spontaneous chronic renal failure in dogs. *J. Am. Vet. Med. Assoc.*, 220: 1163–1170.

Jepson, R. (2013) *Chronic Kidney Disease – More than Just Diets*. North Mymms, Hatfield, Hertfordshire, UK: The Royal Veterinary College.

Mayer-Roenne, B., Goldstein, R.E., and Erb, H.N. (2007) Urinary tract infections in cats with hyperthyroidism, diabetes mellitus and chronic kidney disease. *J. Feline Med. Surg.*, 9: 124–132.

McLeland, S.M., Lunn, K. F., Duncan, C. G. et al. (2014) Relationship among serum creatinine, serum gastrin, calcium-phosphorous product, and uremic gastropathy in cats with chronic kidney disease. *J. Vet. Intern. Med.*, 28: 827–837.

Parkinson, S., Tolbert, K., Messenger, K. et al. (2015) Evaluation of the effect of orally administered acid suppressants on intragastric pH in cats. *J. Vet. Intern. Med.*, 29: 104–112.

Plumb, D.C. (2015) *Plumb's Veterinary Drug Handbook, 8*. Ames, IA: Wiley-Blackwell.

Polzin, D.J. (2011) Chronic kidney disease. In: *Nephrology and Urology of Small Animals* (eds J. Bartges and D.J. Polzin), pp. 433–471. Ames, IA: Wiley-Blackwell.

Quimby, J.M. (2021) Updates on evidence-based management of feline CKD. *VMX (Veterinary Meeting and Expo)*, Orlando, FL. (June 5–9).

Quimby, J.M., Gustafson, D.L., and Lunn, K.F. (2011) The pharmacokinetics of mirtazapine in cats with chronic kidney disease and in age-matched control cats. *J. Vet. Intern. Med.*, 25, 985–989.

Quimby, J.M., Brock, W.T., Moses, K. et al. (2014) Cerenia for the management of vomiting and inappetence associated with chronic kidney disease in cats. 2014 ACVIM Forum Proceedings. *J. Vet. Intern. Med.*, 28: 994.

Sent, U., Gössl, R., Elliott, J. et al. (2015) Comparison of efficacy of long-term oral treatment with Telmisartan and benazepril in cats with chronic kidney disease. *J. Vet. Intern. Med.*, 29: 1479–1487.

Syme, H.M., Barber, P.J., Markwell, P.J. et al. (2002) Prevalence of systolic hypertension in cats with chronic renal failure at initial evaluation. *J. Am. Vet. Med. Assoc.*, 220: 1799–1804.

Tilley, L.P. and Smith, F.W.K. (2011) *Blackwell's Five-Minute Veterinary Consult:* *Canine and Feline*, 5. Ames, IA: Wiley-Blackwell, p. 1095.

Tolbert, K., Olin, S., MacLane, S. et al. (2017) Evaluation of gastric pH and serum gastrin concentrations in cats with chronic kidney disease. *J. Vet. Intern. Med.*, 31: 96.

13

Congestive Heart Failure

Shea Cox, DVM, CHPV, CVPP and Christie Cornelius, DVM, CHPV

In general terms, heart failure is an end-stage clinical syndrome that occurs secondary to severe, overwhelming cardiac disease. Failure occurs because the heart is no longer able to maintain normal venous/capillary pressures, cardiac output, and/or systemic blood pressure and results in the development of edema or effusion significant enough to cause clinical signs. Heart failure is most commonly caused by chronic disease that results in a marked decrease in myocardial contractility, severe regurgitation or shunting, severe diastolic dysfunction, or a combination of one or more of these factors. Congestive heart failure (CHF) will be the focus of this chapter, as this is the most common form of cardiac decompensation encountered in the hospice patient.

Description of Disease

CHF is a sequela to severe cardiac disease and can be due to either right or left-sided heart failure. The most common causes of CHF in dogs are degenerative myxomatous valvular disease and dilated cardiomyopathy, while in cats, hypertrophic cardiomyopathy is considered to be the most common cause, although a variety of cardiomyopathies can be seen (Linney 2015).

Disease Trajectory

Patients with CHF are generally without clinical symptoms until the severity of disease has exceeded the capacity of the body's compensatory mechanisms. With few exceptions, heart failure is not curable; however, most patients with the disease will initially respond well to medication and regain their asymptomatic state when properly managed. Prognosis can range from days to years, and varies with the underlying cause, the severity of disease, time of diagnosis, and individual response to therapies. Patients may present in an acute crisis in critical condition, or may struggle for many weeks with "good days and bad days" or "good moments and bad moments" interspersed throughout each day.

Clinical Manifestations of Disease

Clinical signs observed will vary with the underlying cause, whether due to right- or left-sided failure, the stage of disease, and the species involved.

Dogs with heart disease often have clinical signs that are insidious in onset and slowly progressive. These can include non-specific

Hospice and Palliative Care for Companion Animals: Principles and Practice, Second Edition.
Edited by Amir Shanan, Jessica Pierce, and Tamara Shearer.
© 2023 John Wiley & Sons, Inc. Published 2023 by John Wiley & Sons, Inc.
Companion website: www.wiley.com/go/shanan/palliative

signs such as loss of appetite, lethargy, and a general "slowing down," often attributed by caregivers to normal age-related changes. Because of this, heart failure is often not diagnosed in dogs until more overt signs are observed. In contrast, cats with cardiac disease characteristically remain asymptomatic until very late in the course of the disease, at which time clinical signs are acutely manifested.

As disease progresses, and the body's compensatory mechanisms begin to fail, more significant signs are observed including: coughing (rare in cats), dyspnea, tachypnea, exercise intolerance, cool extremities (ears and paws, especially in cats), crackles and/or wheezes on auscultation (many dogs and cats with CHF have no markedly abnormal lung sounds other than increased bronchovesicular sounds late in the course of the disease), diminished heart sounds on auscultation, delayed capillary refill time due to poor perfusion, cyanosis, weak femoral pulses, appreciation of a jugular pulse, hepatomegaly, preference for sternal recumbency and/or orthopnea, and signs of fluid retention such as pulmonary congestion, pleural effusion, ascites, and peripheral edema. Clinical signs can progress rapidly, and a relatively stable and well-managed pet can have a sudden onset of advanced symptoms with little warning.

Advanced signs that may reflect impending death can include weakness and collapse, changes in the mental status, marked cooling of the skin and extremities, exertional syncope, and Cheyne-Stokes breathing. Although uncommon in animals, there may also be wet, noisy breathing, referred to as "death rattles," which may be palliated by repositioning.

In most cases, heart failure is not considered painful; however, anxiety can arise during periods of respiratory distress when the disease exacerbates, or when death is nearing, and appropriate interventions should be implemented. Although "death rattles" can appear alarming to the caregiver, most human hospice patients report that this is not a painful or distressful symptom.

Palliative Management

For patients with CHF, medications are indispensable for life. Many patients who respond well to therapies can regain their asymptomatic state and good quality of life. Goals of therapy are to: (i) control congestion, (ii) improve cardiac output, (iii) normalize rate and rhythm, and (iv) delay progression. Specific therapies are directed at alleviating clinical symptoms and correcting hemodynamic derangements. While it is ideal to diagnose the specific type of heart disease and monitor for disease progression, it may be in fact more important to treat the body's response to the failing heart. Initial management of CHF is usually treated in a similar manner regardless of the underlying cause and clinical manifestation.

Pulmonary Edema/Cardiac Function

Prevention of pulmonary edema is the mainstay of treatment and includes the use of furosemide, an angiotensin converting enzyme (ACE) inhibitor, and pimobendan (off label for cats). Digoxin (rarely used in cats), beta-blockers, and calcium channel blockers can also be considered based on the type, stage, and severity of disease.

Furosemide, the initial diuretic of choice, is a loop diuretic that blocks sodium, potassium, and chloride reabsorption at the ascending loop of Henle. Furosemide helps to remove excess fluid accumulations. Despite the fact that it has no beneficial effect in terms of improving cardiac output, furosemide is likely the most important therapy in the management of a decompensated CHF patient as it provides immediate symptomatic relief of dyspnea due to pulmonary edema. Although furosemide has a wide therapeutic range (see below) and safety margin, dosing can be challenging because the effective doses vary greatly from patient to patient. A dose too high for a particular patient can have deleterious effects on renal perfusion and electrolytes. Conversely, a dose that is too low can lead to unnecessary hospitalization, expense, and potential euthanasia because of recurrent decompensation (DeFrancesco 2012). Spironolactone can be added as a second diuretic if furosemide alone fails to control signs of CHF (Bernay et al. 2010), or when a chronic furosemide dose is required in excess of 2 mg/kg^{-1} BID. Multimodal therapy can be implemented as the two diuretics work on different parts of the nephron.

The use of ACE inhibitors is predicated on the knowledge that interfering with the activation of the renin angiotensin system leads to diminished plasma levels of angiotensin II and reduced stimulation of aldosterone and, as a result, fluid retention and vasoconstriction are blunted (Rush 2008).

Pimobendan is a calcium-sensitizing drug that is useful as a positive ionotrope in addition to having properties as a phosphodiesterase inhibitor with vasodilating effects (Rush 2008). It produces moderate reductions in systemic and pulmonary vascular resistance, a decrease in left ventricular filling pressure, a moderate increase in heart rate, and a moderate increase in cardiac output. It also increases myocardial blood flow and improves diastolic function (Lombard et al. 2006). It is a part of the "triple therapy" (together with furosemide and an ACE inhibitor) used to manage most causes of canine heart failure. Although not licensed for use in cats, there has been an increased use of pimobendan in the management of feline CHF over the past several years.

Amlodipine can be considered in patients that have a systolic blood pressure greater than 140 mmHg to act as an afterload reducer in refractory heart failure (extra-label use). Owners should be warned of the potential for the development of gingival hyperplasia in dogs.

Due to the number of medications recommended for canine patients in CHF, especially larger dogs, the priority of these medications given in order of importance are furosemide, pimobendan, ACE inhibitor, and spironolactone.

In cats, the cornerstones of chronic CHF management regardless of the underlying etiology are furosemide, clopidogrel, and an ACE inhibitor (enalapril/benazepril). Clopidogrel is recommended to prevent the often devastating and terminal thromboembolic events. The routine use of pimobendin is often made on a case-by-case basis and should be aided by echocardiographic findings (Visser 2018). Cats are often difficult to medicate, so it's important to prioritize medications for caretakers in the following order: furosemide, clopidogrel, ACE inhibitor, and other medications used on a case-by-case basis: pimobendin, and spironolactone.

Diuretics

1) **Furosemide:** dogs and cats, 0.5–2 mg kg^{-1} PO SID–TID; usually administered as a tablet formulation. Human pediatric and higher-concentration veterinary compounded liquid formulations are available and can be useful in pets that are difficult to administer tablets to; liquid formulation also allows more accurate dosing if lower doses are used due to patient size.

2) **Torsemide:** Torsemide can be used off label in dogs and cats, refractory to furosemide; torsemide is given at one-tenth of the daily furosemide dose, divided BID or TID, or 0.2–0.3 mg/kg^{-1} PO q8–24 h.

3) **Spironolactone:** dogs and cats, 0.5–2 mg/kg^{-1} PO SID–BID; may cause facial pruritus in cats.

4) **Thiazide** can be added to furosemide and spironolactone in refractory heart failure cases. This medication can cause severe azotemia and may not be well tolerated.

Ace Inhibitors

1) **Enalapril:** dogs and cats, 0.5 mg/kg^{-1} PO SID for 1–2 weeks followed by an increase to BID if marked azotemia has not occurred (i.e. if creatinine is less than twofold elevated) or when the disease progresses.

2) **Benazepril:** dogs and cats, 0.25–0.5 mg/kg^{-1} PO SID.

Positive Lonotrope, Vasodilator

1) **Pimobendan:** dogs (off label for cats), 0.25–0.3 mg/kg^{-1} PO BID; although an off-label use, many end-stage heart failure dogs respond far better to TID dosing of pimobendan.

Calcium Channel Blocker

1) **Amlodipine:** (as an afterload reducer) dogs, 0.1–0.5 mg/kg^{-1} PO SID. Amlodipine is generally added after ACE inhibitor therapy has been used. Cats, 0.625–1.25 mg per cat SID. In cats that are proteinuric, an ACE inhibitor is added.

The goal of therapy is to gradually titrate to the lowest effective dose of all medications, to minimize the risks of hypotension, prerenal azotemia, and hypokalemia.

Pleural and Abdominal Effusion

CHF may lead to the formation of pleural effusion or abdominal effusion (ascites).

As fluid accumulates in the pleural space, space available for the lungs to inflate is reduced, compromising respiration. If fluid continues to collect, the lungs may eventually collapse, leading to hypoventilation and resulting in hypoxemia and hypercapnia. In patients where pleural fluid has accumulated to a degree that it causes clinical signs, palliative treatment can include relief through thoracocentesis.

Fluid may also collect in the abdominal cavity, leading to significant clinical signs. Respiratory distress may occur due to excessive pressure on the diaphragm, reducing lung capacity. The combination of abdominal discomfort, restlessness, anorexia, renal insufficiency, and other effects of visceral hypoperfusion is referred to as "abdominal compartment syndrome" ("tense ascites"). In patients where ascitic fluid has accumulated to a degree that it causes clinical signs, palliative treatment should include relief through abdominocentesis.

Thoracocentesis and abdominocentesis can be performed in the home setting with the use of a mild sedative and a local block. The sterile use of an appropriately sized IV catheter connected to a three-way stopcock is commonly adopted and provides safe and rapid drainage of the abdominal or pleural space.

Following centesis, it is recommended that caregivers continue to monitor body weight, abdominal girth, and resting respiratory rate to help assess any return of fluid.

Hypokalemia

Furosemide use has been implicated in the development of hypokalemia due to increased urinary loss. Hypokalemia is of concern in animals with heart disease because depletion of this electrolyte can lead to cardiac arrhythmias, decreased myocardial contractility, and muscle weakness. Hypokalemia is generally controlled by concomitant administration of potassium supplementation (Tumil-K) and/or potassium-sparing agents, such as spironolactone.

Prerenal Azotemia

The combination of ACE inhibitors and diuretics can result in prerenal azotemia as well as contribute to the progression of pre-existing renal disease. Renal values should (ideally) be monitored frequently and medication doses adjusted as clinically indicated. Mild azotemia in the absence of clinical signs of chronic kidney disease (CKD) may be acceptable and well tolerated by many patients.

Balancing Renal and Cardiac Disease

A significant number of patients are affected by concurrent cardiac and renal disease, and the interactions between the two systems are referred to as cardiorenal syndrome (CRS). Cardiovascular disease constitutes a significant threat for patients with underlying renal disease as there are important bidirectional functional and pathological interactions between the heart and the kidney, wherein dysfunction of either organ promotes clinical worsening of the other (Schrier 2007). Systemic hypertension occurs in a variable proportion of cases, as a result of mechanisms that also may contribute further to loss of kidney function.

A proposed partial checklist in chronic management of CRS that could be helpful in providing home palliative care to a patient includes the following:

- Verify client compliance with drug administration
- Identify diuretic resistance
- Measure urine-specific gravity
- Have owner measure water intake, confirm >20 cc/lb/day (45 cc/kg/day)
- Identify systemic hypertension and treat it if present and if attributed only to renal disease
- With good client comprehension, taper diuretic to lowest effective dosage.
- Consider dual-diuretic therapy (furosemide + spironolactone – can cause facial dermatitis in cats, specifically the Maine Coon)
- Manage coexistent electrolyte abnormalities, especially hypokalemia
- Differentiate between advanced chronic renal disease and acute-on-chronic disease (e.g. pyelonephritis, occult urinary tract infection (UTI))
- Manage anemia
- Look to the remainder of physical exam to offer clues regarding whether heart or kidney problem is worse at that moment
- Removal of large-volume, recurrent body cavity effusions in chronic states
- Positive inotropes, role still to be defined. Many veterinarians have treated severely ill, "end-stage" cardiorenal patients with pimobendan, resulting in improved azotemia and uremia and prolonged survival due to delay in the owner's decision to euthanize. This response is variable and unpredictable, with some dogs improving dramatically and others deteriorating despite similar therapy. A visible positive response to pimobendan should be observed within the first several days of treatment, an observation that offers the opportunity for a therapeutic trial (Côté 2019).

It is important to note that even with the best efforts to manage patients with CRS, the overall prognosis is poor.

Coughing

Coughing associated with cardiac disease is a finding specific to dogs and generally not observed in cats. The management of coughing in CHF is tied in with the management of heart failure itself; however, coughing can still be noted despite adequate management of disease. In these cases, coughing is generally a result of underlying chronic bronchitis as a comorbidity or cardiomegaly, where the enlarged left atrium puts pressure on the distal trachea, carina, and mainstem bronchi. When coughing affects quality of life, or is itself causing problems such as tussive syncope, antitussives can be utilized for improved patient comfort (Corcoran 2010).

Respiratory Distress

If a quiet environment does not abolish signs of developing stress, sedation should be utilized if a pet is showing significant signs of stress or respiratory distress. In-home oxygen therapy can be considered for short-term use in patients experiencing an acute crisis, and provide additional comfort measures.

1) **Butorphanol:** dogs and cats, $0.2\,mg/kg^{-1}$ SC or IM is an excellent choice due to its sedation effect as well as the fact that it is not an emetic.
2) **Methadone:** (or other mu-opioid such as morphine): dogs and cats, $0.25\,mg/kg^{-1}$ SQ
3) **Acepromazine:** dogs and cats, 0.01–$0.02\,mg/kg^{-1}$ SC or IM.
4) **Oxygen**

Aortic Thromboembolism

Arterial thromboembolism (ATE) is characterized by the migration of a blood clot from the left atrium to the distal aorta in the presence of blood stasis, hypercoagulability, and endothelial damage. While it is infrequently reported in dogs, ATE is a common complication of feline heart disease, eventually occurring in 30–40% of cats. It carries a poor prognosis (Rush 2013). The diagnosis of ATE is usually clinical, using the "five Ps" rule: pulselessness, pallor (bluish or gray toes), polar (cold extremities), pain, and paralysis. Cats with evidence of thrombus formation or severe atrial enlargement are generally treated with a platelet inhibitor, and the author's preference is the use of clopidogrel over standard aspirin therapy.

1) **Clopidogrel (Plavix):** cats, 18.75 mg PO SID with food.

ATE is considered severely painful, and appropriate pain management with injectable opioids is needed.

Dietary Considerations

The ability to easily excrete excess dietary sodium in the urine is diminished in animals with heart disease. Because of this, a moderately sodium-restricted diet is recommended in early disease, and a severe sodium-restricted diet in more advanced disease (Freeman and Rush 2012). The goal should be to avoid excessive sodium intake, as well as to educate the owner about treats and table foods that are high in sodium. Dogs and cats with CHF also commonly have fluctuations in appetite, therefore the primary goal should be to maintain adequate caloric and nutrient intake vs. insisting on a low-sodium diet.

Heart-Gut Interactions in Heart Failure

In humans, it is believed that the gut-heart interactions are contributing to the pro-inflammatory

status found in heart failure through morphological and functional alterations leading to bacterial translocation. It is believed that the intestinal dysfunction contributes to the development of cardiac cachexia, a well-recognized predictor of poor survival (Sandek et al. 2014). In canine cardiac patients, cardiac cachexia has also been associated with decreased survival and perception of poor quality of life by owners, contributing to the decision of euthanasia (Freeman 2012). Omega-3 fatty acids are recommended for their anti-inflammatory and antiarrhythmic properties, although longitudinal and clinical studies assessing its beneficial effects are lacking (Pereira 2017).

Other Considerations

- One of the best ways to evaluate response to therapies is demonstrating a reduction in the sleeping or resting respiratory rate, with a goal being less than 30 breaths per minute.
- In addition to resting respiratory rate, special attention should also be paid to respiratory effort.
- If the caregiver notes sluggishness, dyspnea, or a long time to recover from the activity, then they must understand that the animal has exceeded its capacity and should not be pushed to the same extent again.

Conclusion

Heart disease is a common illness in many geriatric hospice patients. With proper treatment and management of symptoms, many pets are able to sustain a good quality of life for many months to years.

References

Bernay, F., Bland, J.M., Haggstrom, J., et al. (2010) Efficacy of spironolactone on survival in dogs with naturally occurring mitral regurgitation caused by myxomatous mitral valve disease. *J. Vet. Intern. Med.*, 24: 331–341.

Corcoran, B. (2010) Chronic cough: management. *53rd British Small Animal Veterinary Congress*, Birmingham, UK. (April 8-11).

Côté, E. (2019) Managing patients with concurrent cardiac and renal disease. *44th Congress of the World Small Animal Veterinary Association Proceedings Online*, Toronto, Canada (July 16–19).

DeFrancesco, T. (2012) Diagnosis and management of feline congestive heart failure. *International Veterinary Emergency and Critical Care Symposium*, San Antonio, TX. (September 8–12).

Freeman, L.M. (2012). Cachexia and sarcopenia, emerging syndromes of importance in dogs and cats. *J. Vet. Intern. Med.*, 26: 3–17.

Freeman, L.M. and Rush, J.E. (2012) Nutritional management of cardiovascular diseases. In: *Applied Veterinary Clinical Nutrition* (eds A.J. Fascetti and S. Delaney), pp. 301–313. West Sussex: Blackwell.

Linney, C. (2015) How to manage acute congestive heart failure. *Proceedings of the British Small Animal Veterinary Congress*, Birmingham, UK. (April 9–12).

Lombard, C.W., Jons, O., and Bussadori, C.M. (2006) Clinical efficacy of pimobendan versus benazepril for the treatment of acquired atrioventricular valvular disease in dogs. *J. Am. Anim. Hosp. Assoc.*, 42: 249–261.

Pereira, Y.M. (2017) Pathophysiology of Congestive Heart Failure – Beyond the Heart. *American College of Veterinary Internal Medicine Forum*, National Harbor, MD.

Rush, J. (2008) Heart failure in dogs and cats. *Fourteenth International Veterinary Emergency and Critical Care Symposium*, Phoenix, AZ. (September 18–21).

Rush, J. (2013) Cats and cardiac clots: no evidence, no guts, no glory. *Nineteenth International Veterinary Emergency and Critical Care Symposium*, San Diego, CA. (September 7–11).

Sandek, A., Swidsinski, A., Schroedl, W. et al. (2014). Intestinal blood flow in patients with chronic heart failure: a link with bacterial growth, gastrointestinal symptoms, and cachexia. *J. Am. Coll. Cardiol.*, 64: 1092.

Schrier, R.W. (2007) Cardiorenal versus renocardiac syndrome: is there a difference? *Nat. Clin. Pract. Nephrol.*, 3: 637.

Visser, L.C. (2018) Management of congestive heart failure in the cat. *Twenty-fourth International Veterinary Emergency and Critical Care Symposium*, New Orleans, LA. (September 14–18).

14

Respiratory Distress

Cheryl Braswell, DVM, DACVECC, CHPV, CHT-V, CVPP

The upper and lower respiratory tracts of dogs and cats seen in hospice and palliative care practice are affected by a variety of debilitating conditions, often chronic and at times life-threatening. These conditions can be seen as primary problems or as comorbidities or sequellae, adding a significant burden of discomfort and complicating the management of patients with other life-limiting illnesses.

The American Thoracic Society defines dyspnea as "the subjective experience of breathing discomfort that originates from interactions among various physiologic, psychologic, social, and environmental factors." A biopsychosocial model of management is encouraged. This comprehensive approach includes not only the physical but also emotional, social, and spiritual aspect of the patient and their caregivers. Providers are encouraged to determine if the underlying disease has been maximally treated while then providing the best symptom relief.

This chapter will briefly describe several respiratory medical conditions' pathophysiology, their trajectories, and their management as relevant to hospice and palliative care patients. Recommendations for palliation of the suffering of dyspnea are discussed.

Airway Collapse

Description

In dogs, airway collapse is a common cause for coughing. The prototypical condition is collapsing trachea, typically seen in older miniature or toy breed dogs. It is rarely seen in cats. The etiology is unknown but generally attributed to either a congenital (primary) or inflammatory (secondary) process. These patients have a softening of the tracheal cartilage causing a flattening or narrowing of the tracheal lumen. Prolapse of the tracheal membrane occurs, which further compromises the airway diameter (Maggiore 2014).

Collapse of lower airways (bronchomalacia) is a condition of any breed or size of dog. It presents concurrently with a collapsing trachea 45–83% of the time (Maggiore 2014). Additional inflammation, edema, the decreased ability to clear secretions, increased mucous production, and airway obstruction by mucous trapping are sequelae of the dynamically collapsing airway.

Although direct laryngeal examination coupled with bronchoscopy is the gold standard for diagnosis, a good physical examination and detailed history can often lead to a strong

Hospice and Palliative Care for Companion Animals: Principles and Practice, Second Edition.
Edited by Amir Shanan, Jessica Pierce, and Tamara Shearer.
© 2023 John Wiley & Sons, Inc. Published 2023 by John Wiley & Sons, Inc.
Companion website: www.wiley.com/go/shanan/palliative

suspicion of this disease complex. Thoracic radiographs may be helpful if advanced diagnostics are not available, the caregivers are not inclined to pursue them, or the patient's condition is too tenuous.

Trajectory/Prognosis

There is no cure for patients with airway collapse. This condition has a prolonged course of illness with progressive deterioration in some animals. Secondary complications such as infection can be challenging to resolve because of the impaired mucocilliary apparatus. Increasing care over time is required.

Manifestations

Patients with airway collapse initially exhibit paroxysmal respiratory signs (coughing that waxes and wanes), which become more frequent with time. Collapse of the extrathoracic trachea occurs on inspiration and is easily induced on palpation. The cough is classically described as dry, harsh, and "goose honking." It is worse with excitement, drinking/eating, and when pulling against the collar while on a leash.

Collapse of intrathoracic airways (intrathoracic trachea and bronchi) occurs on expiration. These patients have a chronic cough that is not induced by tracheal palpation but is characterized by wheezing and increased expiratory effort. Very severe cases will have a bulging at the thoracic inlet on expiration (cranial lung herniation) (Maggiorie 2014).

Management

The goal of treatment is to manage the severity of symptoms in order to minimize patient discomfort.

Pharmacologic

The mainstay of therapy revolves around the treatment of inflammation and infection, cough suppressants, bronchodilators, and sedation.

1) Secondary infection is addressed with antibiotic therapy. Although best directed by culture and sensitivity testing, this is not always practical. Antibiotics commonly prescribed for the upper airway are the aminopenicillins and macrolides. Amoxicillin/clavulanic acid (13.75 mg/kg q8–12 h) or azithromycin (5–10 mg/kg q24 h) are two examples. For the lower airways, fluoroquinolones and lincosamides are valid considerations, e.g. enrofloxacin (10 mg/kg q24 h) and clindamycin (10 mg/kg q12 h maximum 28 days). If using clindamycin in a dog with hepatic compromise, decrease dose by 50%. Doxycycline (5–10 mg/kg q12 h) is also a good choice for tracheal or lower airway infections.

2) If infection is not present and there is a concern for inflammation, corticosteroids are recommended, e.g. prednisone at 0.5 mg/kg q12–24 h.

3) Over-the-counter (OTC) cough suppressant medications for dogs include dextromethorphan (1–2 mg/kg q6–8 h, as needed), e.g. Robitussin Pediatric Cough Syrup and Vicks Formula 44. Prescription antitussives most commonly used are hydrocodone (0.22 mg/kg q6–12 h) and butorphanol (0.55–1.1 mg/kg q6–12 h as needed). Butorphanol has the added benefit of modest sedation, which helps to relax the patient. Of note, there are holistic and homeopathic products available to relieve coughing. This author has had success with Rescue Remedy® to soothe the pet that is coughing at night.

4) Bronchodilator therapy is helpful in lower airway problems. These include aminophylline (6–10 mg q8 h; this drug is not for long-term therapy) and theophylline (10 mg/kg q12 h). Terbutaline is a beta adrenergic agonist bronchodilator. The recommended dose for small dogs is 0.625–1.25 mg PO q12 h, for medium sized dogs 1.25–2.5 mg PO q12 h, and for large dogs 2.5–5.0 mg PO q12 h.

Physical

Control of environmental factors that cause increased demand for air (increased breathing rate and effort) is beneficial. For example, keeping the patient in a cooler environment, avoiding situations in which the pet becomes over excited, and making sure they do not excessively exercise will decrease the demand for air and subsequently help mitigate episodes of severe coughing. For extrathoracic tracheal collapse, it is helpful to use a harness instead of a collar. For the patient that is in the midst of a significant coughing episode, placing them in front of a fan that is blowing cool air can be very helpful.

Nutritional

Weight loss is a significant component of management if the patient is overweight.

Surgery

As a salvage procedure, when medical management has failed, some caregivers may entertain the possibility of extratracheal rings for extrathoracic tracheal collapse. Laryngeal paralysis may occur postoperatively. Intraluminal stents are recommended for intrathoracic airway collapse of the trachea and mainstem bronchi. Stenting requires extensive medical management postplacement, and complications such as bacterial infection, fracture or migration of the stent, and obstruction of the airway with granulation tissue are not uncommon.

The patient with collapsing airways who is in respiratory distress is a medical emergency. These patients are rescued with oxygen therapy, a cool environment, antitussive medication, and sedation. In severe situations, anesthesia and intubation may be required.

Brachycephalic Airway Obstruction Syndrome

Description

The constellation of genetic abnormalities unique to brachycephalic breeds are stenotic nares, elongated soft palate, everted laryngeal saccules, and hypoplastic trachea (MacPhail 2014). Varying degrees of compromise are noted across the spectrum of individual dogs. Some have minimal problems; others develop serious symptoms with age. These patients have increased airflow resistance requiring them to generate higher negative pressures during inspiration, which is a significant factor in the progression of their disease (MacPhail 2014). Decreasing the diameter of the trachea by 50% will result in a 16-fold increase in resistance. The more compromised the patient's airway, the greater the intraluminal pressure gradient and the more significant the progression of their disease (MacPhail 2014).

The assessment of severity of disease is made by assigning one of three stages. This staging is based on visual inspection of the larynx.

Stage 1: eversion of laryngeal saccules, tissue edema, and inflammation
Stage 2: loss of rigidity and collapse of arytenoid cartilages
Stage 3: fatigued corniculate processes and laryngeal collapse

In these patients, gastrointestinal disease accompanies the respiratory compromise. A linear relationship has been established between respiratory signs and gastrointestinal manifestations such as gastroesophageal reflux, hiatal hernia, and esophagitis/duodenitis, among others (Hoareau et al. 2011; Meola 2013). These gastrointestinal problems can predispose to regurgitation and vomiting, which lead to an increased risk of aspiration. Because of the patients' anatomic abnormalities, resolving an aspiration pneumonia can be extremely challenging (Hoareau et al. 2011).

Trajectory/Prognosis

Patients with brachycephalic airway obstruction syndrome (BAOS) have progressive disease that worsens with time, requiring intensifying support from the caregiver. The time to development of severe disease is variable and uncertain. Secondary aspiration pneumonia is challenging to treat and can be life threatening.

Manifestations

The classic presentation of BAOS is a brachycephalic breed with increased inspiratory effort and audible stertor. While sleeping, these patients are known to snore loudly, which is primarily attributed to their elongated soft palates. Stenotic nares are easily assessed. Radiographs visualize the degree of tracheal hypoplasia. Direct oral examination will confirm arytenoid weakness and laryngeal collapse in advanced cases.

Management

Pharmacologic

1) Controversy currently exists regarding the use of "antacids" and their benefit in patients with regurgitation or vomiting as it relates to potential aspiration pneumonia. One school of thought proposes that a more alkaline stomach pH will encourage bacterial growth. In this scenario, if gastric contents are aspirated, a more severe secondary bacterial infection is potentiated (Dear 2014). This author still uses antacids prophylactically in these patients; specifically, omeprazole 1 mg/kg q12 h. (Please note this is a change from the published dose of once every 24 hours).

2) Sedation may be required in pets that overexert or get too excited and become hyperthermic. Acepromazine 0.01–0.02 mg/kg SC or IM OR butorphanol 0.2–0.3 mg/kg SC or IM are effective.

Physical

Avoiding situations that stress their already compromised airway is important. Cooler environments and preventing overheating are key. Normal daily activity need not be restricted unless the pet has advanced disease. Active cooling (wet hair coat to the skin with tepid water and place in front of a fan) may be necessary in patients that become hyperthermic.

Nutrition

Weight control is an important part of management. Avoiding weight gain in the case of normal body condition and encouraging weight loss in the heavy or obese is recommended. Diets specifically formulated for gastrointestinal disease may be desirable.

Surgery

Corrective airway surgery for brachycephalic patients involves rhinoplasty, resection of the elongated soft palate, and removal of everted laryngeal saccules. Even early stages of laryngeal collapse are amenable to surgery; however, with advanced disease, permanent tracheostomy is often the only option (MacPhail 2014). Surgery may enhance a patients' quality of life by easing respiration, protecting airways in the face of regurgitation or vomiting (providing there is not advanced disease), and relieving comorbid gastrointestinal signs. It is interesting to note that the gastrointestinal signs in these patients resolve in 91–100% following surgical address of their airways (Hoareau et al. 2011; Meola 2013).

BAOS can become a medical emergency when oxygenation and ventilation are impaired. Hospitalization with aggressive medical and/or surgical treatment is needed to rescue these patients from their crisis. For brachycephalics with pneumonia requiring mechanical ventilation, survival to weaning is poor.

Airway Inflammation

Description

Asthma and chronic bronchitis are the most common lower airway conditions in cats (Reinero 2011). Asthma is an allergen-induced hypersensitivity characterized by bronchoconstriction and an eosinophilic inflammation that closely resembles asthma in people. In addition to the inflammation, airway remodeling occurs (Reinero 2011; Schulz et al. 2014). Heartworm-associated respiratory complex and airway parasites can mimic asthma in clinical signs and airway cytology. If in the appropriate geographical area, these conditions should be ruled out in a patient suspected of having asthma. Asthma is rarely diagnosed in canine patients.

Feline chronic bronchitis is a sequela to an insult, most often infection or inhaled irritant (Schulz et al. 2014). The inflammation in bronchitis is neutrophilic with airway edema, excess mucous production, and mucosal hypertrophy. Chronic bronchitis in the dog is considered a syndrome usually seen in the older small breed pet. Narrowing of the airways is caused by airway thickening and excessive mucous production with resultant increased airway resistance.

Trajectory/Prognosis

Inflammatory airway disease is a chronic condition. If properly controlled, it rarely results in the patient's demise but can contribute to decreased activity. Preexisting airway disease becomes a significant comorbidity for any patient concurrently affected by other serious illness.

Manifestations

Wheezing is more often the presenting sign associated with asthma in cats, while fine subtle crackles are associated with chronic bronchitis. This is not true for every case. Both conditions result in occasional coughing. It can be challenging to differentiate these conditions based on history and physical examination alone, and bronchoalveolar lavage is required for definitive diagnosis.

The canine with chronic bronchitis appears generally well but has a chronic productive cough. The inflammatory response perpetuates the cough, and as bronchial walls become thickened and develop malacia, inflammation worsens becoming a vicious cycle. These patients often have increased vagal tone manifest as a pronounced respiratory arrhythmia. One will sometimes observe an increased effort on expiration (Rozanski 2014). Chronic bronchitis patients can develop secondary pulmonary hypertension leading to syncopal episodes. If expiratory airway collapse occurs, hyperinflation and increased work of breathing follows (Rozanski 2014).

Management

Pharmacologic

Feline Asthma This usually responds well to:

1) Oral glucocorticoids (prednisolone 0.51.0 mg/kg PO q24–48 h), or inhaled fluticasone (2 puffs using a chamber and mask q12–24 h).
2) Common bronchodilators are terbutaline (0.312–0.625 mg per cat PO q8–12 h, may be adjusted up to 1.25 mg in larger cats), aminophylline (5 mg/kg q12 h), and theophylline: 20 mg/kg q24 h in the evening. The medications may be used in combination.
3) Inhaled albuterol may be used as a rescue therapy in acute exacerbation.
4) Daily omega-3 polyunsaturated fatty acids (PUFA) in combination with an antioxidant (luteolin) may blunt the production of inflammatory eicosanoids associated with asthma.
5) Recently, lidocaine has received attention as a rescue therapy in feline and human asthma. In one study, lidocaine was nebulized at 2 mg/kg q8 h for up to 2 weeks and did not result in any adverse events in healthy or asthmatic cats (Trzil et al. 2014).
6) If secondary infection is suspected, antibiotics typically considered include clindamycin (10–15 mg/kg q12 h for up to 14 days), marbofloxacin (2.75–5.5 mg/kg q24 h), or azithromycin (5–10 mg/kg PO q24 h for 5 days then q72 h for up to 6 weeks).

Feline Chronic Bronchitis Therapy for this condition includes bronchodilators and omega-3 PUFA/antioxidant. Because this is an inflammatory condition, oral glucocorticoids may be of benefit. Suspected infection should be treated.

Canine Chronic Bronchitis Syndrome Glucocorticoids are the mainstay of therapy (prednisone 0.5 mg/kg q24 h). Cough suppressants are often helpful (Rozanski 2014). In an acute exacerbation, if infection is suspected, antibiotics should be prescribed.

Physical

Eliminate any environmental irritants such as cigarette smoke.

Nutritional

Address obesity as this will significantly worsen any coughing as well as decrease the patient's lung function.

Pneumonia

Description

The broad categories of pneumonia include infectious (bacterial, viral, fungal); aspiration of gastrointestinal contents; and inhaled foreign body (Dear 2014). In both the dog and cat, viral upper respiratory infections can lead to a secondary bacterial pneumonia. Fungal pneumonias are generally associated with the immune compromised patient and specific geographical areas. Aspiration pneumonitis/pneumonia is associated with esophageal disease (regurgitation), chronic vomiting, laryngeal problems, brachycephalic breeds with airway obstruction syndrome, and neurologic disease (particularly seizures) (Dear 2014). Silent regurgitation and aspiration has been documented in some patients after anesthesia. Any condition that compromises the normal swallowing reflex can predispose the patient to aspiration. The acidic pH of gastric contents causes significant lung injury. The inflammation that follows allows the establishment of infection by gastrointestinal bacteria.

Trajectory/Prognosis

If severe, and especially if associated with comorbid respiratory disease such as bronchiectasis or BAOS, pneumonia can lead to hypoxemia and significant impairment. This affects the animal's ability to function and requires an extraordinary amount of supportive care.

Manifestations

Early signs of pneumonia are an increased respiratory rate, decreased activity, and decreased to absent appetite. Modest to severe increase in respiratory effort may also be seen depending on severity. Patients in significant distress, with impending respiratory muscle fatigue, may exhibit paradoxical abdominal breathing. Only half of the patients have a fever (Dear 2014). Breath sounds are not diagnostic and are often described as being "harsh" or "increased." The patient may, or may not, have a cough.

Management

Pharmacologic

Cough suppressants are *not* indicated.

1) Mucolytics such as guaifenesin may be useful.
2) Antibiotics are best chosen based on culture and sensitivity. If that is not feasible, a fluoroquinolone (e.g. enrofloxacin 10 mg/kg q24 h in dogs, 5 mg/kg q24 h in cats) and a lincosamide (e.g. clindamycin 10 mg/kgq12 h for cats and dogs) are good first choices due to their ability to penetrate lung tissue well.
3) Oxygen supplementation will be needed if the oxygen saturation (SpO_2) drops below 93%. In the most severe cases, mechanical ventilation is required to augment oxygenation/ventilation and relieve respiratory muscle fatigue.
4) If the pneumonia is due to aspiration of gastric contents, antiemetic therapy (maropitant 2–8 mg/kg PO q24 h or ondansetron 0.5 mg/kg PO q12 h) and gastroprotectants (sucralfate 0.5–1 g PO as a slurry q8 h and omeprazole 1 mg/kg PO q12 h) are indicated to prevent recurrence.

Physical

Nebulization with sterile saline for 10–12 minutes followed by coupage at least twice daily is indicated to keep airways moist and encourage removal (coughing) of secretions. Minimize the amount of work the patient has to do, keep food and water close, and consider carrying the patient out to the bathroom if feasible.

Nutritional

Patients with significant respiratory difficulty often do not want to eat. Maintaining adequate caloric and fluid intake is important. Particularly tasty, canned foods or home cooked meals, moistened with water, help maintain calories and fluid.

The Suffering of Dyspnea: Palliative Care

The "feeling of breathlessness" is termed dyspnea. This means more than difficulty breathing, more than the inability to oxygenate or ventilate appropriately. The term dyspnea evokes the emotional suffering accompanying the feeling of not being able to get a good breath. Verbal hospice patients state that dyspnea is no less a form of suffering than uncontrolled pain.

In human hospice, pure mu opioid agonists are well known to alleviate dyspnea without hastening death. Reduced doses are used but the dose is repeated every 15 minutes until the patient is more comfortable. This author typically starts with 10–20% of the normal dose, repeating until comfort is noted. Fentanyl (1–2 mcg/kg) or hydromorphone (0.01–0.02 mg/kg) have rapid onset and are both reversible if the need arises. Opioids should not be withheld from the hospice patient suffering from dyspnea.

Patients with dyspnea often have nausea, pain and anxiety. In addition to opioids, benzodiazepines and antiemetics should not be withheld. Midazolam may be given intranasally, oral transmucosally, subcutaneously, intramuscularly, and intravenously. In these fragile patients, start with lower doses such as 0.05 mg/kg. and titrate up to effective dose. The customary doses of maropitant, dolasetron or ondansetron may be administered for nausea.

The administration of steroids may also be considered in the event there is an inflammatory component. The reader is referred to the discussion of feline asthma above which may be applied to canine patients.

Patients with dyspnea may or may not be hypoxic. A trial of oxygen supplementation for three days is recommended. There are various methods to provide oxygen supplementation as well as various concentrations of oxygen to be delivered. Oxygen tanks provide 100% oxygen and oxygen concentrators provide 40% (twice room air). For at home oxygen supplementation, an oxygen concentrator is preferred for a number of reasons. An oxygen tank of 100% oxygen is a potential hazard due to (i) explosion/fire and (ii) oxygen toxicity to the patient if used for too long. Oxygen concentrators are very safe by comparison and equally cost effective. These machines can be rented from a medical supply provider for a monthly fee or purchased outright for approximately $350. Oxygen concentrators avoid the explosion/fire risk as well as the oxygen toxicity risk.

Oxygen can be provided by "flow by," mask, nasal cannula, or oxygen "tent." Flow by is provided by simply holding the end of the oxygen line within 2 inches of the end of the nose. This is fine for immediate need but not practical for long term administration. An oxygen mask covers the end of the muzzle. If the patient is compromised to the point they are laterally recumbent and not moving around, a mask can be sufficient. In larger dogs, an oxygen cage or tent may not be feasible. These patients do well with the placement of a nasal cannula. There are several references for placement of a nasal oxygen catheter. This author recommends the YouTube video by Bernie Hansen titled "Nasal Oxygen Catheter Placement in the Dog" (https://youtu.be/8eJ385APQ3w).

A novel therapy, described in detail in Chapter 19 "Pharmacology Interventions for Symptom Management" in this volume, has recently been introduced for the temporary relief of dyspnea in veterinary patients. Magnesium sulfate followed by furosemide are administered via nebulization (Mellema 2008). This author has successfully used this treatment in a variety of conditions: congestive heart failure, pneumonia, terminal bronchiectasis, and metastatic neoplasia among others. This treatment is strictly a palliative therapy and does not treat the underlying disease.

Most patients are breathing easier, often falling asleep by the time the treatment is finished. Some patients get as much as six hours of relief from one treatment.

As hospice and palliative care providers, it is imperative that we do all we can to alleviate this suffering in our patients.

> Cure sometimes, treat often, comfort always.
> *Hippocrates*

References

Dear, J.D. (2014) Bacterial pneumonia in dogs and cats. *Vet. Clin. Small Anim.*, 44: 143–159.

Hoareau, G.L., Mellema, M.S., and Silverstein, D.C. (2011) Indication, management, and outcome of brachycephalic dogs requiring mechanical ventilation. *J. Vet. Emerg. Crit. Care*, 21: 226–235.

MacPhail, C. (2014) Laryngeal disease in dogs and cats. *Vet. Clin. Small Anim.*, 44: 19–31.

Maggiore, A.D. (2014) Tracheal and airway collapse in dogs. *Vet. Clin. Small Anim.*, 44: 117–127.

Mellema, M. (2008) The neurophysiology of dyspnea. *J. Vet. Emerg. Crit. Care*, 18: 561–571.

Meola, S.D. (2013) Brachycephalic airway syndrome. *Top. Companion Anim. Med.*, 28: 91–96.

Reinero, C.R. (2011) Advances in the understanding of pathogenesis, and diagnostics and therapeutics for feline allergic asthma. *Vet. J.*, 190: 28–33.

Rozanski, E. (2014) Canine chronic bronchitis. *Vet. Clin. Small Anim.*, 44, 107–116.

Schulz, B.S., Richter, P., Weber, K. *et al.* (2014) Detection of feline *Mycoplasma* species in cats with feline asthma and chronic bronchitis. *J. Feline Med. Surg.*, 16: 943–949.

Trzil, J.E., Masseau, I., Webb, T.L. *et al.* (2014) Long-term evaluation of mesenchymal stem cell therapy in a feline model of chronic allergic asthma. *Clin. Exp. Allergy*, 44: 1546–1557.

15

Gastrointestinal Conditions

Shea Cox, DVM, CHPV, CVPP and Christie Cornelius, DVM, CHPV

There are numerous gastrointestinal conditions that can affect animals. It is beyond the scope of this chapter to fully discuss each one of them, and thus the focus will be placed on reviewing three of the more common diseases that hospice care providers encounter. These conditions are inflammatory bowel disease (IBD), pancreatitis, and cholangitis/cholangio-hepatitis syndrome (CCHS).

Inflammatory Bowel Disease

Description of Disease

IBD is a term used to describe chronic inflammation of the gastrointestinal tract, and is one of the most important causes of chronic diarrhea and vomiting in both dogs and cats. IBD is not a single disease entity per se, but the culmination of chronic and sustained inflammation of the gut. Chronic inflammation of the bowel may become uncontrolled and self-perpetuating when loss of mucosal integrity and increased permeability allow bacterial and dietary antigens to enter the lamina propria where they incite ongoing immune stimulation and inflammation (Sherding 2013).

Disease Trajectory

The short-term prognosis for disease control is generally good in most cases; however, long-term prognosis can be more guarded in cases of severe clinical disease. IBD is a disease that is managed, not cured, and relapses are common.

Clinical Manifestations of Disease

The most common clinical signs of IBD include vomiting, diarrhea, weight loss, thickened bowel loops on abdominal palpation, abdominal pain, and fever. Signs can vary with the severity of disease, and they typically wax and wane in their presentation.

Palliative Management

The treatment for IBD is aimed at reducing inflammation and most commonly consists of immunosuppressive therapy, antibiotics, dietary management, and recently fecal microbial transplantation (FMT).

Medical Support

Immunosuppressive Therapy
Corticosteroids are the initial treatment of choice, with the most commonly used medication being prednisone and prednisolone.

Hospice and Palliative Care for Companion Animals: Principles and Practice, Second Edition.
Edited by Amir Shanan, Jessica Pierce, and Tamara Shearer.
© 2023 John Wiley & Sons, Inc. Published 2023 by John Wiley & Sons, Inc.
Companion website: www.wiley.com/go/shanan/palliative

Budesonide, dexamethasone, or methylprednisolone may also be used to treat IBD. Dexamethasone is sometimes more effective than prednisone or prednisolone. Dexamethasone has little to no mineralocorticoid activity, so it is preferable to use in cases where fluid retention is of concern (e.g. dogs with advanced heart disease). In cats that are impossible to medicate orally, periodic injections of methylprednisolone acetate may be substituted for oral treatment. Budesonide is a nonhalogenated glucocorticoid that has a high first-pass effect in the liver resulting in less systemic adverse effects. Budesonide can be an alternative option for management of IBD in both dogs and cats. It can be helpful in cases that are intolerant of corticosteroids, and in severe cases that have proven to be refractory to prednisolone, metronidazole, and dietary management (Tams 2012). In a randomized, controlled trial, budesonide was shown to have similar remission rates to prednisone in the treatment of IBD (78 vs. 69%, respectively Dye et al. 2013). Azathioprine, chlorambucil, and cyclosporine are immunosuppressive agents that are sometimes considered for the management of refractory IBD, but are beyond the scope of this discussion.

Antibiotic Therapy

Metronidazole and Tylosin are two common antibiotics used in the treatment of IBD in combination with corticosteroids. The beneficial effects appear to include an ability to balance intestinal microflora, reduce obligate anaerobe load, and reduce inflammation. In patients with mild disease, a two- to four-week antimicrobial trial may be instituted before starting immune-suppressive therapy (Gaschen 2016). A major advantage of using combination therapy is that the corticosteroid dose may be decreased from the high initial dose sooner, thus decreasing the likelihood of significant corticosteroid-related side effects (Tams 2012).

Special care should be taken in animals that are on long-term metronidazole therapy because of potential risks of neurotoxicosis and hepatotoxicosis. While metronidazole has been popular, its therapeutic margin in cats is narrow and risks of neurological side effects and genotoxicity (with potential to be mutagenic) make it less desirable. Tylosin is a good alternative, although the drug needs to be compounded for use in cats (Gaschen 2016).

Caregivers should be warned that metronidazole tablets have an unpleasant bitter taste and provoke salivation, nausea, and sometimes vomiting. To prevent these adverse reactions, tablets can be split and placed in gel capsules, preventing contact in the mouth. Flavored liquid formulations are sometimes better tolerated but can remain unpalatable to many pets, especially cats.

Additional Support Therapy

Folate and cobalamin levels are frequently abnormal in patients with IBD, and supplementing these vitamins will aid in proper nutrient absorption and digestion (Fogle and Bissett 2007). Cobalamin deficiency can occur with IBD, especially in cats, presumably the result of malabsorption of the vitamin in the ileum. Cobalamin deficiency in turn can impair intestinal mucosal regeneration and cause mucosal atrophy, exacerbating diarrhea and making the patient refractory to the usual anti-inflammatory therapy (Sherding 2013). Subcutaneous fluids should be administered if dehydration develops due to continued vomiting and/or diarrhea.

Cobalamin (if serum cobalamin < 200 ng l^{-1}): cats and small dogs, 250 mcg SC; medium dogs, 500 mcg SC; large dogs, 1000 mcg SC; injections are given weekly for at least 6 weeks, then every other week for 6 weeks, and then monthly. A retrospective study documented that oral supplementation of cobalamin is effective in dogs with chronic enteropathies. There is currently no evidence to support the effect of oral treatment in cats (Gaschen 2016).

Subcutaneous fluid therapy: as needed to maintain appropriate hydration.

Nutritional Support

Dietary therapy for IBD generally involves the use of a limited-ingredient diet with a single, hydrolyzed, or novel protein source. Fish oil can be added to the diet to help reduce intestinal inflammation, and probiotics can be administered to promote overall gastrointestinal heath. If a decision is made to initially manage an animal with dietary therapy alone, the dietary trial should be conducted for a minimum of 3–4 weeks. Some animals require six weeks or more before clinical improvement occurs.

Fecal Microbial Transplantation (FMT): The Ultimate Probiotic

Dysbiosis is a disruption or imbalance in the normal gastrointestinal (GI) microbiota. Significant dysbiosis is found in cases of acute and chronic diarrhea, GI motility disorders, exocrine pancreatic insufficiency (EPI), and the use of antibiotics and gastric acid reducers. Although the research is very limited, dysbiosis appears to be a significant component of canine and feline diarrhea, and the majority of over the counter (OTC) probiotics simply do not live up to label claims.

The fecal microbiotica (actual organisms) and microbiome (genetic material) are essential to the normal development and function of most every system in the body, although most often highlighted with regards to the gastrointestinal tract. The GI tract also houses the largest collection of immune cells anywhere in the body, so it is not surprising that the micribiota has a critical impact on immune function, and FMT might act as an "immunotherapy" (Webb 2020).

Fecal microbial transplantation has been effectively used in people for treatment of *Clostridium difficile* infection. The benefits of FMT are probably not limited to the actual bacteria that are transplanted, but also the bacteriophages and bile acids that are present in feces. Despite dogs being coprophagic in nature, some individual studies suggest FMT may be useful in dogs (Mansfield 2019).

Pancreatitis

Description of Disease

Pancreatitis is defined as inflammation of the pancreas, and it can be broadly categorized as acute, recurrent acute, or chronic. Acute and recurrent acute pancreatitis are characterized by sudden episodes of inflammation, which may resolve after a short time or may continue to cause ongoing inflammation (becoming recurrent acute or chronic). Chronic pancreatitis is characterized by low-grade or subclinical inflammation and may be a factor in the development of diabetes mellitus and EPI in both dogs and cats. Complications such as necrosis and/or abscesses can occur.

The etiology and pathogenesis of pancreatitis is poorly understood. Currently, the majority of both acute and chronic pancreatitis cases in both dogs and cats are considered idiopathic. Some factors that have been implicated in the development of pancreatitis include hereditary causes, drugs or toxins, hypercalcemia, infectious agents, extension of hepatobiliary or intestinal inflammation (cats), duodenal reflux, pancreatic duct obstruction, nutritional factors such as an increase in lipoproteins in the blood, dietary indiscretions, and obesity (Simpson 2012). In a series of studies, severe hypertriglyceridemia is a significant risk factor for acute pancreatitis in dogs (Steiner and Toresson 2020).

Disease Trajectory

Prognosis is generally good for pets with acute, edematous pancreatitis that show response to appropriate therapy. Prognosis is good to guarded for pets with recurrent acute and chronic pancreatitis, because the continued ongoing inflammation of the pancreas can cause scarring and irreversible damage of the organ. A guarded to poor prognosis is given to those pets with necrotizing pancreatitis, especially those with secondary systemic conditions (such as diabetes mellitus).

Clinical Manifestations of Disease

Clinical signs are often vague and non-specific, mimicking many other disease processes. The more common findings in dogs and cats include weight loss, lethargy, abdominal pain, fever, dehydration due to GI losses through vomiting and diarrhea, and icterus. Cats can also present with hypothermia.

Palliative Management

The recommended treatment for acute episodes of pancreatitis often includes hospitalization and aggressive intravenous fluid therapy to address hypovolemia and maintain pancreatic circulation. However, this may not be an acceptable option for families with pets in hospice care. If recommended hospitalization is declined in lieu of home care, the following treatments can be implemented.

Medical Support

Analgesia
Multi-modal analgesia is an essential part of treatment, and opioids, such as buprenorphine or methadone, are generally needed to appropriately manage the level of discomfort caused by pancreatitis.

Antiemetics
Centrally acting antiemetics such as maropitant, metoclopramide, and ondansetron should be used to control signs of nausea and vomiting and further promote patient comfort.

Antibacterials
There is evidence that systemic translocation of bacteria can occur in cases of pancreatitis. Therefore, antibacterials are often used prophylactically. However, the majority of cases are sterile, so there is no need for the routine use of antibiotics unless a secondary infection is identified (e.g. pancreatic abscess).

Immunosuppressants
Based on a suspected immune-mediated etiology, treatment with corticosteroids has been suggested, but clinical trials are lacking. In addition, many feline cases of pancreatitis may be associated with IBD and/or CCHS, and the use of corticosteroids may be helpful in these patients. There may be uneasiness in treating feline patients with chronic pancreatitis with corticosteroids as many of these patients are glucose intolerant or may have diabetes mellitus. However, studies in humans have shown that patients with autoimmune pancreatitis show an overall improved control of diabetes mellitus after treatment with glucocorticoids, and less than 20% of patients develop diabetes mellitus after glucocorticoid therapy has been initiated (Steiner 2020).

Cyclosporine, a calcineurin inhibitor that blocks cytokine production and inhibits T-cell proliferation and activation, is a potential treatment option in cats with chronic pancreatitis. Cyclosporine has the theoretical advantage that it has a less significant impact on insulin resistance than do glucocorticoids (Steiner and Toresson 2020).

Subcutaneous Fluid Therapy
For pets treated at home, subcutaneous fluid therapy is an important component of treatment and should be given once to twice daily, depending upon the patient's hydration status, severity of clinical signs, and tolerance to treatment.

Nutritional Support
Acute pancreatitis, especially when severe, is a highly catabolic disease and early caloric support is essential for treatment success. Therefore, there should be attempts to recommence feeding as soon as vomiting subsides. Percutaneous jejunostomy placement can be considered in pets that are unable or unwilling to eat despite supportive measures. Jejunostomy tube placement is preferred to that of an esophagostomy tube as it allows for enteral nutrition while promoting rest of the pancreas. When a pet is able to eat, it is recommended that they be fed small, frequent meals of a high-carbohydrate, low-fat diet. Protein

sources should be of high biologic value, such as cottage cheese or lean meat. A low-fat diet is usually recommended long term, although this may be less essential in cats than in dogs.

Cholangitis/Cholangiohepatitis Syndrome

Description of Disease

CCHS is a group of disorders that affect either the biliary tree, or more commonly, the biliary tree and the liver. CCHS is relatively rare in dogs, but is common in cats, with the non-suppurative form being most prevalent (Scherk 2011). The non-suppurative form is believed to involve immune-mediated mechanisms, while the suppurative form involves an ascending bacterial infection. There is often coexistent IBD and low-grade pancreatitis in these cats, and thus the caregiver should be educated about these disease processes as well.

Disease Trajectory

Regardless of whether a cat suffers from acute suppurative CCH or chronic non-suppurative CCH, survival time is good (Scherk 2011). With suitable therapy, a good long-term prognosis may be expected. Suppurative CCHS may be cured. Non-suppurative CCHS is generally a chronic disease with possibility of remission.

Clinical Manifestations of Disease

Most cats affected with nonsuppurative CCHS are middle aged or older and present with a chronic, often episodic (several weeks or more) history of vague illness. The disease may be occurring for several months before a diagnosis is made. The clinical presentation can include periods of inappetence/anorexia *or* polyphagia, lethargy, nausea, vomiting, diarrhea, and weight loss. On physical examination, signs of dehydration, weight loss, muscle wasting, icterus, salivation, palpable liver

margins, and cranial abdominal tenderness or firmness may be present.

Cats with suppurative CCHS, on the other hand, generally appear more acutely ill as the disease is associated with an ascending bacterial infection. The signalment includes males and younger cats more commonly than the nonsuppurative form. These patients have a history and clinical signs of vomiting, diarrhea, lethargy, fever, dehydration, jaundice, and abdominal pain.

Palliative Management

Determining what form of CCHS is present enables the veterinarian to begin the appropriate therapy. However, many families of pets in hospice decline the measures needed to obtain a diagnosis, and treatment recommendations may need to be based on the level of suspicion of disease being present, the history and physical examination findings, and response to initial therapies implemented. The following nonspecific treatment strategies are aimed at slowing progression and improving patient comfort.

Medical Support

Antimicrobial Therapy

Because enteric bacteria are often associated with disease, antibiotics can be a critical part of the therapy. If there is suspicion of CCHS and a definitive diagnosis remains open, it is recommended that an antibiotic trial be started and continued for at least 4–6 weeks while monitoring for improvement or decline. Ampicillin, ampicillin–clavulanic acid, and cephalosporins have been suggested as effective antibiotics. Cefovecin is also an option in cats that cannot take oral medications.

Immunosuppressive Therapy

If a pet fails to respond to antibiotic therapy, or if clinical decline is occurring despite antibiotic therapy, immunosuppressive therapy can be implemented. If there is a confirmed diagnosis of the chronic form of CCHS and bacterial infection has been ruled out, the traditional therapy for the chronic form recommends using anti-inflammatory or immunosuppressive therapy starting with prednisolone at $2\text{--}4\,mg/kg^{-1}$ daily, and then slowly tapering over 6–8 weeks to $0.5\text{--}1\,mg/kg^{-1}$ given once or every other day. This therapy does not appear to resolve this chronic disease, but generally slows the progression and may minimize the clinical signs.

Analgesia
Abdominal discomfort may be associated with hepatobiliary pain and analgesics should be administered.

Antiemetics
Antiemetics are indicated for nausea and vomiting. In the case of significant liver disease, the dose of antiemetics that are metabolized by the liver (such as maropitant) should be halved.

Support Therapy
Antioxidant therapy is indicated to help protect against inflammation-induced free radicals. Antioxidant agents that can be used include zinc, glutathione, S-adenosyl-L-methionine (SAMe), vitamin E, vitamin C, beta-carotene, coenzyme Q10, and super oxide dismutase (Scherk 2010).

Ursodeoxycholic acid (ursodiol) is also suggested for treatment of CCHS, dosed at $10\text{--}15\,mg\,/kg^{-1}\,day^{-1}$. Concerns that ursodiol may exacerbate the condition of patients with a bile duct obstruction are unfounded. Ursodeoxycholic acid is not a prokinetic and will not cause a gallbladder rupture (Twedt 2020).

Subcutaneous Fluid Therapy
Subcutaneous fluids should be given as needed to maintain appropriate hydration.

Nutritional Support
A limited-antigen diet is often recommended as part of the general supportive treatments.

Conclusion

Gastrointestinal diseases are common in geriatric canine and feline patients. A definitive diagnosis is frequently not pursued in hospice patients. Therapies are directed to the palliative management of clinical symptoms and/or based upon suspicion of disease presence. Much can be done to provide comfort and quality of life to patients with gastrointestinal diseases during the hospice relationship, even when a definitive diagnosis cannot be reached.

References

Dye, T.L, Diehl, K. J., Wheeler, S. L. et al. (2013) Randomized, controlled trial of budesonide and prednisone for the treatment of idiopathic inflammatory bowel disease in dogs. *J. Vet. Intern. Med.*, 27: 1385–1391.

Fogle, J. and Bissett, S. (2007) Mucosal immunity and chronic idiopathic enteropathies in dogs. *Compendium*, 29(5): 290–306.

Gaschen, F. (2016). Feline IBD vs. alimentary lymphoma – which one is it? *Pacific Veterinary Conference*, San Francisco, CA. (June 23–26).

Mansfield, C. (2019). The gut microbiome in GI diseases: how and when to manipulate it? *World Small Animal Veterinary Association Congress Proceedings*, Toronto, Canada. (July 16–19).

Scherk, M. (2010) Cholangitis/cholangiohepatitis complex. *Western Veterinary Conference*, Las Vegas, NV. (February 16–19).

Scherk, M. (2011) Understanding cholangitis/cholangiohepatitis in the cat. *Atlantic Coast Veterinary Conference*, Atlantic City, NJ. (October 12–14).

Sherding, R. (2013) Inflammatory bowel disease – etiology and diagnosis. *Atlantic Coast Veterinary Conference*, Atlantic City, NJ. (October 12–14).

Simpson, K. (2012) An update on pancreatitis in dogs and cats. *Western Veterinary Conference*, Ithaca, NY.

Steiner, J. (2020) Feline Pancreatitis: More Common Than You Think (SO8C). *Western Veterinary Conference*, Las Vegas, NV. (February 16–19).

Steiner, J. and Toresson L. (2020) Updates on Treatment of Pancreatitis in Dogs and Cats. *European College of Veterinary Internal Medicine-Companion Animals Online Congress*. Online. (September 2–5).

Tams, T. (2012) Inflammatory bowel disease and intestinal lymphoma in cats. *Atlantic Coast Veterinary Conference*, Atlantic City, NJ. (October 12-14).

Twedt, D. (2020) Canine Chronic Hepatitis: Diagnostic Keys and the Latest Therapies. *Western Veterinary Conference*, Colorado State University, Las Vegas, NV. (February 16-19).

Webb, C. (2020). Fecal Microbiota Transplantation: What's Coming Down the Pipline (SA173). *Western Veterinary Conference*, Las Vegas, NV. (February 16-19).

16

Musculoskeletal Disorders

Tamara Shearer, MS, DVM, CCRP, CVPP, CVA, MSTCVM

Musculoskeletal disorders involve the interaction between the body's muscles, bones, ligaments, tendons, fascia, and joints. These are common comorbidities seen in hospice and palliative care patients. They result in such profound disability that drastic decisions have to be made because of decline in quality of life. In 2011, musculoskeletal disorders were considered the second most common cause of death because of organ system change in adult and juvenile dog patients, according to a retrospective study of over 75 000 dogs that died at 27 North American veterinary teaching hospitals (Fleming et al. 2011). However, in a pilot study (Shearer and Marchitelli 2015) musculoskeletal cause for euthanasia or death in dogs moved from second, as observed in the Flemming study, to eighth in frequency for a practice offering physical medicine. Cats also struggle with musculoskeletal disorders that can affect quality of life, but documentation of incidence is more difficult because of the nature of their behaviors.

A special note: when fragile patients present for investigation of musculoskeletal conditions, practitioners should be mindful that an aggressive examination may leave some individuals profoundly painful and even debilitated. A gentle approach is recommended.

The following are a few of the more common musculoskeletal problems seen in hospice and palliative care patients.

Osteoarthritis

Description

Osteoarthritis (OA) is a common condition seen in patients enrolled in hospice and palliative care. Like other diseases where pain is a symptom, the incidence of OA is probably under reported. It has been estimated that 20% of dogs suffer from osteoarthritis (Marcellin-Little et al. 2014). A study of 100 client-owned cats, equal to or older than 6 years of age, found a 61% incidence of OA in one joint and a 48% incidence of OA in more than one joint (Slingerland et al. 2011). Osteoarthritis is often secondary in nature and may be the result of genetic predisposition, past injury or overuse, developmental changes, and inflammatory processes. Conditions like osteochondrosis dissecans, angular limb deformities, past trauma, and hip dysplasia are examples of problems that increase the risk of OA.

The mechanism behind the development of osteoarthritis is complex and has been

Hospice and Palliative Care for Companion Animals: Principles and Practice, Second Edition.
Edited by Amir Shanan, Jessica Pierce, and Tamara Shearer.
© 2023 John Wiley & Sons, Inc. Published 2023 by John Wiley & Sons, Inc.
Companion website: www.wiley.com/go/shanan/palliative

discussed extensively by Fox (2012) and others (e.g. Henderson and Millis 2014). Simply put, the cartilage undergoes a series of physiological changes that include decreased proteoglycan concentration, increased water content, collagen fibril disruption, and degradation of macromolecules. Loss of articular cartilage is exacerbated in areas bearing increased load. As a result of these changes, sclerosis of the subchondral bone, osteophytes, and synovitis develop, all of which can contribute to the joint pain.

Trajectory/Prognosis

Osteoarthritis has a type 3 disease trajectory. It is a condition with a prolonged course of decline that would require increasing care over time if proactive measures are not offered to the patient or if the OA is at end stage. The chronicity of this disorder predisposes pets to complicated pain issues and to comorbidities related to muscle and joint disuse.

Manifestations

The cardinal signs of OA are lameness of varying degrees and other mobility impairments; however, it is often preceded by a subclinical phase. Early, subtle clinical signs of pain may include changes in body posture and in facial expression, decreased activity, decreased social interaction, restlessness, and other changes in behavior. In cats, often times only behavioral signs are noted, like decreased activity and increased incidence of house soiling. In some cases the early symptoms of OA are only evident after a patient has fallen or participated in a rigorous activity that overexerted the joints. As the disease progresses pain or periods of stiffness may become more noticeable. Over time, the patient may be hesitant to participate in the normal exercise routine. The pet may also resist sitting, lying down, or even standing for long periods of time. They may avoid climbing steps and jumping onto furniture or into vehicles.

Depending on the individual, some patients with OA progress to develop profound lameness and severe debilitation. They are reluctant to move or are incapable of moving.

Examination findings may include painful joints, joint effusion, joint inflammation, and crepitus in the joint. A decrease in a joint's range of motion may result from pain or from physical changes to various joint structures. Thickening of the joint capsule may be present. Atrophy of the affected limbs may be seen with hypertrophy of the other limbs or muscles used to compensate for the OA changes. Comorbidities seen with OA include, but are not limited to, muscle wasting/weakness, urinary tract infections, and decubitus ulcers.

Noninvasive diagnostic methods for hospice or palliative care patients include taking a complete history and conducting a complete orthopedic examination. As mentioned above, practitioners should be mindful about overexerting a fragile pet during an orthopedic examination. Radiographs can be helpful but it is important to remember that radiographic evidence of osteoarthritis may not correlate with the level of pain that a patient experiences (Gordon et al. 2003). Because radiographs are better at demonstrating bony changes, the changes in the cartilage and synovial surfaces can be difficult to assess with plain radiographs. However, increased synovial fluid, thickened joint capsules, periarticular osteophytes, subchondral bone sclerosis, and bone remodeling may be recognized or confirmed radiographically. Because these symptoms and findings are not specific to osteoarthritis, other differentials need to be considered, including immune-mediated conditions, neoplasia, and infectious processes that may require different palliative management. When performing radiographs with fragile patients, care must be taken not to exacerbate pain that leaves the pet painful and debilitated as a consequence of a diagnostic intervention. Clients should be educated about this potential risk.

Management

At this time, there is no treatment method resulting in perfect healing of articular cartilage. Once the cartilage is degraded it can never fully recover. The body's efforts to self-repair degraded cartilage result in the development of fibrocartilage. Unfortunately, fibrocartilage does not function effectively under weight-bearing loads, lacking the flexibility and durability of hyaline cartilage.

Palliation of OA symptoms is similar in many ways to palliating other musculoskeletal conditions. In general, the types of interventions available for helping hospice and palliative care patients with impaired mobility include:

1) management of pain and inflammation;
2) environmental modifications;
3) activity modifications;
4) use of assistive devices, rehabilitation, or physical modalities;
5) use of nutraceuticals, chrondroprotectants, and other supplements.

The first priority in palliative care should be to manage the pain associated with the disorder and then work to restore function. Relieving the pain and applying rehabilitation techniques will provide enough relief for some pets to resume some or all of the activities of daily living (Millis and Levine 1997). One of the mainstays of managing pain and slowing the progression of OA and other musculoskeletal conditions is to attain an optimal weight because excess weight produces increased stress on joints. This may not be an attainable goal for pets that are at the end stage of their disease trajectory and moving into hospice care. Weight loss is, however, important for patients that are in long-term palliative care such as pets with debilitating osteoarthritis secondary to cruciate ligament disease.

Pain management can be accomplished by the administration of nonsteroidal anti-inflammatory drugs (NSAIDs), corticosteroids, opioids, and osteoarthritis-modifying agents.

The use of intra-articular corticosteroids may also improve joint comfort. A unique intra-articular elbow joint injection, Synovetin OA® by Exubrion Therapeutics, is a veterinary device consisting of a tin colloid that emits low energy conversion electrons to reduce synovitis. The injected colloid is confined and retained in the joint space. Apoptosis and reduction in inflammatory cells occur when the particles are absorbed by the cells in the synovium. Special handling and disposal of materials are required because of the radioactive nature of the product. Despite the special handling, the safety profile of Synovetin OA and efficacy look promising at this point in time. For a more detailed discussion of pain management techniques see Chapters 19 and 20.

Solensia™ (frunevetmab) is a cat-specific monoclonal antibody that is administered to cats by a once monthly subcutaneous injection. It is designed to treat pain from osteoarthritis by attaching to nerve growth factor that is involved with the pain regulation. It was approved by the US Food and Drug Administration (FDA) for this use on January 13, 2022, but had been used in other countries with success prior to this date. Librela® (bedinvetmab) is the is the monoclonal antibody developed for dogs, not yet approved in the United States.

Optimizing the animal's environment is very important in managing patients with mobility impairment. To prevent trauma, the environment should be modified to provide nonslip flooring and low incline ramps to bypass steps. Stairways should be blocked off to prevent falls. Modifications to facilitate access to food and water may include placing them in additional locations and/or raising existing bowls.

Modification of the activities that the patient was once involved in can often improve comfort. Because this component of care may cause a profound disruption in the human-animal bond, it may be one the most difficult parameters of care to implement. In some cases, if a pet avoids strenuous exercise the symptoms of pain are less apparent or prevented. Low-impact exercises, like walking and swimming, are safer choices than more rigorous exercise. For example, chasing a ball down a hill for 15 minutes may need to be modified to pitching the ball to the dog for 5 minutes on a flat surface. Play with a feline companion may avoid jumping up and twisting to catch a feather.

The use of assistive devices, rehabilitation, and physical treatment modalities can also improve the comfort of hospice and palliative patients with musculoskeletal disorders. Modalities such as laser therapy, extracorporeal shock wave therapy, hydrotherapy, therapeutic ultrasound, electrotherapy, pulsed signal therapy, and targeted pulsed electromagnetic therapy help manage pain and improve recoveries in patients (See Chapter 20 for details on physical medicine options for hospice and palliative care patients).

There are a large number of foods, nutraceuticals, chrondroprotectants, and other aids to support a patient with OA and other musculoskeletal issues. Disease-modifying osteoarthritic agents are a favorite among pain practitioners. Injectable polysulfated glycosaminoglycans (PSGAGs) are used to improve the health of the affected joints by promoting the development of fibrocartilage, inhibiting collagenase and metalloproteinases (Altman et al. 1989). Adequan® (Luitpold Animal Health, Shirley, NY) is the only FDA-approved PSGAG drug for dogs. In the original studies, the product was administered by intramuscular injection, but it is now being widely used subcutaneously with reproducible results. Although not approved for use in cats, it is widely used in this species. When used for palliative care, common off-label use includes the administration of subcutaneous injections in the following manner: 1 induction twice weekly for 4 weeks, then one injection every 10 days to 4 weeks depending on the patient. If the injections were discontinued for various reasons, reinduction or an increased dose frequency should be considered working up to a maintenance level. Acupuncturists often divide the dose and inject acupoints to accomplish additional benefits.

The availability of products advertised to support patients with osteoarthritis is overwhelming. It is important to choose supplements and herbal formulas that have scientific research to support their efficacy. Supplements to support OA might include a combination of the following. Avocado/soybean unsaponifiables help to maintain joint health (Dasuquin; Nutramax Laboratories Veterinary Sciences, Inc., Lancaster, SC) (Boileau et al. 2009). Elk antler velvet powder (Qeva, Calgary, Alberta Canada) may improve a dog's gait, activities of daily living, and vitality (Moreau et al. 2004). Duralactin® (Veterinary Products Laboratories, Phoenix, AZ), a milk protein concentrate from hyperimmunized cows helps to manage inflammation (Gingerich and Strobel 2003). Actistatin® (GLC Direct, Paris, KY), a blend of supplements, helps to support musculoskeletal conditions (Montgomery 2011). Omega-3 fatty acids, S-adenosylmethionine, turmeric, boswellia, and willow bark (extract contains parent compound of aspirin – do not use with NSAIDs) are other favorites of practitioners (Raditic and Bartges 2014).

More practioners turn to Traditional Chinese veterinary medicine to support and manage osteoarthritis in hospice and palliative care patients. Because of the low risk of side effects and the scientific evidence now available, the use of herbal formulas, acupuncture, *Tui-na* (massage), and nutritional management are nice options over some conventional medicine choices (DiNatale 2014). For example, Astragalus (*Huang Qi*), a common Chinese herb, has over 10 000 references on PubMed describing its use ranging from its anti-inflammatory to immunostimulatory effects.

Platelet-rich plasma (PRP) has a role in palliative care as an adjunctive therapy, when conservative treatment has failed and the next treatment option is an invasive surgical procedure. It is a type of regenerative medicine that is less invasive than mesenchymal stem cell therapy. PRP uses tissue engineering and molecular biology to assist the body's own repair mechanisms to help restore cartilage health (Kazemi and Fakhrjou 2015). This technique harnesses growth factors found in platelets to help initiate new connective tissue, blood vessels, and bone regeneration, improving recovery. The PRP is injected into the patient's affected joints under a local anesthetic and/or a light sedative. The process is well tolerated by pets.

Cranial Cruciate Ligament Pathology

Description

Besides osteoarthritis, cranial cruciate ligament (CCL) pathology is one of the most common orthopedic conditions seen in dogs. In this author's experience, clients are often desperate to seek palliative care for lameness associated with CCL pathology especially when an older pet with comorbidities is affected or if there are financial constraints that limit therapy options. In addition to the ligament rupture, 45% of dogs may also experience a meniscal tear. This may occur with the initial injury or later in the recovery process and present as an acute lameness (Davidson and Kerwin 2014). Fortunately for cats, CCL rupture is seen less frequently. The origin of the problem in cats is often traumatic injury; whereas in dogs, the rupture is usually attributable to degenerative changes.

Trajectory/Prognosis

In dogs, even though the origin of the disorder is usually degenerative in nature, there is often an acute exacerbation of lameness that leads to the diagnosis of a CCL rupture. Clients often report weeks to months of intermittent mild lameness that waxes and wanes in severity. Because CCL rupture in cats is caused by trauma in most cases, the onset of symptoms is nearly always acute. When the cruciate ligament is partially or completely torn, the stifle becomes mechanically unsound; lameness

may improve with time but the health of the joint is compromised. Depending upon the degree of cartilage damage, the condition follows a type 3 disease trajectory, where there is a prolonged course of decline that would require increasing care over time if proactive measures are not offered to the patient to slow the progression of secondary osteoarthritis.

Manifestations

The clinical signs of the disease vary according to the severity of the damage to the cruciate ligament, from a grade 1, or mild subtle lameness, with partial weight bearing to a persistent, full non-weight-bearing lameness (grade 4). Bilateral cruciate disease can make it difficult for a patient to stand or walk. Without close scrutiny, bilateral cruciate disease can be mistaken for a neurologic or intervertebral disk disease based on the presentation of the patient. Diagnosis is made by careful palpation of the knees. An anterior drawer sign, tibial thrust, and/or joint effusion may be present. As the condition progresses, a medial buttress or periarticular thickening may be palpated on the medial side of the stifle.

Management

In some patients, surgery may be the treatment of choice to stabilize the stifle joint after a cruciate ligament tear; however, patients in hospice or palliative care may not be good candidates for surgery because of other preexisting health disorders. Also some pet owners lack the financial resources to invest in a surgical intervention. This group often become palliative care patients. Depending upon the extent of the injury, many cats do well with medical management. An alternative plan needs to be developed for patients that cannot undergo surgery, consisting of pain management, mobility assistance, and focus on supporting cartilage health. It is paramount that good client education includes what are realistic goals and that there may be a prolonged recovery for the patient. They need to be reassured that the patient will be supported in a way to reduce any distress associated with the condition during this process.

Medical Management

Medical management consists of pain management, mobility assistance, and a focus on supporting cartilage health. Medical management for patients that are not candidates for surgery includes restricting activity for at least – weeks. Pain management can be accomplished by administration of NSAIDS, opioids, and pain-modifying agents. See Chapters 19 and 20 for a more detailed discussion of pain management techniques.

Non-weight-bearing activities are preferred early on in the medical management of CCL rupture, like performing range of motion exercises of the affected joints and swimming. Assisted walking, with the caregiver bearing part of the dog's weight by use of a sling, can unload the affected knee and minimize the instability when walking. A dynamic brace may help provide support to the leg allowing the dog to be more active. The long-term benefit of using a dynamic brace allows added support for increased activity (Fleming et al. 2000). Practioners can check for local professionals that can create an on-sight orthotic. Top Dog Bracing (www.topdogbracing.com; telephone 865-219-3280) provides on-sight help for pet owners near the Knoxville, Tennessee area. Orthopets of Denver, CO (orthopets.com; telephone 303-953-2545) provide long distance orthotic services for practitioners and pet owners. The use of other therapeutic rehabilitation modalities like laser therapy, extracorporeal shock wave therapy, pulsed signal therapy, and targeted pulsed electromagnetic therapy helps manage pain and improves recovery.

There are a large number of nutraceuticals, chrondroprotectants, and other aids to support a patient with tendon and ligament damage by helping to preserve cartilage health. The supplements used for patients with osteoarthritis (see Section Osteoarthritis in this chapter) should also be used for animals with cruciate ligament injuries. Traditional Chinese veterinary medicine also helps to support and manage cruciate ligament rupture patients through the use of herbal formulas, acupuncture, *Tui-na* (massage), and nutrition (Pozzi 2015). One example of a veterinary research study where 181 dogs with complete CCL rupture received the Chinese herbal formula HipGuard (www.naturalsolutionsvet.com). These dogs showed statistical improvement with their lameness (Wen et al. 2016). The study demonstrated that this formula was a safe and effective alternative for individuals that could not have surgery for various reasons. Tendon Ligament Formula® (Jing Tang Herbal, tcvm-herbal.com; telephone 800-891-1986) is another common Chinese herbal formula to support tendon and ligament health and that can be added as an adjunctive therapy (Vargus 2015).

Platelet rich plasma (PRP) has a role in palliative care in cruciate ligament rupture, especially when a surgical procedure is not an option. As mentioned in the Section Osteoarthritis, PRP is a regenerative medicine procedure that uses tissue engineering and molecular biology to assist the body's own repair mechanisms. It has been shown to reduce pain and improve function in cruciate ligament impairment (Cook et al. 2015).

Prolotherapy is another option for palliative care patients that cannot have surgery. A sclerosing agent is injected into the affected tendon. This is has been shown to increase blood supply to the area, resulting in stimulation of osteoblasts and fibroblasts that promote healing. This technique has been used to treat ligament or tendon injuries, boney changes, patellar luxations, and sprains (Gladstein 2012).

Surgical Management

Surgical interventions may be considered in the older, healthy pet if any comorbidities that have been found do not to pose a risk to a good surgical outcome. The choice of surgical intervention (tibial plateau leveling osteotomy vs. tibial tuberosity advancement vs. extracapsular stabilization) should be at the discretion of the surgeon.

Strains, Sprains, and Myofascial Pain

Description

Common soft tissue conditions including muscle strains, sprains, and myofascial pain syndrome are often under reported and under diagnosed in hospice and palliative care patients.

A muscle strain involves an injury to a muscle or to a tendon, which connects the muscle to a bone, whereas a sprain involves the bands of tissue that connect bone to bone. Depending on the severity of the injury, either involve overstretching of only a few fibers of the muscle or tendon, or it can result in a partial or complete tear. A common cause of muscle strains/sprains in weakened patients is associated with the trauma of a fall. A common area of pathology is the iliopsoas muscle, which should always be checked when there is restricted hip extension, rear limb lameness or kyphosis, or hunched posture where the spine curves upward.

Myofascial pain is usually considered a chronic disorder. It affects the fascia by generating pain within the muscle, called trigger points. Trigger points are painful areas located in the muscles or fascia that will palpate as hard nodules of various sizes ranging from 3 mm to 5 cm. Interestingly, biopsies of these nodules show cellular changes including the formation of contraction knots and giant muscle fibers (Starlanyl and Copeland 2001). In addition to interfering with muscle function, these nodules in the muscle can trap or compress nerves, resulting in pain. The pain can be referred to a location distant from the trigger point. There are two types of trigger points, latent and active. Latent trigger points cause pain only when they are touched but prevent proper functioning of

the muscle. Active trigger points evolve when there is overuse or injury to the body. These points can cause pain during activity and/or at rest. Some active points are a consequence of muscle overuse to compensate for pathology in another part of the musculoskeletal system, which is common in older patients with musculoskeletal pathology.

Trajectory/Prognosis

Soft tissue disorders are often manageable conditions that should have a good outcome if palliated. Untreated trigger points can create pain and dysfunction even though the original injury has healed. If left untreated, the condition would be considered chronic and would follow a type 3 disease trajectory, where there is a prolonged course of decline that would require increasing care over time.

Manifestations

The clinical signs of the disease vary according to the location and severity of muscle strain or trigger point involvement. Patients may be sensitive to palpation over affected areas. Clinical symptoms may range from weakness to a mild, subtle lameness with partial weight bearing (grade 1 lameness) to a persistent, full non-weight-bearing lameness (grade 4 lameness). Muscle strains and trigger points may affect the patient's range of motion, including the ability to assume the normal posture to defecate and the ability to turn the head from side to side.

Management

Similar to what was mentioned above for other musculoskeletal disorders, the types of interventions available for helping hospice and palliative care patients with muscle strains and myofascial disorders includes the following:

1) management of pain and inflammation;
2) environmental modifications;

3) activity modifications;
4) use of assistive devices, rehabilitation, or physical modalities.

Many strains can be treated with rest and supportive care. Where there is a complete rupture of the supportive fibers, surgery might be a treatment option for the correct candidate. For patients that are not candidates for surgery, palliative care of rest, pain management, environmental enhancement, use of physical modalities, and the use of braces or splints (preferably dynamic in nature) may aid in providing comfort, stabilization, or recovery. Adjunctive therapies that may aid in healing include acupuncture, pulsed signal therapy, extracorporeal shock wave therapy, laser therapy, and regenerative medicine techniques.

It is important to treat all trigger points associated with any type of musculoskeletal problem. Trigger points can be treated with a combination of acupuncture, laser, massage, and extracorporeal shock wave therapies. New techniques using kinesiology taping may be used to treat trigger points or muscle pain that are too sensitive to receive dry needles or other forms of care. Dogan (2019) compared the effectiveness of the kinesiology taping and dry needling methods in human patients with trigger-point-related myofascial pain syndrome of the upper trapezius muscle. Results showed improvement in pain and cervical range of motion ($p < 0.05$) with no significant difference between the dry needling and the taping patients. When indicated, trigger point pain should also be managed through the use of appropriate medications.

Coxofemoral Luxation

Description

Dislocation of the coxofemoral joint or hip dislocation is a condition that is usually a result of trauma and is seen more often in dogs than in cats. In a hospice or palliative care setting, it is unfortunately often reported after an aging dog has taken a fall on a slippery surface and/or with patients that have preexisting hip dysplasia The force generated by a fall when the legs splay out causes the luxation of the coxofemoral joint. Many times this condition can be prevented by being proactive with all geriatric consults by recommending nonslip flooring in areas of the home with poor traction.

Trajectory/Prognosis

Coxofemoral subluxations are a manageable condition that should have a good outcome if palliated. If left untreated, the condition would be considered chronic and would follow a type 3 disease trajectory, where there is a prolonged course of decline that would require increasing care over time because of biomechanical challenges that cause secondary conditions like muscle atrophy and pain.

Manifestations

Patients may be sensitive to palpation over the affected hip. Clinical symptoms may range from subtle lameness with partial weight bearing (grade 1 lameness) to a persistent, full non-weight-bearing lameness (grade 4 lameness). Upon examination, the affected leg with a craniodorsal subluxation will be shorter than the normal leg.

Management

Conservative treatment consists of manipulation of the dislocated femoral head (with sedation) back into its place in the acetabulum. The patient should wear an Ehmer sling for two weeks with careful monitoring for tightness and pressure sores. The patient should also rest for 4–6 weeks and, of course, receive therapy to manage pain and inflammation concurrently with other physical modalities.

If conservative management fails, a femoral head ostectomy (FHO) or total hip replacement are two options if the patient is a candidate for surgery. The total hip replacement is more invasive, has a longer recovery time, and has a higher risk of complications compared to the FHO. Again, patients that cannot have surgery should be palliated with pain management and rehabilitation modalities.

Fractures

Description

Fractures associated with falls or bone pathology are often associated with a high level of stress and/or guilt experienced by the client. Fractures can occur because of trauma or secondary to a variety of diseases including neoplasia, osteomyelitis, secondary hyperparathyroidism, etc. Aging pets are more prone to trauma when they must navigate steps, steep inclines, climb into vehicles, or jump onto and off of furniture, but even simple activities may cause a fracture in a patient with bone pathology. It is imperative to provide appropriate emotional support for clients with a beloved pet that has experienced a catastrophic fracture.

Trajectory/Prognosis

The trajectory and prognosis for patients with fractures varies according to the general health of the animal, the cause, and location of the fracture.

Manifestations

Pain and lameness are the most common clinical signs when a fracture occurs with the limbs, spine, or pelvis. The degree of pain and lameness depends on the amount of trauma and the location of the fracture. Fractures of the maxilla, mandible, or skull may result in pain and challenge the patient's ability to masticate.

Management

Palliative care for fractures includes aggressive pain management with pharmaceuticals and stabilization of the fracture:

1) management of pain;
2) reduce movement;
3) stabilize fracture;
4) seek consultation with orthopedic specialist.

Making use of the acronym of "PRICE," which stands for protect, rest, ice, compress, elevate (keep fracture side up), is helpful in supporting a patient with a fracture while arrangements for long-term care are investigated.

While waiting for a referral or an important family decision, the use of a Robert Jones bandage may reduce swelling and provide temporary stabilization of fractures below the elbow and stifle. A Schroeder Thomas splint may also provide stabilization for fractures below the elbow and stifle and in the past were often used for fracture fixation. Spica splints can be used for temporary stabilization for fractures of the shoulder and hips.

The palliation of fractures of the mandible, maxilla, and skull will vary depending upon the location of the break. In these locations it is paramount to manage pain and provide proper nutrition for the patient.

It is important to have a consultation with an orthopedic, rehabilitation specialist, or veterinary dentist to investigate all options and to assess the ability of the fracture to heal. For geriatric patients, it is important to utilize adjunctive therapies that aid in the healing of fractures, like targeted pulsed electromagnetic field therapy (tPEMF), pulsed signal therapy, extracorporeal shock wave therapy, laser therapy, and regenerative medicine techniques. Utilizing management options listed for the OA patient may be helpful to decrease the progression of osteoarthritis as a comorbidity/sequel to any fracture. In the geriatric population, it is important to note that not all fractures are capable of healing. Some may have delayed healing. The practitioner needs to prepare the client for these possibilities and discuss what options are available to mitigate suffering.

Conclusion

As described above, there are many disorders of the musculoskeletal system that interfere with the interaction between the body's muscles, bones, ligaments, tendons, fascia, and joints.

Because some patients with musculoskeletal conditions are not candidates for surgical interventions, it is important to become familiar with how to palliate conditions when surgery is not an option. Like most medical conditions, an integrative approach to caring for patients provides the best opportunity to minimize side effects and promote quality of life.

References

Altman, R., Dean, D.D., Muniz, O.E. *et al.* (1989) Therapeutic treatment of canine osteoarthritis with glycosaminoglycan polysulfuric acid ester. *Arthritis Rheum.*, 32: 1300–1307.

Boileau, C., Martel-Pelletier, J., Caron, J., *et al.* (2009) Protective effects of total fraction of avocado/soybean unsaponifiables on the structural changes in experimental dog osteoarthritis: inhibition of nitric oxide synthase and matrix metalloproteinase-13. *Arthritis Res. Ther.*, 11: R41.

Cook, J., Smith, P.A., Bozynski, C.C., *et al.* (2015) Multiple injections of leukoreduced platelet rich plasma reduce pain and functional impairment in a canine model of ACL and meniscal deficiency. *J. Orthop. Res.*, 25: 607–615.

Davidson, J. and Kerwin, S. (2014) Common orthopedic conditions and their physical rehabilitation. In: *Canine Rehabilitation and Physical Therapy* (eds D.L. Millis and D. Levine), 2. Philadelphia: Elsevier, p. 566.

DiNatale, C. (2014) Geriatric medicine. In: *Practical Guide to Traditional Chinese Veterinary Medicine* (eds H. Xie, L. Wedemeyer, *et al.*). Reddick, FL Chi Institute Press, pp. 924–930.

Dogan, N. (2019) Kinesio taping versus dry needling in the treatment of myofascial pain of the upper trapezius muscle: a randomized single blind (evaluator) prospective study. *J. Back Musculoskelet. Rehabil.*, 32: 819–827.

Fleming B., Renstrom, P.A., Beynnon, B.D., *et al.* (2000) The influence of functional knee bracing on the anterior cruciate ligament strain biomechanics in weight bearing and non-weight bearing knees. *Am. J. Sports Med.*, 28: 815–824.

Fleming, J., Creevy, K.E., and Promislow, D.E. (2011) Mortality in North American dogs from 1984 to 2004: an investigation into age-, size-, and breed related causes of death. *J. Vet. Intern. Med.*, 25: 187–198.

Fox, S. (2012) Painful decisions for senior pets. *Vet. Clin. North Am. Small Anim. Pract.*, 42: 727–734.

Gingerich, D. and Strobel, J. (2003) Use of client-specific outcome measures to assess treatment effects in geriatric, arthritic dogs: controlled clinical evaluation of a nutraceutical. *Vet. Ther.*, 4: 376–386.

Gladstein, B. (2012) A case for prolotherapy and its place in veterinary medicine. *J. Prolother.*, 4: e870–885.

Gordon, W., Conzemius, M.G., Riedesel, E., *et al.* (2003) The relationship between limb function and radiographic osteoarthritis in dogs with stifle osteoarthrosis. *Vet. Surg.*, 32, 451–453.

Henderson, A. and Millis, D. (2014) Tissue healing: tendons, ligaments, bone, muscle, and cartilage. In: *Canine Rehabilitation and Physical Therapy* (eds D.L. Millis and D. Levine), 2. Philadelphia: Elsevier, pp. 79–89.

Kazemi, D. and Fakhrjou, A. (2015) Leukocyte and platelet rich plasma (L-PRP) versus leukocyte and platelet rich fibrin (L-PRF) for articular cartilage repair of the knee: a comparative evaluation in an animal model. *Iran. Red Crescent Med. J.*, 17: e19594.

Marcellin-Little, D., Levine, D., and Millis, D.L. (2014) Physical rehabilitation for geriatric and arthritic patients. In: *Canine Rehabilitation and Physical Therapy* (eds D.L. Millis and D. Levine), 2. Philadelphia: Elsevier, p. 635.

Millis, D. and Levine, D. (1997) The role of exercise and physical modalities in the treatment of osteoarthritis. *Vet. Clin. North Am. Small Anim. Pract.*, 27: 913–930.

Montgomery, M. (2011) Evaluation of the safety and efficacy of the dietary supplement Actistatin® on established glucosamine and chondroitin therapy in the horse. *Intern. J. Appl. Res. Vet. Med.*, 9: 100–105.

Moreau, M., Dupuis, J., Bonneau, N.H. *et al.* (2004) Clinical evaluation of a powder of quality elk velvet antler for the treatment of osteoarthrosis in dogs. *Can. Vet. J.*, 45: 133–139.

Pozzi, R. (2015) Comparison between CCL surgery and acupuncture treatment in dogs. In: *Traditional Chinese Veterinary Medicine for the Diagnosis and Treatment of Lameness and Pain in Dogs, Cats, and Horses* (eds H. Xie and L. Trevisanello). Reddick, FL: Chi Institute Press, pp. 59–63.

Raditic, D. and Bartges, J. (2014) The role of chondroprotectants, nutraceuticals and nutrition in rehabilitation. In: *Canine Rehabilitation and Physical Therapy* (eds D.L. Millis and D. Levine), 2. Philadelphia: Elsevier, pp. 254–276.

Shearer, T. and Marchitelli, B. (2015) *Death Statistics from Database of Western Carolina Animal Pain Clinic and 4 Paws Farewell: Mobile Pet Hospice and Home Euthanasia.* Sylva, NC: Shearer Pet Health Services.

Slingerland, L., Hazewinkel, H.A., Meij, B.P., *et al.* (2011) Cross-sectional study of the prevalence and clinical features of osteoarthritis in 100 cats. *Vet. J.*, 18 304–309.

Starlanyl, D. and Copeland, M. (2001) *Fibromyalgia and Chronic Myofascial Pain.* Oakland: New Harbinger Publications Inc., p. 26.

Vargus, M. (2015) Aquapuncture and herbal medicine for medical management of ACL in dogs. In: *Traditional Chinese Veterinary Medicine for the Diagnosis and Treatment of Lameness and Pain in Dogs, Cats, and Horses* (eds H. Xie and L. Trevisanello). Reddick, FL: Chi Institute Press, pp. 65–75.

Wen J.J., Johnston K., and Gucciardo D. (2016) Chinese herbal medicine for dogs with complete cranial cruciate ligament rupture: 181 cases. *Am. J. Trad. Chin. Vet. Med.*, 11: 41–48.

17

Nervous System Disease

Tamara Shearer, MS, DVM, CCRP, CVPP, CVA, MSTCVM

Changes in the nervous system are common among dog and cat patients in hospice and palliative care. Neurologic organ system change was ranked highest as the cause of death in adult dogs. In juvenile dogs, it ranked third as the cause of death (Fleming et al. 2011).

As patients age, the hospice practitioner should be aware that there are physical changes that may interfere with interpretation of the neurologic examination findings. Many of these changes are associated with non-neurogenic comorbidities. For example, cataract formation or iris atrophy can result in a decreased to absent menace response and poor pupillary light response. Chronic musculoskeletal changes that include fibrotic myopathies and infraspinatus contracture may mimic a neurologic gait. Pain or range of motion changes associated with osteoarthritis can also interfere with the pet's posture, gait, reflex, and proprioceptive testing. Older pets with heightened anxiety or fear may also experience an adrenaline surge that could alter behavior when away from home.

Often with hospice and palliative care patients, a definitive diagnosis is not possible, and a tentative diagnosis must be made based on the clinical signs and the progression of disease. For example, some neoplastic conditions present with the clinical signs associated with neurologic changes. These conditions are often progress despite palliative intervention. The conditions chosen for review here are some of the more common neurologic problems that are seen in hospice or palliative care practice and may present unique challenges.

Intervertebral Disc Disease

Description

Intervertebral disc disease (IVDD) is one of the most common neurologic changes seen in veterinary medicine. It is a condition in which the discs that separate the spinal vertebra become displaced and create pressure on the spinal cord, meninges, or nerve roots.

It is important to note that there are two common types of disc changes that help explain symptom differences between different breeds and individuals. Hansen type I disc, or chondroid metaplasia protrusion, affects younger dogs of the chondrodystrophic breeds, but there are exceptions with age and breed. Onset may occur between three and six years of age and is more acute in nature. In this type of disc protrusion, the annulus fibrosis (fibrous outside part of the disc) becomes weak, and the nucleus pulposus (gelatinous center of

Hospice and Palliative Care for Companion Animals: Principles and Practice, Second Edition.
Edited by Amir Shanan, Jessica Pierce, and Tamara Shearer.
© 2023 John Wiley & Sons, Inc. Published 2023 by John Wiley & Sons, Inc.
Companion website: www.wiley.com/go/shanan/palliative

disc) pushes through to cause compression of the spinal cord and nerve roots.

The fibrous metaplasia, or Hansen type II disk protrusion, occurs in an older population of dogs, averaging 5–12 years of age. It is more common in non-chondrodystrophic dogs like German Shepherds and Labrador Retrievers. The onset of type II disk protrusion is gradual. Here, the disc undergoes a fibroid metaplasia, where the nucleus pulposus is contained within a degenerating annulus. The nucleus pulposus pushes on the annulus causing compression of the spinal cord.

IVDD is often overwhelming to clients because their pet may present with mobility dysfunction and/or pain. This is especially true when there is an acute onset of clinical signs. A good understanding of IVDD by the practitioner will help guide clients along this difficult journey with their pet.

Trajectory/Prognosis

IVDD is a unique condition because of the type of disc disease, severity of the insult, and the location of the lesion in the spinal cord play a role in the outcome. All of these variables make the disease trajectory and prognosis difficult to determine. One study showed that patients with cervical disc disease have a 48.9% chance of a successful recovery; however, 33% go on to have a recurrence. A little over 18% failed to recover (Levine et al. 2007). Many patients go on to have good recoveries, but some have a trajectory type 3, where there is a prolonged course of disease that would require increasing care over time, especially for patients that experience long-term paresis or paralysis. Some patients may require ongoing efforts to maintain good hygiene to prevent skin irritation from feces or urine.

Of interest, it was found that dogs that get one hour or more of daily exercise were less likely to have acute IVDD compared to dogs not allowed to jump on and off furniture and who got less than 30 minutes of exercise (Packer et al. 2016).

Manifestations

Clinical symptoms also vary by the type of disk disease, severity of the insult, and what part of the spinal cord is affected. The signs of IVDD range from paralysis to paresis, and the degree of pain is contingent upon how much pressure or injury occurs around the nerve roots, meninges, and spinal cord. Diagnosis for hospice and palliative care patients is usually based on a complete history and a neurologic examination. Plain radiographs may not show all lesions, and advanced imagining is usually necessary for a definitive diagnosis.

The most common sign for disc disease in the cervical region is pain. Approximately 90% of patients with cervical disk protrusion experience pain without neurologic deficits (Thomas et al. 2014). The vertebral canal in the cervical vertebrae is larger than in the thoracolumbar area, resulting in less pressure on the spinal cord when a disk protrudes and, hence, fewer neurologic changes. In addition to pain, a change in head position, posture change, reluctance to move, and muscle spasms may be observed. A front limb lameness may be present if there is compression of a nerve root. The most common breeds affected by cervical IVDD are Beagles and Dachshunds, and the most common location is between C2 and C3.

The most common symptom with thoracolumbar disease is a change in posture with a hunched back. Pets may also have difficulty jumping or climbing steps. There may be varying degrees of pain, ataxia, paraplegia, urinary incontinence, and fecal incontinence. Approximately 10% of dogs experience back pain without neurologic deficits (Thomas et al. 2014). The most common location for IVDD in the thoracolumbar area is between discs T12–13 and L1–2. Dachshunds, Cockers, Beagles, and other chondrodysplastic dogs are the breeds most affected by thoracolumbar IVDD.

Myelomalacia is a severe complication of disc disease in which necrosis of the spinal cord occurs as a result of profound damage to the spinal cord. Signs of myelomalacia include urinary and fecal incontinence, hypoalgesia, and ascending paralysis. There is loss of abdominal tone and the cutaneous trunci reflex. As the condition ascends, it may cause respiratory failure. Caregivers need to be prepared to transition from palliative care to hospice care if this complication occurs.

Sequelae to IVDD include urinary tract infections, muscle atrophy, decubitus ulcers or pressure sores, contractures of the ligaments and tendons with disuse, and respiratory infections. An elevated level of nursing care for these individuals is important.

Management

A manuscript (Moore et al. 2020) provides the most current information on thoracolumbar IVDD based on a review of research studies. Some of the generalizations should help provide a better standard of care for patients with IVDD. This information may offer additional insight into other areas of the spine in dogs that may also experience IVDD.

The goals of IVDD management is to restore function and mitigate pain. These goals are accomplished though minimizing spinal cord injury such as ischemia, inflammation, and free radical production. Conservative management and surgical interventions are the two options for patients with IVDD. Unfortunately, there are no studies to compare the outcomes between medically managed and surgically managed patients with documented conservative management. There are only a small number of published conservative management cases of 113 compared to over 1500 cases of surgical publications (Moore et al. 2020).

Typically palliative or conservative treatment for pets that cannot have surgery consist of strict rest for a minimum of three to eight weeks to prevent worsening of disc protrusion and protect an ataxic pet from falling and minimize pain; however, there was only one retrospective study that showed that the duration of rest did not predict the outcome for the patient (Levine et al. 2007). The duration of rest should be based on the individual's condition and behavior associated with confinement.

Patients should be treated concurrently for pain and inflammation. Common choices include gabapentin and corticosteroids or nonsteroidal anti-inflammatory drugs (NSAIDS). Although there is controversy over utilization of an NSAID versus corticosteroid, this author chooses corticosteroids as a first choice; however, there are some considerations to analyze before reaching for the corticosteroid. Corticosteroid use can interfere with the ability to confirm a diagnosis that might be time sensitive, in addition, immediate improvement with administration followed by a decline after the use may deter a client to move forward with any diagnostics (Nichols 2014). Many clients that seek hospice or palliative care have communicated that they are not pursuing diagnostics. Currently, there is no study comparing NSAIDS versus corticosteroids. Of interest, dogs receiving corticosteroids had a lower incidence of myleomalacia (Castel et al. 2017). It is important to communicate the side effects of short- and long-term use of corticosteroids before their use. Muscle relaxants like methocarbamol and diazepam may also help with medical management. Acetaminophen (dogs only), opioids, and amantadine can be added if needed as an adjunct to treat severe pain. Studies now show that the use of methylprednisolone sodium succinate and polyethylene glycol did not have any treatment effect (Olby et al. 2016) for acute IVDD. See Chapter 19 for more details on pain management.

Electroacupuncture may improve the outcome of IVDD (Joaquim et al. 2010). Other examples of physical modalities that may promote recovery include laser therapy, targeted pulsed electromagnetic field therapy (tPEMF), and electrotherapy. Assisted standing and range-of-motion exercises are important to maintain muscle tone in patients that are experiencing paresis during their period of restricted activity.

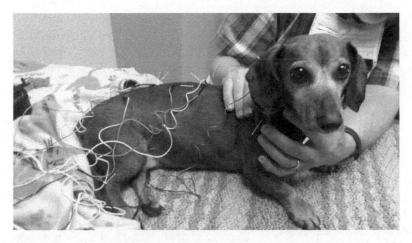

Figure 17.1 Belle receiving electroacupuncture. She began walking three weeks after starting therapy.

Another conservative, minimally invasive option for certain dogs with Hansen type II disc protrusion is the use of an epidural infiltration of methylprednisolone acetate at the lumbosacral space. In a 38 dog study, there was a 79% improvement with the methylprednisolone acetate injection (Janssens et al. 2009). Surgery could be considered for patients that are good candidates and are experiencing profound pain and/or severe or progressing neurologic change. Controversy exists between the time interval between the association of deep pain loss, diagnosis, and surgery (Moore et al. 2020). There is no evidence that recovery is not possible for dogs with loss of deep pain is greater than 48 hours; however, studies show that a delay in decompression of greater than 12 hours increased the incidence of myleomalacia (Castel et al. 2017). There are, of course, many exceptions to this correlation depending on the individual and the nature of ongoing therapy. One example of an exception from this author's practice is Belle, a 13-year-old, female spayed dachshund with paralysis of the rear limbs with complete loss of deep pain for several days. She was given a grim prognosis, and surgery was not recommended by a neurology specialist. Based on this prognosis, euthanasia was considered. With therapy, within three weeks, Belle started to regain her mobility with multimodal support including laser therapy, tPEMT

(Assisi LOOP®), Chinese herbal formulas, electroacupuncture, corticosteroids, gabapentin, and methocarbamol (Figure 17.1).

Concurrent nursing care for patients should be provided 24/7 to prevent or treat urinary tract infections, muscle atrophy, decubitus ulcers or pressure sores, contractures of the ligaments and tendons, and respiratory infections. Patients that suffer from a neurogenic bladder may require assistance in their urinations through manual expression or catheterization.

Cervical Spondylomyelopathy

Description

Cervical spondylomyelopathy (CSM) is a condition in which progressive compression of the cervical spinal cord occurs. It may sometimes have a similar presentation as IVDD. The compression of the caudal cervical cord may be caused by stenosis of the vertebral canal or by abnormalities in size, shape, or position of articular processes leading to malarticulation. Other possible causes include vertebral instability and proliferation of soft tissues like the interarcuate ligament, dorsal longitudinal ligament, and dorsal annulus. This is one type of neurologic condition where a younger patient may need to be admitted into a hospice or palliative care program. The condition is most prevalent in younger, giant breed dogs like Bernese Mountain Dogs, Great Danes, Mastiffs, Rottweilers, and Swiss Mountain Dogs. It is also seen in middle-aged to older Doberman Pinschers.

Trajectory/Prognosis

There is often a progressive deterioration of patients with CSM that would require increasing care over time. The rate of change varies among individuals. Sequelae may include injuries from falling, decubitus ulcers, and urinary tract infections, which are common in patients that have become recumbent.

Manifestations

The symptoms range from mild gait changes to complete paralysis. Ataxia can affect all limbs with hind limb changes being most profound. A wide-based stance of the forelimbs, with elbows rotated out and inward pointed toes, is a posture that helps some dogs with their balance. A hypermetric gait may be observed with the forelimbs. Not all dogs show neck pain; however, discomfort may be exhibited upon extension of the neck.

Advanced imaging is needed to confirm a definitive diagnosis, but this is not always possible for patients that are in hospice or palliative care. In the absence of advanced imaging, a tentative diagnosis is made based on the history, a complete neurologic examination, and progression of the condition.

Management

Palliative medical treatment of an acute exacerbation of symptoms consists of managing pain and providing rest. Like with IVDD management, patients should be treated concurrently for pain and inflammation. Common choices include gabapentin and corticosteroids or NSAIDS. As mentioned above with IVDD, there is controversy over utilization of an NSAID versus corticorticosteroid use. This author chooses corticosteroids as a first choice, with mindful considerations knowing that the use can interfere with the ability to confirm a diagnosis that might be time sensitive. Currently, there is no study comparing NSAIDS versus corticosteroids. Again, many clients that seek hospice or palliative care have communicated that they are not pursuing diagnostics. Before using corticosteroids, it is important to communicate the side effects of short- and long-term use. Acetaminophen (dogs only), opioids, and amantadine can be added if needed as an adjunct to treat severe pain. See Chapter 19 for more details on pain management.

Electroacupuncture and herbal therapies may be helpful in regaining mobility (Hayashi 2015). Another study showed that dogs receiving electroacupuncture improved by 85%, compared to 20% for patients not receiving electroacupuncture (Sumano and Mateos 1999). Other physical modalities used to promote recovery include laser therapy, tPEMF, and electrotherapy. Assisted standing and range-of-motion exercises are important to maintain muscle tone in patients that are experiencing paresis.

Surgical treatment may be considered for patients that are good candidates and are experiencing pain or worsening of symptoms. Surgery can improve the patient's comfort by improving cervical stability and relieving compression of the spinal cord. A retrospective study showed that 81% of dogs that underwent surgery experienced improvement with their symptoms, compared with 54% of patients that receive medical treatment only. Interestingly, the overall survival time was similar, and even slightly longer, for the medical intervention group (36–48 months) compared to the surgical group (36–46.5 months) (da Costa et al. 2008).

Fibrocartilagenous Embolic Myelopathy

Description

Fibrocartilagenous embolic myelopathy (FCEM) is a debilitating neurologic event where an embolus of fibrocartilage is lodged in the spinal cord arteries or veins, causing an infarction of the spinal cord. It is uncertain as to how the fibrocartilage, which is presumed to come from the nucleus pulposis of the intervertebral disc, enters the circulation. It affects both dogs and cats. It is the most common type of myelopathy in Miniature Schnauzers. There is also a breed predilection in large to giant breed dogs.

Trajectory/Prognosis

FCEM has a trajectory type 4 because often there is a sudden, severe neurologic insult. This condition may cause anywhere from a mild to extreme impairment of the pet's ability to function and requires an extraordinary amount of supportive care during the initial event. Typically, this condition is nonprogressive, and patients have a good prognosis for return to function. In a retrospective study, 88% of non-ambulatory dogs with FCEM regained the ability to walk (Dunie-Merigot et al. 2007).

Manifestations

The acute disease may progress only for the first one to two hours, but then symptoms stabilize. The severity of the changes can range from ataxia to complete paralysis. Typically, the disease is not painful, and symptoms are somewhat asymmetric. Conditions like hypothyroidism and hypertension, which may predispose patients to vascular occlusion events, should be ruled out or treated to prevent recurrence.

Management

Palliative medical treatment consists of rest, good nursing care, rehabilitation modalities, and close monitoring for pain and urinary tract infections. The same therapeutic modalities that support IVDD patients are useful for FCEM. Patients that suffer from a neurogenic bladder may need assistance in their urinations through manual expression or catheterization. Assisted standing and range-of-motion exercises are important to maintain muscle tone in patients that are experiencing paresis. Like other debilitating conditions, good client education on how to support their pet is paramount. Typically, with FCEM a patient should show small signs of improvement every few days.

Vestibular Disorders

Description

Vestibular disorders (VDs) are common in both dogs and cats. Because of the acute onset and the profound clinical signs exhibited by the patient, it is a condition that is alarming to the pet owners. Idiopathic vestibular disease is one the most common forms of peripheral vestibular disorders seen in dogs with an incidence of 39% and in cats with an incidence of 43% (Schunk and Averill 1983; Negrin et al. 2010). In dogs, idiopathic disease is mostly seen in animals over the age of five and geriatric patients. In cats, it can occur in all ages with a predisposition for outdoor cats occurring more in the summer.

The vestibular system is responsible for perception of body position and maintaining balance in respect to gravity. Lesions that cause this disorder can involve components of the vestibular system in the peripheral or central nervous system, including the receptor organs of the inner ear, vestibular portion of the eighth cranial nerve, petrous portion of the temporal bone, and the brainstem. Interestingly, the condition causes inhibition of the extensors on the same side as the lesion and activation of the extensors on the affected side resulting in a patient listing/leaning toward the lesion. Idiopathic vestibular disorders, frequently referred to as "vestibular syndrome," are acute but nonprogressive. When older patients are affected, it is often referred to as "geriatric vestibular syndrome." In contrast to the idiopathic condition, vestibular disorders with other etiologies (e.g. neoplasia in the brainstem) can be progressive in nature.

Of special note, drug toxicity associated with the administration of metronidazole should be ruled out as a cause of vestibular clinical signs. It is often prescribed to geriatric patients with diarrhea. Signs can develop weeks after starting the drug.

Trajectory/Prognosis

In most patients, vestibular disorders have a sudden onset with a type 4 trajectory. A trajectory type 4 is seen when there is a sudden, severe neurologic or circulatory injury or insult and results in extreme impairment of the pet's ability to function, often requiring an extraordinary amount of supportive care. Typically, feline and canine idiopathic vestibular syndrome are nonprogressive conditions after their initial onset, with the most severe symptoms lasting approximately 72 hours, and a near full recovery seen in 2–3 weeks. Patients with vestibular disorders caused by other etiologies such as neoplasia or unmanaged otitis interna or media may progress over time.

Manifestations

The symptoms of vestibular disorders include a head tilt, ataxia, leaning, falling, rolling, circling, and nystagmus (horizontal, rotary or vertical, or positional). To help understand prognosis, there are some signs that help distinguish central vestibular disorders from peripheral change. Non-ambulatory tetraparesis is significantly more common in dogs with central nervous system disease, and veering and leaning are significantly more common in dogs with peripheral disease. The rate of resting nystagmus may also be useful in distinguishing the two conditions (Troxel et al. 2005). A rate of nystagmus greater than 66 beats per minute is a significant indicator of peripheral disease (Platt 2013). Lesions in the central nervous system may also be associated with other symptoms like changes in mentation, paresis, proprioceptive deficits, and vertical or positional nystagmus.

Management

Concurrent with treatment, dogs should be screened for hypothyroidism because it is thought that it can predispose a dog to physiologic changes that result in vestibular changes if left untreated. All treatments should be targeted at the cause of the disorder when possible, especially if otitis interna or media is suspected. Unfortunately, it may be difficult to obtain a definitive diagnosis with some patients.

Palliative care for patients with suspected otitis interna or media and uncertain tympanic membrane integrity include topical ear preparations with Tris-EDTA, chlortrimazole/ miconazole, enrofloxacin, and dexamethasone. These treatments are considered to have less risk (Jurney 2020).

For all etiologies, palliative medical treatment consists of rest, good nursing care, rehabilitation modalities, and close monitoring for pain and urinary tract infections. Patients will most likely need assistance in eating and drinking. Most patients may require extra efforts to maintain good hygiene to prevent skin irritation from feces or urine. A helpful tip in caring for patients is to move them slowly with good support and provide a quiet, well lighted environment during their recovery with nonslip flooring.

Although there are currently no randomized, blinded clinical studies; this author feels that physical modalities in the form of acupuncture, laser and tPEMF help to speed recoveries compared to patients in her practice not receiving this type of support.

Antiemetics such as maropitant (Cerenia®) can help manage nausea that may be a consequence of the motion sickness associated with the disorder. Meclizine, which is available over the counter, can also be helpful in the management of nausea associated with motion sickness. For anxiety and sedation, diazepam or other benzodiazepines and/or trazadone may help calm a patient.

Laryngeal Paralysis/ Geriatric Onset Laryngeal Paralysis Polyneuropathy

Description

Laryngeal paralysis is a peripheral nervous system disorder that affects dogs and cats and can disrupt quality of life. Laryngeal paralysis involves the loss of function of the recurrent laryngeal nerve resulting in the paralysis of the laryngeal muscles that can be unilateral or bilateral. The paralysis has a number of causes including a heredity predisposition in Bouvier des Flandres, Siberian Huskies, Dalmatians, Rottweilers, and Bull Terriers (Costello 2009). It is also seen frequently acquired in Golden Retrievers and Labrador Retrievers. Laryngeal paralysis is often idiopathic in nature but may also be the result of neoplasia, or develop secondary to trauma to the neck, exposure to toxins, and infections in the pharyngeal area. Current thought is that laryngeal paralysis that occurs in the geriatric population is part of a polyneuropathy, so a more progressive and descriptive term for laryngeal paralysis in older patients is geriatric onset laryngeal paralysis polyneuropathy (GOLPP) (Bryden 2018).

Trajectory/Prognosis

Laryngeal paralysis may follow a type 2 trajectory. Most patients with laryngeal paralysis have a gradual onset that may result in a respiratory crisis, especially when exposed to stressors like exercise and increased temperature or humidity. Increased care is required over time because of the incidence of comorbidities including aspiration pneumonia. At times, the disease may wax, wane, or even stabilize, but the patient rarely reclaims the original level of health.

Manifestations

Early signs of laryngeal paralysis include changes in the volume and tone of the animal's voice. Inspiratory noise becomes present and is exacerbated by exercise. In cats, there is less weakness, respiratory distress, and exercise intolerance reported compared to dogs (Lam et al. 2012). When a patient cannot compensate, dyspnea and collapse may result. Dogs with laryngeal paralysis are prone to heatstroke and pneumonia. When evaluating a patient, it is important to remember that laryngeal paralysis may be a sign of a generalized polyneuropathy and could be accompanied by esophageal dysfunction or other signs of nerve dysfunction associated with subtle changes in posture and ambulation.

Typically, the diagnosis of laryngeal paralysis is confirmed by visualizing the absence of laryngeal fold's movement with the patient under anesthesia. During normal inspiration, the arytenoid cartilages should move laterally or abduct. In patients that are at a high risk for complications associated with anesthesia, diagnosis may be based on the history and symptoms of the disease.

Management

Unfortunately, there is no curative treatment for this condition. The main goal of management is prevention of respiratory distress by being proactive with client education. A patient can get relief from the clinical manifestations of laryngeal paralysis through a surgical intervention or medical management. Again, medical management or palliative care is often chosen because of age, preexisting comorbidities, or financial constraints.

Emphasis should be placed on lifestyle change to prevent distress by modifying a pet's exercise routine and providing an indoor controlled environmental temperature. Pets that choke or cough when drinking water may benefit from the addition to their drinking water of an over-the-counter product called Thick-It®

(Kent Precision Food Group: St. Louis, MO), which contains a xanthan gum-based agent that thickens the consistency of liquids. Because of concurrent esophageal changes, feeding various textures of foods to determine which is best tolerated and having a patient sit for 10–15 minutes after eating may mitigate some complications like coughing, choking, and regurgitation after eating. Having the patient eat from an elevated bowl where the pet must also stand with their front feet on a step may be helpful. Promotility drugs such as metoclopramide and cisapride may also help with regurgitation or throat clearing.

Diagnosis and treatment of endocrinopathies that could cause additional polyneuropathies is important when palliating a pet with laryngeal paralysis.

The use of a therapy laser over the ventral and lateral throat area may help to reduce the symptoms of laryngeal paralysis by reducing inflammation (Shearer 2013). In this author's experience, placement of an Assisi Loop utilizing tPEMF therapy treating the laryngeal area may also reduce inflammation associated with the disorder. There are acupuncture protocols and Chinese herbal formulas that help to palliate patients with laryngeal paralysis (Xie and Preast 2007; Chrisman 2011). Relief from episodes of mild respiratory distress can also be obtained by providing supplemental oxygen at home.

If a patient is presented in severe respiratory distress, oxygen should be administered, and dexamethasone given intravenously to reduce laryngeal inflammation and edema. Sedation with acepromazine may be indicated for hemodynamically stable patients. If acepromazine cannot be used or the patient requires additional therapy, butorphanol can be given to act as a sedative and antitussive (Costello 2009). If the patient is experiencing hyperthermia, their temperature should be reduced using a cold bath.

Pharmaceutical interventions to manage the anxiety caused by shortness of breath, such as the use of a benzodiazepine, can improve quality of life. In a recent double blind, randomized study, it was found that doxepin, a tricyclic antidepressant, did not improve the perceived quality of life by pet owners, contradicting the trend of its past usage for laryngeal paralysis. The additional use of bronchodilators may only be helpful when there is coughing associated with concurrent lower airway disease.

Some clients with medically managed patients may change their minds and decide to choose surgery if the respiratory distress becomes unmanageable and euthanasia is one of the final options. A unilateral arytenoid lateralization is a common surgical procedure in which the arytenoid cartilage is fixed in a lateral position using a suture to open the airway. Owners need to be informed of the risks and benefits of a surgical intervention, which include but are not limited to seroma formation at the surgical site and aspiration pneumonia.

Degenerative Myelopathy

Description

Degenerative myelopathy (DM) is a progressive neurodegenerative disorder, most commonly affecting dogs eight years of age and older. The incidence in dogs is approximately 0.19%, with certain breeds and crossbreeds more affected (Coates et al. 2007). In this author's opinion, the incidence is much higher because of the difficulty in obtaining a definitive diagnosis. It is recognized in the following breeds: Pembroke and Cardigan Welsh Corgis, German Shepherd Dogs, Siberian Huskies, Miniature Poodles, Boxers, Chesapeake Bay Retrievers, and Rhodesian Ridgebacks. DM is considered a central and peripheral axonopathy (a disruption of the normal functioning of axons). Histologic lesions include degeneration and nerve fiber loss in the ascending and descending motor pathways of the mid to caudal thoracic spine.

Interestingly, DM shares some features with the human disease, amyotrophic lateral sclerosis (ALS or Lou Gehrig's disease). Studies are being conducted to determine if DM can be useful as a model for ALS for the purpose of developing therapies for both diseases (Morgan et al. 2014). Both DM and the upper neuron form of ALS share a mutation in a gene called superoxide dismutase 1 (SOD1) (Awano et al. 2009).

Trajectory/Prognosis

DM is a challenge to manage because of its type 3 trajectory, where there is progressive deterioration of the mobility of the patient. A pet with DM has a prolonged course of disease that requires increasing care over time with a poor long-term prognosis.

Manifestations

The first signs of the disease may be subtle and involve the occasional scraping of rear toenails when walking. General proprioceptive ataxia with upper motor neuron spasticity of rear limbs may appear asymmetrical then later change to a more symmetrical pattern. Over a course of months the condition progresses causing a flaccid paraplegia. The pelvic limbs develop lower motor neuron signs with possible decreased patellar and flexor reflexes, profound rear limb muscle atrophy; and later, the development of fecal and urinary incontinence. In the late stages of DM, respiration and cranial nerves can be affected and swallowing can become difficult. DM itself is not painful; however, many of the sequela like abrasions, muscles strains, urinary tract infections, and decubitus ulcers do create discomfort.

For patients in hospice and palliative care, advanced imaging to rule out other problems is not always a desirable and/or practical option. In these cases diagnosis can be aided by taking a good history, watching the progression of symptoms, and monitoring for pain. Diagnosis is based on ruling out other conditions like Hansen type II disk disease and FCEM. Testing negative for the SOD1 gene mutation rules out DM; however, not all dogs that have the mutation will develop clinical signs of the disease. Information about test kits and submission can be found at www.ofa.org.

Management

Physiotherapy may be the most important tool used to maintain mobility and quality of life for dogs with DM (Kathmann et al. 2006). Dogs that underwent extensive physical therapy lived an average of 255 days; in contrast, dogs that had no therapy lived an average of 55 days. Dogs receiving therapy also remained ambulatory longer. Another study showed that dogs that received photobiomodulation with a wavelength of 980 and treatment time of 25–26 minutes compared to a wavelength of 904 and 5 minutes applied over the spinal column and paraspinal muscles had a delay from the time of onset to becoming non-ambulatory, and the time between onset of signs and euthanasia was also increased in the group receiving the 980 wavelength (Miller et al. 2020).

Depending upon the patient, a physiotherapy protocol might include:

1) Passive range-of-motion exercises and stretching
2) Assisted standing on flat surfaces
3) Placement of feet on a low balance disk
4) Weight shift to improve proprioception and core strength
5) Leash walking over various textured surfaces
6) Stepping over low obstacles
7) *Tui-na* (Chinese manipulation/massage) or other massage techniques
8) Acupuncture
9) Swimming or underwater treadmill therapy
10) tPEMF therapy and/or photobiomodulation

More details on physical medicine therapies and assistive devices that can be used to help DM patients can be found in Chapter 20.

Besides physical medicine and exercise, proper nutrition rich in antioxidants and supplements may also help to support any individual with a debilitating disease. Offering balanced home-cooked meals or premium dog foods may be helpful to maintain weight and support the immune system. Some patients may require extra efforts to maintain good hygiene to prevent skin irritation from feces or urine. Like other debilitating diseases, support and good communication with the client are important to maintaining a good quality of life for the patient and the pet owner.

To date, reliable scientific evidence or studies of specific treatments for DM are lacking; however, major universities and foundations have ongoing research, so it is important to revisit any new treatment options on a regular basis.

Disorders of Micturition/ Urination

Description

Neurologic disorders of micturition or urination are common in aging dogs and cats, and they pose a huge concern for the pet owner and often present a challenge for the practitioner to find a time-sensitive remedy to solve the problem. It is important that patients in hospice and palliative care be monitored closely for regular urinations and that the bladder is prevented from getting over distended. Over distention disrupts the tight junctions between muscle fibers and interferes with nerve impulse transmission through the bladder, which can disrupt its motor function. Repeated overdistention may cause muscle fibrosis and prevent the bladder muscle from producing effective contractions.

Changes in the ability to urinate can be caused by an increased or decreased urethral sphincter tone and/or by changes in detrusor muscle function. Localization of neurologic disorders affecting micturition is important as they may reflect dysfunction of peripheral nerves, the spinal cord, and/or the brain.

Trajectory/Prognosis

The trajectory is dependent upon the cause of the micturition disorder, but typically, chronic conditions would follow a type 3 trajectory, where a patient would have a prolonged course of disease that would require increasing care over time. The outcome or prognosis is dependent on the cause, the comorbidities encountered, and the availability of reliable nursing care.

Manifestations

Clinical signs depend on the cause of the micturition disorder. These signs may range from straining to urinate without any voiding of urine to urinary incontinence with continual dribbling without control. Urinary tract infections are commonly seen as sequelae in patients with disorders of micturition. Patients that leak urine, or patients that need manual expression of the bladder, pose nursing care challenges, so good education is important for supporting the caregiver and patient. More details of the manifestations commonly seen with hospice and palliative care patients are listed below.

Management

For the best comfort of the patient, treatment should be targeted at the origin of the micturition dysfunction. Palliative care should include making sure the bladder is emptied at least four times per day. The patient should be catheterized if pharmacologic intervention for emptying the bladder and manual expression both fail or cannot be performed with comfort. It is beyond the scope of this chapter to describe urinary catheter placement, but multiple references can be found online and in veterinary technique text books (www.cliniciansbrief. com/article/urinary-catheter-placement-dogs; "VIN: Urinary Catheters Made Easy," Amy Newfield. 41st Annual Ontario Association of Veterinary Technicians (OAVT) Conference).

At the time of this printing, phenoxybenzamine, a commonly used drug in the past and an alpha-adrenergic blocker, has become cost prohibitive to use, so it will no longer be mentioned as a viable treatment option. Any concurrent urinary tract infections should be treated based on culture and sensitivity results. Some conditions may require extra efforts to maintain good patient hygiene in order to prevent skin irritation from urine contact. Treatment options for the various situations are listed below:

Bladder Is Difficult or Cannot Be Expressed

Nursing care of hospice and palliative care patients is most challenging when the bladder is difficult or cannot be expressed. Great caution must be exercised when attempting to express the bladder to avoid iatrogenic trauma to the abdomen and urinary tract. This challenging condition may occur when detrusor areflexia is combined with sphincter hypertonus caused by lesions from the brain to the L7 spinal cord segment. This disorder is most often seen as a complication of intervertebral disk protrusion.

Prazosin, an alpha-adrenergic blocker, may be used to decrease sympathetic tone and thus urethral sphincter tone. Diazepam can be used as a striated sphincter muscle relaxant to aid in manual expression. The use of oral diazepam in cats is somewhat controversial because of the risk of hepatotoxicity associated with felines; however, a decision needs to be made if the possibility of liver disease outweighs the risk of urine retention and discomfort associated with it (Plumb 2015). When possible, the shorter course and lowest dose possible should be considered. Cats prescribed diazepam should be monitored for hepatic changes.

Bethanechol is a cholinergic parasympathomimetic drug that can increase detrusor contractile input. It may be used in some situations to help stimulate bladder contraction but should not be used if a physical obstruction is suspected (Macintire et al. 2006). Cats should be monitored closely for side effects of the drug.

Bladder Can Be Expressed with Effort

Bladders that can be expressed but require some effort may be experiencing detrusor areflexia with normal sphincter tone. The detrusor muscle does not respond to stimuli, but the sphincter is functioning normally. This condition can occur when there is a spinal cord or brain stem lesion or when there has been trauma to the pelvis that spares the pudendal nerve.

Manual expression can be performed with careful effort for bladders that are difficult to express. Prazosin, an alpha-adrenergic blocker may be used to decrease sympathetic tone and thus urethral sphincter tone. Diazepam may help reduce the sphincter tone to make expression less difficult. As mentioned earlier, the use of oral diazepam in cats is somewhat controversial because of the risk of hepatotoxicity. If used in cats, when possible, the shorter course and lowest dose possible should be considered and they should be monitored for hepatic changes.

Straining to Urinate with Spurts of Urine Produced

Reflex dyssynergy is a condition where a normal first stream of urine is followed by short spurts or cessation of voiding. The patient may also be seen straining to urinate. The disorder is more common in males than in females. It occurs when there is a miscommunication between the detrusor muscle and the urethral sphincter muscle and the muscle contracts instead of relaxing during voiding. This may be a result of a functional loss of the reflexive inhibition of the pudendal nerve that normally occurs during micturition.

Prazosin, an alpha-adrenergic blocker may be used to decrease sympathetic tone and thus urethral sphincter tone. Diazepam can be used as a striated sphincter muscle relaxant to aid in manual expression Cats prescribed diazepam should be monitored for hepatic changes. As mentioned earlier, the use of oral diazepam in cats is somewhat controversial because of the risk of hepatotoxicity. If used in cats, when possible, the shorter course and lowest dose possible should be considered.

Bladder Easily Expressed with Continuous Leakage

Bladders that can be easily expressed but have continuous leakage may occur when detrusor areflexia is combined with sphincter areflexia. Both the detrusor muscle and the urethral sphincter do not respond to stimuli in these pets. This condition may occur when there are lesions in the sacral spinal cord and/or nerve roots L6–L7 and is most often seen as a result of trauma to this area.

For a pet that cannot produce a voluntary void, manual expression of the bladder is a requirement to provide complete emptying of the bladder at least four times daily. Phenylpropanolamine (PPA) may be used to increase urethral tone to help control leakage. Low-dose hormone replacement and herbal formulas may also be helpful.

Urine Leakage when Urine Accumulates

Urine leakage may also occur after a patient empties the bladder when there is normal detrusor reflex with decreased sphincter tone. The most frequent cause of this condition is hormone-responsive incontinence. However, this may also be caused by a structural lesion, loss of sympathetic innervation to the urethra, or loss of pudendal innervation.

Like above, PPA may be used to increase urethral tone. And low-dose hormone replacement and/or herbal formulas may also be helpful.

Ancillary Therapies for Micturition Disorders

In addition to the recommendations above, acupuncture and Chinese herbal formulas can promote better urinary function (Roger-Swaney 2014) and can be a stand-alone treatment to resolve micturition dysfunction. A number of other complimentary therapies have been recommended to support urinary tract health (Raditic 2015). In the human literature there is published scientific studies documenting the effects of the use of cranberry extracts and D-mannose to help manage urinary tract infections that may complicate micturition issues (Zhuxuan et al. 2017; Lenger et al. 2020).

Conclusion

Neurologic organ system change was ranked highest as the cause of death in adult dogs and is common in cats. Basic understanding of common neurologic conditions and their trajectory and management is paramount for good hospice and palliative care. A multimodal approach is often beneficial to minimize the consequences of neurologic conditions, aiding both the patient and caregiver. It is important to incorporate physical medicine in the management of any neurologic condition that interferes with ambulation. A sound knowledge of neurologic conditions will improve the quality of life of hospice and palliative care patients.

References

Awano, T., Johnson, G.S., Wade, C.M., et al. (2009) Genome-wide association analysis reveals a SOD1 mutation in canine degenerative myelopathy that resembles amyotrophic lateral sclerosis. *Proc. Natl. Acad. Sci.*, 106: 2794–2799.

Bryden, S.J., *Geriatric Onset Laryngeal Paralysis Polyneuropathy*. (2018) ACVIM.

Castel, A., Olby, N.J., Mariani, C.L., et al., (2017) Clinical characteristics of dogs with progressive myelomalacia following acute intervertebral disc extrusion. *J. Vet. Intern. Med.*, Available at: https://pubmed.ncbi.nlm. nih.gov/28961348 (Accessed: Feb. 2022).

Chrisman, C. (2011) Peripheral cranial nerve disorders. In: *Traditional Chinese Veterinary Medicine for Neurological Disease* (eds H. Xie, C. Chrisman and L. Trevisanello). Reddick, FL: Jing Tang Publishing, pp. 197–205.

Coates, J.R., March P.A., Oglesbee M., et al. (2007) Clinical characterization of a familial degenerative myelopathy in Pembroke Welsh Corgi dogs. *J. Vet. Intern. Med.*, 21: 1323–1331.

da Costa, R., Parent, J.M., Holmberg, D.L., et al. (2008) Outcome of medical and surgical treatment in dogs with cervical spondylomyelopathy: 104 cases (1988–2004). *J. Am. Vet. Med. Assoc.*, 233: 1284–1290.

Costello, M. (2009) Upper airway disease. In: *Small Animal Critical Care Medicine* (eds D. Silverstein and K. Hopper). St. Louis: Saunders, pp. 68–69.

Dunie-Merigot, A., Huneault, L., and Parent, J. (2007) Fibrocartilaginous embolic myelopathy in dogs: a retrospective study. *Can. Vet. J.*, 48: 63–68.

Fleming, J., Creevy, K.E., and Promislow, D.E. (2011) Mortality in north American dogs from 1984 to 2004: an investigation into age-, size-, and breed related causes of death. *J. Vet. Intern. Med.*, 25: 187–198.

Hayashi, A. (2015) Electroacupuncture for neuropathic pain and tetraparesis due to wobbler syndrome in a Doberman pinscher dog. In: *Traditional Chinese Veterinary Medicine for the Diagnosis and Treatment of Lameness and Pain in Dogs, Cats and Horses* (eds H. Xie and L. Trevisanello). Reddick, FL: Chi Institute Press, pp. 83–86.

Janssens, L., Beosier, Y., and Daems, R. (2009) Lumbosacral stenosis in the dog. The results of epidural infiltration with methylpre-dnisolone acetate: a retrospective study. *Vet. Comp. Orthop. Traumatol.*, Available at:

https://pubmed.ncbi.nlm.nih.gov/19876516 (Accessed: February 2022).

Joaquim, J., Luna, S.P., Brondani, J.T. et al. (2010) Comparison of decompressive surgery, electroacupuncture, and decompressive surgery followed by electroacupuncture for the treatment of dogs with intervertebral disk disease with long-standing severe neurologic deficits. *J. Am. Vet. Med. Assoc.*, 236: 1225–1229.

Jurney, C. (2020) Don't let vestibular disease spin you around. Pacific Veterinary Conference, San Francisco, CA. (June 18–21).

Kathmann, I., Cizinauskas, S., Doherr, M.G. et al. (2006) Daily controlled physiotherapy increases survival time in dogs with suspected degenerative myelopathy. *J. Vet. Intern. Med.*, 20: 927–932.

Lam, A.L., Betty, J.A., Moore, L. et al. (2012) Laryngeal disease in 69 cats: a retrospective multicenter study. *Aust. Vet. Pract.*, 42: 321–326.

Lenger, S.M., Bradley, M.S., Thomas, D.A. et al. (2020) D-mannose vs other agents for recurrent urinary tract infection prevention in adult women: a systemic review and meta-analysis. *Am. J. Obstet. Gynecol.*, 2: 223.

Levine, J., Levine, G.J., Johnson, S.I. et al. (2007) Evaluation of the success of medical management for presumptive cervical intervertebral disk herniation in dogs. *Vet. Surg.*, 36: 492–499.

Macintire, D., Drobatz, K., Haskins, S.C. et al. (eds) (2006) *Manual of Small Animal Emergency and Critical Care Medicine*. Ames, IA: Blackwell, pp. 276–277.

Miller, L.A., Torraca, D., De Taboada, L. (2020) Retrospective observational study and analysis of two different photobiomodulation therapy protocols combined with rehabilitation therapy as therapeutic interventions for canine degenerative myelopathy. *Photobiomodul. Photomed. Laser Surg.*, 38: 195–205.

Moore, S.A., Tipoid, A., Olby, N.J. et al. (2020) Current approaches to management of acute thoracolumbar disc protrusion in dogs. *Front.*

Vet. Sci., Available at: https://pubmed.ncbi.nlm.nih.gov/33117847/ (Accessed: Feb. 2022).

Morgan, B., Coates, J.R., Johnson, G.C. et al. (2014) Characterization of thoracic motor and sensory neurons and spinal nerve roots in canine degenerative myelopathy, a potential disease model of amylotrophic lateral sclerosis. *J. Neurosci. Res.*, 92: 531–541.

Negrin, A., Cherubi, G.B., Lamb, C. et al., (2010). Clinical signs, magnetic resonance imaging findings and outcome in 77 cats with vestibular disease: a retrospective study. *J. Feline Med. Surg.*, 12: 291–299.

Nichols, J.D. (2014) Corticosteroid use in small animal neurology. *Vet. Clin. North Am. Small Anim. Pract.*, 44: 1059–1074.

Olby, N.J., Muguet-Chanoit, A.C., Lim, J.H. et al. (2016) A placebo-controlled, prospective, randomized clinical trial of polyethylene glycol and methylprednisone sodium succinate in dogs with intervertebral disc herniation. *J. Vet. Intern. Med.*, Available at: https://pubmed.ncbi.nlm.nih.gov/26520829 (accessed February 2022).

Packer, R.M., Seath I.J., O'Neill, D.M. et al. (2016) DachsLife 2015: an investigation of lifestyle associations with the risk of intervertebral disc disease in dachshunds. *Canine Genet. Epidemiol.*, Available at: https://pubmed.ncbi.nlm.nih.gov/27826450 (accessed Feb 2022).

Platt, S. (2013) Vestibular disease: has my dog had a stroke? British Small Animal Veterinary Congress. Birmingham, UK. (April 4-7).

Plumb, D. (2015) *Plumb's Veterinary Drug Handbook*, 8. Ames, IA: Wiley.

Raditic, D. (2015) Complementary and integrative therapies for lower urinary tract diseases. *Vet. Clin. North Am. Small Anim. Pract.*, 45: 857–878.

Roger-Swaney, S. (2014) Kidney and bladder diseases. In: *Practical Guide to Traditional Chinese Veterinary Medicine* (H. Xie, L. Wedemeyer, C. Chrisman, and L. Trevisanello). Reddick, FL: Chi Institute Press, pp. 857–875.

Schunk, K.L. and Averill, A.R. (1983) Peripheral vestibular syndrome in the dog: a review of 83 cases. *J. Vet. Med. Assoc.*, 182: 1354–1357.

Shearer, T. (2013) *How to Improve Quality of Life Using Laser Therapy*. Whittier, NC: Shearer Pet Health Services, p. 68.

Sumano, H. and Mateos, G. (1999) Treatment of wobbler syndrome in dogs with electroacupuncture. *Am. J. Acupunct.*, 27: 5–14.

Thomas, W., Olby, N., and Sharon, L. (2014) Neurologic conditions and physical rehabilitation of the neurologic patient. In: *Canine Rehabilitation and Physical Therapy*, (A.L. Millis and D. Levine), 2. Philadelphia, PA Elsevier, pp. 611–613.

Troxel, M., Drobatz, K.J., and Vite, C.H. (2005) Signs of neurologic dysfunction in dogs with central versus peripheral vestibular disease. *J. Am. Vet. Med. Assoc.*, 227: 570–574.

Xie, H. and Preast, V. (2007) Acupuncture for the treatment of musculoskeletal and neurologic disorders. In: *Xie's Veterinary Acupuncture* (eds H. Xie and V. Preast). Ames, IA: Blackwell, p. 262.

Zhuxuan, F., Liska, D., Talan, D. et al. (2017) Cranberry reduces the risk of urinary tract infectin recurrence in otherwise healthy women: a systematic review and meta-analysis. *J. Nutr.*, 147: 2282–2288.

18

Cognitive Dysfunction

Tamara Shearer, MS, DVM, CCRP, CVPP, CVA, MSTCVM

Description

Cognitive dysfunction (CD) is a neurodegenerative condition experienced by both cats and dogs. This condition commands its own chapter because of its high incidence and the disruption that it causes in the quality of life of the patient and the caregiver. CD results in a progressive decline of conscious mental activities including the ability to think, learn, and remember. The decline in mental activities is manifested in changes in behavior and the animals' daily routines which causes disturbances in what once was household norms. Behavioral changes associated with cognitive decline occurred in 28% of dogs 11–12 years of age and 68% of dogs 15–16 years of age (Neilson et al. 2001). The incidence in cats also increased with age: in 135 cats over the age of 11, there was a 35% incidence of clinical signs associated with CD (Landsberg et al. 2010).

Cognitive dysfunction has become an intriguing condition to study in dogs and cats because it shares some characteristics of Alzheimer disease (AD) in humans (Vite and Head 2014). As people and pets age, anatomical and physiological changes take place in the brain that predispose it to additional insults, resulting in neuronal degeneration with synaptic dysfunction. Some of the biological changes include brain atrophy and neuron loss. Like in AD, β-amyloid (Aβ) plaques are found within the brain in both dogs and cats (Gunn-Moore et al. 2006). These plaques are considered a biomarker for cognitive dysfunction. Vascular changes secondary to deposition of Aβ protein in the brain may also result in microhemorrhages that affect cognition.

Other age-related changes include the presence of phosphorylated tau epitopes, which are defective tau proteins. They are found in the aging brains of people, dogs, and cats and are common in AD patients. Oxidative damage also contributes to the aging changes in the brain secondary to production of free radicals (Vite and Head 2014). Ultimately, there is also impaired neuronal glucose metabolism and disruption of the mitochondria, microglial cells, and astrocytes (Landsberg et al. 2010).

CD has a profound effect on the relationship between the family and the pet because of the overwhelming behavioral components of the disease. Because the disease does not shorten life expectancy, it can be a challenge for the hospice practitioner to manage the patient as the disease progresses. Early recognition, proactively implementing supportive care, and treating symptoms, sequelae, and comorbidities will help to maintain the animal's quality of life.

Hospice and Palliative Care for Companion Animals: Principles and Practice, Second Edition.
Edited by Amir Shanan, Jessica Pierce, and Tamara Shearer.
© 2023 John Wiley & Sons, Inc. Published 2023 by John Wiley & Sons, Inc.
Companion website: www.wiley.com/go/shanan/palliative

Trajectory/Prognosis

Cognitive dysfunction follows a type 3 trajectory. A pet with cognitive dysfunction may have a prolonged course of disease that might require increasing care over time, especially because the disease may not shorten life expectancy. Unlike AD, dogs and cats with CD do not lose the ability to eat and drink, and it is not associated with early death (Nagga et al. 2014). In a long-term study of CD in Denmark, clinical characteristics, survival, and risk factors were documented in dogs enrolled in 2008 and 2009 and followed through 2012. Of the 94 dogs older than 8 years that were enrolled in the study, 44 were categorized in the CD group, 27 in the pre-CD group, and 23 in the non-CD group. At the time of follow-up, 74 dogs had died. Only six owners reported CD to be the primary cause for euthanasia. It was found that the median survival time for the non-CD group was 12.6 years (range, 9.7–15.0), for the pre-CD group 13.5 years (range, 9.3–17.0), and for the CD group 13.9 years (range, 10.0–17.0). The results suggest that dogs with CD are likely to live their full life expectancy (Fast et al. 2013).

Manifestations

During the subclinical phase of cognitive dysfunction, functional and morphologic changes can be documented in the brain, but clinical signs cannot yet be recognized by the caregiver. In dogs, memory task studies show changes as early as six years of age, and brain Aβ proteins have been found in eight- to nine-year-old dogs (Landsberg et al. 2012). The Siamese breed may have a higher incidence of CD than domestic short-haired felines. The youngest cat reported to have Aβ in the central nervous system was 7.5 years old (Brellou et al. 2005). The symptoms associated with cognitive dysfunction, known as DISHA, include disorientation, altered interactions, sleep–wake pattern disruption, house soiling, and the development of anxiety (Figure 18.1). In dogs, the most

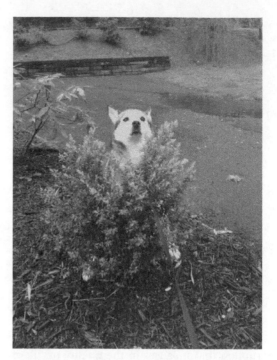

Figure 18.1 "Prince" experiencing disorientation: getting stuck in a bush.

common signs were anxiety, night waking, and vocalizing. Other clinical signs might include compulsive circling, resistance to restraint, transient vestibular episodes, and seizure activity especially when there are lesions in the forebrain (Dewey et al. 2019). In cats, the most common signs were vocalization at night and house soiling (Landsberg et al. 2012).

Sequelae to CD may be direct or indirect, and coping with them can be challenging for caregivers. Indirectly, exacerbations of preexisting conditions may be precipitated by the additional stressors associated with CD, like decreased sleep and obsessive walking resulting in fatigue and dehydration. Direct sequelae include frequent episodes of dogs that wander, get stuck, and then collapse between or behind furniture or the bathroom toilet bowl while the caregiver is away. When they are found, they are frequently anxiety ridden, painful, and/or lying in urine and feces.

Another important consideration is the impact that CD has on the caregiver's quality of life due to frequent sleep disruptions caused by the animals' nighttime waking and vocalization. Disruption of sleep habits in caregivers of human patients with AD results in reports of poor quality of life for caregivers (Cupidi et al. 2013). When parents care for children with disabilities that interfere with the caregivers' sleep, both parents report poor health, psychological exhaustion, and increased nighttime wakefulness (Morelius and Hemmingsson 2014). It is very likely that sleep interruption impacts caregivers of animals with CD in similar ways.

Studies show that cognitive dysfunction in pets is underdiagnosed. An epidemiological study of companion dogs with an average age of 11.67 years showed a prevalence rate of 14.2% in comparison to the 1.9% diagnosed by veterinarians (Salvin et al. 2010). Cats too are most likely underdiagnosed with CD. One proposed reason for the underdiagnosis may be the reluctance of some pet owners to opt for diagnostic testing when seeking hospice or palliative care. Because CD is a condition diagnosed by exclusion, diagnostic testing would be necessary to rule out other conditions that could affect mentation. Those conditions may include, but are not limited to, changes in internal organ function, hormone imbalances, decreased vision and hearing, brain tumors, and pain. Prescribed medications may also have side effects that might include restlessness, dysphoria, or somnolence, so it is also important to rule out drug side effects as a cause of CD-like clinical signs.

Management

Palliative care for cognitive dysfunction may be very challenging with some patients, requiring 24/7 supervision to keep them safe and comfortable. This is especially true of those patients that are awake at night, suffer from anxiety, and wander aimlessly. There are six components of care that help to mitigate the clinical signs of cognitive dysfunction: (i) client education and prevention, (ii) behavior modification and environmental enhancement, (iii) diet modification, (iv) supplements (v) alternative care and (vi) pharmaceutical interventions.

Client Education and Prevention

Clients with senior pets should be educated about the clinical signs associated with cognitive decline and reminded that there is a pathology, and not just aging, associated with the changes in behavior. Clients often misinterpret behaviors of cognitive decline to the misconception of aging changes or "acting senile." These reported changes include having difficulty with navigating stairs, narrow passageways, and door openings or getting stuck in small spaces and getting lost in familiar surroundings. Some report increased sleeping, while others report pacing and vocalizing.

Suggesting that the caregiver be proactive and show patience toward their pet is of utmost importance. Because there is a subclinical phase to CD, an emphasis should also be placed on preventative measures to slow the disease process. A practitioner should consider recommending early interventions for dogs and cats starting at age 5–7 years, based on the earliest lesions found in the brains of these species (Landsberg et al. 2012). Because cognitive dysfunction is common but difficult to diagnose, practitioners should consider recommending that all older pets be supported with behavior modification, wholesome diets, appropriate supplements, and environmental enrichment. Besides slowing down the progression of CD, these measures may also improve overall physical and emotional health.

Behavior Modification and Environmental Enhancement

Before or while instituting pharmaceutical management to palliate the effects of CD described in this section, it is recommended to institute concurrent behavior modification programs to attain the best outcome. It is important to note that CD patients are sometimes unable to send the proper social signals, and this behavior change may trigger aggression toward them by other animals in the household. In these circumstances, it is important to keep the other pet safe through better structure and ultimately separation as a last resort.

Depending on the individual, behavior modification may include mental stimulation in the form of increasing interactive play time with the introduction of new toys for pets that like to play. For pets that do not play, increasing the frequency of exercise may be helpful. The introduction of new smells, sounds, and/or encouragement of tactile change (for example, by having pets walk over novel surfaces like bubble wrap, foam cushions, sand, mulch, or smooth pebbles) may be stimulating. Food puzzles may help preserve problem-solving behavior for the patients. A physical medicine consultation for a patient may support the mental stimulation for the cognitive dysfunction patient by creating new exercise routines.

The Calmer Canine®, created by Assisi Animal Health (New Vernon, NJ; assisianimalhealth.com), is a device that delivers targeted pulsed electromagnetic field (tPEMF) to the area of the brain to help manage anxiety. This modality has no known side effects associated with its use. This author recommends its use to help mitigate clinical signs of separation anxiety for senior dogs. Two, 15-minute treatments daily for 4–6 weeks is the recommended frequency and duration.

Environmental enrichment should be provided to ensure that the pets are not isolated. Bird feeders and keeping the window blinds open may help to entertain cats and dogs. Cats should have easy litter box accessibility. Dogs should have at least four or five opportunities per day to go outdoors to exercise, urinate, and defecate. The environment should also be modified for safety. To prevent trauma, the environment should be modified by providing nonslip flooring and blocking off stairways to prevent falls. Doors should be shut to decrease access to areas of the house that could pose dangers to pets that exhibit aimless wandering. Using heavy cardboard, a palliative care client designed a circular track to protect and contain her wandering Maltese when unsupervised (author's patient). Modifications should be made to make food and water more available by placing bowls in additional locations and/or by raising existing bowls. Adding pheromones to the environment (e.g. Adaptil® and Feliway Optimum®) may reduce anxiety (Kim et al. 2010).

Diet Modification

Studies have shown that good nutrition is important in managing CD. Special diets and supplements, including diets that are high in antioxidants, long-chain omega-3 fatty acids, and medium-chain fatty acids, may be beneficial to CD patients (Laflamme 2012). A good option to consider is NC NeuroCare™, a Purina Pro Plan Veterinary Diet, includes medium-chain fatty acid vegetable oil, antioxidants, a high level of vitamin E, and omega fatty acids with EPA and DHA. Another consideration is to provide home-cooked meals for senior pets tailored to meet medical and nutritional needs through consultation with a nutritionist or through the BalanceIT website (secure.balanceit.com).

The following foods and supplements are recommended to enhance the nutrition for Alzheimer's patients and may also be utilized in supporting animal patients. They include fish, fruits, and vegetables, whole grains, soybeans, nuts, medium-chain fatty acids found in coconut oil, omega-3-fatty acids, probiotics, and antioxidants. Foods that may contribute to CD include processed foods, over consumption of red meat, dairy products high in fat, and refined sugars (Solfrizzi et al. 2017).

Supplements

Many supplements and herbal formulas recommended for managing CD are rich in antioxidants and therefore may have other benefits for the patient. The following have been recommended by veterinary behaviorists to help preserve cognition (Landsberg et al. 2012):

- Alpha-casozepine (Zylkene® from Vetoquinol) showed efficacy in controlling anxiety similar to selegiline (Beata et al. 2007). Zylkene can be used in dogs and cats.
- Apoequorin is a supplement that is associated with a greater improvement of spatial memory and attention tasks compared to selegiline (Milgram et al. 2015). This supplement helps to support memory and cognition and has been shown to experimentally protect against neuronal death.
- Senilife®, by CEVA Animal Health, is a supplement that contains phosphatidylserine, pyroxidine, *Ginkgo biloba* extract, resveratrol, and D-alpha-tocopherol to help support brain health. It improved short-term memory performance in older Beagles (Araujo et al. 2008). It is labeled for use in dogs.
- Solliquin® (Nutramax Laboratories Veterinary Sciences, Inc., Lancaster, SC), is another supplement that may be helpful in palliating CD in dogs. It includes a natural blend of L-theanine, *Magnolia officinalis*, and *Phellodendron amurense* and helps to reduce stress-related behaviors (DePorter et al. 2012).
- *S*-adenosylmethionine (SAMe) and L-theanine also target cognitive decline. SAMe supplementation has been clinically proven to decrease age-related behavior problems (Reme et al. 2008). Purified l-theanine may be helpful to reduce anxiety. It is a compound found in green tea leaves, which have been found to help humans calm and relax (Rao et al. 2015). Both supplements can be used in dogs and cats.
- Phytochemicals such as curcumin, resveratrol, and green tea may be considered to help improve cognition.
- Calming Care Pro Plan® Veterinary Supplements for cats and dogs is a probiotic designed to help manage anxiety.
- CogniCaps, a supplement that contains both Chinese herbs and Western supplements,

was developed by Dr. Cutis Dewey and Dr. Terry Fossum. It contains curcumin, zinc, *S*-adenosylmethionine, Salvia, BioCog, vitamin E, Polygala, phosphatidylserine, and coenzyme Q10.
- Traditional Chinese veterinary medicine herbal formulas may also help support the patient exhibiting clinical signs of CD. There are clinical studies that show that some herbal formulas reduce inflammation, inhibit Aß production, and act as antioxidants. This author often prescribes Shen Calmer™ or Stasis in the Mansion of the Mind™ by Jing Tang Herbals.

Alternative Care

Consultation with a practitioner of traditional Chinese veterinary medicine may provide other options for patients with CD. Specific acupuncture points, herbal formulas, food therapy, massage techniques, and *Qi Gong* (a method of self-care for caregivers) may be helpful (DiNatale 2014). Acupuncture has been shown to enhance neuronal glucose utilization and increase neuronal stem cells and neurotrophic factors and decrease Aß accumulation (Park et al. 2017). Helpful acupoints in treating CD may include ST-36, ST-40, SP-6, SP-9, SP-10, HT-7, HT-9, BL-14, BL-15, BL-17, KID-3, PC-6, PC-9, GV-20, GV-14, CV-12, CV-17, and *An-shen*. Interestingly, acupuncture at *Yin-tang* and LI-20 has been shown to decrease Aß proteins and increase brain-derived neurotrophic factor (BDNF). The memory and cognition centers of the cerebrum are activated when LI-4 and LIV-3 were stimulated. Other benefits seen with acupuncture include suppression of oxidative stress and apoptosis but enhancement of neurotrophin, increased expression of synaptophysin, and cholinergic neural transmission (Leung et al. 2014).

Pharmaceutical Interventions

Pharmaceutical therapy for CD includes the use of selegiline, a monoamine oxidase inhibitor. Anipryl® (Pfizer Animal Health) is a selegiline that is approved by the US Food and Drug Administration (FDA) for the treatment of CD in dogs. The dosage for dogs is 0.5–1 mg/kg^{-1} PO once daily. It can be used in cats (extralabel) at 0.25–1 mg/kg^{-1} PO once daily. It may take up to 2–6 weeks to see an effect. It needs to be used with caution because of the number of drug interactions and the number of side effects associated with the drug (Plumb 2015). It is worth noting that the studies supporting the use of selegiline did not include comparative cognitive testing but only pet owner questionnaires (Dewey et al. 2019).

Additional drugs may be needed to help manage anxiety and night waking. Lorazepam, a benzodiazepine, can be used in dogs and cats. The dosage in dogs is 0.02–0.2 mg/kg^{-1} PO one to three times daily. The dose for cats is 0.025–0.08 mg-kg^{-1} PO once or twice daily (Plumb 2015).

The use of trazodone for anxiety or tramadol for sedation can help palliate the symptoms of CD but should be avoided if the patient is given selegiline. Both drugs are serotonin reuptake inhibitors, and their concomitant use with selegiline or at higher doses together may precipitate a serotonin syndrome in the patient. The trazodone dose ranges from 1.7 to 19.5 mg/kg^{-1}/day^{-1} with an average of 7.25 mg/ kg^{-1}/day^{-1} divided into once to twice daily (Plumb 2015).

Levetiracetam has been shown to improve central nervous system mitochondrial function and inhibits astrocyte glutamate release, thus improving cognitive dysfunction in human and animal models (Sanchez et al. 2012).

Pentoxyfyllin, a methylxanthene, may be used to improve peripheral blood flow by decreasing blood viscosity and enhancing red blood cell deformability, which may have benefit for some CD patients where decreased brain perfusion contributes to clinical signs. It is commonly used for the treatment of ischemic dematopathies, vasculitis, and other conditions where increased perfusion would be of benefit. A related drug, propentofylline (Vivitonin) is approved for use in Europe for age-related behavior changes associated with CD by improving demeanor. Pentoxyfylline is contraindicated in patients with bleeding disorders.

Melatonin is a pineal gland hormone that may be used for sleep disorders. It should be given 30 minutes prior to bedtime to help with night waking at a dose of 3–9 mg for dogs and 1.5–6 mg for cats (Landsberg et al. 2012).

Proactive pain management is recommended for CD patients because under-managed pain can contribute to restlessness (Muir 2009). Gabapentin, a neuropathic pain analgesic and anticonvulsant medication, may be of benefit to help a pet rest and to manage pain. See additional information in Chapter 19 for additional information on pain management.

Antihistamines or anticholinergic drugs, like diphenhydramine, hydroxyzine, and chlorpheniramine, may help some patients with night waking. Be mindful that aging individuals are more likely to experience adverse reactions to these drugs due to age-related cholinergic decline.

The use of cannabinoids (CBD) can be tried to mitigate the clinical signs of CD. There are anecdotal reports of a reduction in anxiety and more peaceful sleep when administered. It is important for the practitioners to be familiar with the purity and safety of the product being used. In older pets, it is recommended to start with a lower dose and increase based on the patient's response.

Conclusion

Cognitive dysfunction (CD) is an often undiagnosed, progressive condition of dogs and cats that results in decline of conscious mental activities and often does not shorten life expectancy. Proactive care may preserve the quality of life for the patient with CD and his or her caregiver. There is a subclinical phase to the disease, so early preemptive intervention is warranted in all aging patients. To achieve optimal quality of life for CD affected dogs and cats, the use of an integrative approach to care for patients includes providing client education, behavior modification, environmental enhancement, diet modification, use of supplements, alternative care options, and pharmaceutical interventions.

References

Araujo, J., Landsberg, G.M., Milgram, N.W. et al. (2008) Improvement of short-term memory performance in aged beagles by nutraceutical supplement containing phosphatidylserine, Ginko bilobo, vitamin E and pyridoxine. *Can. Vet. J.*, 49: 379–385.

Beata, C., Beaumont-Graff, E., Diaz, C. et al. (2007) Effects of alpha-casozepine (Zylkene) versus selegiline hydrochloride (Selgian, Anipryl) on anxiety disorders in dogs. *J. Vet. Behav.*, 2: 175–183.

Brellou, G., Vlemmas, I., Lekkas, S. and et al. (2005) Immunohistochemical investigation of amyloid-β (Aβ) in the brain of aged cats. *HistolHistopath*, 20: 725–731.

Cupidi, C., Realmuto, S., Lo Coco, G. et al. (2013) Sleep quality in caregivers of patients with Alzheimer's disease and Parkinson's disease and its relationship to quality of life. *Int. Psychogeriatr.*, 11: 1827–1835.

DePorter, T., Landsberg, G.M., Araujo, J.A. et al. (2012) Harmonease chewable tablets reduces noise-induced fear and anxiety in a laboratory canine thunderstorm simulation: a blinded and placebo controlled study. *J. Vet. Behav.*, 7: 225–232.

Dewey, C.W., Davies, E.S., Xie, H. et al. (2019) Canine cognitive dysfunction pathophysiology, diagnosis and treatment. *Vet. Clin. North Am. Small Anim. Pract.*, 49: 477–499.

DiNatale, C. (2014) Geriatric medicine. In: *Practical Guide to Traditional Chinese Veterinary Medicine* (eds H. Xie, L. Wedemeyer, C. Chrisman, L. Trevisanello). Reddick, FL: Chi Institute Press, pp. 920–924.

Fast, R., Schutt, T., Toft, N. et al. (2013) An observational study with long term followup of canine cognitive dysfunction: clinical characteristics, survival, and risk factors. *J. Vet. Intern. Med.*, 4: 822–829.

Gunn-Moore, D., McVee, J., Bradshaw, J.M. et al. (2006) Aging changes in cat brains demonstrated by beta-amyloid and AT-8-immunoreative phosphorylated tau deposits. *J. Feline Med. Surg.*, 8: 234–242.

Kim, Y., Lee, J.K., Abd el-Aty, A.M. et al. (2010) Efficacy of dog appeasing pheromone (DAP) for ameliorating separation-related behavioral signs in hospitalized dogs. *Can. Vet. J.*, 4: 380–384.

Laflamme, D. (2012) Nutritional care for aging cats and dogs. *Vet. Clin. North Am. Small Anim. Pract.*, 42: 769–791.

Landsberg, G., Denenberg, S., and Araujo, J.A. (2010) Cognitive dysfunction in cats. A syndrome we used to dismiss as old age. *J. Feline Med. Surg.*, 12: 837–848.

Landsberg, G., Nichol, J., and Araujo, J.A. (2012) Cognitive dysfunction syndrome. *Vet. Clin. North Am. Small Anim. Pract.*, 42: 749–768.

Leung, M.C., Yip, K.K., Ho, Y.S. et al. (2014) Mechanisms underlying the effect of acupuncture on cognitive improvement: a systematic review of animal studies. *J. Neuroimmune. Pharmacol.*, 9: 492–507.

Milgram, N., Landsberg G., Merrick, D. et al. (2015) A novel mechanism for cognitive enhancement in aged dogs with the use of a calcium-buffering protein. *J. Vet. Behav.*, 10: 217–222.

Morelius, E. and Hemmingsson, H. (2014) Parents of children with physical disabilities-perceived health in parents related to the child's sleep problems and need for attention at night. *Child Care Health Dev.*: 40, 412–418.

Muir, W. (2009) Pain behaviors. In: *Handbook of Veterinary Pain Management* (eds J. Gaynor and W. Muir), 2. St. Louis: Mosby, pp. 62–77.

Nagga, K., Wattmo, C., and Zhang, Y. et al. (2014) Cerebral inflammation is an underlying mechanism of early death in Alzheimer's disease: a 13 year cause specific multivariate mortality study. *Alzheimers Res. Ther.*, 6: 41.

Neilson, J., Hart, B.L., Cliff, K.D. et al. (2001) Prevalence of behavioral changes associated with age-related cognitive impairment in dogs.

Park, S., Lee, J.H., and Yang, E.J. (2017) *Effects of acupuncture on Alzheimer's disease in animal-based research*. Evid Based Complement Altern. Med., Available at: https://pubmed.ncbi.nlm.nih.gov/29234418/ (Accessed: February 2022).

Plumb, D. (2015) *Plumb's Veterinary Drug Handbook*, 8. Ames, IA: Wiley.

Rao, T., Ozeki, M., and Juneja, L.R. (2015) In search of a safe natural sleep aid. *J. Am. Coll. Nutr.*, 34: 436–447.

Reme, C., Dramard, V., Kern, L. et al. (2008) Effect of S-adenossylmethionine tablets on the reduction of age related mental decline in

dogs: a double-blind placebo-controlled study. *Vet. Ther.*, 9: 69–82.

Salvin, H., McGreevy, P.D., Sachdev, P.S. et al. (2010) Under diagnosis of canine cognitive dysfunction: a cross-sectional survey of older companion animals. *Vet. J.*, 184: 277–281.

Sanchez, P.E., Zhu, L., Verret, L. et al. (2012) Levetiracetam suppresses neuronal network dysfunction and reverses synaptic and cognitive deficits in an Alzheimer's disease model. *Proc. Natl. Acad. Sci. U.S.A.*, 109: E2895–E2903.

Solfrizzi, V., Custodero, C., Lozupone, M. et al. (2017) Relationships of dietary patterns, foods, and micro- and macronutrients with Alzheimer's disease and late life cognitive disorders. *J. Alzheimer's Dis.* 59: 815–849.

Vite, C. and Head, E. (2014) Aging in the canine and feline brain. *Vet. Clin. North Am. Small Anim. Pract.*, 44: 1113–1129.

19

Pharmacology Interventions for Symptom Management

Shea Cox, DVM, CHPV, CVPP

Introduction

Patients who have advanced, progressive illness generally present with multiple symptoms that require simultaneous assessment and management. Symptoms do more than cause suffering directly; when there are multiple symptom burdens present, they affect a patient's distress level, quality of life, and survival (Vachon 1995). Therefore, a core function of animal hospice and palliative care is the alleviation of the symptoms that accompany life-limiting illness and the advanced stages of disease. Although not the exclusive form of intervention offered to patients and their families, symptom management is an essential part of the skills required in providing palliative care, and it is often the primary focus of the palliative care team.

Pain

Clinical Signs of Pain

Behavioral expression of pain is species-specific and is influenced by age, breed, individual temperament, and the presence of additional stressors such as anxiety or fear. Additionally, the presence of debilitating disease can dramatically reduce the range of behavioral indicators of pain that the animal would otherwise express (Matthews et al. 2014).

Anticipating, controlling, and preventing pain in the hospice patient is of paramount importance and comprises a cornerstone in the quality of care we can provide. Effective and appropriate pain management considers the following: (i) early recognition and understanding of the clinical signs of pain; (ii) anticipating the perceived level of pain experienced based on the disease process present; (iii) implementing a multimodal pain management plan; and (iv) continued evaluation and reassessment of the response to treatments administered. Due to the complexity and scope of information available from other sources, this chapter provides only a brief overview of pain management.

Behavioral Indicators of Pain

An extensive discussion of the behavioral indicators of pain is included in this volume in Chapter 5, "Recognizing Distress." A more extensive summary is available in the *Handbook of Veterinary Pain Management* (Gaynor and Muir 2015). The following is a brief summary of the changes in animals' behavior that may indicate the presence of pain, listed in the Handbook:

1) **Attitude**: Deviations from the animal's normal including lethargy, depression, hiding or reclusiveness, decreased social interaction with family and/or other pets in the

Hospice and Palliative Care for Companion Animals: Principles and Practice, Second Edition.
Edited by Amir Shanan, Jessica Pierce, and Tamara Shearer.
© 2023 John Wiley & Sons, Inc. Published 2023 by John Wiley & Sons, Inc.
Companion website: www.wiley.com/go/shanan/palliative

household, agitation, fearfulness, or development of submissive behaviors.

2) **Body posture and facial expression**: Body postures including a tense or rigid posture, stiffness, trembling, low tail carriage, resting in an abnormal position, a crouched stance or arched back, a wide-based stance or "praying position" (dogs), or a tucked up "meatloaf" position (cats). Facial expressions including a "distant appearance" or dullness in the eyes, a wide-eyed expression, squinting or furrowed brow, flattening of the ear carriage, or lowering of the head.

3) **Activity level and activities of daily living**: Reduced activity, reluctance to move or lie down, restlessness, frequent changes in body position, circling or making multiple attempts to lie down, reduced weight bearing or limping, shifting weight carriage, or making no attempts to remove themselves from the area of elimination. Decreased grooming behaviors are often noted in the presence of pain, especially in cats, resulting in the development of a dull and unkempt hair coat. Elimination habits may change due to pain directly caused by elimination, or indirectly caused by posturing to urinate or defecate or discomfort with ambulation.

4) **Focused attention or response to touch**: Focused attention to a painful area can be expressed by staring, self-mutilation, rubbing, excessive licking, chewing or excessive grooming of a particular area on the body, or guarding behavior of a painful area. Petting or manipulation of a painful area may evoke a response such as irritability or aggression, including growling, hissing, tail flicking (cats), attempting to bite, or withdrawing and moving away from touch.

5) **Appetite**: Hyporexia, anorexia, and less commonly polyphagia.

6) **Vocalization**: Vocalization can include whining, whimpering, groaning, crying, or howling. It is important to note that vocalization can also be an attempt to communicate needs or feelings other than pain such as anxiety, frustration, need to urinate or defecate, or desire for food or water intake.

Visit the Companion Website for access to the BEAP Pain Scale. BEAP is short for Breathing, Eyes, Ambulation, Activity, Appetite, Attitude, Posture, and Palpation. This pain scale is available for both canine and feline species and is an excellent education and communication tool. The BEAP Pain Scale helps caregivers recognize signs and severity of pain based on common behaviors exhibited by their pet.

Pharmacology for Pain Management

When managing pain, a preemptive, multimodal approach should be implemented. With this approach, pharmacologic and non-pharmacologic therapies complement one another, working better together than any single therapy can provide on its own. This allows for intervention at multiple places along the nociceptive pathway, increases the effectiveness of any given analgesic drug, and allows efficacious use at lower drug doses (Gaynor and Muir 2015). Preemptive therapy should be implemented if pain is anticipated, and pain medications should be given around the clock rather than waiting for overt signs of pain to be present. The use of a pain management algorithm can help aid in pain identification, prevention, and management.

A multimodal pain management approach can include the use of anti-inflammatories, non-opioid analgesics, opioids, tricyclic antidepressants (TCAs), serotonin-norepinephrine reuptake inhibitors (SNRIs), anticonvulsants, *N*-methyl-D-aspartate (NMDA) receptor antagonists, nutraceuticals, and adjunctive physical modalities.

Nonsteroidal Anti-Inflammatory Drugs

Nonsteroidal anti-inflammatory drugs (NSAIDs) are a part of a balanced multimodal analgesic plan and are effective in the reduction of pain associated with tissue inflammation. NSAIDs reduce peripheral sensitization, and COX-2-specific NSAIDs may assist in reducing central sensitization as well. There is no compelling evidence to suggest that NSAIDs can be ranked by efficacy, and the best NSAID for a particular patient is the NSAID that is the most effective for that patient while providing minimal or no adverse effects (Downing 2011).

Glucocorticoids

Glucocorticoids, like NSAIDs, are anti-inflammatory agents that can be used to manage pain and are available in both oral and injectable formulations.

Acetaminophen

Acetaminophen (paracetamol) can be used extra-label in dogs, but is lethal in cats and should never be considered for administration in this species. When appropriately dosed, it has a good safety record and can be helpful in the treatment of chronic pain in dogs, particularly those that cannot tolerate NSAID use.

Acetaminophen has antipyretic and analgesic properties, yet differs from the NSAIDs and inhibitors of prostaglandin-H-synthase-2 (PGHS) by exhibiting little effect on platelets or inflammation (Boutaud 2002); because of this, acetaminophen can be used concurrently with NSAIDs for improved pain management. While the precise mechanism of action for the analgesic effect of acetaminophen remains uncertain, evidence suggests that its activity resides primarily in the central nervous system, while the site of action for the analgesic effect of NSAIDs is predominantly peripheral within injured or inflamed tissue. Several controlled clinical studies among patients with musculoskeletal conditions, dental pain, or postoperative pain have shown that combinations of acetaminophen and NSAIDs provide additive pain-relieving activity, thereby leading to dose-sparing effects and improved safety (Altman 2004).

Acetaminophen is also often coadministered with opioids and is found in combination formulas with codeine, hydrocodone, and oxycodone. Although the bioavailability of the opioid component is reported to be low due to a robust first-pass effect, these combination medications are useful.

Acetaminophen: Dog (extra-label), 10–15 mg kg^{-1} PO q8 h; if using long term (>5 days) consider giving q12 h at the lower end of dosing range. *Lethal in cats.*

Acetaminophen/opioid combinations: calculated on the basis of the acetaminophen dose; a general recommendation for acetaminophen 325 mg/hydrocodone 10 mg is 1 tablet per 20 kg of body weight BID–TID.

Opioids

Opioids remain the most efficacious systemic means of controlling moderate to severe acute pain.

Morphine is a pure mu-agonist and an effective opioid choice for dogs and cats receiving palliative and hospice care, for both short-term and long-term use. Dogs, 0.5–2 mg/kg^{-1} IM, SC, or IV (slowly): lower dosages may be necessary in geriatric or severely debilitated animals, and higher dosages required for severe to excruciating pain. Duration of effect can vary, and often re-dosing is needed after two hours. Cats, morphine is sometimes used in cats, but it does not appear to be as effective as in dogs and alone it does not produce good sedation; doses range from 0.05 to 0.4 mg/kg^{-1} IM, SC every 3–6 hours as needed. Duration of effect can vary and often re-dosing is needed after 3 hours.

Methadone acts similarly to morphine with regard to its degree of analgesia and duration of action, and is a mu-receptor agonist that is also a noncompetitive inhibitor of NMDA receptors. Methadone can reduce reuptake of norepinephrine and serotonin, which may further contribute to its analgesic effects. Due to these other actions, methadone may be more efficacious than other mu agonists (e.g. morphine), particularly for neuropathic or chronic pain (Plumb 2015). Dogs, 0.1–0.5 mg/kg^{-1} IV, IM, SC q2–4 h; 0.5 mg/kg^{-1} PO BID–QID. Although this is a published dose in the *Handbook of Veterinary Pain Management* (Gaynor and Muir 2015), oral methadone appears to have a low oral bioavailability (<20%, compared with >70% in humans) and rapid clearance in dogs (KuKanich et al. 2005); until more is understood about the pharmacokinetics and pharmacodynamics of oral methadone in dogs, its use cannot be recommended. Cats, 0.1–0.25 mg/kg^{-1} IV, IM, SC q2–4 h; 0.1–0.3 mg/kg^{-1} buccally BID–TID, and 0.25–0.5 mg/kg^{-1} PO BID–QID. Of note, in cats, efficacy can be expected to last at least two hours after IV administration and at least four hours after oral transmucosal (OTM) administration (Ferreira et al. 2011).

Hydromorphone has the same efficacy as morphine in dogs and may produce better analgesia than morphine in cats. Duration is shorter than morphine in dogs, 1–2 hours after IV administration and up to 2 hours after IM or SC administration. In cats, hydromorphone may have a longer duration of action (potentially up to 7 hours). Hydromorphone is associated with less histamine release, nausea, and sedation compared to morphine. In cats, hydromorphone is implicated more than other opioids in episodes of hyperthermia (Gaynor and Muir 2015). Dogs (extra-label), recommendations are generally 0.1–0.2 mg/kg^{-1} IV, IM, or SC q2–4 h, and 0.2–0.6 mg/kg^{-1} PO q6–8 h. Cats (extra-label), recommendations are generally 0.05–0.1 mg/kg^{-1} IV, IM, or SC q2–6 h.

Fentanyl is a potent pure mu-agonist opioid with a very short duration of action, approximately 30 minutes after a single injection. Absorption of fentanyl from transdermal patches has been shown to be highly variable in dogs and cats; therefore, not a good first choice for controlling escalating pain in animal hospice and palliative care patients.

Additionally, they carry the risk of being ingested by the patient, potentially raising liability issues for the veterinarian.

Buprenorphine is a partial mu-agonist and therefore does not produce the same level of analgesia as morphine. Buprenorphine has a ceiling effect, meaning neither adverse side-effects nor analgesia become more pronounced at higher doses (Slingsby et al. 2011). The advantage to buprenorphine is its relatively long duration (6–12 hours) and good data to support its use in cats. Dosages for dogs, 0.005–0.03 mg/kg^{-1} IV, IM, or SC q6–12 h; cats, 0.01–0.03 mg/kg^{-1} IM, IV, SC, OTM q6–8 h.

Zorbuim is a new transdermal formulation of buprenorphine that allows veterinarians to provide pain relief to their feline patients for up to 4 days with a single application. Currently, Zorbium is only indicated for the control of postoperative pain associated with surgical procedures in cats, but can have a place in hospice and end-of-life patients with proper clinical assessment. Zorbium is intended to be administered topically as the entire tube contents based on body weight range provided in the insert (dose ranges from 2.7-6.7mg/kg).

Butorphanol is a mu-agonist/antagonist agent described in the past for use in chronic maladaptive and malignant pain. However, its short duration of action and the lack of significant analgesia make butorphanol a poor pain management choice. Some animal hospice and palliative care patients can, however, benefit from its sedating effect to resolve restlessness and assist in achieving continuous sleep at night (Downing 2011).

Commercial oral opioid preparations are available, and although pharmacokinetic data exist for some formulations, pharmacodynamic (efficacy) data is currently lacking. However, they are not without usefulness in the hospice and palliative care setting.

Morphine: oral absorption can be very low (less than 20% bioavailable in the dog) and sustained-release oral products have been shown to have highly variable absorption rates: however, oral products can be tried for palliative care. One recommendation in dogs is 1 mg/kg^{-1} PO q4–6 h and in cats 0.5 mg/kg^{-1} BID–TID. Sustained-release morphine is used in dogs at $2–5 \text{ mg kg}^{-1}$ PO twice a day, and when using be sure to educate pet owners not to break or crush the tablets under any circumstances because crushing turns sustained-release morphine into immediate release and can result in overdose and death (Downing 2011).

Oxycodone has been subjectively shown to be efficacious in dogs at a dose of $0.1–0.3 \text{ mg/kg}^{-1}$ PO twice to three times a day and may induce less sedation and dysphoria than morphine. Oxycodone dose has not been described in cats.

Hydrocodone has approximately 50% of the bioavailability found in humans (KuKanich and Paul 2010).

Codeine in dogs does not significantly metabolize into morphine, as it does in humans; however, dogs do produce another mu-agonist metabolite, codeine-6-glucuronide in significant quantities, and this metabolite is thought to render an analgesic effect in this species (Vree et al. 2000).

Tramadol: The opioid effect of tramadol is believed to be related to its major metabolite, O-desmethyltramadol (M1), which is considerably more potent than the parent compound. In humans and in cats, most of the opioid-mediated analgesic effects of tramadol are derived from the active M1 metabolite. In multiple pharmacological studies, however, it has been discovered that dogs make very negligible amounts of the Ml metabolite and instead mainly make the metabolites N,O-di-desmethyltramadol (M5) and N-desmethyltramadol (M2). This leads to the conclusion that, in this species, most of tramadol's activity is actually derived from its serotoninergic and noradrenergic activity, not from its opioid activity (Giorgi 2009). While the dosing interval in the cat is 12 hours, tramadol has been shown to have an exceptionally short half-life in the dog (about 1.7 hours), and therefore must be dosed frequently to be efficacious. For this reason tramadol may lend itself best for use with breakthrough pain. In this context, tramadol can be used effectively as a periodic add-on analgesic during a time of increased discomfort. Dogs may benefit from tramadol administered $4–10 \text{ mg kg}^{-1}$ PO three times a day. It should be noted that maximum analgesic effects may not occur immediately and may be delayed up to 14 days for chronic pain conditions such as cancer and degenerative joint disease. Additionally, long-term efficacy of tramadol may decrease with time. Some data support tramadol use in clinical veterinary patients, but more studies need to be conducted to confirm its efficacy and safety (KuKanich 2010, 2013). Cats (extra-label), at present there is no clear dosage for tramadol based upon prospective studies and most current recommendations for dosing are $1–2 \text{ mg/kg}^{-1}$ PO q12 h. Some suggest that some cats may only need once-daily doses; others suggest going as high as 4 mg/kg^{-1}. It has an unpleasant taste and dose avoidance may be an issue. Neurologic and opioid adverse effects can be seen, particularly at doses higher than 2 mg/kg^{-1}.

Tricyclic Antidepressants

TCAs are the main group of antidepressants used for the management of neuropathic pain syndromes. They have a postulated action via serotonin and norepinephrine reuptake inhibition at nerve endings in the spinal cord and brain. The most commonly used TCA in animal patients is amitriptyline.

Amitriptyline: Amitriptyline is frequently used off label for the treatment of chronic pain, especially when the pain has a neuropathic component. It is most often combined with other analgesics because it is not efficacious when used alone. Dogs (extra-label), $1-2\,mg/kg^{-1}$ PO q12–24 h; if discontinuing, taper off slowly. Cats (extra-label), 2.5–12.5 mg per cat PO once daily.

Serotonin-Norepinephrine Reuptake Inhibitors

Although not specifically intended to treat chronic pain, SNRIs may be helpful in the management of chronic pain conditions. While the analgesic effects are not fully understood, it is thought that SNRIs may increase neurotransmitters in the spinal cord that reduce pain signals. While duloxetine has a chronic pain label indication for humans, evidence is lacking for its use in veterinary medicine.

Duloxetine (Cymbalta): Dogs only (extra-label), $1.5-3\,mg/kg^{-1}$ PO divided BID–TID.

Anticonvulsants

Anticonvulsants (antiepileptic drugs [AEDs]) are traditionally used in the management of neuropathic pain. Gabapentin is the gold standard drug in this category. Sedation is a noted side effect that can be reduced by starting therapy at a low dose and titrating upward to the desired pain-relieving effect. Newer agents in this class include pregabalin.

Gabapentin: Dogs and cats (extra-label), recommended starting dose is $5-10\,mg/kg^{-1}$ PO BID–TID. However, given the frailty of our patient population, the author recommends starting with a dose of $3\,mg/kg^{-1}$ PO once nightly for three nights, then increasing to $3\,mg/kg^{-1}$ PO BID for an additional three days, then increasing the dose and frequency as clinically indicated. Higher doses and frequency of administration (every 6 hours) are often needed.

Pregabalin: Dogs, recommended starting dose is $2\,mg/kg^{-1}$ PO q12 h to minimize sedation, followed by titrating the dosage upwards in $1\,mg/kg^{-1}$ increments per week to $3-4\,mg/kg^{-1}$ PO q8–12 h. Cats (extra-label), anecdotal reports of pregabalin use in cats; $1-2\,mg/kg^{-1}$ PO q12 h is most commonly mentioned (Munana 2010).

N-methyl-ᴅ-aspartate Receptor Antagonists

NMDA receptor antagonists can also be used when pain does not respond well to standard analgesics (steroid or NSAID plus an opioid) together with an antiepileptic (gabapentin) and/or an antidepressant (amitriptyline). The NMDA receptor provides a specific target in managing maladaptive pain and often allows use of a lower dose of opioids by increasing the analgesic effect of the opioid. NMDA antagonists are effective adjuncts to NSAIDs, especially in canine patients with osteoarthritis or osteosarcoma.

Amantadine: Dogs and cats (extra-label), $2-5\,mg/kg^{-1}$ PO once daily; start at lower end of dosing range and increase slowly if needed. Because amantadine has a significantly shorter half-life in dogs and cats when compared to humans, twice-daily dosing may be more effective.

Methadone: Methadone is an attractive opioid because of the mild to moderate NMDA receptor antagonist activity and evidence of effectiveness in rodent models of neuropathic pain, adding another pain-modifying effect, and possibly helping to prevent opioid tolerance (Erichsen et al. 2005). Dog and cat doses are listed above. An oral methadone hydrochloride solution is available; however, pharmacokinetic data in dogs and cats is lacking and it is anecdotally reported to be bitter tasting (Gaynor and Muir 2015). The parenteral injectable formulation can be delivered orally or OTM.

Ketamine: The growing body of literature recommending ketamine for the management of chronic pain has led to an increase in its utilization, which has considerably outpaced the development of any kind of clinical standards governing the practice of its use. Given the parallels between chronic pain and central sensitization in both humans and lab animals, it is promising to think that ketamine could be used to address chronic pain issues for our veterinary patients. Dogs and cats, $0.5\,mg/kg^{-1}$ SQ every 1–4 weeks for chronic pain management and $0.5\,mg/kg^{-1}$ SQ SID for acute pain management. It can also be administered as a CRI at subanesthetic doses to address allodynia and hyperalgesia, 60 mg ketamine added to 1 l of lactated Ringer's solution (LRS) administered at a rate of $2\,ml/kg^{-1}/h^{-1}$ to deliver $2\,\mu g/kg^{-1}/min^{-1}$ of ketamine for ideally a minimum of six hours. An initial bolus of $0.25–0.5\,mg/kg^{-1}$ IV needs to be given to rapidly reach plasma levels.

Visit the Companion Website for access to the Subanesthetic Ketamine Guide.

Monoclonal antibodies

Monoclonal antibodies are a class of drug that can be used to treat an array of conditions, including inflammatory disorders such as arthritis. Frunevetmab (Solensia) is a new felinized monoclonal antibody that targets Nerve Growth Factor (NGF) to reduce pain signals and effectively control feline osteoarthritis pain (Isola et al., 2011).

- Frunevetmab (Solensia): Cats should be dosed by weight range according to the dosing chart. Cats are given the full content of 1 or 2 vials based on body weight to target a minimum dosage of 1.0 mg/kg body weight, administered subcutaneously once a month. Aseptically withdraw the total dose into a single syringe and administer immediately.

Pharmacologic Protocols

Pharmacologic protocols can be devised based upon the anticipated and/or perceived level of pain that is expected to be associated with

Table 19.1 Examples of pain severity based on common diseases seen in hospice patients.

Pain severity	Disease
Mild	Dental disease, mild cystitis, osteoarthritis
Moderate	Cystitis, osteoarthritis
Moderate to severe	Osteoarthritis, capsular pain due to organomegaly, intervertebral disc disease, oral cancer, corneal abrasion/ulceration, pleuritis, hollow organ distension, trauma, peritonitis, hemoabdomen, pancreatitis
Severe to excruciating	Thrombosis/ischemia, inflammation (cellulitis), neuropathic (nerve entrapment, inflammation, disc herniation), bone cancer/pathologic fracture, CNS infarction/tumors, necrotizing pancreatitis, aortic saddle thrombus

a specific disease. Typical levels of pain associated with specific disease conditions commonly seen in hospice patients are presented in Table 19.1. It should also be noted that the designation of pain level based upon the disease process present is intended to serve only as a guide. Pain will vary according to many factors outside of disease: thus, each patient should be assessed individually. The choice of drug(s) used to treat pain will depend upon the underlying cause, the severity, and the duration of time that pain is present. From this perspective, the practitioner can layer treatment modalities that work synergistically together to provide optimal patient comfort. Adjunctive physical modalities can, and should be, incorporated at any level in the pain management plan. These modalities, including acupuncture, chiropractic adjustments, therapeutic massage, physiotherapy, heat and cryotherapy, therapeutic laser, and others are described in detail in Chapter 20.

The following summary outlines potential pharmacologic pain management strategies based on increasing severity of pain.

For mild to moderate pain, consider:

- nonsteroidal anti-inflammatory drugs
- non-opioid analgesics
- neuropathic pain analgesics, such as gabapentin
- monoclonal antibodies
- herbal therapies and nutraceuticals

For moderate pain, consider the above *plus* the addition of:

- NMDA antagonist, such as amantadine
- opiate-like (mu-receptor) agonist, tramadol
- opioids, such as buprenorphine

For moderate to severe pain, consider the above *plus* the addition of:

- tricyclic behavior/neuropathic pain modifier, such as amitriptyline
- mild opioids, such as buprenorphine or hydrocodone/acetaminophen combination (*dogs only!*)
- topical and/or local analgesia, such as lidoderm patches
- administration of ketamine subcutaneously
- for moderate to severe osteoarthritis in dogs, targeted therapy such as Synovetin OA, administered via intraarticular injection while under sedation, can be considered to address the pain of synovial inflammation

For severe to excruciating pain, consider the above *plus* the addition of:

- strong opioids, such as morphine, hydromorphone, methadone
- consider continuous rate infusion of opioid plus NMDA antagonist, such as ketamine
- bisphosphonates for bone tumors
- palliative radiation

The algorithm given in Figure 19.1 illustrates an approach to pain management in the hospice patient.

Assessing Response to Treatment

In addition to assessing the level of pain, appropriate management also includes assessing the response to interventions on a frequent basis and using the outcomes of these assessments to guide ongoing care (Matthews et al. 2014).

Key principles of assessing response to treatment include:

- Educating and involving all caregivers in the assessment of pain; owners are the mainstay of the ongoing assessment of pain and are often best suited at assessing gradual or subtle changes.
- Establishing and documenting a baseline assessment of the level of pain present.
- Reassessing and documenting pain level on a frequent basis, paying particular attention to the response to therapies at the appropriate time frame (i.e. assessing improvement in the level of pain one hour following administration of an oral medication versus 20 minutes following administration of a subcutaneous medication).
- Adopting a standardized protocol, with all team members using the same assessment tools, for evaluating pain severity and response to care.

When assessing pain, a pain measurement scale should be utilized to communicate and assess the effectiveness of therapeutic interventions given. All pain scales require the user to record a subjective score for pain intensity and, because of this, pain measurement scales have a degree of built-in variability due to the observer's personal judgment and experiences. However, when caregivers adopt a standardized protocol, and apply the protocol to an individual pet in a consistent manner, the pain measurement scale can be an effective way to communicate and evaluate pain.

Anxiety

Animals can experience anxiety for a variety of reasons. For the hospice patient, anxiety can be a symptom of an underlying medical issue, such as pain or dyspnea, or an unmet physical need, such as the need for elimination. Psychosocial factors can also contribute to anxiety and can include separation from family or

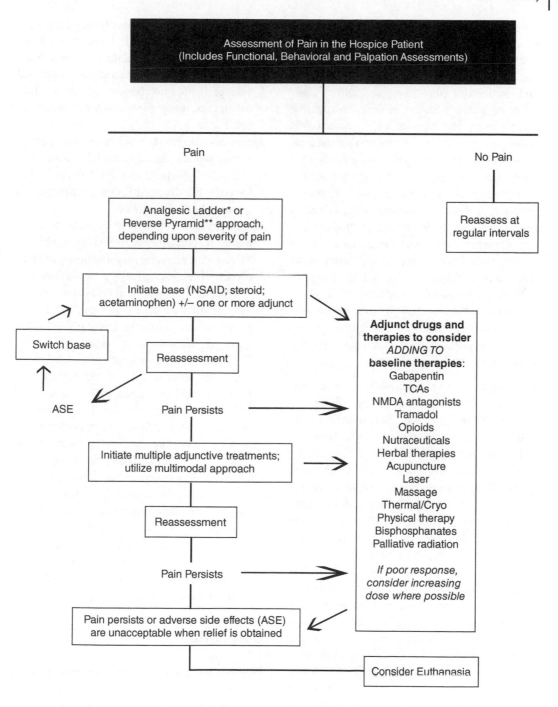

* Analgesic ladder: gradual addition of analgesic medications until adequate comfort is achieved
** Reverse pyramid: initial, aggressive multimodal approach with systematic removal of analgesic medications (or a reduction in their dose) as pain is managed

Figure 19.1 Algorithm for an approach to pain management in the hospice patient.

a change in social situation involving both people and other pets in the home.

With regards to pain, anxiety can further increase a patient's perception of discomfort, and anxiolytics may have an indirect pain-relieving effect. Because anxiety and distress can increase the level of pain perceived, it should be included in the clinician's considerations when formulating a symptom management plan. Management of anxiety can include non-pharmacologic measures such as touch, massage, and using a calming voice, as well as pharmacologic interventions, including the use of benzodiazepines (lorazepam, alprazolam, diazepam), serotonin antagonists (trazodone), TCAs (amitriptyline, doxepin), central alpha-2 agonist (clonidine), and gabapentin. Phenothiazine tranquilizers (acepromazine, chlorpromazine) do not reduce anxiety but may be useful given at a low dose in combination with other medications.

Lorazepam: Dogs (extra-label), anecdotal dosage recommendations usually range from 0.02 to $0.2 \, \text{mg/kg}^{-1}$ one to three times a day or on an as-needed basis. However, dosages ranging from 0.02 to $0.5 \, \text{mg/kg}^{-1}$ q8–24 h have been noted. It is suggested to start therapy at the lower end of the dosing range and to choose a practical dose for the patient that is closest to half or one 0.5-mg or 1-mg tablet (per dog); titrate upwards if necessary. Cats (extra-label), anecdotal dosage recommendations range from 0.025 to $0.08 \, \text{mg/kg}^{-1}$ one or two times a day or on an as-needed basis. However, dosages ranging from 0.025 to $0.25 \, \text{mg/kg}^{-1}$ q8–24 h have been noted. It is suggested to start therapy at the lower end of the dosing range, choosing a practical dose for the patient that is closest to one-quarter or one-half of a 0.5-mg tablet (0.125–0.25 mg per cat); titrate upwards if necessary.

Alprazolam: Dogs (extra-label), 0.02–0.1 mg/kg^{-1} (usually $0.02–0.05 \, \text{mg kg}^{-1}$ initially) PO two to four times daily as needed. Cats (extra-label), 0.125–0.25 mg per cat one to three times a day.

Diazepam: Dogs (extra-label), $0.5–2 \, \text{mg/kg}^{-1}$ PO as needed. Cats (extra-label), 0.2–0.5 mg/kg^{-1} PO one to three times a day. *Note:* Because of concerns associated with oral diazepam and rare idiosyncratic hepatic failure in cats, many clinicians avoid diazepam use in cats.

Trazodone: Dogs only, based on empirical effect, recommended dosing schedule involves a three-day initiation dose ($1.25–5 \, \text{mg/kg}^{-1}$), followed by the therapeutic dose ($3–10 \, \text{mg/kg}^{-1}$) (Gruen and Sherman 2008).

Amitriptyline: Dogs (for adjunctive treatment of behavior disorders amenable to TCAs, with behavior modification and anxiolytics if necessary; extra-label), initially, $1–2 \, \text{mg/kg}^{-1}$ PO q12 h for two to four weeks. May gradually increase by $1 \, \text{mg/kg}^{-1}$ as tolerated to a maximum of $4 \, \text{mg/kg}^{-1}$ PO twice daily. If discontinuing, taper off slowly. Cats (for adjunctive treatment of behavior disorders amenable to TCAs, extra-label), $0.5–1 \, \text{mg/kg}^{-1}$ PO once daily (or divided twice daily). Practically, 2.5–12.5 mg per cat once daily. Start at lower end of dosing range and gradually increase as tolerated. If discontinuing, gradually taper off dosage.

Clonidine: Dogs only (as an adjunctive treatment with other medications and behavioral therapy for situational use for fears, phobias, and separation anxiety, extra-label), $0.01–0.05 \, \text{mg/kg}^{-1}$ PO approximately 1.5–2 hours prior to the triggering event. A 0.1 mg tablet given to a 10-kg (22-lb) dog would be a dose of $0.01 \, \text{mg/kg}^{-1}$.

Dysphoria

Dysphoria is a potential adverse effect following the administration of opioid analgesics, especially pure mu agonists. Veterinary reports indicate that dysphoria is frequently opioid total-dose related (Becker et al. 2013). It is of utmost importance to determine whether an agitated pet is dysphoric or has continued unmanaged pain. Pain should always be ruled out prior to assuming other causes of behavior.

If pain is suspected, slowly titrate up the dose of the chosen opioid (fentanyl, hydromorphone, methadone, morphine) in very small increments, while watching for a change in behavior. A dysphoric patient's behavior may become worse, or the sedative effects of the opioid may settle them for only a short period of time. If the behavior resumes within 30 minutes, dysphoria should be suspected. If the patient settles and sleeps for greater than 30 minutes, then pain is the problem.

If dysphoria is suspected, administration of an agonist–antagonist (such as butorphanol) may effectively antagonize the excitatory effects of a pure agonist (such as morphine) without antagonizing analgesia.

Another general rule of thumb is that animals in pain will generally respond to human interaction, whereas animals with dysphoria will not.

Weakness or Fatigue

Weakness is a multidimensional syndrome, often with multiple contributing causes including, but not limited to, pain, sleep disturbances, malnutrition or anorexia/cachexia, anemia, and endocrine or metabolic derangements. Optimal management involves comprehensive symptom assessment and treatment of reversible or manageable causes, when possible.

Interventions can include appropriate pain management, maintaining appropriate nutrition, subcutaneous fluids for dehydration, erythropoiesis stimulating therapy for anemia (erythropoietin, darbepoetin), and correction of endocrine and metabolic disorders (e.g. thyroid replacement; potassium supplementation). In human medicine, preliminary studies have shown that corticosteroids administration can reduce symptoms such as weakness and fatigue, pain, poor appetite, and nausea, thus improving the overall quality of life in patients with advanced cancer (Yennurajalingam and Bruera 2007).

Respiratory Symptoms

Respiratory symptoms can be due to a myriad of disease processes including, but not limited to, anemia, infection, ascites, pleural effusion, heart failure, pulmonary edema, pulmonary hypertension, pulmonary thromboembolism, metabolic acidosis, and neoplasia. Palliative treatment is aimed at management of the underlying cause, which influences the type of care needed. The two most common respiratory symptoms observed in hospice patients, regardless of the underlying etiology, are dyspnea and cough.

Dyspnea

Dyspnea is the unpleasant sensation of being unable to breathe easily and can be a distressing symptom not only for the patients, but also for the caregivers. Management of dyspnea should be individualized, with treatment being aimed at managing the underlying etiology.

Oxygen can be a nonspecific treatment for dyspnea and can serve as a short-term palliative measure for a select population of our animal hospice patients. Oxygen can be delivered in a home setting via the use of oxygen concentrators, providing approximately 40% F_iO_2 (Figure 19.2).

Opioids can be effective as a first-line therapy for the symptomatic relief of dyspnea. Unfortunately, the mechanism of this action is not well understood.

Anxiolytics are frequently administered for anxiety that often coexists with dyspnea and can be safely used as an adjunct to opioid therapy.

Bronchodilation can be achieved with inhaled bronchodilators (such as albuterol) or nebulization, and can provide additional palliative relief. One such protocol for bronchodilation via nebulization is to use 1 ml of magnesium sulfate ($MgSO_4$) added to 6 ml of sterile water, using approximately half of the mixture in a nebulizer, which will allow for approximately 10 minutes of

(a)

(b)

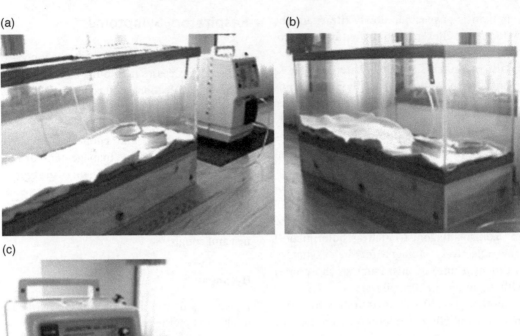

(c)

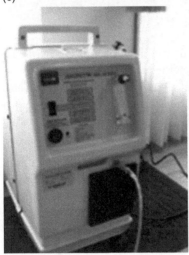

Figure 19.2 (a, b) Example of fish tank set up (85 gallons in this photograph; another suitable container for instance might be a large Rubber Maid storage container with lid) for oxygen delivery for a small animal that is oxygen dependent. It is important to monitor chamber temperature and humidity to prevent hyperthermia – ideally keeping these at less than 60% humidity and 75 °F. For patients with severe lung disease, pulmonary hypertension, etc., this may allow 6–8 or more hours per day of relief and treatment of potential hypoxic vasoconstriction and secondary adverse cardiac effects. Other homemade or similar chambers may be used. It should not be completely airtight and should be large enough to allow the animal to move around, have food and water etc. (c) The oxygen concentrator is available through respiratory stores/outlets (a prescription is needed). It is electric, quiet and can deliver up to 4–5 L/min O_2. Insert the tubing into a small hole at one end of the chamber and have one or two, 1-inch holes at the opposite end for the air to exit. A veterinarian will need to write a prescription for this. *Source:* Brendan C. McKiernan, University of Illinois.

nebulization time. Magnesium has a direct effect by relaxing contraction of smooth muscle, as occurs in bronchoconstriction. In the pulmonary system, ketamine causes bronchodilation that appears to be due to circulating catecholamines, and with that,

there is the potential to utilize this side effect to our advantag. Because there remains a lack of evidence for its use in our veterinary patients, the dose, frequency, and efficacy continue to be explored. Recommended doses are similar to pain management doses, 0.25–0.5 mg/kg^{-1} SQ PRN for both dogs and cats.

MgSO$_4$ followed by furosemide is a novel nebulization treatment protocol in which MgSO$_4$ nebulization 1 ml of magnesium sulfate (MgSO$_4$) added to 6 ml of sterile water, using approximately half of the mixture in a nebulizer, which will allow for approximately 10 minutes of nebulization time as described above, is followed by nebulization with furosemide at 5 mg kg^{-1}, diluted in enough sterile water or sterile saline to make approximately 3.5 ml of liquid. A diuretic effect is not expected because the patient absorbs systemically only approximately 20% of the nebulized furosemide. Furosemide used this way "resets" slow and rapid adapting receptors in the airways and pulmonary parenchyma causing them to fire in such a way that neural signals tell the brain a "good breath" has been taken (Mellema 2008).

Cool, moving air, such as through the use of a floor fan, can help provide symptomatic relief and improvement of clinical signs.

Cough

Pathological cough is common in both malignant and non-malignant disease, and can be classified in various ways; several causes may coexist in one patient. Examples include a malignant disease causing mechanical distortion of the airway leading to a dry cough or infectious disease causing accumulation of material in the airway causing a productive cough of mucus or purulent sputum. Management should be based on the type and cause of the cough and should be combined with appropriate symptomatic measures.

Cough suppressants are generally used to manage dry coughs or nocturnal coughing, such as occurs with chronic bronchitis. The most effective antitussive agents are opioids, such as butorphanol or hydrocodone.

Steroids can be used to relieve a cough related to endobronchial tumors, lymphangitis, or pulmonary neoplasia. Inhaled steroids, such as fluticasone, can offer additional palliative relief for cough caused by chronic or inflammatory airway disease.

Mucolytic treatments may be of benefit to patients with a wet unproductive cough. Use of nebulized saline or steam inhalation can result in the production of sputum (note: this measure would be unsuitable for compromised patients who are unable to expectorate).

Maropitant is an NK-1 receptor antagonist which has been anecdotally reported to decrease the frequency and severity of coughing in dogs with chronic bronchitis. Although this medication does not have a significant effect on inflammation, its potential role as an antitussive may be helpful.

Nebulized or inhaled bronchodilators, such as albuterol, can be used to address bronchospasm, which can occur.

Antibiotics can be used to treat suspected infection.

Nausea and Vomiting

Nausea and vomiting are common symptoms in patients in palliative and hospice care. Pharmacological management of nausea and vomiting includes the use of drugs to block the emetogenic reflex in the brain stem (antiemetics such as maropitant, ondansetron, and dolasetron), drugs to promote peristalsis in the upper gastrointestinal (GI) tract (prokinetic agents such as metoclopramide or cisapride), and adjuvant drugs such as H2 antagonists (famotidine, ranitidine, cimetidine) and proton pump inhibitors (omeprazole); adjunct therapies such as acupuncture should also be considered. It is also important to continually reassess; if nausea still persists, there may be additional triggers that have not been identified. Continue one antiemetic while introducing a second antiemetic that acts at a different site in the brain, continually reassessing. It should also be noted that gastric emptying is reduced in the presence of nausea, and therefore, oral antiemetic drugs may be unreliably absorbed; because of this, injectable formulations should be considered.

Maropitant: Dogs and cats, SC 1 mg/kg^{-1} (recommend giving in subcutaneous fluid line during administration to reduce injection discomfort) q24 h PRN. 2 mg/kg^{-1} PO (dogs) and 1 mg/kg^{-1} PO (cats) q24 h PRN. Although recommended for up to 5 days, may be used long term (extra-label). A Good Laboratory Practice (GLP) compliant study in dogs revealed no adverse effects after repeated oral doses of 5 mg/kg^{-1} q24 h for 93 days.

Ondansetron: Dogs (extra-label), 0.5–1 mg/kg^{-1} PO, SQ, or IV (slowly over 2–15 minutes) q12 h; however, IV dosages of 0.1–0.2 mg/kg^{-1} have been noted and are closer to human pediatric recommendations. Cats (extra-label), 0.1–1 mg/kg^{-1} IV (slowly), IM, SC, or PO q6–12 h; based upon a recent pharmacokinetic study (Quimby et al. 2013), oral dosages may need to be toward the high end and given more frequently than IV or SC.

Dolasetron: Dogs and cats (extra-label), 0.6 mg kg^{-1} PO, IV, or SC q24 h. Some recommend giving higher dosages up to 1 mg/kg^{-1} to treat active vomiting disorders. Because it is given once a day, the injectable form of dolasetron is often preferred over ondansetron, a similarly effective antiemetic. However, for oral use in small animals, dolasetron tablets are too large (50 and 100 mg) to be practically administered.

Metoclopramide: Dogs and cats, 0.2–0.4 mg kg^{-1} PO or SC q8 h.

Cisapride: Dogs (extra-label), most recommend initially dosing between 0.1 and 0.5 mg/kg^{-1} PO q8–12 h and some gastroenterologists recommend giving 30 minutes before feeding. Some sources state that dosages (gradually increased) up to 1 mg/kg^{-1} PO q8 h may be required (if tolerated). Cats (extra-label), initially, 2.5 mg per cat PO twice daily, preferably 15–30 minutes before food. Dosages may be titrated upwards, if tolerated, to as high as 7.5 mg per cat PO three times daily in large cats. Cats with hepatic insufficiency may need the dosage intervals extended.

Famotidine: Dogs and cats (extra-label), recommended dosages are generally 0.5–1.1 mg/kg^{-1} PO q12–24 h. Rounding doses to the nearest 5 mg increment (e.g. 5 mg per cat) is reasonable. Once-daily administration is most often recommended in patients with significantly diminished renal function. Recommended doses for parenteral use are generally 0.5 mg kg^{-1} IV (slowly), IM, or SC q12–24 h.

Ranitidine: Dogs and cats, 0.5–2.0 mg/kg^{-1} PO q12 h.

Cimetidine: Dogs and cats (extra-label), 5–10 mg/kg^{-1} PO q6–8 h.

Omeprazole: Dogs (extra-label), usually dosed at 0.5–1 mg/kg^{-1} PO once daily, practically rounding to the nearest 10 mg within this range. For severe esophagitis some have recommended giving twice a day (up to 2 mg/kg^{-1}). Cats (extra-label), usually dosed at 0.5–1 mg/kg^{-1} PO once daily.

Anorexia and Cachexia

Anorexia is defined as a loss of normal appetite while cachexia is characterized by involuntary weight loss, regardless of nutritional intake or appetite. The anorexia/cachexia syndrome occurs when there is catabolism of lipid stores and proteins, especially that of muscle tissue, coupled with defects in anabolism, and is characterized by progressive nutritional changes, weakness, and wasting, and can become debilitating over time, potentially affecting quality of life. Anorexia and cachexia are most frequently seen in the later stages of disease, especially with tumors of the GI tract, pancreas, and lungs, and other advanced noncancer illnesses such as congestive heart failure and end-stage renal disease. The treatment of anorexia and cachexia focuses mainly on stimulation of appetite and alleviation of the causative factors, when possible. With regards to cachexia, families should be educated that increasing caloric intake will not necessarily result in a weight gain or functional improvement, and that continued weight loss, despite caloric intake, is essentially a byproduct of disease and is to be expected. It should also be discussed that a cachectic appearance does not necessarily equate that the pet is experiencing a poor quality of life.

Cyproheptadine: typical feline dosing is 2 mg per cat SID–BID.

Mirtazapine: typical feline dosage is 3.75 mg PO every 3 days; however, smaller more frequent dosing appears to have less side-effects while remaining effective; the author recommends using 1.88 mg SID or EOD (compounded formulations allow for ease of dosing). Canine dose, 0.6 mg/kg^{-1} PO q24 h not to exceed 30 mg day^{-1}. Alternatively, dogs <9 kg = 3.75 mg PO q24 h; 9.5–22.5 kg = 7.5 mg PO q24 h; 22.5–34 kg = 15 mg PO q24 h; >34 kg = 15 mg PO BID or 30 mg PO q24 h.

Owners should be aware that mirtazapine and cyproheptadine cannot be administered concurrently.

Capromorelin: (Entyce®) for appetite stimulation in dogs: 3 mg/kg^{-1} PO once daily.

In cats (extra-label) 1–2 mg/kg^{-1} PO once daily for up to 21 days. Elura® is US Food and Drug Administration (FDA) approved for the management of weight loss in cats with CKD; 2 mg/kg^{-1} PO q24h.

Non-pharmacologic interventions can also be considered to help improve appetite and can include such measures as the modification of the types of foods offered and the times they are offered, decreasing the portion size, proper oral care, and managing pain.

Dehydration

A vast majority of patients in the terminal phase of disease experience dehydration, generally due to a reduced oral intake of fluids, or an increased loss of fluids through the disease process (e.g. chronic kidney disease). Dehydration may occur in spite of a seemingly adequate intake of oral fluids. Signs of dehydration can include dry mucous membranes, decreased skin turgor, decreased urine output, weakness, lethargy, weight loss, mental dullness, tachycardia, and hypotension. For those pets treated at home, subcutaneous fluid therapy becomes an important component of treatment and should be given once to twice daily depending upon the patient's hydration status and severity of clinical signs.

Constipation

Constipation is the infrequent and difficult passage of hard feces, which can be small or large in diameter. The most important causes of constipation are patient immobility or decreased mobility, poor fluid and nutritional intake, and opioid use. Constipation may cause or aggravate underlying nausea. Subcutaneous fluids, offering a canned diet in place of dry, increasing dietary bulk, stool softeners, and motility enhancers (in cats) can be considered if straining or pain when defecating is repeatedly observed, or whenever the average frequency of defecation falls significantly below the pet's normal elimination habits. If these measures are not enough to control clinical signs, an intestinal motility enhancer such as cisapride can be considered. Enemas may also need to be considered if obstipation develops.

MiraLax: One-quarter teaspoon in food BID, titrating upwards as clinically indicated.

Lactulose: Dogs, 1 ml/4.5 kg body weight PO q8 h initially then adjust as needed. Cats, 0.5 ml/kg^{-1} PO BID–TID with dosage adjusted to obtain stool quality desired.

Psyllium husk (bulk-forming GI laxative): In dogs prone to constipation, 2% psyllium was added as part of diet; 80% of studied dogs had easier defecation process (Tortola et al. 2009). Cats (extra-label), one-quarter teaspoon per meal added to canned cat food, adjusting the amount as clinically indicated. Be sure the cat is properly hydrated (Washabau 2001).

Cisapride: Dogs, 0.1–0.5 mg/kg^{-1} PO BID–TID given 30 minutes before meals (higher doses of 1 mg kg^{-1} may be required in some cases). Cats, 2.5–5 mg per cat for cats up to 4.5 kg and 5 mg for cats 5 kg or heavier SID–TID given 30 minutes before meals.

Lactulose as an in-home enema: 5–10 ml/cat administered slowly with a well-lubricated 10–12 Fr rubber catheter.

Oral Health

Ulcers

Patients with advanced renal disease may develop oral ulcerations associated with uremia. Symptomatic management includes addressing the underlying disease and uremic state, as well as the management of associated pain.

Famotidine: used to reduce gastric hyperacidity and nausea. Dogs, 0.5–1.0 mg/kg^{-1} PO q24 h. Cats, 5 mg/cat PO q24–48 h; if difficulty administering medication orally, consider 0.5–1.0 mg/kg^{-1} SC q24 h; when possible, give in subcutaneous fluid line during administration.

Sucralfate (Carafate): Dogs, 0.5–1 g PO BID–TID. Cats, 0.25–0.5 g PO per cat PO BID–TID.

Buprenorphine: Small dogs and cats, 0.005–0.03 mg/kg^{-1} transmucosally for oral ulcer pain.

"**Magic mouthwash**": Recipe for dogs and cats to provide topical pain relief from oral ulcers, can be applied every 6 hours, combine 1 part viscous lidocaine 2% + 1 part Maalox + 1 part diphenhydramine 12.5 mg/5 ml elixir. Dogs, 2–5 ml; cats, 2 ml; aim to limit the dosing to less than 2.5 ml/kg^{-1}/day^{-1}. In addition to topical anesthetics, topically applied morphine can be effective for painful ulcers. Information is based on its use in human medicine.

"**Morphine gel recipe**": using a sterile technique, mix 1 mg morphine per 1 g of hydrogel or 1 g of 0.75–0.8% metronidazole gel to produce a 1% solution. Apply thin layer using sterile swab SID–TID. Mixture is stable for up to 28 days.

Dry Mouth (Xerostomia)

Xerostomia is a condition that occurs when saliva production is decreased and can be associated with oral discomfort, difficulty chewing, difficulty swallowing, and an increased risk of oral infection and ulceration. Signs of a dry mouth can include interest in eating but turning away as if the food does not taste good, lip smacking, and excessive tongue thrusting when trying to eat. Discomfort experienced from dry mouth can be alleviated by simple measures such as oral care including moistening the oral cavity with water or implementing the use of artificial saliva substitutes; wetting the food may also help. If using an artificial saliva substitute, ensure that it does not contain xylitol or other ingredients toxic to pets.

Conclusion

In hospice practice, patients present with multiple symptoms that require simultaneous assessment and management. Our obligations to the animal patient include preventing and relieving pain, managing symptoms of disease, and maximizing comfort and quality of life through appropriate, targeted, and comprehensive medical management strategies.

References

Altman, R.D. (2004). A rationale for combining acetaminophen and NSAIDs for mild-to-moderate pain. *Clin. Exp. Rheumatol.*, 22: 110–117.

Becker, W.M., Mama, K.R., Rao, S. et al. (2013) Prevalence of dysphoria after fentanyl in dogs undergoing stifle surgery. *Vet. Surg.*, 42: 302–307.

Boutaud, O, (2002) Determinants of the cellular specificity of acetaminophen as an inhibitor of prostaglandin H_2 synthases. *Proc. Natl. Acad. Sci. U.S.A.*, 99: 7130–7135.

Downing, R. (2011) Pain management for veterinary palliative care and hospice patients. *Vet. Clin. North Am. Small Anim. Pract.*, 41: 531–550.

Erichsen, H.K., Hao, J.X., Xu, X.J. et al. (2005) Comparative actions of the opioid analgesics morphine, methadone, and codeine in rat models of peripheral and central neuropathic pain. *J. Pain*, 116: 347–358.

Ferreira, T.H., Rezende, M.L., Mama, K.R. et al. (2011) Plasma concentrations and behavioral, antinociceptive, and physiologic effects of methadone after intravenous and oral transmucosal administration in cats. *Am. J. Vet. Res.*, 72: 764–771.

Gaynor, J. and Muir, W. (2015) Handbook of Veterinary Pain Management, 3. St. Louis, MO: Elsevier, pp. 67–82.

Giorgi, M. (2009) Biopharmaceutical profile of tramadol in the dog. *Vet. Res. Commun.*, 33(Suppl. 1): 189–192.

Gruen, M.E. and Sherman, B.L. (2008) Use of trazodone as an adjunctive agent in the treatment of canine anxiety disorders: 56 cases (1995–2007), *J. Am. Vet. Med. Assoc.*, 233: 1902–1907.

Isola, M., Ferrari, V., Miolo, A. et al. (2011) Nerve growth factor concentrations in the synovial fluid from healthy dogs and dogs with secondary osteoarthritis. *Vet Comp Orthop Traumatol.*, 24: 279–284.

KuKanich, B. (2010) Managing severe chronic pain: maintaining quality of life in dogs. American College of Veterinary Internal Medicine Forum. Aneheim, CA (June 9–12). Veterinary Information Network, vin.com.

KuKanich, B. (2013) Outpatient oral analgesics in dogs and cats beyond nonsteroidal antiinflammatory drugs: an evidence-based approach. *Vet. Clin. North Am. Small Anim. Pract.*, 43: 1109–1125.

KuKanich, B. and Paul, J. (2010) Pharmacokinetics of hydrocodone and its metabolite hydromorphone after oral hydrocodone administration in dogs.

American College of Veterinary Internal Medicine Forum. Aneheim, CA (June 9–12). Veterinary Information Network, vin.com.

KuKanich, B., Lascelles, B.D., Aman, A.M. et al. (2005) The effects of inhibiting cytochrome P450 3A, p-glycoprotein, and gastric acid secretion on the oral bioavailability of methadone in dogs. *J. Vet. Pharmacol. Ther.*, 28: 461–466.

Mathews, K., Kronen, P.W., Lascelles, D. et al. (2014). Guidelines for recognition, assessment and treatment of pain: WSAVA global pain council members and co-authors of this document: *J. Small Anim. Pract.*, 55(6): 10–68.

Mellema, M. (2008) The neurophysiology of dyspnea. *J. Vet. Emerg. Crit. Care*, 18: 561–571.

Munana, K. (2010) Current approaches to seizure management. Proceedings American College of Veterinary Internal Medicine Forum. Aneheim, CA (June 9–12). Veterinary Information Network, vin.com.

Plumb, D.C. (2015) Plumb's Veterinary Drug Handbook, 8. Stockholm, WI: PharmaVet Inc.

Quimby, J.M., Lake, R.C., Hanson, R.J. et al. (2013) Oral, subcutaneous and intravenous pharmacokinetics of ondansetron in healthy cats. *J. Vet. Intern. Med.*, 27: 749–750.

Slingsby, L.S., Taylor, P.M., and Murrell, J.C. (2011) A study to evaluate buprenoprhine at 40 µg kg$(^{-1})$ compared to 20 µg kg$(^{-1})$ as a post-operative analgesic in the dog. *Vet. Anaesth. Analg.*, 38: 584–593.

Tortola, L., Zaine, L., Vasconcellos, R.S. et al. (2009). Psyllium (*Plantago psyllium*) uses in the management of constipation in dogs. World Small Animal Veterinary Association (WSAVA) World Congress Proceedings. São Paulo, Brazil (July 21–24). Available at: Veterinary Information Network, https://www.vin.com/apputil/content/defaultadv1.aspx?id=4253105&pid=11290 (Accessed: September 2016).

Vachon, M.L.S. (1995) Staff stress in hospice/palliative care: a review. *Palliat. Med.*, 9: 91–122.

Vree, T.B., van Dongen, R.T., and Koopman-Kimenai, P.M. (2000) Codeine analgesia is due to codeine-6-glucuronide, not morphine. *Int. J. Clin. Pract.*, 54: 395–398.

Washabau, R. (2001) Feline constipation, obstipation and megacolon: Prevention, diagnosis and treatment. World Small Animal Association World Congress Proceedings Online. Available at: Veterinary Information Network, https://www.vin.com/apputil/content/ defaultadv1.aspx?id=3843763&pid=8708 (Accessed: September 2016).

Yennurajalingam, S. and Bruera, E. (2007) Palliative management of fatigue at the close of life: "It feels like my body is just worn out." *J. Am. Med. Assoc.*, 297: 295–304.

20

Physical Medicine and Rehabilitation for Hospice and Palliative Care Patients

Tamara Shearer, MS, DVM, CCRP, CVPP, CVA, MSTCVM

Providing physical medicine and rehabilitation modalities is often an underutilized tool that can benefit hospice and palliative care patients in multiple ways. Most importantly, this extension of care may maintain or strengthen the human–animal bond. This is especially true when other activities shared with the patient have decreased because of illness or disability. Although not a perfect substitute for the lost activities, some forms of physical medicine can be taught to the caregiver, which helps to replace time otherwise spent doing a favorite activity. This helps to promote the emotional well-being of the pet and allows the caregiver to participate in the patient's care. Physical medicine may also help to manage or decrease pain, reducing the amount of medication that could have adverse effects. It also aids in earlier and better recoveries from surgery or traumas. In some situations, it may allow a patient to reclaim the activities of daily living. The benefits of using physical medicine in the treatment of hospice and palliative care patients are summarized in Box 20.1.

Physical Medicine vs. Physical Rehabilitation

Physical medicine is the branch of medicine that includes all techniques and technologies that use physical means to treat and prevent disease, such as manual therapy, therapeutic exercise, mechanical devices, thermal modalities, and hydrotherapy. Physical medicine helps to prevent and relieve distress in patients with a broad variety of conditions often seen in hospice and palliative care practice. The terms physical medicine and rehabilitation need to be used mindfully when caring for hospice patients because the connotations differ. Physical rehabilitation is a term used for patients in palliative care whose compromised musculoskeletal or neurological functioning can be restored. For example, one would use physical rehabilitation to describe restoring the mobility of a dog with an anterior cruciate ligament rupture. The term physical medicine is a more appropriate term when addressing the care of a pet in hospice care when a recovery is not expected. For example, laser therapy would be a good physical medicine choice to relieve pain in a hospice patient with an active trigger point secondary to osteosarcoma.

Considerations for Physical Medicine with Hospice and Palliative Care Patients

The goals of physical medicine in hospice and palliative care are often different than the goals of rehabilitation therapy for other patients. It is important to discuss the goals with the pet's

Hospice and Palliative Care for Companion Animals: Principles and Practice, Second Edition.
Edited by Amir Shanan, Jessica Pierce, and Tamara Shearer.
© 2023 John Wiley & Sons, Inc. Published 2023 by John Wiley & Sons, Inc.
Companion website: www.wiley.com/go/shanan/palliative

Box 20.1   Benefits of Physical Medicine Use for Hospice and Palliative Care

1) Promotes emotional well-being of the pet and allows caregivers to participate in care
2) Manages or decreases pain
3) Decreases the amount of medication needed to maintain comfort
4) Faster and better recoveries from surgery or trauma
5) Assists in weight management for pets that have become less active
6) Reclaims activities of daily living
7) Carries a low risk of adverse effects

---

caregiver because a return to function may not be achievable. In cases in which return to function is not likely to be achieved, the goals of physical medicine should be the enhancement of both physical and emotional aspects of the quality of life, including pain management.

When providing physical medicine to a hospice patient, it is important to consider the type of disease trajectory of the pet's condition. Some physical medicine tools take a longer time to see improvement than others and may be a poor choice for a patient that might not live long enough to benefit from that particular treatment. For example, platelet-rich plasma therapy is appropriate for medical management of an anterior cruciate rupture, but it may take several weeks for its benefits to materialize. Therefore, it would not be the best choice for a patient in late-stage kidney failure. Other treatment options such as the use of a dynamic brace or assisted walking techniques should be suggested.

Physical medicine is often most efficacious when initiated as soon as possible after the patient's diagnosis. Starting treatment early helps to minimize the adverse consequences of the disuse of the affected body part. Disuse is a significant problem when encountered in hospice and palliative care patients because it contributes to weakness, pain, muscle atrophy, and/or joint contracture (Gillette and Dale 2014), all of which further compromise the patient's mobility. Decreased mobility is known to be associated with emotional distress and, in extreme cases, may lead to development of decubitus ulcers. Starting physical modalities early in the course of care may slow the progression of a disorder and provide additional pain relief (Kathmann et al. 2006). This is particularly significant when the patient's discomfort is severe and life expectancy is limited.

The hospice and palliative care practitioner must be familiar with precautions and contraindications of all treatment modalities. Additional safety measures must be taken when providing physical medicine to aid hospice and palliative care patients to ensure that the treatment doesn't cause emotional distress or physical discomfort. For example, extreme precaution must be used when applying thermal modalities in patients with decreased sensation. Percussing massage or therapy should not be used with patients with bleeding disorders. Certain modalities carry a lower risk of side effects, therefore may be better suited for hospice and palliative care patients. Patients must always be carefully observed during treatment for development of any respiratory distress, abrasions, pinched skin, or pressure sores. Most modalities should not be applied over neoplastic lesions.

Lastly, it is important to assess a pet's willingness to accept each specific therapy and the patient's comfort level with the modalities that will be applied to them. Older patients are at an increased risk of developing anxiety issues and may be more sensitive to change (Landsberg et al. 2012). For example, a patient that does not like water may not be a good candidate for hydrotherapy.

Ideally, treatment options should be a shared responsibility between the medical profession and the home caregiver. With good communication, many techniques can be taught to the caregiver to be performed on a regular basis at home.

Box 20.2 Physical Medicine Guidelines for Hospice and Palliative Care Patients

1) Define and discuss goals for the pet and family
2) Determine the disease trajectory and choose appropriate therapies
3) Start physical modalities as soon as possible after diagnosis
4) Be familiar with precautions and contraindications of all modalities
5) Assess the patient's willingness to accept each specific therapy
6) Define caregiver delivered techniques versus professionally delivered techniques

Box 20.2 summarizes the considerations for the use of physical medicine that are of special importance in hospice and palliative care patients.

Assistive Devices: Priority in Hospice Care

One of the most challenging mental and physical aspects to caring for a debilitated pet is how to improve the patient's ability to move while minimizing the stress and effort involved in doing so. Simple solutions are often overlooked that can reduce caregiver fatigue.

Concurrent with providing support using assistive devices, it is an important principle to insure that the flooring at home or in a clinic provides good footing. Patients that continually slip, slide, or fall are at risk for further injury and will derail any healing progress.

No matter what the equipment, it is important to introduce it gradually to minimize aversion to the device, which may develop secondary to fear or anxiety. Gradual introduction also helps to ensure the proper fit of a device. New devices should be removed at designated intervals to allow examination for pressure sores. No matter what device is used

to support the patient, observing the pet for pain, pressure sores, swelling of limbs, discomfort, and respiratory distress is a must. All devices should only be worn when supervised to prevent accidental injury and kept clean daily to prevent localized infections.

Many types of assistive devices are available to make caring for debilitated pets less burdensome. An important role of the practitioner and/or hospice care team is to utilize the proper assistive devices and educate the clients on the safe use of each device. This is especially important for owners of medium to large dogs where moving the pet can be very difficult. The assistive device can have an enormous effect on quality of life by improving mobility and minimizing risk of injury to the caregiver and patient. Another benefit of assistive devices is that they extend exercise time and comfort by preventing fatigue and pain.

The equipment most commonly used to assist hospice and palliative care patients with lifting and walking includes slings and harnesses, straps and bands, protective footwear, braces or splints, and mobility carts.

Slings and Harnesses

There are a variety of slings and harnesses available, ranging from the simple use of a towel sling placed under the abdomen to elaborate systems that distribute weight equally and minimize any pinching. There are advantages and disadvantages to most harnesses, which includes a diverse range of prices. Some questions to ask when considering which choice to invest in are: does the pet need total body support or is the area affected just the front limbs or rear limbs? Are there any comorbidities, like iliopsoas pain or urinary/fecal incontinence, which would suggest picking a sling that would not impinge on problem areas? This author prefers the Help 'Em Up Harness® for most patients that experience some degree of front and rear limb pathology (Figure 20.1). Simple under the abdomen slings can be equally useful for patients that

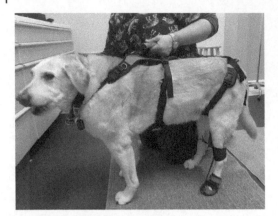

Figure 20.1 Help 'Em Up® Harness.

need limited assistance to get up or to slightly unweight a limb or limbs.

Straps and Bands

A variety of straps and bands can be protective and also assist in ambulation. A few examples of therapeutic devices include Biko Progressive Resistance Bands, dorsiflex devices/toes-up straps for the tibial tarsal area, and forelimb/rear limb hobbles (see Figure 20.2).

Biko Progressive Resistance Bands (www.animotionproducts.com) is a unique device made for dogs that have moderate ataxia, hind limb weakness, and knuckle over, but are still able to stand (Figure 20.3). The device has elastic straps that run from a dorsal midline harness connecting to the tarsus. It assists with the elevation and forward movement of the feet and, in this manner, prevents knuckling. Because the device prevents knuckling, it is also a good option to protect the feet from abrasions while walking.

Protective Footwear

The goal of providing protective footwear is to avoid slipping and prevent abrasions on the feet and toes while walking. There are various brands of socks and boots available to protect the feet, many of which have advantages and disadvantages. Like trying to find the best pair

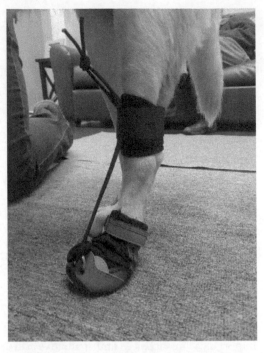

Figure 20.2 Dorsi-flex device protects toes from dragging.

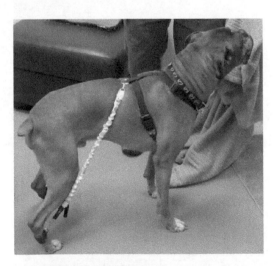

Figure 20.3 The use of Biko Progressive Resistance Bands to assist with ataxia and proper foot placement.

of shoes, some boots or socks do not fit properly or may be too bulky. An alternative to boots for some patients are ToeGrips® rubberized grips that fit onto a dog's nail. It helps dogs from slipping and sliding on smooth surfaces such as hardwood floors and tile, plus they can protect the nails from wear if a patient drags their toes. Another great aid are the Loobani Paw Protector Anti-slip Grip Pads that are applied to the bottom of the feet to improve traction. They are hypoallergenic, soft, and breathable with rubber spots on the surface to provide better traction between the feet and the floor. Active dogs may need the pads replaced every couple days. Kinesiology tape can also be used to protect the feet by applying it over the toes (see Kinesiology Taping in this chapter).

Support of Joints: Orthotic Devices

An orthotic device provides support to help align, protect, and correct the function of the limbs. An orthotic brace is indicated to assist in walking when a pet's mobility is impaired due to an instability of a particular joint (Figure 20.4). A splint or brace provides protection and stabilization of the affected joint, thus minimizing the pet's discomfort when bearing weight on the affected limb and preventing further injury. Some patients only require a soft wrap made of neoprene and nylon straps that can be splinted for additional support to aid in pathology of the carpus and tarsus. Other hinged or dynamic braces give more support while allowing the joint to bend,

which helps to prevent muscle atrophy due to disuse and helps to strengthen the limb. Practioners can look for local professionals that can create an on-site orthotic. Top Dog Bracing (www.topdogbracing.com; telephone 865-219-3280) provides on-site help for pet owners near the Knoxville, TN, and other areas of the country. Orthopets of Denver, CO; (orthopets.com; telephone 303-953-2545) provide long-distance orthotic services for practitioners and pet owners.

Gaining more popularity, prosthetic devices may help restore normal function and prevent future orthopedic and neurologic problems by maintaining better posture for patients that must undergo amputation. A prosthetic device, is typically, an artificial limb that replaces the missing limb that may have been lost because of a birth defect, disease, or trauma. It is of paramount importance to discuss whether a patient is a candidate for a prosthetic limb *before* an amputation procedure because the surgical technique will need to be modified to accommodate the device. Many pets cope well with a missing limb; however, the support of a prosthetic device to restore function after amputation may allow for a more normal posture and gait. The concept is not a new one considering the devices can be documented in early photographs from the early 1900s (Figure 20.5).

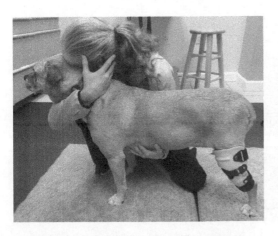

Figure 20.4 Dynamic brace for stifle support.

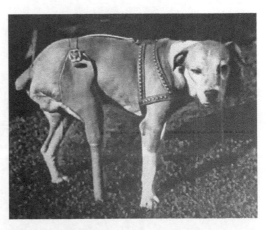

Figure 20.5 Sparky, a 14-year-old from 1937, and his prosthetic limb.

Support for Paralysis/Pararesis: Carts and Drag Bags

Mobility carts can be used to assist with walking and should be introduced early on to patients with mobility decline when possible. Carts allow the pet to retain and regain their mobility to move about, which can improve the pet's quality of life. They are available for pets with paraparesis/paralysis and tetraparesis/tetraparalysis. A variety of carts are available to fit all sizes, shapes of patients, and financial needs of clients (Figure 20.6). Some retired carts can be repurposed to fit new patients in need.

Drag bags protect disabled pets from abrasions while they scoot around their homes. Once the pet is placed into the bag, it anchors around the neck and chest preventing it from sliding off when the pet moves forward. A modified drag bag with a platform with attached roller ball castors allows pets to move about with more ease and any direction (Walkin' Scooter by Walkin' Pets, handicapped-pets.com).

Like other assistive devices, carts and drag bags should be monitored closely for discomfort and respiratory distress and removed at designated intervals to allow examination for pressure sores.

Four Simple but Important Manual Therapies and Therapeutic Exercises

Some physical medicine treatments require minimal training but have significant benefits when caring for hospice and palliative care patients. For example, mobility assistance and simple exercises may preserve remaining strength, improve respiratory function, and prevent decubitus ulcers (Hamilton et al. 2004). The following techniques are easy to learn and can also be taught to the caregiver.

Range of Motion

Range of motion (ROM) is a manual therapy that is simple to learn and can provide many benefits (Figure 20.7). The two types of ROM used in hospice and palliative care are passive ROM and active-assisted ROM. Passive ROM is used when a patient cannot initiate a voluntary muscle contraction and is often used in the treatment of paralyzed pets. It does not increase strength but will help to improve the movement of joints by increasing flexibility and the extensibility of soft tissues. Passive ROM will also increase the flow of blood, lymphatic, and synovial fluid (Millis et al. 2004).

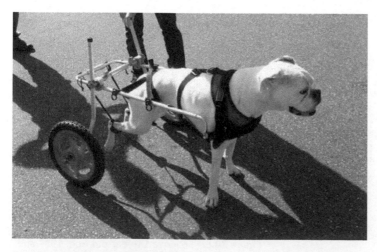

Figure 20.6 The use of a cart to assist Harper with her mobility.

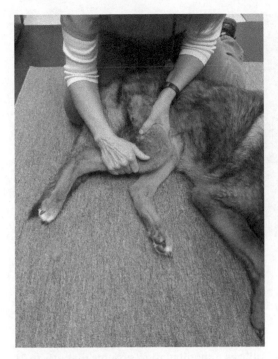

Figure 20.7 Range of motion.

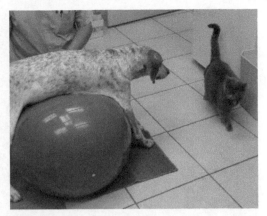

Figure 20.8 Assisted standing using a therapy ball.

Active-assisted ROM is utilized when a pet is able to assist in muscle activity. It may improve strength and also aid in the nerve reeducation, proprioceptive training, and gait training. With both passive and assisted-active ROM, the technique is started by gently flexing and extending the joints through their comfortable range of motion. This is accomplished by stabilizing the limb proximal and distal to the joint being treated. This exercise should be done for all affected joints, including those in the distal extremities. ROM exercises may be performed up to 6 times daily, 10–30 repetitions each time (Millis et al. 2004).

Assisted Standing and Walking

Assisted standing is a technique that helps hospice and palliative care patients in several regards. Not only does it improve mental contentment, but it may also improve circulation, respiration, balance, and proprioception (Hamilton et al. 2004). It relieves pressure over joints that could result in decubitus ulcers. It

can also be used to maintain strength and slow muscle atrophy.

If a pet cannot support its body weight without effort, the use of slings and therapy balls can make this task more manageable. When the pet is assisted into a standing position by use of a sling, or supported over a therapy ball, the pet's feet should be on the ground in the normal position (Figure 20.8). The duration of assisted standing is determined on a case-by-case basis. If the pet is comfortable, the technique should be repeated 3–6 times or more per day (Hamilton et al. 2004).

Walking is a great exercise regularly performed by most caregivers. Some patients, however, may need extra assistance and the aid of assistive devices described above. Short multiple walks, even if inside the house, have benefits. It provides mental contentment, helps to maintain strength, and may also help define circadian cycle by promoting being awake during the day and resting peacefully at night. Starting with a simple two-minute walk, five times a day is better than remaining sedentary. When possible, time can be increased by one to two minutes every few days.

Proprioceptive and Balance Techniques

Various methods have been created to assist pets suffering from loss of conscious proprioception and/or balance. Weight shifting is one

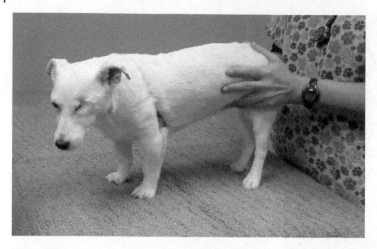

Figure 20.9 Weight shifting for balance training.

type of proprioceptive and balance training that helps to maintain core strength and balance (Millis and Levine 2014). This author prescribes this technique to most geriatric patients seen in her practice. When standing next to or over the pet while it is standing, the hands are placed on each side of the pet's hips (Figure 20.9). The pet is gently nudged using the hands to cause the animal to gently sway from side to side. These motions disrupt the pet's center of gravity and require the pet to shift weight by engaging core muscle activity to recenter its balance. Where applicable, placement of front feet then rear feet on a balance disk or soft surface and performing weight shifting can magnify the intensity of the exercise.

Massage and/or *Tui-na*

Massage helps hospice and palliative care patients by increasing blood flow to the massaged area, improving tissue perfusion, oxygenation, and removal of metabolic wastes. Massage also increases release of endorphins and improves lymphatic and venous return (Bochstahler 2004). There are many forms of massage that can be tailored to the individual's comfort and needs.

In addition to conventional massage techniques, *Tui-na* is a form of manipulative therapy and massage. This therapy is a form of traditional Chinese veterinary medicine that draws upon the use of specific techniques to manage pain and improve function. *Tui-na* utilizes 6 manipulation systems that utilize 21 different techniques, many of which focus on the treatment over the meridians and acupoints. Because of this close relationship to the meridians and acupoints, the benefits are compounded. The textbook, *Application of Tui-na in Veterinary Medicine* by Xie, Ferguson, and Deng is a good reference to learn more about the technique.

The Role of Acupuncture for Hospice and Palliative Care Patients

One of the most misunderstood, overlooked, and underutilized tool in physical medicine is acupuncture, as well as the four other forms of traditional Chinese veterinary medicine (TCVM): herbal formulas, nutrition, *Tui-na*, and *Gi-gong* (self-care of exercise and mediation). They all should be considered for supporting patients in need of rehabilitation for primary problems and comorbidities. Acupuncture offers a treatment option that is well tolerated, effective, and has a low risk of side effects (White 2004). The goals of

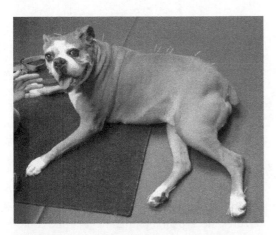

Figure 20.10 A patient receiving acupuncture.

acupuncture in the treatment of hospice and palliative care patients include decreasing pain, minimizing discomfort from other symptoms such as nausea and anxiety, and helping to improve organ function. Thus, acupuncture can address pain and improve function in a mobility-impaired patient but also help manage vomiting due to comorbidity in the same patient. Acupuncture is often used to treat conditions that did not respond satisfactorily to other therapies (Figure 20.10).

Acupuncture has evolved over thousands of years. Zhao Fu and Bo Le were veterinary acupuncturists that practiced in China around 947–928 BC and 659–621 BC (Xie and Chrisman 2009). Through careful observation, the ability to achieve consistent responses to acupuncture treatment has been established. Modern science is now documenting the treatment's reliability and illuminating the mechanisms behind these historic observations. Evidence-based research has confirmed the efficacy of acupuncture therapy, and those conditions can be found listed by the World Health Organization (Xie and Wedemeyer 2012).

In its simplest form, acupuncture is administered at any of 361 acupoints located along a meridian system, which is a series of channels that run throughout the body. In addition, there are 44 acupoints not associated with a meridian system (Xie and Priest 2007). In

TCVM theory, each acupuncture point is associated with an internal organ or function. Current research has validated some TCVM theories and confirmed the efficacy of acupuncture. For example, when acupuncture points were injected with an MRI contrast agent, the contrast material was found within the target organs according to TCVM theory (Kim et al. 2009). Acupuncture points have been shown to be located in areas where there are high densities of free nerve endings, arterioles, lymphatic vessels, and mast cells. Some are located near nerve bifurcations and where nerves penetrate into fascia. These areas are characterized by high conductivity and low electrical resistance. A number of theories have been proposed to explain acupuncture's mechanism of action, including the counter irritant theory, the gate theory, release of endorphins, and release of signaling molecules plus activation of T-cell lymphocytes (Xie and Ortiz-Umpierre 2006).

Based on the patient's condition, a certified veterinary acupuncturist develops an acupuncture prescription to address the patient's needs. Common methods of acupuncture delivery include dry needles, electroacupuncture, aquapuncture, moxibustion, pneumoacupuncture, hemoacupuncture, laser stimulation, gold or titanium implants, and acupressure. The method selected depends upon the condition and the patient treated. Techniques that use alternatives to needles (laser stimulation, moxibustion, or acupressure) can be used for clients that are worried about any discomfort associated with needling or if the patient experiences hyperalgesia or allodynia associated with needles. The frequency of acupuncture treatments depends on the condition being treated, the delivery system (for example, electroacupuncture treatments have a longer duration of action than dry needle treatments), and the patient's response to the treatment.

Acupressure can be a popular technique to assign to the caregiver for at home therapy. It is a technique used to stimulate acupuncture points by applying digital or manual pressure.

The caregiver can perform acupressure once the points to be treated have been identified by a professional acupuncturist. Those points can then be marked on the animal's body using a marker, by trimming hair away from the area, or by marking an acupuncture point diagram. Anatomic descriptions of some points use a unit of measure called the *cun*. One *cun* equals the width of the last rib of the patient and is used as a proportional unit of measurement for all sizes of individuals.

Listed below are 10 examples of commonly used acupoints used to treat clinical signs in hospice and palliative care patients. Most points have multiple applications but are beyond the scope of this section to include a complete list.

LU-9. This point is the Master Point for the head and neck. It treats cervical pain as well as respiratory conditions. Other benefits include, but are not limited to, forelimb pain and seizure control. This author also uses it to treat dental pain. LU-9 is located on the medial aspect of the forelimb in the depression just proximal to the radial styloid process.

LI-11. This point has many applications that include managing local elbow pain, cervical pain, and thoracic paresis. It is also helpful in the treatment of dermatological conditions and autoimmune disorders. LI-11 is also known for its ability to dissipate heat and to regulate constipation or diarrhea. It is located on the lateral side of the elbow in the cubital crease halfway between the lateral epicondyle and the biceps tendon.

ST-36. This point is the Master Point for the abdomen and gastrointestinal tract. It is known for its ability to support any digestive issue. In addition, it can be used to support an animal's *Qi* (vital energy). The acupoint also supports hindlimb weakness and is a local point for stifle disorders. ST-36 is located 3 *cun* distal to the patella, 0.5 *cun* lateral to the tibial crest in the *tibialis cranialis* muscle.

KID-1. A common use of this point in physical medicine is to manage pelvic limb paresis/paralysis and weakness or collapse as well as supporting kidney health. This point is located on the palmar surface of the hindlimb just beneath the central metatarsal pad.

PC-6. This point is the Master Point for the chest and cranial abdomen. It can be used to treat multiple purposes including nausea/vomiting, heart problems, and chest/cranial abdominal pain and helps manage anxiety. PC-6 is located between the flexor carpi radialis and the superficial digital flexor 3 *cun* proximal to the transverse carpal crease.

GB-20. This point is commonly used to treat seizures, neck pain, ophthalmic and otic conditions, and epistaxis. It may also help with patients that night wake to sleep. GB-20 is located in the depression caudal to the occipital protuberance and medial to the cranial edge of the atlas.

LIV-3. This point is commonly used for generalized pain relief as well as liver conditions and seizures. The point is located between the 2nd and 3rd metatarsal bones.

GV-14. This point also has multiple functions including, but not limited to, managing thoracic and cervical pain, dissipating heat, stimulating an immune response and treating respiratory conditions. GV-14 is located along the dorsal midline between C7 and T1.

Ding-chuan. This point is a Classical Point that is used to treat respiratory conditions that include dyspnea, asthma, and cough. It can also be used to treat cervical pain. *Ding-chuan* is located 0.5 *cun* off of the dorsal midline at the cervicothoracic junction.

Shen-gan. This is a Classical Point that it used to stimulate appetite and can aid in resuscitation. *Shen-gan* is located on the dorsal midline of the nose at the junction where the hair meets the non-haired area of the nasal planum.

Innovative and Noninvasive Techniques

Kinesiology Taping

Kinesiology taping is an additional therapeutic option that helps to improve quality of life through mitigating pain and promoting healing. The low cost of materials, the ease of application, and the physical benefits make kinesiology taping a good treatment option. Kinesiology taping was developed in the 1970s by Dr. Kenzo Kase of Japan and is used widely with human athletes and patients.

The term kinesiology is defined as "the study of movement." Medical kinesiology deals with the functional anatomy of an individual in conjunction with biomechanics, which differs from the concept of applied kinesiology recognized for its muscle testing technique.

Kinesiology tape is different from other types of medical tape because it has the properties needed to provide tissue decompression. It is made of a latex-free medical-grade adhesive that is embedded onto the tightly woven cotton tape in a wave-like pattern to allow better movement for the patient. The tape only stretches in one direction and has approximately a 10% pre-stretch to the material. Unlike conventional tape, it contours around body parts and allows for a full ROM, so it promotes movement. It is also porous and breathable but water resistant, so a patient can swim once it is applied.

Even though the tape can be used to help support joints, its main principle is not for stabilization. Taping materials and techniques employ the theory of tissue decompression in relation to the mechanics of body movements to achieve its therapeutic effect (Figure 20.11). In general, the tape provides a subtle lift of the underlying tissues allowing for this

compartment to expand to help dilation of capillaries and lymphatics, resulting in improved circulation. It is proposed that this local effect cascades into the deeper tissues thus providing a more generalized affect. This reduction of pressure can also reduce pain because swelling can put pressure on pain receptors. The tape stimulates sensory nerves in the skin as well as altering the afferent signals transmitted to the brain (Kase et al. 2013). Some examples of conditions that can be treated include taping for flexor tendon pathology, back pain, tendonitis, postoperative recovery from intervertebral disk surgery, scar tissue reduction, postoperative care of cruciate ligament surgery, cauda equina syndrome, muscle spasm, hematomas, and taping for posture modification.

Kinesiology taping can be utilized to enhance care in several ways. First, it can be used to treat trigger points or acupoints in patients that are too sensitive to receive dry needles as a treatment. In 2019, Dogan compared the effectiveness of kinesiology taping and dry needling methods in human patients with trigger-point-related myofascial pain syndrome of the upper trapezius muscle. Results showed improvement in pain and cervical ROM ($p < 0.05$) with no significant difference between dry needling and the taping patients (Dogan et al. 2019). Second, it can be used on the patient's body to mark or identify acupoints or areas to massage, so the animal caregiver can provide care at home.

The tape can be applied to the patient's body to provide noninvasive care for pain

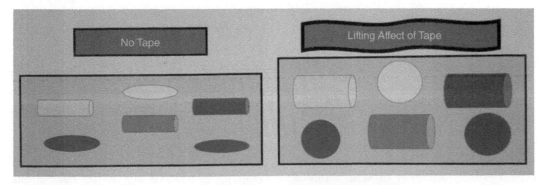

Figure 20.11 Schematic of tissue decompression before and after taping.

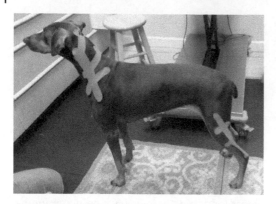

Figure 20.12 Kinesiology taping of six-year-old female-spayed Doberman Pincher with Wobbler's syndrome and Achilles tendon pathology.

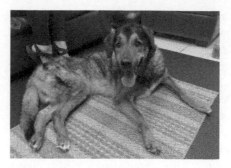

Figure 20.13 A simple patch of kinesiology tape for neurosensory awareness.

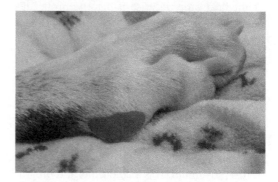

Figure 20.14 Kinesiology tape used for protection of decubital ulcers or abrasions.

management as part of a multimodal plan (Figure 20.12). The tissue decompression techniques, often by the use of a fan-like tape pattern, can reduce subcutaneous edema by facilitating lymphatic drainage by taping near the lymph node center closest to the area of pathology. Lastly, for pets that have proprioceptive deficits, the tape can also be applied for neurosensory awareness by stimulating proprioceptors and mechanoreceptors by lifting the skin in the areas being taped. A simple patch or a pattern over the effective area provides stimulation (Figure 20.13). Because of the unique physical qualities of the tape being porous, yet water resistant, it can be used to protect the toes from abrasions in patients that drag their feet or can be used over pressure points to protect from decubital ulcers in animals that are debilitated (Figure 20.14).

Precautions, complications, and challenges with animals include the length of the hair coat and aversion to the tape itself. A haircoat length of less than or equal to 2 cm is best suited for taping. For animals with longer hair coats, the hair needs to be shaved before application. Removal of the tape in the direction of the hair pattern while holding the skin tight can help to minimize discomfort. Contraindications of kinesio taping include avoiding use over areas of skin pathology and near or over neoplastic masses. It should

not be used over the abdomen of pregnant animals. There is the potential that ingestion of large amounts of tape could cause obstructions. A rare complication would be hypotension if a large amount of tissue is decompressed.

Cross tape is a type of kinesiology tape that differs from the standard tapes because it is statically charged and has minimal decompressive properties. It is used primarily to treat acupoints and small trigger points in human patients. It can also be used in veterinary medicine by being applied after an acupuncture treatment or for patients that do not tolerate acupuncture needles.

For more information on taping techniques, an excellent resource is *Kinesiology Taping for Dogs*, which provides step-by-step instructions on application (Bredlau-Morich 2020).

Extracorporeal Magnetotransduction Therapy: EMTT

Extracorporeal Magnetotransduction Therapy (EMTT) is a new tool to the veterinary market that provides a novel, noninvasive treatment option for patients with a multitude of musculoskeletal and neurological problems. Because of its noninvasive nature, it is an ideal device for hospice and palliative care patients. Its application in the human market has resulted in healing and symptom relief with various musculoskeletal conditions and tendinopathies that are typically challenging to treat (Krath et al. 2017). This modality shows equal promise in veterinary medicine. This author has used EMMT for the treatment of neuropathies, Achille's tendinopathy, IVDD, myofascial pain, cranial cruciate rupture, and osteoarthritis (Figure 20.15).

EMTT uses a form of magnetic energy producing a magnetic field strength of 80–150 militesla (mT). Its uniqueness is thought to lie in the ability to balance cellular metabolism through the sodium-potassium ion pump and possibly other mechanisms of action. EMTT differs from PEMF therapy by producing a higher oscillation frequency (100–300 kHz). It also provides a large treatment area of 5.5 inches with good depth of penetration of 7 inches.

Besides being noninvasive, other benefits of the EMTT device include that it is easy to learn how to operate, treatment times are short (under five minutes per region depending on the frequency), and it has a great safety profile. The short treatment time provides an added advantage with geriatric pets that may experience heightened anxiety when they are in a clinic setting. This modality also penetrates through hair and bandages, so no coupling agent is needed for the magnetic field to penetrate tissues.

Electronic devices that can be affected by magnetic fields should be removed from close proximity of ongoing therapies. Other precautions include avoiding pacemakers and metal implants other than titanium. The use of this device over the brain has not been studied, so treatments of the head should be avoided at this point in time.

EMTT has great potential to change the landscape of symptom management in veterinary medicine, especially for hospice and palliative care patients that suffer from complicated conditions.

Extracorporeal Shockwave Therapy

Extracorporeal shockwave therapy (ESWT) has many benefits for the palliative care patient, including analgesia, improved healing of tendons and ligaments, wound healing, and bone healing (Durant and Millis 2014). It is a good tool to use as a primary modality, or if the patient is refractory to other modalities, used as combined adjunctive therapy. Studies show its efficacy in the treatment of forelimb lameness and improved limb use after tibial plateau leveling osteotomy (Leeman et al. 2016; Barnes et al. 2019). Studies to explore ESWT use in lower back pain are ongoing.

ESWT utilizes acoustic waves to treat a variety of musculoskeletal problems. The pressure

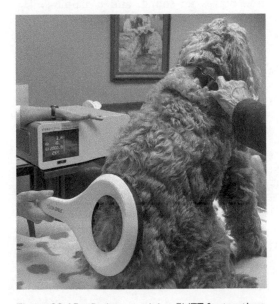

Figure 20.15 Patient receiving EMTT for treating lumbosacral pain.

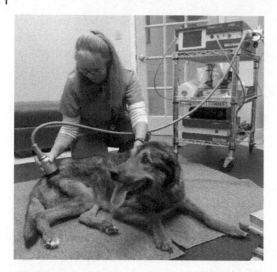

Figure 20.16 Patient receiving extracorporeal shockwave therapy.

waves are applied to a clipped treatment site using a probe with a water-soluble coupling agent. When a focal point at a tissue interface is encountered, sound wave energy is released. The extracorporeal sound waves are of lower frequency than ultrasound sound waves, and they do not produce heat in the target tissue. It is noninvasive and has few side effects. There are precautions and contraindications unique to ESWT: it should not be used over gas-filled cavities or over lung fields and should not be used in pets with unstable fractures, bleeding disorders, or inflammatory conditions such as infectious or immune-mediated arthritis.

Depending on the patient, the machine, and the condition being treated, patient sedation may be unnecessary, unlike ESWT units of the past (Figure 20.16).

Targeted Pulsed Electromagnetic Field Therapy

Targeted pulsed electromagnetic field therapy (tPEMF) is a very important modality for the care of multiple conditions seen in hospice and palliative care patients. tPEMF is a noninvasive physical modality that utilizes low-power electromagnetic currents to aid in healing. The

technology has been in use since the 1970s when bone growth stimulators were developed to aid in fracture repair. Since then, the tPEMF therapies have evolved to manage pain and aid in healing (Pilla 2013).

It has been theorized that tPEMF acts through the targeting of microcurrents that activate the binding of calcium to calmodulin. The bound molecule then binds to endothelial nitric oxide synthases and neuronal-nitric oxide synthases, increasing nitric oxide production. The end result is growth factor production through cyclic guanosine monophosphate signaling (Nelson et al. 2013). To date, veterinary studies look promising. In a study (Zidan et al. 2018), tPEMF reduced incision-associated pain in dogs post-surgery for IVDD and may reduce the extent of spinal cord injury and enhance proprioceptive placing. In another study (Alvarez et al. 2019), pain medications were administered less frequently in dogs receiving tPEMF treatment during a seven-day postoperative hemilaminectomy period compared with the control treatment group.

The Assisi Loop® (www.assisianimalhealth.com) is an example of a device used for providing tPEMF therapy (Figure 20.17). It is easy to use, makes no sound, and is painless. The center of the circular device is placed over the area of pathology that might include a soft

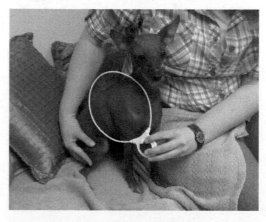

Figure 20.17 Patient in a pulsed signal therapy unit.

tissue injury, incision, wound, or painful joint. The treatment times vary, depending on the condition; on average, a 15-minute, 4 times daily protocol is recommended for acute conditions. There are two versions of the device: one with an automatic timer that delivers a treatment every two hours without manually resetting it (Assisi Auto-Cycle), and a manual version that must be turned on and off for therapy sessions. In addition to the Loop, a Loop Lounge has the technology inserted into a padded bed that provides full body coverage from nose to tail and from toes to ears. Respond Systems Incorporated also makes a therapeutic bed for small animals and provides additional products for horses (respondsystems.com/ pemf). Because of the ease of use and its effectiveness, this tool is ideal for hospice and palliative home care.

Other Therapeutic Modalities for Hospice and Palliative Care Patients

The following is a brief description of treatment modalities that have beneficial applications for many hospice and palliative care patients. Additional information can be found in rehabilitation and physical medicine literature, including the references listed at the end of this chapter.

Thermal Modalities

The use of thermal modalities is an often forgotten, simple technique to support patients. Thermal modalities include the application of cold (cryotherapy) and heat (thermotherapy). These have been used for centuries to relieve pain and improve function. Care must be taken when using thermal modalities in debilitated pets. Thermoregulation is not efficient in the older patient and also in the very young. Patients with sensory or cognitive compromise are at higher risk of complications because they cannot move away from the thermal

source or indicate that they are in discomfort. In addition, thermal modalities should be used cautiously over superficial nerves and over metal implants.

A common question is when does one use cold versus heat? The main use of cryotherapy is after an acute injury or immediately postoperatively to minimize edema and inflammation. The physiologic effects of cold include hemodynamic changes associated with vasoconstriction, delayed reactive vasodilation, and decreased acute inflammation. The neuromuscular affects include slowed nerve conduction velocity, decreased firing rates of muscle spindles making them less excitable, and the reduction in muscle spasticity in some patients (Weber and Brown 2004). The benefits of cryotherapy include pain relief, vasoconstriction and decreased blood flow, decreased swelling, and reduced enzyme-mediated tissue damage. In general, a severely hypertensive patient should not be vasoconstricted using cold. An average guideline, depending on the patient and condition, is for cold therapy to be applied for 15–20 minutes every 2–4 hours, if needed (Dragone et al. 2014). Care should be taken not to allow the tissues being treated to become too cold resulting in tissue damage.

The main use of heat is for chronic conditions and may be useful in treating patients with osteoarthritis, tense muscles, contractures, and chronic inflammatory conditions. The hemodynamic changes associated with heat therapy include vasodilation, increased blood flow, decreased chronic inflammation, increased acute inflammation, increased edema, and increased bleeding. The neuromuscular effect is increased nerve conduction velocity. Heat also causes increased collagenase activity and increased joint flexibility (Weber and Brown 2004). Heat applications can result in improved pain relief, increased circulation, increased soft tissue extensibility, and reduction of muscle spasm.

Heat should not be applied until the acute phase of an injury has resolved, no sooner than 48 hours after an insult for the best results. The vasodilatory effects of heat can actually exacerbate bleeding and edema in the acute phase of tissue trauma. Heat therapy should be used with caution in patients that are hypotensive because of the vasodilatory effects. Heat is contraindicated for active inflammation, over contaminated wounds, and over neoplastic masses.

Heat can be provided through hot packs, hydroculator pads, and dampened, microwaved towels. The use of methods that lose heat over time is preferred over the use of electric heating pads and infrared lights because the latter carry a higher risk of causing burns. One tip to avoid overheating and burns is for the caregiver to place their hand between the heat source and the patient to monitor the temperature. An average guideline, depending on the patient and condition, is that heat may be applied for 15–30 minutes and repeated every 6–8 hours (Dragone et al. 2014). Treatment should be stopped immediately if there is any doubt about overheating.

Photobiomodulation Therapy (also known as Laser Therapy)

Photobiomodulation therapy (PBMT) (also known as laser therapy) offers another effective treatment option for hospice and palliative care patients that is noninvasive and has a low risk of side effects. PBMT improves quality of life by minimizing pain and expediting the healing process. It is well tolerated by pets because there is typically no discomfort associated with the treatment when administered properly. The marketplace is inundated by laser options that range from Class 2 to Class 4 lasers, so it is not unusual to have pet owners ask about the therapy or to get the practitioner's opinion about a purchase of a laser for home use.

The term "laser" stands for light amplification by stimulated emission of radiation. Laser diodes produce energy-rich photons of a specific wavelength that cause changes in the body at the cellular level.

A laser's efficacy is effected by a number of variables including the laser class, wavelength, power output, beam (focus/dispersion), duration of exposure, and variability of the tissue exposed. All of these variables need to be taken into account when designing a treatment plan.

Numerous studies have shown that therapy lasers affect cells in a variety of ways on the molecular level, increasing cellular receptor activity, influencing cell membrane permeability, increasing production of ATPase and activation of cAMP, increasing procollagen synthesis in fibroblasts, stimulating cell membranes' Na/K pump, promoting endogenous opiate production, and inhibiting release of bradykinin and leukotrienes. Exposure to laser's high-energy photons results in activating macrophages and promotes biostimulation and photostimulation of cells. As a result of these cellular changes, lasers may reduce inflammation, increase tendon and wound strength, reduce pain, increase lymphatic drainage, improve healing time, relax tight muscles, increase mobility, reduce swelling, reduce scarring, and speed bone repair (Pryor and Millis 2015). In a study at the University of Florida, postoperative, low-level laser therapy reduced time to ambulation in dogs after a hemilaminectomy procedure (Draper et al. 2012). Multiple studies about PBMT are available for review on the PubMed® website (pubmed.ncbi.nlm.nih.gov).

Lasers are classified by the US Food and Drug Administration (FDA) based on their safety to eye exposure, not their efficacy. Class 1 has the lowest risk, whereas Class 4 can cause serious injury to the eyes. Devices that are most efficacious in veterinary medicine include the Class 3B and Class 4 lasers. Power outputs may vary from 5–500 mW for class 3B lasers and higher than 500 mW for Class 4 lasers. In general, higher wavelengths are needed to treat deeper structures like joints. Superficial conditions like wounds require less penetration and are most effectively treated with a lower wavelengths (Pryor and Millis 2015). Treatment protocols may vary from 1–$5\,\mathrm{J\,cm^{-2}}$ for more superficial problems, 8–$10\,\mathrm{J\,cm^{-2}}$ for treatment of deep tissues, and 15–$35\,\mathrm{J\,cm^{-2}}$ for complex or chronic conditions (Riegel and Godbold 2017). It is beyond the scope of this chapter to review treatment parameters. A wonderful resource for more detailed information on PBMT and various protocols is *Laser Therapy in Veterinary Medicine Photobiomodulation* by Riegel and Godbold.

Precautions and contraindications for PBMT use vary by the type and class of laser device. One should refer to the user's manual for safety guidelines and for details on the protective eyewear required for safely operating the device. Typically, laser devices should be used with care near any reflective surfaces. Caution should be exercised when using PBMT through hair, over darkly pigmented skin, or over tattoos. The laser device should not be applied over the patient's eyes or over an open fontanelle or over the abdomen of a pregnant animal. Again, it is important to refer to the owner's manual for the specific safety protocols.

Pulsed Signal Therapy

Pulsed signal therapy (PST) is a technology widely used in Europe and Canada to provide pain relief for people suffering from arthritis and/or various injuries. It is now being used in the United States to help pets experiencing pain caused by various conditions including osteoarthritis and tendonitis (Figure 20.18).

PST is a painless, noninvasive therapy that promotes new bone and cartilage growth through the generation of a low-powered electrical field (2 mT at 30 Hz). This mimics the body's streaming potentials during weight bearing. A randomized, blinded study at the University of Illinois evaluated the efficacy of the PST in 60 dogs with osteoarthritis. The PST group of dogs performed better than the control group (Sullivan et al. 2013). One study found the effects of the PST are due to upregulation of transforming growth factor (TGF)-pi,

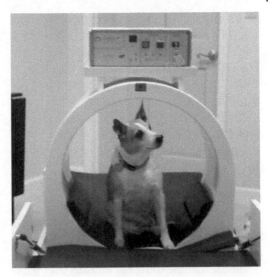

Figure 20.18 Use of an Assisi Loop for pain management.

which stimulates collagen II synthesis and proteoglycan deposition (Ciombor et al. 2003).

In-hospital and portable units are available for administration of PST therapy. Portable units are useful for treating pets that are difficult to transport to a veterinary facility or suffer from anxiety when away from home. PST is delivered in 9 consecutive 30-minutes treatments to achieve the best results.

Electrotherapy

Transcutaneous electrical nerve stimulation (TENS) and neuromuscular electrical stimulation (NMES) are two methods of therapy that may be used to manage pain and/or to strengthen muscles. This a great modality, but sometimes challenging to use because of interference of the hair coat and difficulty getting good contact with electrodes.

TENS is used to help manage pain by placing the electrodes directly over the painful area. There is a choice of three common settings: sensory, motor, or mixed, with each delivering a specific combination of various frequencies and intensities to treat the patient. Different theories have been postulated for the TENS mechanism of action, varying from stimulating the gate control mechanism to producing counter irritation to release endogenous opioids. Recommended treatment time ranges from 15 to 60 minutes up to several times per day (Levine and Bochstahler 2014).

NMES is used to cause muscle contraction in patients postoperatively, patients with spinal cord injuries, and patients with other conditions resulting in muscle atrophy. The electrodes are placed over a motor point and a muscle-tendon junction to elicit muscle contraction. Recommended treatment time ranges from 15 to 20 minutes once daily (Levine and Bochstahler 2014).

Electrotherapy must not be used over pacemakers, over the heart or carotid sinus, and over areas with thrombosis. In patients with a history of seizures, electrotherapy should not be used around the head and neck.

Therapeutic Ultrasound

Therapeutic ultrasound is a physical treatment modality that utilizes high-frequency acoustic energy to produce deep thermal and nonthermal effects. Currently, it is less commonly used because other modalities like photobiomodulation, tPEMF, and ESWT are being utilized more often. It can, however, help hospice and palliative care patients that are struggling with musculoskeletal pain, osteoarthritis, and other chronic inflammatory conditions, as well as enhancing wound healing (Hanks et al. 2015). Safe and effective use of this modality requires advanced, specialized training.

Therapeutic ultrasound requires shaving the hair coat over the affected area, and a water-soluble coupling gel needs to be applied to provide good contact between the ultrasound probe and skin during the procedure.

Precautions and contraindications for therapeutic ultrasound use include avoiding application over laminectomy sites, near pacemakers, over acutely inflamed areas, and over physeal areas of growing pets. Caution must be used when treating over bony prominences and

fractures. Tissue overheating is a risk and can cause a burning injury. Excessive heating can also cause periosteal pain.

Manual Therapy/Medical Manipulation/Chiropractic Care

Many clients seek out manual therapies like chiropractic care because of good experiences they have had with this type of therapy and are looking for the same type of relief for their pets. Manual therapy, chiropractic care, and/or medical manipulation is based on the theory that mechanical disorders of the musculoskeletal system affect comfort and general health. Medical manipulation or chiropractic care employs techniques for manipulation and adjustment of the spinal column and musculoskeletal structures.

Chiropractic care should only be performed by Doctors of Veterinary Medicine that have acquired specialized training and certification or by licensed Doctors of Chiropractic that have acquired special training that focuses on animals. The American Veterinary Chiropractic Association (AVCA) has stringent requirements for its certification. A list of national and international institutions that provides continuing education in chiropractic care can be found on the AVCA website.

The Integrative Veterinary Medical Institute, part of Chi University, offers courses to become a Certified Veterinary Medical Manipulation Practitioner. This program provides 107 hours of American Association of Veterinary State Boards (AAVSB) Registry of Approved Continuing Education (RACE)-approved curriculum on medical manipulation.

The University of Tennessee offers two types of continuing education for manual therapies. Certified Canine Manual Therapists can provide skilled manual therapy techniques to joints and soft tissues. The goals of combining traction, massage, and joint mobilizations is to modulate pain, manage inflammation, and improve range of motion. Certified Small Animal Myofascial Practitioners can also provide a form of manual therapy to help support hospice and palliative care patients.

Conclusion

Integrating physical medicine techniques into treatment plans for hospice and palliative care patients gives the hospice team another tool to help to improve or maintain a good quality of life for its patients. The low risk of adverse effects and the many benefits of different modalities make this discipline of care extremely useful in the treatment of patients struggling with a chronic condition or at the end of life. In addition, it is a tool that can help preserve the human–animal bond for the caregivers.

References

Alvarez, L.X., McCue, J., Lam, N.K. et al. (2019) Effect of targeted pulsed electromagnetic field therapy on canine postoperative hemilaminectomy: a double-blind, randomized, placebo-controlled clinical trial. *J. Am. Anim. Hosp. Assoc.* 55: 83–91.

Barnes, K., Faludi, A., Takawira, C. *et al.* (2019) Extracorporeal shock wave therapy improves short-term limb use after canine tibial plateau leveling osteotomy. *Vet. Surg.* 48: 1382–1391.

Bochstahler, B. (2004) Massage therapy. In: *Essential Facts of Physiotherapy in Dogs and Cats* (eds B. Bochstahler, D. Levine, and D. Millis). Babenhausen, Germany: BE VetVerlag, p. 46.

Bredlau-Morich, K. (2020) *Kinesiology Taping for Dogs*. North Pomfret, Vermont: Trafalgar Square Books.

Ciombor, D., Aaron, R.K., Wang, S. et al. (2003) Modification of osteoarthritis by pulsed electromagnetic field-a morphologic study. *Osteoarthr. Cartil.*, 11: 455–462.

Dogan, N., Sengul, I., Akcay-Yabuzdag, S. *et al.* (2019) Kinesio taping versus dry needling in the treatment of myofascial pain of the upper trapezius muscle: a randomized, single blind (evaluator), prospective study. *J. Back Musculoskelet. Rehabil.*, 32: 819–827.

Dragone, L., Heinrichs, K., Levine, D. *et al.* (2014) Superficial thermal modalities. In: *Canine Rehabilitation and Physical Therapy* (eds D. Millis and D. Levine), 2. Philadelphia, PA: Elsevier, p. 321–325.

Draper, W., Schubert, T.A., Clemmons, R.M. et al. (2012) Low-level laser therapy reduces time to ambulation in dogs after hemilaminectomy: a preliminary study. *J. Small Anim. Pract.*, 53: 465–469.

Durant, A. and Millis, D. (2014) Applications of extracorporeal shockwave in small animal rehabilitation. In: *Canine Rehabilitation and Physical Therapy* (eds D.L. Millis and D. Levine), 2. Philadelphia, PA: Elsevier, pp. 381–389.

Gillette, R. and Dale, R. (2014) Basics of exercise physiology. In: *Canine Rehabilitation and Physical Therapy* (eds D.L. Millis and D. Levine), 2. Philadelphia, PA:Elsevier, p. 159.

Hamilton, S., Millis, D., Taylor, R. *et al.* (2004) Therapeutic exercise. In: *Canine Rehabilitation and Physical Therapy* (eds D. Millis, D. Levine, and R. Taylor), 1. Philadelphia: Saunders, p. 244–263.

Hanks, J., Levine, D., and Bockstahler, B. (2015) Physical agent modalities in physical in physical therapy and rehabilitation of small animals. *Vet. Clin. North Am. Small Anim. Pract.*, 4, 33–37.

Kase, K., Wallis, J., Kase, T., (2013) *Clinical Therapeutic Applications of the Kinesio Taping Method*, 3. Tokyo: Ken Ikai Co Ltd, pp.13–23

Kathmann, I., Cizinauskas, S., Doherr, M.G. *et al.* (2006) Daily controlled physiotherapy increases survival time in dogs with suspected degenerative myelopathy. *J. Vet. Intern. Med.*, 20: 927–932.

Kim, J., Bae, K.H., Hong, K.S. *et al.* (2009) Magnetic resonance imaging and acupuncture: a feasibility study on the migration of tracers after injection of acupoints of small animals. *J. Acupunct. Meridian Stud.*, 2: 152–158.

Krath, T., Kluter, T., Stukenberg, M. *et al.* (2017) Electromagnetic transduction therapy in non-specific low back pain: a prospective randomized controlled trial. *J. Orthop.*, 3: 410–415.

Landsberg, G., Nichol, J., and Araujo, J.A. (2012) Cognitive dysfunction syndrome. *Vet. Clin. North Am. Small Anim. Pract.*, 42: 749–768.

Leeman, J.J., Shaw, K.K., Mison, M.B. *et al.*, (2016) Extracorporeal shockwave therapy and therapeutic exercise for supraspinatus and biceps tendinopathies in 29 dogs. *Vet. Rec.*, 15: 385.

Levine, D. and Bochstahler, B. (2014) Electrical stimulation. In: *Canine Rehabilitation and Physical Therapy* (eds D.L. Millis and D. Levine), 2. Philadelphia, PA: Elsevier.

Millis, D., Lewelling, A., and Hamilton, S. (2004) Range of motion and stretching exercises. In: *Canine Rehabilitation and Physical Therapy* (eds D. Millis, D. Levine, and R. Taylor), 1. Philadelphia, PA Saunders, p. 229.

Millis, D. and Levine, D. (2014) Exercises for proprioception and balance. In: *Canine Rehabilitation and Physical Therapy* (eds D. Millis and D. Levine), 2. Philadelphia, PA: Elsevier, p. 486.

Nelson, F., Zvirbulis, R., and Pilla, A.A. (2013) Non-invasive electromagnetic field therapy produces rapid and substantial pain reduction in early knee osteoarthritis: a randomized double-blind pilot study. *Rheumatol. Int.*, 33: 169–173.

Pilla, A. (2013) Nonthermal electromagnetic fields: from first messenger to therapeutic applications. *Electromagn. Biol. Med.*, 32: 123–136.

Pryor, B. and Millis, D. (2015) Therapeutic laser in veterinary medicine. *Vet. Clin. North Am. Small Anim. Pract.*, 45: 45–56.

Riegel, R.J. and Godbold, J.C. (2017) Fundamental information. In: *Laser Therapy in Veterinary Medicine Photobiomodulation*, (eds R. Riegel and J Godbold), West Sussex, UK: Wiley Blackwell, pp. 9–16.

Sullivan, M., Gordon-Evans, W.J., Knap, K.E. et al. (2013) Randomized, controlled clinical trial evaluating the efficacy of pulsed signal therapy in dogs with osteoarthritis. *Vet. Surg.*, 42: 250–254.

Weber, D. and Brown, A.(2004) Physical agent modalities. In: *Handbook of Physical Medicine and Rehabilitation* (eds R. Braddom et al.), 1. Philadelphia, PA: Saunders:, pp. 291–301.

White, A. (2004) A cumulative review of the range and incidence of significant adverse events associated with acupuncture. *Acupunct. Med.*, 22: 122–133.

Xie, H. and Chrisman, C. (2009) Equine acupuncture: from ancient art to modern validation. *Am. J. Trad. Chin. Vet. Med.*, 4: 1–5.

Xie, H. and Ortiz-Umpierre, C. (2006) What acupuncture can and cannot treat. *J. Am. Anim. Hosp. Assoc.*, 42, 244–248.

Xie, H. and Priest, V. (2007) *Xie's Veterinary Acupuncture*, Ames, IA: Blackwell. p 15.

Xie, H. and Wedemeyer, L. (2012) The validity of acupuncture in veterinary medicine. *Am. J. Trad. Chin. Vet. Med.*, 7: 35–43.

Zidan, N., Fenn J., Griffith, E. et al. (2018) The effect of electromagnetic fields on post-operative pain and locomotor recovery in dogs with acute, severe thoracolumbar intervertebral disc extrusion: a randomized placebo-controlled, prospective clinical trial. *J. Neurotrauma*, 35:1726–1736.

21

Integrative Medicine in Animal Hospice and Palliative Care

Kristina August, DVM, GDVWHM, CHPV

Caring for animals nearing the end of life requires flexibility and adaptation to the individual needs of the patient. A multimodal approach enhances the ability to observe the patient and monitor changes while adjusting treatments based on multiple factors that improve treatment outcomes and quality of life. Integrative medicine brings together the advantages of conventional and pharmaceutical diagnosis and treatment, physical therapies, botanical medicines, nutritional support and supplements, behavioral and emotional support, and other modes of care to provide the best possible patient comfort. This is especially applicable during the final phases of life.

The National Institute for Health (NIH) describes integrative medicine as "Bringing conventional and complementary approaches together in a coordinated way" (NCCIH 2021). Doctor Andrew Weil, founder of the University of Arizona Center for Integrative Medicine, takes it a few steps further stating that integrative medicine (for humans) is "healing-oriented medicine that takes account of the whole person, including all aspects of lifestyle. It emphasizes the therapeutic relationship between practitioner and patient, is informed by evidence, and makes use of all appropriate therapies" (AzCIM 2022). This definition is in very close alignment to the comprehensive, inclusive, evidence-based, and patient-centered approach of hospice and palliative care.

Terms

The terminology used to describe complementary and integrative medicine is often inadequate and confusing. A few common terms will be discussed here to improve understanding and communication between conventional and integrative practitioners.

Holistic or Wholistic: The two spellings are used interchangeably, some add the "W" to emphasize the "Whole." Based on the view that the "whole is greater than the sum of its parts," holistic medicine strives to consider as many influences as possible that may affect patient wellness. A holistic approach to medical care generally involves an extensive intake exam including detailed patient history of diet, patterns of elimination, environmental influences, behavioral characteristics, and much more. This term can be used very loosely as an overarching description for "complementary," "alternative," and even "integrative" medicine. Although interpretations vary, in the modern world the "whole" may also include pharmaceutical or conventional treatments as appropriate to provide the best patient care.

Complementary: The term complementary has been used to describe therapies that were not accepted by the modern medical community but could be used in a supportive manner to improve patient outcomes. The next section will give examples of several therapies that were once considered "complimentary" or "alternative" that have gained enough evidence to now be readily recommended and prescribed.

Alternative: The word "alternative" is often used interchangeably with "complementary," though it infers an "either/or" choice for therapies. Alternative treatments, by definition, would be used in place of other more conventional treatments. Integrative medicine opens the possibilities to combine therapies, within reasonable consideration of their actions, without having to choose between alternatives.

Traditional/Modern: Words such as "traditional" or "modern" are sometimes used to describe conventionally accepted medicine. Both can also describe "complementary" or "alternative" therapies that may come from a cultural tradition such as Traditional Chinese Medicine (TCM) or conversely use modern technologies such as laser therapy. It is important to understand that the use of these terms may be confusing.

Allopathic: This term is often used to describe "conventional" or "pharmaceutical" medicine. Literally, it means "different than disease" or "opposing disease." This treatment method employs medicines that counter disease conditions such as anti-inflammatory or anti-nausea medications. Many herbal and other therapies often use a similar approach, so this is not really an appropriate term to distinguish pharmaceutical medicine. Interestingly it originates as an antithetical descriptor of the homeopathic philosophy (see below) of treatment, which treats "like with like" or "same as disease."

Homeopathic: This word is often confused with or used to describe "holistic" and "complementary" medicine, in general, but actually describes a very specific branch of energy medicine where remedies are significantly diluted and "succussed" (shaken in a specific way) to create the final treatment in which "like treats like."

Conventional: "Conventional" refers to the most commonly accepted form of medicine, also described as "mainstream." Though still less than perfect, this will be the primary term used in this chapter.

Western and Eastern: Historically these terms distinguish the origins of medical thinking with "Western" referring to the development of medicine through Ancient Greece and Hippocrates throughout Europe and into North America. "Eastern" medicines would include traditional approaches from China (TCM), India (Ayurveda), Persia (Unani Tibb), and other Asian and Middle Eastern countries. Again, these are challenging and imprecise designations. Indigenous cultures of the Americas also have a history of medicine as do those of Australia, the rest of Africa, and essentially every place inhabited by humans over time. The division between West and East is a simplistic view in modern times.

Going Mainstream

The use of many therapies that were once considered "alternative" or untested are now commonly seen in human as well as veterinary medicine. Much of this change has been patient- or client-driven as the popularity of integrative care grows and the benefits are seen in practice. A review by Kligler et al. found significant evidence in human patients for the primary treatment use of acupuncture for chronic low-back pain, *Ginkgo biloba* for dementia, St. John's wort (*Hypericum perforatum*) for depression, fish oil for hypertriglyceridemia, probiotics for antibiotic and *Clostridium difficile*-associated diarrhea, and coenzyme Q_{10} for adjunctive treatment for heart failure (Kligler et al. 2016). In human medicine, complementary and integrative medicine is increasingly used to support patients with cancer, neurological conditions, musculoskeletal pain, and other conditions (Shalom-Sharabi et al. 2017; Wells et al. 2017). Human medical, hospice, and veteran support programs are increasingly including acupuncture, massage, herbs and supplements, reiki, music therapy, meditation, yoga, and other physical and mental health assistance in a patient-centered multi-modal approach to care (Schwartz et al. 2021; Zeng et al. 2018; Reed et al. 2022).

Overall, the benefits of complementary therapies appear to outweigh the risks when low-toxicity products are chosen. Madeline Leong et al. at Johns Hopkins Hospital, reviewed the use of a number of herbs and supplements in elderly human palliative care patients: "Low-risk solutions to pain are even more important in an elderly population because the clinician must consider polypharmacy, altered metabolism of medications, and increased neuropsychiatric sensitivity to medications" (Leong et al. 2015). Leong's review lists massage, acupuncture, herbs, and other supplements that may be helpful in the treatment of pain, nausea, constipation, diarrhea, restlessness, insomnia, and cough. For example, in addition to massage and acupuncture, two commonly recommended herbal treatments for pain are turmeric (*Curcuma longa*) and its isolated chemical constituent curcumin, as well as ginger (*Zingiber officinalis*). These herbs, which are considered safe for use as spices in food, have anti-inflammatory activity and a growing body of evidence points to their efficacious use in pain management. Some of the human-derived information in Leong's review and others can be extrapolated for beneficial use in animal patients, keeping in mind their individual and species differences in metabolism and physiology.

Safety and Adverse Reactions

A survey by the NIH in 2012 found that 33.2% of adults in the United States used complementary medicine to supplement their healthcare (Clarke et al. 2015). Many of these people also seek to provide this care for their animals and may not offer information on their use of complementary therapies if they perceive resistance or lack of understanding from their veterinary care providers. It is important for clients to feel comfortable having an open discussion about the use of complementary therapies. This communication allows the veterinary team to identify goals of treatment, explore possible interactions and contraindications, and assist in the selection of reliable providers, products, and resources with the highest probability of beneficial effect.

There are some legitimate concerns, of course, in the use of complementary therapies. If a treatment has significant medical effects on the body, there will also be concerns for adverse events. Just as proper training is needed in surgery or pharmaceutical medicine, education is required to safely provide laser therapy or botanical medicine. Referral to a qualified professional, skilled in the chosen treatment modality, is in the best interest of patient well-being.

The popularity of integrative medicine may derive from a desire for gentler treatment and reduced side effects; perceived harm or invasiveness of some conventional treatments; or the simple wish of caregivers to provide additional supportive measures. Many pharmaceutical drugs may cause adverse effects such as nausea, diarrhea, liver damage, kidney damage, or gastrointestinal bleeding and may have known interactions with other specific drugs. These are often the reasons that caregivers and veterinarians turn to complementary medicine, particularly at the end of life when the discomfort of adverse effects may result in a decision to euthanize more quickly.

Adverse effects and drug interactions are also occasionally seen with herbal medicines, essential oils, and dietary supplements and should be addressed during the treatment of patients for end-of-life support similarly to any other life phase. Herb–drug interactions can be *synergistic* or *additive* allowing for the efficacious use of lower dosages of pharmaceutical drugs (Wagner 2011; Williamson 2001). Examples include herbs with hypoglycemic effects that may help to lower insulin dosages, or herbs with sedative effects that might allow the reduction of pharmaceutical antianxiety or anesthetic medications. The herb Saint John's wort (SJW) (*H. perforatum*), used for the treatment of depression, is a significant example of additive effect as it increases serotonin and is therefore a risk for serotonin syndrome when used in combination with other antidepressant drugs, particularly selective serotonin reuptake inhibitors (SSRIs), tricyclic antidepressants (TCAs), and monoamine oxidase inhibitors (MAOIs) (Russo et al. 2014).

Herb–drug interactions may also be *antagonistic*, interfering with the absorption or pharmacologic action of prescribed drugs. SJW can increase the metabolism of some drugs in the liver by cytochrome P450 enzymes, thereby decreasing their effect. Drugs that are known to be affected by SJW include warfarin (coumadin), some antibiotics and antifungal drugs, NSAIDs, corticosteroids, and opioids (Russo et al. 2014). For these reasons, St. John's wort is not recommended to be used with pharmaceutical drugs except under expert management. Fortunately, this significant interaction is unusual for most commonly prescribed phytotherapeutics, and this information is readily available in professional herbal resources (Wynn and Fougere 2007; Stansbury 2020)

Knowledge of appropriate herbal selection, dosing, and administration intervals in relation to other medications is essential. The most concerning reactions occur when using pharmaceuticals having narrow therapeutic windows and strong effect. Drugs that affect the cardiovascular and central nervous systems, including warfarin, digoxin, and MAOI, are of particular concern for herb–drug interactions (Tsai et al. 2012; Gurley 2012; Gurley et al. 2012).

Collaboration between care providers with different expertise provides the framework to address specific areas of concern such as drug interactions, toxicity, hemorrhagic risk, or other issues. Open communication with clients and colleagues in assessing realistic risks facilitates the ultimate goal of supporting animals in health, longevity, and good quality of life.

Healing Philosophies

In holistic medicine, various medical paradigms from around the world may be used in diagnostic and treatment practices. Bodies of knowledge developed in other cultures, including TCM and Ayurvedic medicine, may approach diagnosis and treatment in a way unfamiliar to Western-trained professionals. They use concepts and language that can be difficult to translate without extensive study. The meridians used to identify acupuncture points have been found to relate to the nervous system as we now understand it, though many continue to find success using the more nuanced diagnostic and treatment techniques of the traditional system. Treatments, including botanicals, may be chosen not only for their specific medical action such as antinausea or gastrointestinal (GI) protectant, but also based on other characteristics such as warming (ginger, *Zingiber officinale*), cooling (marshmallow, *Althaea officinalis*), or calming (chamomile, *Matricaria chamomilla*) effects. These systems, blended with current scientific understanding, continue to offer new insight to patient care and medical discovery.

A core principle of holistic medicine is to support the body's inherent processes of healing and repair. Therapies that provide necessary nutritional and chemical constituents, enhance circulation, protect vital organ function, and other biological processes support complex body systems present in all living organisms.

As it is not within the scope of this text to offer a complete review of all possible complementary therapies, a few key points have been selected for discussion.

Nutritional Supplements

Often referred to as "nutraceuticals," many supplements have been found to be beneficial including omega-3 fatty acids, vitamins and minerals, pre- and probiotics, amino acids and enzymes, glucosamine/chondroitin, and others. Herbs and mushrooms, generally placed in this category, will be covered separately. At the end of life, it is important to weigh the potential benefits of these products, as some may be more supportive of wellness goals that are no longer relevant.

Omega-3 fatty acids are known for their benefits for many conditions including support of dermatological conditions, retinal healing, diabetes and lipid metabolism, gastrointestinal, renal, neurological, and joint health. Their anti-inflammatory effects benefit multiple organ systems. Clinical trials indicate significant improvement with human patients treated with omega-3 fatty acids for rheumatoid arthritis and osteoarthritis (Akbar et al. 2017). As mentioned earlier, probiotics can be useful in supporting digestion, particularly with diarrhea induced by antibiotic therapy and overgrowth of pathogenic bacteria (*C. difficile*) (Goldenberg et al. 2013, 2015; Kligler et al. 2016). Additional supplements are covered in Chapters 11, 16, 18, and 19.

Herbal Medicine

Also known as phytotherapy or botanical medicine, the origins of herbal medicine parallel the evolution of humankind. From basic nutrition to food preservation, therapeutic remedies, tools, and clothing, plants have been a part of human existence from the beginning. Every culture developed a medicinal system based on the plants in their area. Although these approaches may be diverse, analogous plant chemical constituents (phytochemicals) are found worldwide and often used for similar medical conditions. Many of our modern drugs originated as plant chemicals that were either extracted or synthesized into the medicines we know today.

Phytotherapy uses whole plants and plant extracts in various forms (liquid, pill, dried herb) as "simples" (single herb) or combined into formulas. These plant medicines can offer distinct benefits in treatment and prevention. Botanical medicines can provide nutritional and biochemical support for the liver (Greenlee et al. 2007), kidney (Jeyanthi and Subramanian 2009; Ojha et al. 2014), gastrointestinal system (Gadekar et al. 2010; Leong et al. 2015), and other organs. Immune support can help in fighting infections, reducing antimicrobial resistance, as well as reducing certain cancers (Luo et al. 2019). Herbs with anti-inflammatory and analgesic effects can be combined with sedative, muscle relaxant, anxiety reducing, circulatory supportive, and other herbs to create multimodal pain support that works well in combination with pharmaceutical pain medications.

A few specific herbs are highlighted here as examples.

Milk Thistle (*Silybum marianum*): Milk thistle, commonly used either as a whole plant extract or isolated constituents (primarily the silymarin complex), has been found to be protective of the liver, kidneys, heart, and pancreas and is supportive against damage caused by anesthesia, chemotherapy, and other drug treatments. It has potential therapeutic value in liver diseases, cancer, diabetes, and other conditions (Greenlee et al. 2007; Wang et al. 2012; Hackett et al. 2013; Polachi et al. 2016; Surai 2015).

Ginger (*Z. officinale*): Used in the treatment of pain, nausea, and general inflammation, including respiratory as seen in the study below, ginger can be a very spicy, hot herb and may need to be used in lower doses. Studied extensively as an antinausea agent, especially in human chemotherapy patients, the effect appears to be most beneficial when used regularly and prior to the onset of clinical signs (Marx et al. 2013; Nikkhah Bodagh et al. 2018). Gingerols and shogaols, phenolic compounds of ginger, have been found to inhibit the NF-kB pathway and other inflammatory processes (Dugasani et al. 2010; Luettig et al. 2016). In a randomized controlled double-blinded clinical study of human patients with acute respiratory distress syndrome (ARDS) in an ICU setting, enteral ginger supplementation resulted in significantly increased oxygenation levels, reduced inflammatory markers (serum IL-1, IL-6, TNF-α, and leukotriene B4), reduced time on mechanical ventilation, and reduced stay in ICU (Shariatpanahi et al. 2013).

Turmeric (*C. longa*): Known for its anti-inflammatory effects, turmeric also offers liver protection and has many antineoplastic actions. Often used as an isolated chemical, the constituent curcumin targets various cell signaling pathways including growth factors, cytokines, transcription factors, and genes that modulate cellular proliferation and apoptosis (Giordano and Tommonaro 2019). Many other constituents of the turmeric root have demonstrated significant effects on signaling pathways (NF-kB, TNF), enzymes (COX-2, protein kinase, cytokines), and disrupting cancer cell proliferation while also increasing cell uptake of constituents helping them to act synergistically with curcumin. This supports the herbalist experience that the whole plant is potentially more beneficial than the isolated chemical curcumin (Nair et al. 2019). Turmeric, among other herbs, has been found to work synergistically with chemotherapy agents, showing evidence that it assists in reversing multidrug resistance (Luo et al. 2019).

Ashwagandha (*Withania somnifera*): Commonly used for general support in convalescing and palliative patients, ashwagandha has been shown in animal studies and in vitro testing to be anti-inflammatory, antioxidant, an inhibitor of nuclear factor kappa B (NF-kB) activation and MAPK signaling pathways, and in various cancer cell lines to induce apoptosis, inhibit

angiogenesis and inhibit cell proliferation (Dar et al. 2015; Berghe et al. 2012).

Hawthorn (*Crataegus spp.*): Hawthorn leaf and flower extract has been shown to reduce signs of heart failure, increasing functional capacity, and improving quality of life in clinical trials while demonstrating positive safety profiles with concurrent cardiac medications (Holubarsch et al. 2018).

Calendula (*Calendula officinalis*): Used as a salve topically for wound healing and protection against decubital ulcers, calendula significantly decreases healing time while increasing connective tissue growth factor (CTGF) and wound granulation (Dinda et al. 2016). In studies of human patients having radiation therapy, calendula was found to decrease the incidence of dermatitis, including inflammation, pruritis, and radiation-induced pain resulting in fewer interruptions of treatments (Rosenthal et al. 2019).

Astragalus (*Astragalus propinquus/membranaceus*): Important in long-term immune support, general organ support, as well as bone marrow support during chemotherapy, astragalus has been shown in mice to improve the hematopoietic microenvironment by enhancing bone marrow stromal cell survival and proliferation of colony forming unit fibroblasts (CFU-F) among other cell parameters promoting myelopoiesis (Zhu and Zhu 2007). Astragalus extracts and a primary chemical constituent, astragaloside IV, demonstrated protective effects on the cardiovascular, immune, digestive, nervous, and renal systems through various mechanisms, including antioxidant, anti-inflammatory, and antiapoptotic effects (Han et al. 2016; Shahzad et al. 2016; Li et al. 2017).

Medicinal Mushrooms: Turkey tail (*Trametes versicolor*), reishi (*Ganoderma lingzh*), maitake (*Grifola frondosa*), and many other medicinal and edible mushrooms are known for their immune supportive and antineoplastic effects, such as apoptosis, stimulating natural killer cells, enhancing cytotoxicity of chemotherapeutic agents, inhibiting cancer cell proliferation, migration, and angiogenesis. Many medicinal mushrooms are also beneficial for diabetes, liver support, cardiovascular disease, and other conditions (Saleh et al. 2017; Rossi et al. 2018; Cor et al. 2018). Beta glucans, found in the highest concentration in the fruiting body of most species, are the primary active compounds in medicinal mushrooms, although they contain many other chemical constituents and nutrients as well. When choosing a mushroom product, it is important to know how the product is grown and processed. The constituents and quality will vary depending on the individual species and whether mycelium or fruiting body is harvested. Certain constituents are extracted more readily in hot water, while others are released by alcohol extraction. A double extraction uses both methods. It is important to understand that raw, powdered mushroom sprinkled on food will not provide the medicinal benefits that an extracted powder contains. For more details of specific mushroom therapies, see Chapter 11, "Integrative Therapies for the Palliative Care of the Veterinary Cancer Patient."

Before prescribing herbal medications, dosing and safety precautions must be reviewed (Wynn and Fougere 2007). When using these therapeutics, especially in patients with reduced organ function, it is important to consult with veterinarians trained in the actions and appropriate use of both pharmaceutical and botanical medicines in order to develop an optimal multimodal treatment plan, minimizing the potential for side effects, and offering the best control possible for clinical signs that may affect patient quality of life.

Essential Oils

Essential oils, also known as volatile oils, are metabolic end-products of plant metabolism stored in glandular cells, oil cells, and resin ducts of various plants. They are particularly concentrated in plants that we consider "aromatic" such as lavender, thyme, certain citruses, and flowers. The final product after extraction is highly potent and for most essential oils this "neat" (undiluted) product can cause caustic reactions and sensitization upon contact with skin or by ingestion. Extraction methods vary depending on the plant material. Contaminants, adulterants, and decomposition products are common in poor quality, often inexpensive products. Due to intensive marketing, high-volume production, and use in cosmetics, the public is exposed to and may use essential oils in the home on or near their animals. The high concentration of active chemical compounds and questionable quality make sourcing and education in their use paramount for patient safety.

Essential oils have potential healing benefits including antianxiety, antioxidant, anti-inflammatory, antimicrobial, and antineoplastic effects (Lesgards et al. 2014; de Lima et al. 2014). Generally, the safest essential oil and most commonly used is lavender (*Lavandula angustifolia*), not to be confused with spike lavender (*Lavandula latifolia*) essential oil that has a high camphor concentration and is more stimulating and less calming. The best way to use lavender essential oil is to put 1 or 2 drops in an aromatherapy diffuser and place it away from the animal. Dogs and cats have a much stronger sense of smell than humans and can easily be offended or overwhelmed by essential oils. Only run diffusers for an hour or two spread out over a day, and never leave an animal in a position that they cannot move away to another room. This is particularly important with immobile patients.

Dilution of essential oils is key to their therapeutic use. This can be accomplished through diffusion (aromatherapy), hydrosols (essential oils suspended in water during processing), or carrier oils (coconut oil, almond oil, and olive oil are commonly used). As a general guideline for essential oils diluted in a carrier oil (assuming safe selection of specific plant product), 1% dilutions are used for animals, children 5–12 years of age, people over 65, pregnant people, chronic illness, immune disorders, and other sensitivities (Butje 2017). Animal patients at the end of life should be considered even more sensitive, and extreme care should be taken if essential oils are used. Dilutions are created by adding drops of essential oil to a container of carrier oil. A 1% concentration is approximately 5–9 drops in 30 ml of carrier oil (drop size can vary, so this may be imprecise). This demonstrates the very low dosing of essential oil therapy. Species sensitivities must be considered along with the age and fragility of the patient. Use should be limited to aromatic diffusers and highly diluted topical if at all. Ingestion should be avoided. If accidental application occurs, a carrier oil (olive oil or other) can be used immediately to dilute on contact and reduce skin reaction and absorption of chemicals.

The potential for toxicity of these highly concentrated oils must be considered (Bakkali et al. 2008), especially when unintended oral ingestion may occur. Cats and patients with renal or liver insufficiency are at a higher risk for toxicity from certain oils. Cats have decreased UDP-glucuronosyl transferase, the enzyme which allows for hepatic metabolism (glucuronidation) of many chemicals including terpenes and phenols present in many essential oils (Little 2011). The unique respiratory system of birds makes them especially sensitive, and any animal that self-grooms (cats, rabbits, guinea pigs, rodents) is at risk of ingestion of essential oils. Clinical signs of toxicity include weakness, ataxia, muscle tremors, depression, vomiting, diarrhea, and hypothermia, as well as increases in liver enzymes and potential liver failure.

Depending on the plant, it can require 50–3000 pounds of plant material to extract 1 pound of essential oil. Particularly with the growing popularity in the lay public, this can have a significant environmental impact. Essential oils present within whole plants used as herbal medicine occur in safer, diluted concentrations when used in teas and other simple forms of administration, improving safety and maintaining the efficacy of whole plant medicine.

Other Therapies

Some modalities of complementary therapy, such as homeopathy, homotoxicology, reiki, *Qi-gong*, and other forms of energy medicine, defy our current scientific ability to explain their efficacy. However, positive results are commonly reported and concern for toxicity is minimal. A legitimate concern has been raised that clients are vulnerable, especially when facing life-threatening illness, and may be taken advantage of by unethical practitioners. Unfortunately, this can be true at any time with complementary or conventional medicine and caregivers must ultimately make their own decisions regarding the ethical constitution of the providers they choose to help them care for their animals.

As long as appropriate veterinary care ensures that measures are taken to support quality of life and consider the animal's needs for the control of pain and other distressing clinical signs, pursuit of additional therapies need not be discouraged and may be beneficial to the animal as well as the caregiving family. Reducing anxiety levels of the caregivers using these methods may result in transfer of feelings of calm and well-being to their animal companions; this by itself may reduce the incidence and/or intensity of stress-enhanced clinical signs including pain, gastrointestinal, cardiovascular, and respiratory distress. Dogs are especially known to look to their owners for reassurance (Merola et al. 2012). Many complementary therapies have been used in human hospice and palliative care to reduce anxiety, including music therapy, meditation, reiki, essential oils, and herbal medicines (Berger et al. 2013; Vandergrift 2013; Leong et al. 2015).

Further discussion of complementary therapies commonly used in veterinary medicine can be found in Chapter 20 Physical Medicine and Rehabilitation.

Ensuring Quality of Life

There are times when complementary therapies are not enough to maintain animal comfort and the integration of both pharmaceutical and complementary therapies is required. This integration may be provided by a single veterinarian or by multiple care providers working cooperatively. The use of complementary therapies should not preclude adequate and timely provision of highly efficacious medications that are important in maintaining patient quality of life. Inadequate control of pain or other signs of animal discomfort is a grave concern. Caregivers, veterinarians, and other animal hospice team members must be proficient in identifying and responding to animal pain and discomfort promptly and effectively.

Reliable Choices and Client Education

When facing a terminal diagnosis in a beloved animal, there can be a desire to grasp at treatments that might be lifesaving. Products can be sold on the Internet and through other sources that have exaggerated marketing claims, and this can be very appealing to vulnerable clients. While these products may offer hope and potential for remission of disease signs, it is important to discuss realistic expectations. By using integrative medicine it can be possible for patients to live comfortably with their disease for longer than expected, cures are even experienced at times, but death is inevitable and preparation for that decline is also part of the hospice experience. Enjoying a good life for as long as possible is the goal – hospice is truly about living well until death. Many clients and veterinary practitioners find that using additional therapies can add comfort, relaxation, and wellness for the time remaining. Overuse of these therapies may also be a concern, and as with any treatment plan, weighing the benefits of the treatments with the burdens felt by the animal in receiving them is crucial to good end-of-life care (See Chapter 6).

There is a plethora of information on complementary therapies available on the Internet, in printed publications, in health food stores, and elsewhere; some are reliable and some not. Herbs and supplements are considered food products and are not stringently regulated as pharmaceuticals, making it difficult to be fully confident in the quality of these products. Therefore, it is very important to provide caregivers with information and products that are as reliable as possible. Botanicals must be properly identified and processed, and all supplements should be free of contaminants. In the United States, labeling such as NSF (certified by the National Sanitation Foundation) (NSF 2022) and USPC (certified by the United States Pharmacopeial Convention) (USP 2022) indicates a higher quality product, as does company membership in the American Herbal Products Association (AHPA 2022) for human products and the National Animal Supplement Council (NASC 2022) for veterinary products. All companies should use GMP (good manufacturing practices) and be able to supply information on their quality control and testing methods.

When researching a company's quality control practices, certain information indicates a higher attention to detail. Established protocols for plant/product identification and verification are absolutely necessary, including sourcing information such as whether it is organically grown or wildcrafted and use of animal or mineral products. Appropriate processing needed for the specific plant part or chemical extracted should be known. Chemical analysis of the final product from independent laboratories testing for contaminants or adulterants as well as expected chemical constituents helps to verify quality. Certificates of

Analysis should be available upon request with lot numbers, dates, and tracking information. An adverse event reporting system, such as the one through NASC, helps to track products of concern. Reputation of a company over time is used as an indicator that they have produced reliable quality products but should be verifiable with some of these other methods.

Conclusion

With a growing interest in research on complementary medicine, the quality of the studies is improving. As new evidence comes forth, and the actions of various complementary and integrative medicine therapies are better understood, more educated decisions about the efficacy and risks of treatment can be made. Therapy decisions should be made on a case-by-case basis with the ultimate decision for patient care being one that is efficacious, ensures patient comfort with the fewest side-effects, and does not overwhelm the patient or the caregiving family with medications, treatments, or financial burden.

As many previously considered "complementary" or "alternative" therapies join the ranks of "conventional" medicine, the lines between these terms become blurred. Integrative medicine describes a container for all of these potential treatment modalities each with their pros and cons, appropriate in different situations. Consultations and cooperative relationships with integrative veterinarians help to determine optimal treatment strategies to address varying needs. The knowledge and perspective given by different traditions and approaches to patient care can open pathways to empathy and understanding for our caregiving families and their beloved animals. When used in combination with current information including recognition of animal pain and distress, advances in diagnostics, treatment, and emergency care, integrative medicine can blend the best of all worlds.

Educational Opportunities

The following organizations provide advanced learning opportunities combining traditional and current scientific knowledge in various topics:

American Holistic Veterinary Medical Association (AHVMA): www.ahvma.org
Chi University of Traditional Chinese Veterinary Medicine: www.tcvm.com
College of Integrative Veterinary Therapies (CIVT): www.civtedu.org
CuraCore: www.curacore.org
International Veterinary Acupuncture Society (IVAS): www.ivas.org
Purple Moon Herbs and Studies: www.purplemoonherbstudies.com
Veterinary Botanical Medicine Association (VBMA): www.vbma.org

References

Akbar U, Yang M, Kurian D et al. (2017) Omega-3 fatty acids in rheumatic diseases: a critical review. *J. Clin. Rheumatol.*, 23: 330–339
American Herbal Products Association (AHPA) (2022) American Herbal Products Associateion. Available at: www.ahpa.org (Accessed: March 2022).
Bakkali, F., Averbeck, S., Averbeck, D. et al. (2008) Biological effects of essential oils—a review. *Food Chem. Toxicol.*, 46: 446–475.
Berger, L., Tavares, M., and Berger, B. (2013) A Canadian experience of integrating complementary therapy in a hospital palliative care unit. *J. Palliat. Med.*, 16: 10.

Berghe, W.V., Sabbe L, Kaileh M. et al. (2012). Molecular insight in the multifunctional activities of Withaferin A. *Biochem. Pharmacol.* 84: 1282–1291

Butje, A. (2017). The Heart of Aromatherapy. New York: Hay House.

Clarke, T.C., Black, L.I., Stussman, B.J. et al. (2015) Trends in the Use of Complementary Health Approaches Among Adults: United States, 2002–2012. National health statistics reports; no 79. Hyattsville, MD: National Center for Health Statistics. Available at: https://www.nccih.nih.gov/research/10-most-common-complementary-health-approaches-among-adults2012 (Accessed: September 2016).

Cor. D., Knez. Z., Hrncic, M.K. (2018) Antitumour, antimicrobial, antioxidant and antiacetylcholinesterase effect of *Ganoderma Lucidum* terpenoids and polysaccharides: a review. *Molecules*, 23: 649

Dar, N.J., Hamid, A., and Ahmad, M. (2015) Pharmacologic overview of *Withania somnifera*, the Indian Ginseng. *Cell. Mol. Life Sci.*, 72: 4445–4460.

Dinda, M., Mazumdar, S., Das, S. et al. (2016) The water fraction of *Calendula officinalis* hydroethanol extract stimulates in vitro and in vivo proliferation of dermal fibroblasts in wound healing. *Phytother. Res.* 30: 1696–1707.

Dugasani, S., Pichika, M.R., Nadarajah V.D. et al. (2010) Comparative antioxidant and anti-inflammatory effects of [6]-gingerol, [8]-gingerol, [10]-gingerol and [6]-shogaol. *J. Ethnopharmacol.* 127(2): 515–520.

Gadekar, R., Singour, P.K., Chaurasiya, P.K. et al. (2010) A potential of some medicinal plants as an antiulcer agents. *Phcog. Rev.*, 4: 136–146.

Giordano, A. and Tommonaro, G. (2019) Curcumin and cancer. *Nutrients*, 11(10): 2376.

Goldenberg, J.Z., Ma, S.S., Saxton, J.D., et al. (2013) Probiotics for the prevention of *Clostridium difficile*-associated diarrhea in adults and children. *Cochrane Database Syst. Rev.*, 5.

Goldenberg, J.Z., Lytvyn, L., Steurich, J., et al. (2015) Probiotics for the prevention of pediatric antibiotic-associated diarrhea. *Cochrane Database Syst. Rev.*, 12.

Greenlee, H., Abascal, K., Yarnell, E. et al. (2007) Clinical applications of *Silybum marianum* in oncology. *Integr. Cancer Ther.*, 6: 158–165.

Gurley, B.J. (2012) Pharmacokinetic herb-drug interactions (part 1): origins, mechanisms, and the impact of botanical dietary supplements. *Planta Med.*, 78: 1478–1489.

Gurley, B.J., Fifer, E.K., and Gardner, Z. (2012) Pharmacokinetic herb-drug interactions (part 2): drug interactions involving popular botanical dietary supplements and their clinical relevance. *Planta Med.*, 78: 1490–1514.

Hackett, E.S., Twedt, D.C., and Gustafson, D.L. (2013) Milk thistle and its derivative compounds: a review of opportunities for treatment of liver disease, *J. Vet. Intern. Med.*, 27: 10–16.

Han, R., Tang, F., Lu, M. et al. (2016) Protective effects of *Astragalus* polysaccharides against endothelial dysfunction in hypertrophic rats induced by isoproterenol. *Int. Immunopharmacol.* 38: 306–312.

Holubarsch, C.J.F., Colucci, W.S., and Eha, J. (2018) Benefit-risk assessment of *Crataegus* extract WS 1442: an evidence-based review. *Am. J. Cardiovasc. Drugs*, 18:25–36.

Jeyanthi, T. and Subramanian, P. (2009) Nephroprotective effect of *Withania somnifera*: a dose-dependent study. *Ren. Fail.*, 31: 814–821.

Kligler, B., Teets, R., and Quick, M. (2016) Complementary/integrative therapies that work: a review of the evidence. *Am. Fam. Physician* 94(5): 369–374.

Leong, M., Smith, T., and Rowland-Seymour, A. (2015) Complementary and integrative medicine for older adults in palliative care. *Clin. Geriatr. Med.*, 31: 177–191.

Lesgards, J.F., Baldovini, N., Vidal, N. et al. (2014) Anticancer activities of essential oils constituents and synergy with conventional therapies: a review. *Phytother. Res.*, 28: 1423–1446.

Li, L., Houb, X., Xub, R. et al. (2017). Research review on the pharmacological effects of astragaloside IV. *Fundam. Clin. Pharmacol.* 31(1): 17–36.

de Lima, V.T., Vieira, M.C., Kassuya, C.A. et al. (2014) Chemical composition and free radicalscavenging, anticancer and anti-inflammatory activities of the essential oil from Ocimum kilimandscharicum. *Phytomedicine*, 21: 1298–1302.

Little S. (2011) The Cat: Clinical Medicine and Management. Elsevier p. 926

Luettig, J., Rita Rosenthal, R., Lee, I.M. et al. (2016). The ginger component 6-shogaol prevents TNF-α-induced barrier loss via inhibition of PI3K/Akt and NF-kB signaling. *Mol. Nutr. Food Res.*, 60(12): 2576–2586.

Luo, H., Vong, C.T., Chen, H. et al. (2019) Naturally occurring anti-cancer compounds: shining from Chinese herbal medicine. *Chin. Med.*, 14: 48.

Marx, W.M., Teleni, L., McCarthy, A.L. et al. (2013) Ginger (*Zingiber officinale*) and chemotherapy-induced nausea and vomiting: a systematic literature review. *Nutr. Rev.*, 71(4): 245–254.

Merola, I., Prato-Previde, E., and Marshall-Pescini, S. (2012) Dogs' social referencing towards owners and strangers. *PLoS One*, 7: e47653.

Nair, A., Amalraj, A., Jacob, J. et al. (2019) Non-Curcuminoids from turmeric and their potential in cancer therapy and anticancer drug delivery formulations. *Biomolecules*, 9(1): 13.

National Animal Supplement Council (NASC) (2022) The NASC Quality Seal. Available at: http://nasc.cc (Accessed: March 2022).

National Center for Complementary and Integrative Health (NCCIH) (2021) Complementary, alternative, or integrative health: what's in a name? NCCIH. Available at: https://www.nccih.nih.gov/health/complementary-alternative-or-integrative-health-whats-in-a-name (Accessed: March 2022).

National Sanitation Foundation (NSF) (2022) NSF. Available at: www.nsf.org (Accessed: March 2022).

Nikkhah Bodagh, M., Maleki, I., and Hekmatdoost, A. (2018) Ginger in gastrointestinal disorders: a systematic review of clinical trials. *Food Sci. Nutr.*, 7(1): 96–108.

Ojha, S., Alkaabi, J., Amir, N. et al. (2014) Withania coagulans fruit extract reduces oxidative stress and inflammation in kidneys of streptozotocin-induced diabetic rats. *Oxid. Med. Cell. Longev.*, 2014: 201436.

Polachi, N., Bai, G., and Li, T., et al. (2016) Modulatory effects of silibinin in various cell signaling pathways against liver disorders and cancer - a comprehensive review. *Eur. J. Med. Chem.*, 123: 577–595.

Reed, D.E., Bokhour, B.G., Gaj, L. et al. (2022) Whole health use and interest across veterans with co-occurring chronic pain and PTSD: an examination of the 18 VA medical center flagship sites. *Glob. Adv. Health Med.*, 11: 21649561211065374.

Rosenthal, A., Israilevich, R., and Moy, R. (2019) Management of acute radiation dermatitis: a review of the literature and proposal for treatment algorithm. *J. Am. Acad. Dermatol.*, 81(2): 558–567.

Rossi, P., Difrancia, R., Quagliariello, V. et al. (2018) B-glucans from *Grifola frondosa* and *Ganoderma lucidum* in breast cancer: an example of complementary and integrative medicine. *Oncotarget*, 9(37): 24837–24856.

Russo E, Scicchitano F, Whalley BJ, et al. (2014) Hypericum perforatum: Pharmacokinetic, Mechanism of Action, Tolerability, and Clinical Drug–Drug Interactions. *Phytotherapy Research* 28 pp 643–655.

Saleh, M.H., Rashedi, I. and Keating, A. (2017) Immunomodulatory properties of *Coriolus versicolor*: the role of polysaccharopeptide. *Front. Immunol.*, 8: 1087.

Schwartz, M.R., Cole, A.M., Keppel, G.A. et al. (2021) Complementary and integrative health knowledge and practice in primary care settings: a survey of primary care providers in the northwestern United States. *Glob. Adv. Health Med.*, 10: 21649561211023377.

Shahzad, M., Small, D., Morais, C. et al. (2016) Protection against oxidative stress-induced apoptosis in kidney epithelium by Angelica and Astragalus. *J. Ethnopharmacol.*, 179: 412–419.

Shalom-Sharabi, I., Samuels, N., Lev, E. et al. (2017) Impact of a complementary/integrative medicine program on the need for supportive cancer care-related medications. *Support. Care Cancer*, 25(10): 3181–3190.

Stansbury, J. (2020) Herbal Formularies for Health Professionals, Volumes 1-5. Chelsea Green Publishing.

Shariatpanahi, Z.V., Mokhtari, M., Taleban, F.A. et al. (2013) Effect of enteral feeding with ginger extract in acute respiratory distress syndrome. *J. Crit. Care*, 28: 2171–2176.

Surai, P. (2015) Silymarin as a natural antioxidant: an overview of the current evidence and perspectives. *Antioxidants*, 4(1): 204–247.

Tsai, H.H., Lin, A., Pickard, S. et al. (2012) Evaluation of documented drug interactions and contraindications associated with herbs and dietary supplements: a systematic literature review. *Int. J. Clin. Pract.*, 66: 1056–1078.

United States Pharmacopeia (USP) (2022) The USP Convention (USPC) https://www.usp.org/about/usp-convention (Accessed: March 2022).

University of Arizona Andrew Weil Center for Integrative Medicine (AzCIM). (2022) What is integrative medicine? Andrew Weil Center for Integrative Medicine Available at: https://integrativemedicine.arizona.edu/about/definition.html (Accessed: March 2022).

Vandergrift, A. (2013) Use of complementary therapies in hospice and palliative care. *Omega*, 67: 227–232.

Wagner, H. (2011) Synergy research: approaching a new generation of phytopharmaceuticals. *Fitoterapia*, 82: 34–37.

Wang, Q., Liu, M., Liu, W-W. et al. (2012) In vivo recovery effect of silibinin treatment on streptozotocin-induced diabetic mice is associated with the modulations of sirt-1 expression and autophagy in pancreatic b-cell. *J. Asian Nat. Prod. Res.*, 14(5): 413–423.

Wells, R.E., Baute, V., and Wahbeh, H. (2017) Complementary and integrative medicine for neurologic conditions. *Med. Clin. North Am.*, 101(5): 881–893.

Williamson, E.M. (2001) Synergy and other interactions in phytomedicines. *Phytomedicine*, 8: 401–409.

Wynn, S., and Fougere, B. (2007) Veterinary Herbal Medicine. Mosby.

Zeng, Y.S., Wang, C., Ward, K.E. et al. (2018) Complementary and alternative medicine in hospice and palliative care: a systematic review. *J Pain Symptom Manage.*, 56(5): 781–794.e4.

Zhu, X-L. and Zhu, B-D. (2007) Mechanisms by which Astragalus membranaceus injection regulates hematopoiesis in Myelosuppressed mice. *Phytother. Res.*, 21: 663–667.

22

Nursing Care for Seriously Ill Animals: Art and Techniques

Shea Cox, DVM, CHPV, CVPP and Mary Ellen Goldberg, CVT, LVT, SRA-retired, CCRVN, CVPP, VTS-lab animal-retired, VTS-Physical Rehabilitation-retired, VTS-anesthesia/ analgesia-Honorary

Unless we are making progress in our nursing every year, every month, every week, take my word for it we are going back.

Florence Nightingale 1914

Introduction

The American Veterinary Medical Association's (AVMA) policy on the human–animal bond states, "The bond includes, but is not limited to emotional, psychological, and physical interactions of people, animals, and the environment" (AVMA 2015). Hospice care begins when the veterinarian diagnoses a family pet as "seriously ill" and recognizes that the bond between the animal and its human caregivers is threatened. The care for the animal hospice patient is determined by the goals and preferences of the family with support and guidance from the hospice team (Shanan 2015). Palliative care is defined as, "An approach that improves the quality of life (QOL) of patients and their families facing serious illness, through the prevention and relief of suffering" (WHO 2022). Maintaining the highest standards for the patient's comfort and treatment is the ultimate goal of the pet's caregiving family and hospice and palliative care (HPC) providers. Animal

HPC seek to accomplish this goal, utilizing a collaborative and supportive approach with the pet's caregiver. The goals of animal hospice are perfectly aligned with the veterinary oath and the fundamental reasons veterinary teams do what they do (Shanan et al. 2016). The AVMA recommends that a team approach be used when addressing the needs for veterinary hospice patients (AVMA 2016). A key member in the hospice team is the veterinary technician nurse.

The veterinary hospice nurse's role can be divided into three core competencies:

1) *Medical*: This role requires the veterinary nurse to be able to assess the level of pain and discomfort, to intervene to keep the patient comfortable, and know when and how to use other healthcare resources.
2) *Educator*: In this role, the veterinary nurse delivers information from the medical team to the animal's caregivers, to ensure the best care for the patient.
3) *Advocate*: The veterinary nurse can be the bridge between patient, family, and the hospice team. The veterinary nurse intervenes on the patient's and caregiver's behalf, taking on the role of communicator and translator of information and feelings. As an

advocate, the veterinary nurse provides guidance and support to the human members of the family during that final journey with their pet, utilizing knowledge, communication skills, intuition, and empathy. Nurses are also advocates for maintaining an effective interdisciplinary team, and can play essential roles in building and promoting team coordination in the context of palliative care.

Nurses' Medical Roles

Nurses are in the right position to integrate palliative care practices into their patients' care plans throughout the disease trajectory and ensure that the palliative care needs of the patients and those of their families are appropriately met (Ogunkorode 2019).

Veterinary nurses assess, treat, and maintain adequate symptomatic control for their patients during all phases of the HPC process: starting at the initial contact between caregiver, animal, and the hospice team, through planning and delivery of medical and nursing care, assessments of patient's progress or decline, revisions of plans of care, and including participation in end-of-life decisions.

Intake

The veterinary nurse will conduct an extensive interview about the patient and the family's history. While history taking is a medical task, empathy for the patient and caregiver must be communicated for a compassionate and family-centered atmosphere.

Planning of Care

The family, attending veterinarian, and veterinary hospice team meet to develop an individualized plan of care, taking into consideration the family's background, challenges, resources, and preferences.

Ongoing Monitoring and Assessments

Patient monitoring and assessment may be the veterinary hospice nurse most important medical role. The function of the nurse as "the doctor's eyes and ears" is invaluable and essential to the delivery of high-quality patient care. Once the patient has been placed in an HPC program, continued monitoring and assessments must be carried out regularly. Monitoring is best done by a combination of Shanan (2015):

- progress reports from the caregivers, communicated to the hospice team in person, by phone, or electronically
- recheck examinations by veterinary nurses
- recheck examinations by veterinarians (required when a change in the patient's condition has occurred)
- repeated collection of laboratory data, as deemed necessary

Frequency of Assessments

Providing adequate nursing care for hospice cats and dogs requires periodic assessments. The frequency of assessments should be determined by the pet's current condition, an understanding of potential complications associated with the patient's illnesses, and an appreciation for the risk of medication adverse effects. Assessments can be performed daily, weekly, monthly, or on a flexible schedule.

Parameters of Assessments

Assessments of HPC patients must be timely and comprehensive, including monitoring of the animal's degree of pain and severity of other symptoms, his or her mobility and mental status, and the caregiver's competence in medication administration and maintenance of the patient's hygiene and comfort. Below is a brief description of the main components of the veterinary nurse's patient assessment.

Assessment of Pain

Pain is a complex, multidimensional experience involving sensory and affective components. The physiology and pathophysiology of pain are remarkably similar across mammalian species. Some pain-related physiological changes are listed in Box 22.1.

The capacity of animals to suffer as sentient creatures is well established and enshrined in law in many countries (McKune et al. 2015), and pain assessment is an essential part of every animal patient evaluation. A change in behavior is the most common sign of pain, so understanding a patient's normal behavior is important in identifying changes and making an appropriate choice to intervene (AAFP 2010). Detailed information about assessment of pain and pain management can be found in several important sources (e.g. Goldberg and Shaffran 2015; Gaynor and Muir 2015; AAHA/AAFP 2015). For an extensive discussion of the behavioral indicators of pain in dogs and cats see Chapter 5 in this book. A species-specific table has been created by M.E. Goldberg to explain various behavioral signs of pain (Table 22.1).

Box 22.1   Pain-related physiologic changes can include the following,

Cardiovascular
- Hypertension
- Tachycardia, tachyarrhythmia
- Peripheral vasoconstriction (pale mucosa)

Respiratory
- Tachypnea
- Hypoxemia
- Shallow breathing (abdominal or thoracic guarding)
- Exaggerated abdominal component
- Panting (dogs)
- Open-mouth breathing (cats)
- Pulmonary edema
- Respiratory acid–base imbalance

Gastrointestinal
- Ulcers
- Ileus
- Nausea and vomiting
- Anorexia

Ophthalmic
- Mydriasis

Metabolic
- Cachexia
- Increased oxygen demand
- Negative nitrogen balance

Immune function
- Hemorrhage

Sleep pattern
- Behavior changes

Source: Kata et al. 2015. Reproduced with Permission of Wiley.

Pain Scales

A sound approach to pain management favors anticipation of the severity and duration of pain that is likely to occur with any procedure, condition, or surgery (Shaffran and Grubb 2010). Pain assessment is an essential part of every patient evaluation, regardless of presenting complaint.

Pain scales are a useful tool for categorizing the degree of pain experienced by humans and animal patients. Following types of pain scales are helpful and practical for use by veterinary nurses in assessing the degree of pain in their HPC patients:

1) Subjective verbal scales (SVSs): assign simple descriptive words and a corresponding serial number to qualify pain, e.g. no pain, 0; mild,1; moderate, 2; and severe, 3 (Gaynor and Muir 2015, p. 83)
2) Visual analog scales (VASs): a line with no markings is used, numbers are at each end, 0 being no pain and 100 being worst (Figure 22.1)
3) Numerical rating scales (NRSs): a number line with individual numerical markings (1–10), which are chosen as the score (Figure 22.2)

Table 22.1 Species-specific behavioral signs of pain.

Species	Vocalizing	Posture	Locomotion	Temperament
Dog	Whimpers, howls, growls	Cowers, crouches; recumbent	Reluctant to move; awkward, shuffles	Varies from chronic to acute; can be subdued or vicious; quiet or restless
Cat	Generally silent; may growl or hiss	Stiff, hunched in sternal recumbency; limbs tucked under body	Reluctant to move limb, carry limb	Reclusive
Primate	Screams, grunts, moans	Head forward, arms across body; huddled crouching	Favors area in pain	Docile to aggressive
Mice, rats, hamsters	Squeaks; squeals	Dormouse posture; rounded back; head tilted; back rigid	Ataxia; running in circles	Docile or aggressive depending on severity of pain, eats neonates
Rabbits	Piercing squeal on acute pain	Hunched; faces back of cage	Inactive; drags hind legs	Apprehensive, dull, sometimes aggressive depending on severity of pain; eats neonates
Guinea pig	Urgent repetitive squeals	Hunched	Drags hind legs	Docile, quiet, terrified, agitated
Horses	Grunting, nicker	Rigid; head lowered	Reluctant to move; walk in circles "up and down" movement	Restless, depressed
Chickens	Gasping	Stand on one foot, hunched huddled	None	Lethargic, allows handling
Cows, calves, goats	Grunting; grinding teeth	Rigid; head lowered; back humped	Limp; reluctant to move the painful area	Dull, depressed; act violent when handled
Sheep	Grunting; teeth grinding	Rigid; head down	Limp; reluctant to move the painful area	Disinterested in surroundings; dull, depressed
Pigs	From excessive squealing to no sound at all	All four feet close together under body	Unwilling to move; unable to stand	From passive to aggressive depending on severity of pain
Birds	Chirping	Huddled, hunched	From excessive movement to tonic immobility depending on severity of pain	Inactive; drooping, miserable appearance
Fish	None	Clamped fins; pale color; hiding; anorexia	None unless forced; if a schooling fish, will separate itself from others	First sign to occur is anorexia; lethargic; stressed easily
Amphibians	None	Closed eyes; color changes; rapid respirations	Immobility; lameness	Anorexia; aggressive
Reptiles	Hiss; grunting	Hunched; hiding; color change	Immobility unless forced	Anorexia; aggressive; lethargic; avoidance

This chart is meant to display some of the different signs that species may exhibit if in pain. Individuals may not show any of these signs or show signs not listed. This is meant as a general guide.

Source: Goldberg 2010. Reproduced with permission of NAVTA Journal.

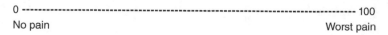

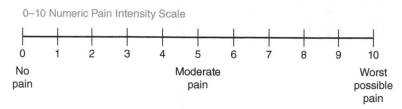

Figure 22.1 Visual analog scale.

Figure 22.2 Numerical rating scale.

4) Simple descriptive scales (SDSs): numbers are assigned to descriptions that categorize different levels of pain intensity
5) Pain scales such as VAS, NRS, and SDS are thought to be unidimensional. A pain scale should ideally be multidimensional, in that several aspects of pain intensity and pain related disability are included and question especially the dynamic aspects. The Glasgow CPS is thought to be Multidimensional (Reid et al. 2007, 2017).

Assessment of Other Signs of Discomfort

Clinical signs that affect QOL, other than pain, may influence decisions about palliative care and euthanasia. Digestive discomfort, dyspnea, pruritus, thermoregulatory difficulty, incontinence, blindness, and cognitive dysfunction are examples of conditions that may cause discomfort and should be addressed (Jones 2014).

Assessment for Dehydration

Assessment for dehydration is challenging in emaciated and geriatric patients because they have poor skin elasticity, which can mimic dehydration. It is commonly reported that 5% dehydration is not detectable, while 12–15% dehydration leads to a completely moribund animal and imminent death. It has been shown that the response to dehydration varies markedly between dogs. Similar studies have not been performed in cats. In emaciated or geriatric patients, when compatible history and physical examination findings are present, it is reasonable to assume 7% dehydration and treat accordingly. Regular reassessment followed by adjustment of therapy is required to safely rehydrate the patient (Goggs et al. 2008).

Assessment of Medication Administration

The veterinary nurse should review the list of medications the pet is receiving in addition to making sure the dosages are correct. Another important role of the nurse is questioning the owner about medication side effects, as well as ensuring the caregivers understand what to watch for once a pet begins a new medication. For pets that are receiving injections (such as insulin or subcutaneous fluids) the nurse should observe the caregiver's technique when administering the injection to ensure that the procedure is being done properly (Todd-Jenkins and Bentz 2013).

Assessment of Mobility

Mobility refers to the patient's ability to use voluntary muscles, coordinated and activated by central nervous system (CNS) activity, to perform most activities of daily living. Mobility contributes to the patient's QOL by enabling movement to accommodate the patient's preferences for location and body position. Villalobos comments that the importance of mobility seems to be dependent on the weight and species of the patient. Cats and small lap dogs can and do enjoy life with much less need for handling their own mobility than large and giant breed dogs (Villalobos 2011a).

Shearer lists five common categories of mobility impairment (Shearer 2011, p. 611):

1) can stand to support self with minimal lameness, paraparesis, or ataxia
2) can stand to support self but frequently stumbles and falls with mild lameness, mild paraparesis, or ataxia
3) unable to stand to support self, but when assisted moves limbs yet stumbles and falls frequently with moderate lameness, paraparesis, or ataxia
4) unable to support self, has slight movement when supported, with severe lameness or paraparesis
5) absence of purposeful movement secondary to disease or near death.

Shearer developed a questionnaire (Shearer 2011, p. 610) for owners to assign a grade to various aspects of their pet's mobility impairment, on a 0–3.5 scale (0–0.5 normal; 1.0–1.5 mild; 2.0–2.5 moderate; 3.0–3.5 severe impairment) (Box 22.2).

The assessment of mobility should include information about the pet's living conditions. Owners should be asked questions such as whether the patient is an indoor or outdoor pet. How many steps does the patient have to navigate? Does the patient sleep in the owner's bed? Is the patient able to travel in a car? What is the flooring in the home? What is the terrain outside? Questionnaires regarding mobility help determine how much care the pet may need to maintain QOL (Box 22.3).

Assessment of Mental and Emotional Status

Frank McMillan, in his discursive article on stress, distress, and emotions in animals (McMillan 2005), concludes that "distress

---

Box 22.2 Mobility questionnaire.

Owners should assign a grade to each question based on the rating scale.
  Rating system: 0–5 none; 1–1.5 mild; 2–2.5 moderate; 3–3.5 severe

Question	0	1	2	3
Any problem with walking?				
Can your pet move from lying down to stand?				
Can your pet move from stand to lying down?				
Can your pet move from sit to stand?				
Can your pet move from stand to sit?				
Can your pet hold posture to defecate?				
Can your pet hold posture to urinate?				
Can your pet ascend stairs?				
Can your pet descend stairs?				
Can your pet jump?				
Can your pet run?				
Can your pet climb inclines?				
Can your pet lose weight?				
Can your pet gain weight?				
Does your pet have trouble with endurance?				

Source: Shearer 2011. Reproduced with permission of Elsevier.

Box 22.3 Questionnaire on activities of daily living.

Questions:

Does your pet stay outside or inside?

What type of ground does your pet use: rocky, hills, flat?

What is the flooring like in your home?

Does your pet climb steps? How many? Inside or outside?

Does your pet sleep in your bed?

Does your pet ride in a car?

Does your pet walk long distances?

Source: Shearer 2011. Reproduced with permission of Elsevier

---

shares many attributes with suffering in that both are *mental states* attributable to an underlying unpleasant affect." McMillan goes on to state that "distress is a function of how the animal copes with the unpleasant affect elicited by aversive events rather than the quantity of aversive stimulation it actually receives." Coping and adaptation are the psychological and mental processes enabling humans and animals to function despite pain, distress, or suffering; animals experiencing a gradual progression of respiratory dysfunction, for example, may manifest unchanged mood despite their increasing physical discomfort. Assessing the patient's mental status must include tracking of the balance between negative emotional states and positive emotional states experienced by the patient, which is critical to assessing overall QOL.

An extensive discussion of QOL, pain, distress, and suffering is included in Chapter 4 in this volume.

Geriatric hospice patients, as well as ones with CNS disease, require special consideration. Anxiety and cognitive function may be compounded by a variety of medical conditions, medications, changes in sensory perception, and previous learning. Because behavior may be the only way to recognize signs of pain, illness, and cognitive decline, family members may

need assistance in recognizing the significance of behavior changes and the importance of reporting them promptly to the hospice team. Medical causes of behavioral signs of pain, illness, or cognitive decline are listed in Table 22.2 (Landsberg and DePorter 2011).

Delivery of Care: Nursing Care Considerations

Comfort for the Patient

The most important goal of palliative care and hospice is to help patients achieve a good QOL. Patients may suffer if a symptom is out of control or overwhelming, so controlling symptoms forms the foundation of comfort care for patients in palliative care and hospice. It is the veterinarian's responsibility to ensure that appropriate, aggressive, and comprehensive symptom management therapies are in place and continuously updated as the pet's disease progresses. Therapeutic goals for animals receiving palliative care are most effective when they are as specific as possible, as realistic as possible, and as relevant as possible for the individual patient. When a pet cannot effectively escape or minimize the ongoing stress of unmitigated pain and/or discomfort, a state of distress develops in which biologic functions are disrupted (Downing 2011). The adverse consequences of the pet's uncontrolled pain are determined by the severity and duration of the pain experience. *The number one priority for working with animals receiving palliative care is managing their pain.* All other therapeutic goals in palliative care are secondary to this one (Downing and Gaynor 2015).

Oral and Ocular Comfort

Mucous membranes are rich in nerve endings, and when affected, may be a source of significant discomfort for the HPC patient. The mucous membranes of the oral cavity and the eyes are relatively easy to monitor and to access with topical treatments to alleviate discomfort.

Table 22.2 Medical causes of behavioral signs of pain, illness, or cognitive decline.

Medical condition/medical presentation	Examples of behavioral signs
Neurologic: central (intracranial/extracranial), particularly if affecting forebrain, limbic/temporal, and hypothalamic areas; rapid eye movement, sleep disorders	Altered awareness, response to stimuli, loss of learned behaviors, house soiling, disorientation, confusion, altered activity levels, temporal disorientation, vocalization, soiling, change in temperament (fear, anxiety), altered appetite, altered sleep cycles, interrupted sleep
Partial seizures: temporal lobe epilepsy	Repetitive behaviors, self-traumatic disorders, chomping, staring, alterations in temperament (e.g. intermittent states of fear or aggression), tremors, shaking, interrupted sleep
Sensory dysfunction	Altered response to stimuli, confusion, disorientation, irritability/aggression, vocalization, house soiling, altered sleep cycles
Endocrine: hyperthyroid or hypothyroid, hyperadrenocorticism or hypoadrenocorticism, insulinoma, diabetes, testicular or adrenal tumors	Altered emotional state, irritability/aggression, lethargy, decreased response to stimuli, anxiety, house soiling/marking, night waking, decreased or increased activity, altered appetite, mounting
Metabolic disorders: hepatic/renal	Signs associated with organ affected: may be anxiety, irritability, aggression, altered sleep, house soiling, mental dullness, decreased activity, restlessness, increased sleep, confusion
Pain	Altered response to stimuli, decreased activity, restless/unsettled, vocalization, house soiling, aggression/irritability, self-trauma, waking at night
Peripheral neuropathy	Self-mutilation, irritability/aggression, circling, hyperesthesia
Gastrointestinal	Licking, polyphagia, pica, coprophagia, fecal house soiling, wind sucking, tongue rolling, unsettled sleep, restlessness
Urogenital	House soiling (urine), polydipsia, waking at night
Dermatologic	Psychogenic alopecia (cats), acral lick dermatitis (dogs), nail biting, hyperesthesia, other self-trauma (chewing/biting/sucking/scratching)

Source: Landsberg and De Porter 2011. Reproduced with permission of Elsevier.

Oral comfort is known to be important to human patients (Wrigley and Taylor 2012; Jucan and Saunders 2015). It is important in palliative care for pets to keep the mouth moist. Oral ulcers are painful and when they occur, a small amount of topical lidocaine gel or benzocaine gel (e.g. Orajel Mouth Sore Medicine™) can be used to reduce discomfort. Home dental care for pets in palliative care should be used only if significant oral pain is not present and the pet is receptive. Suitable products include children's or infant's soft toothbrushes, veterinary toothbrushes, finger toothbrushes, gauze pads, and other products designed for plaque removal. Oral hygiene products are available as toothpastes, liquids, gels, and sprays (Hoskins 2004).

Ocular diseases that can affect geriatric patients are keratoconjunctivitis sicca (KCS), cataracts, and retinal disease (Senior Care Guidelines Task Force 2005).

KCS is a condition caused by an aqueous tear deficiency or increased tear film evaporation, frequently resulting in persistent, mucopurulent conjunctivitis, and corneal ulceration and scarring. KCS occurs infrequently in cats but has been associated with chronic feline herpes-virus-1 infections. Topical therapy for KCS consists of artificial tear solutions, ointments, and, if there is no corneal ulceration, antibiotic–corticosteroid combinations. Canine KCS requires long-term topical lacrimogenic therapy. Puralube® Vet Ophthalmic Ointment, made by Pharmaderm Labs, provides a protective barrier and is used to provide relief from irritation as well as to protect the surface of the eye when tear production is decreased.

Nutrition

It is "ordinary care" to provide oral nutrition to the patient who wants to eat. That includes bringing food to the patient's mouth (using a spoon, syringe, or finger) if he or she is too weak to eat independently. For the pet who needs assistance, food and water can be moved closer and placed on a raised surface for easy access. Special attention to appearance, color, smell, and consistency may be needed to make food more appetizing (Villalobos 2011b).

Monitoring the patient's weight is essential. Malnutrition, weight loss, and cachexia develop quickly in anorectic animals. Educating pet owners regarding the pet's minimum caloric intake or resting energy requirement (RER) may help them recognize when their pet's nutritional intake is less than adequate. Appetite stimulants, such as mirtazapine or cyproheptadine, along with coaxing or encouraging intake by hand-feeding flavorful foods, might restore and maintain adequate nutrition intake. Box 22.4 offers information for calculating pets' daily caloric requirements.

IER should be adjusted according to body condition, and comparing weight loss or gain to target weight.

It is unethical and illegal to force a human patient to eat if the patient declines to do so, and animals in HPC should not be force fed when they are actively resisting. Administration of nutrition by an alternate route should be considered if the patient is refusing oral food intake. Feeding tubes may improve patient QOL and should be considered for anorexic animals as a treatment option. Feeding tubes should not, however, be offered because anorexic patients are "suffering from starvation" or "starving to death" (see discussion below). A balanced discussion with caregivers of the realities of artificial nutrition – pros and

---

Box 22.4   Calculating daily kilocalories (kcal) needed for dogs and cats.

Linear formula can be used for animals larger than 2 kg:

$$RER\, kcal\, /\, day^{-1}\left[(BWkg \times 30) + 70\right]$$

Allometric formula can be applied to dogs and cats of all weights:

$$RER\left(kcal\, /\, day^{-1}\right)70\left(BWkg^{0.75}\right)$$

RER is multiplied by 1–1.5 in dogs, and 1–1.2 in cats, to allow for increased nutritional demands of illness, stress, and healing. The end result is IER (Illness Energy Requirement).

Rough estimate is:

60–80 kcal/kg^{-1}/day^{-1} for tiny pets (less than 5 lb)

45–60 kcal/ kg^{-1}/day^{-1} for small dogs and cats (5–20 lb)

40–55 kcal/ kg^{-1}/day^{-1} for medium dogs (20–50 lb)

35–50 kcal/ kg^{-1}/day^{-1} for large dogs (50–100 lb)

30–45 kcal/ kg^{-1}/day^{-1} for giant dogs (>100 lb)

Source: Adapted from Mitchell 2010

cons – should precede any decision to place a feeding tube in an HPC patient.

Esophagostomy tubes are often well tolerated by animals, well managed by caregivers, and may result in improved patient QOL. For example, one of the authors treated a cat with liver cirrhosis and another cat with cystic liver tumors, whose families elected to place feeding tubes to manage medication administration and meet caloric needs. As a result, the cats felt better, resumed eating, and enjoyed good QOL for several months. Once a feeding tube has been placed, most patients can be discharged to home care. It is appropriate to teach the animal's caregiver tube management, the feeding protocol, the strategy for managing tube patency, and monitoring the entry site for infection (Marrelli 2005).

Considerable data are available from studies on physiological changes that occur during anorexia experienced by human patients with cancer and those that are in the early and final phases of active dying. Comparable data for animal patients is nonexistent. In the authors' opinion, the data available from human studies can serve as a guide in caring for animals in HPC until species-specific data become available.

There is no evidence that artificial nutrition alone improves functional ability or energy, relieves fatigue, or improves survival or symptom control in human cancer patients. The consequences of anorexia depend on the composition of what continues to be ingested. The patient who takes in no calories develops ketosis as fats and proteins are metabolized to an energy source. Anorectic ketosis, in contrast to diabetic ketoacidosis, is experienced as a mild euphoria or sense of well-being and analgesia. Supplemental carbohydrates or other foods interfere with this process.

Common reasons cited for instituting enteral nutrition in anorectic patients include to improve fatigue or "strength" and to avoid "starving to death." Patients, family, and some clinicians erroneously believe that the patient is weak because he or she is not eating. Further, they erroneously believe that if the patient does not eat, he or she will die suffering from starvation.

In contrast with conventional wisdom, there is no evidence that enteral nutrition improves energy level or survival in patients with progressive cancer. The pathophysiology underlying the causes of cancer cachexia and anorexia is not reversible. No study has demonstrated improved outcome of enteral feeding over oral feeding alone. Furthermore, in contrast to original expectations, percutaneous endoscopic gastrostomy (PEG) tubes increase the risk for aspiration in human patients rather than reduce it. The use of feeding tubes is associated with infection, obstruction, edema, ascites, aspiration pneumonia, and increased mortality.

In summary, there is no evidence that enteral nutrition improves survival or improves QOL for the advanced human cancer patient, and there are reasons to believe that the patient with anorexia associated with advanced cancer is not suffering because of it.

Hydration

One of the most common treatments associated with medical care is an intravenous infusion of fluids, indicated to maintain fluid and electrolyte balance when the patient is temporarily unable to drink adequate volumes. The administration of isotonic fluids subcutaneously is an equally efficacious way to administer fluids to HPC patients that are not in hypovolemic crisis. The most common *inappropriate* reason to consider intravenous fluids in the setting of symptom control is to prevent or treat thirst and to prevent "dehydrating to death"

Treating Fluid Deficit (Dehydration)

Treating dehydration is critical for stabilizing hypovolemic patients and to replace fluid losses due to acute or chronic diarrhea, vomiting, polyuria, third-space losses (e.g. into the gut), or insensible losses due to panting, pyrexia, or hyperthermia. As mentioned above, assessing dehydration in emaciated and geriatric patients may be challenging. When compatible history and physical examination findings are present, it is reasonable to assume 7% dehydration and treat accordingly. Regular reassessment followed by adjustment of therapy is required to safely rehydrate the patient.

Maintenance Fluids Administration

Maintenance fluid therapy is widely used in HPC to maintain patients in a normal state of hydration. Maintenance fluids administration should only be considered once a patient has been stabilized by volume replacement. Subcutaneous administration is equally efficacious to intravenous administration of maintenance fluid therapy and more suitable for home and outpatient care. Maintenance fluids administration makes a huge difference in many HPC patients' QOL.

If a feeding tube is placed, fluid therapy can be administered enterally.

Calculating Fluid Deficit

Replacement fluids are used to replace body water and electrolyte deficits. Their electrolyte balance is similar to extracellular fluid. It is important to remember that fluids administered intravenously equilibrate quickly with interstitial fluids and only 15–25% are left in the intravascular space within an hour of administration (Humm et al. 2008).

To calculate body fluid deficits and rates of maintenance fluid administration see Table 22.3.

Hygiene

Hygiene is of primary importance to QOL for the patient. Preventing urine and fecal skin irritation and preventing transmission and spread of infection are the primary health benefits for the animal. It is commonly presumed

Table 22.3 Dehydration assessment.

Dehydration	Physical exam findings
Normal	Normal skin elasticity
Mild (~5%)	Minimal loss of skin elasticity, slightly dry mucus membranes, eyes normal
Moderate (~8%)	Moderate loss of elasticity, mucus membranes are dry, pulses are rapid and weak, eye is sinking in orbital cavity
Severe (>10%)	Considerable loss of elasticity, severe sinking in orbital cavity, Increased heart rate, extremely dry mucous membranes, pulse is weak and rapid, low blood pressure, altered level of consciousness

Source: Davis et al. 2013. Reproduced with permission of Journal of the American Animal Hospital Association.

that there is always psychological benefit to maintenance of hygiene, by preventing the "loss of dignity" associated with the loss of life-long toileting habits, and preventing the unpleasant affect associated with the sensations and odors of uncleanliness. However, experience suggests that the psychological importance of hygiene varies greatly from patient to patient. Most hygiene maintenance tasks can be taught and delegated to the animals' caregivers (see discussion in the section in this chapter entitled "Nurses' Role as Educators").

Bedding

Clean, comfortable bedding adds to the patient's comfort level and QOL. Bedding should be changed daily (at least). Cages or runs should be cleaned daily as well. It has been well documented that frequent position changes and ample bedding decrease the incidence of pressure sores, edematous limbs, and joint and muscle stiffness. If the patient is unable to sit sternal, foam rolls, pads, wedges, or rolled-up towels can be placed beside the patient to help it maintain a sternal position and prevent it from falling over (Drum et al. 2014).

Bedding options can include:

- pet bed wrapped in a trash bag or a child's mattress cover, then covered with blankets
- old towels
- old bathmats (great because of rubber back lining)
- cheap fleece fabric/blankets

Check local garage sales and thrift stores for inexpensive items for pet bedding. Sometimes you can also find fleece fabric on sale. Buy several yards and cut it into bed-blanket size.

Environment

HPC treatments are primarily delivered at home or on an outpatient basis. In-home and outpatient treatments allow pets to spend time with their families in a comfortable low-stress environment, preserving the human–animal bond. Providing for the safety and comfort of patients in palliative and hospice care means focusing on the big picture of their lives at home and within the home environment, and detailed questioning of caregivers is critical to success. A home visit provides invaluable insights into the day-to-day life of the pet and his or her family.

A safe and comfortable environment consists of nonskid floor surfaces, such as area rugs, yoga mat runners, or interlocking foam tiles, which provide the additional traction that is often needed for independently getting up and getting around (Downing et al. 2011); gated staircases help to prevent falls; room temperature and humidity controlled to the patient's preference; background sounds or music (leaving the television or radio on at low volume) to minimize loneliness; and as much human and/or animal companionship for the patient as possible and as desired by the patient.

It is important to remember that HPC patients may experience episodic decompensation, necessitating occasional hospitalization (Jones 2014).

Mobility

Mobility allows HPC patients to perform most activities of daily living. Mobility contributes to QOL by enabling the patient to be where he wants and with whom he wants to be. It enables the patient to accommodate his or her preferences: for location, for interaction with the family and the world, for finding a comfortable body position. As described above, veterinary nurses make a significant contribution to maintaining pets' mobility by skillfully monitoring for any changes in functioning and strength, providing support to ensure correct pain medication administration, questioning caregivers, and observing for medication side effects.

Pets who become weaker and more unsteady as they reach their end of life deserve to have secure footing available to them. Nurses guide caregivers in making changes in the pet's environment such as providing nonskid floor surfaces and the use of "booties" or "toe grips," which provide additional traction (Villalobos 2011b).

An assistive device is a type of rehabilitation equipment designed to perform a particular function that makes caring for the mobility-impaired pet easier. Regardless of the type of device, any new piece of equipment must be introduced gradually to avoid complications such as aversion to the device secondary to fear of the novelty of the apparatus (Shearer 2011).

Veterinary HPC nurses are skilled at fitting assistive devices and performing some therapeutic exercises. They also train caregivers to perform the exercises and use the devices appropriately on their own. Below is a brief description of some therapeutic exercises and assistive devices veterinary nurses use to maximize patients' comfort. For additional information, see Chapter 20 and the references listed at the end of that chapter.

Range of Motion (ROM)

Range of motion (ROM) exercises are useful for diminishing the effects of disuse and immobilization. To maintain ROM, joints must be periodically moved through their available ranges, which also helps to maintain flexibility of associated muscles. Movement may be passive, active assisted, or active. In each situation a load is produced on soft tissues to help maintain articular cartilage, muscle, ligaments, and tendons in a healthy state. Be certain that the entire limb is supported to avoid any undue stresses to the involved joint (Starr 2013). ROM exercises are suitable for patients when recommended by a licensed veterinarian following a thorough physical examination and pain assessment.

Transitions
Providing support to help a patient that appeared to be incapable of rising up from a down position (a transition). The support needed to make the transition may be light or amount to almost full body support (Millis et al. 2014).

Standby Assisted Standing
The animal has the strength and motor control necessary to support itself against gravity in a standing position. It may still experience ataxia or weakness and have an occasional loss of balance, requiring standby assistance. The caregiver should be behind the animal or at the animal's side, ready to guard against a fall caused by a loss of balance. The caregiver does not assist the dog unless support is needed to prevent a fall (Millis et al. 2014).

Weight Shifting Exercises
Exercises performed to challenge the animal's balance while walking include encouraged weight shifting, manual uploading of a single limb, balance board, and exercise balls and rolls. The goal is to disturb the animal's balance just enough so the animal can recover, being careful not to force the animal to fall (Fox 2014).

Assisted Standing Exercises
The purpose of assisted standing is to encourage neuromuscular function, develop strength and stamina of supporting postural muscles, and enhance proprioception. Assisted standing is one of the first exercises prescribed for animals that are unable to independently rise from a recumbent position or support their own body weight. These exercises are only appropriate for patients with pain adequately controlled and physiologically stable. Animals with unstable injuries or that are in pain may further injure themselves (or the care provider) while struggling (Calvo 2012b).

Aids for Assisted Standing
Mobility slings and harnesses can be used to move pets more comfortably while minimizing injury to the pet and the pet owners (Shearer 2011). Slings and harnesses are designed to accommodate forelimbs, hind limbs, or all four legs. When choosing a sling, ease of use should be considered. Proper padding is also important for comfort. The skin should be inspected after each session in the sling to identify areas of potential skin irritation or breakdown (Millis et al. 2014).

Mobility Carts
These may be necessary for the palliative care patient as it continues to decline. This will enable the patient to continue with basic independence and provide stimulation to combat depression, common during end-of-life decline. The home environment may need to be altered to allow the animal to freely ambulate in the cart without encountering dangerous conditions. The animal's exercise area should be free of obstructions that could hinder the animal's ability to safely ambulate in the cart. Caution should be taken to prevent falls downstairs (Millis et al. 2014).

Nursing Care for Recumbent Patients

Recumbency is the inability to get up from a laying down position. It may be caused by ataxia or weakness. Recumbent patients require a nonslip floor surface for traction, soft bedding throughout to avoid decubital ulcers ("bed sores"), impeccable hygiene – keeping the skin clean from urine or feces – as well as frequent turning to help avoid complications such as hypostatic pneumonia or atelectasis (Olby 2010; Calvo 2012a).

Urination

Some recumbent patients cannot or will not urinate voluntarily and require bladder catheterization or manual expression. It is important to teach those caring for the patient how to palpate the bladder and assess bladder function.

Assessment of the bladder includes:

- palpation to assess bladder size before and after urination (training in palpation of bladders is important)
- recording of all urination in the medical record noting whether voluntary, expressed manually, or via a catheter
- preferably, urinalysis on admission and testing urine with a dipstick every two to four days for the presence of white blood cells and protein

Appropriate bladder management in recumbent patients includes:

- regular walks outside to encourage the patient to urinate, at least three times daily
- if unable to urinate, three bladder management options are available: manual expression every 4–6 hours (depending on bladder size), intermittent catheterization every 4–6 hours (depending on bladder size), or placement of indwelling catheter (urine bag to check every 4–6 hours and record output)
- keep the patient clean and dry at all times
- clip long hair if necessary to enable hygiene management and to allow accurate assessment of urine scalding developing/progressing.

Defecation

It is important to keep the patient clean and dry at all times. Stool softeners may be used to aid defecation if constipation is suspected.

Patients receiving opioid analgesia should be monitored closely for constipation.

Note: For dogs and cats that have trouble with holding their urine or bowels, it may be helpful to utilize items like disposable baby diapers or adult protective overnight briefs. These aid the owner in helping to protect the household from frequent soiling with urine and feces.

Respiration

Recumbency can lead to complications, including atelectasis and aspiration pneumonia, unrelated to the primary disease process. Patients with generalized lower motor neuron disease affecting the laryngeal and pharyngeal muscles and the esophagus (e.g. myasthenia gravis) are particularly predisposed to aspiration pneumonia, and preventative nursing care is crucial in the outcome of these patients.

Assessment of respiration in recumbent patients includes:

- Regular assessment and recording of the resting respiratory pattern, rate, and effort (degree of abdomen "pulling in" or retractions; nares and/or cheeks flaring) as often as every four to six hours in severely affected patients and less often in stable patients.
- If there is a suspicion of aspiration pneumonia, the temperature should be taken at least twice daily to monitor for pyrexia.

Measures to prevent respiratory complications include:

- Regular turning of the patient (every four to six hours) with adopting a sternal position as often as possible using appropriate padding. (Record each time the position was changed: e.g. from sternal to left lateral to sternal to right lateral to sternal.)
- Only offering water and food when the patient is in a sternal position. Someone should sit with the patient while eating. It is beneficial for the patient to adopt an upright position maintained for 30 minutes after

feeding to decrease the risk of regurgitation and aspiration pneumonia.

- If aspiration or hypostatic pneumonia is suspected and the patient can tolerate it, coupage should be performed each time the patient is turned.
- Thoracic auscultation should be performed at least once daily to identify abnormalities; these should be reported to the veterinarian immediately.
- Postural physiotherapy techniques can also be implemented to aid removal of excess secretions in combination with nebulization and coupage.

Skin Care

Recumbent patients are at risk of developing dermatitis secondary to urine scald and fecal soiling, and of developing decubital ulcers over pressure points. In addition, skin abrasions can develop if the patient is dragging her or his trunk or limb over rough ground.

Complications can be prevented by:

- Bedding that absorbs the liquid. This includes the use of incontinence pads, taking care to *avoid placing the pad directly against the patient's skin* because urine will disperse across the pad. This results in increased contact area and contact time, leading to urine scald. Acrylic absorbent bedding, such as synthetic fleece, should be placed between the patient and the incontinence pad, to allow for wicking of urine away from the skin and down into the pad.
- Appropriate soft padding around pressure points. Perform systematic bony point checks twice daily to monitor for skin redness or early development of decubital ulcers.
- Turning the patient from side to side regularly (every 4–6 hours). Massage pressure points to increase local blood flow.
- Clipping the hair in the perineal region if necessary.
- Prompt removal of soiled bedding.
- Appropriate bladder management.

- Keeping the patient dry and clean.
- Treatment of skin complications includes:
- Cleaning of dermatitis with a dilute chlorhexidine solution followed by thorough drying and application of a barrier cream.
- A dilute solution of bicarbonate of soda and cooled boiled water is very effective on urine scalds or irritation of testes. The area should be doused and left to dry at room temperature. This can be repeated three to four times daily.
- If decubital ulcers develop, ensure that pressure is no longer placed over that region. This can be done by creating a cushion for decubital ulcers ("doughnut").
- Debridement of dead tissue.
- Elizabethan collars to prevent the patient licking or chewing the region.

Mobilizing the Recumbent Patient

Efforts should be made to encourage patients to do as much as possible for themselves. Promoting independence increases confidence and early mobilization of patients. Patients who are unable to support themselves stand can be assisted using appropriate slings and harnesses while eating and drinking. This promotes strength and is an excellent opportunity for weight bearing or weight shifting exercise. Encouraging patients to ambulate and stretch for "cookies" (treats) is an easy early mobility exercise. For patients that are lacking proprioception, placing food near their paws and limbs can increase body awareness.

Nurses as Advocates and Educators

In addition to their medical roles, veterinary hospice nurses' responsibilities as educators and advocates are critical to the hospice team's success. In these roles, nurses act as a communication hub, connecting and facilitating understanding among all stakeholders in the animal HPC process. Nurses are charged with communicating the veterinarian's treatment recommendations to caregivers, ensuring caregivers understand the recommendations and are motivated to actively participate in carrying them out. Nurses are charged with interpreting the patient's condition for the caregivers ("Ms. Jones, Fifi is definitely experiencing some pain, even if she's not crying") and reporting it to the rest of the hospice team ("Last time I saw Fifi, Ms. Jones reported administering gabapentin only when Fifi whines"). Last but not least, nurses are in charge of communicating to the hospice team the caregivers' goals for their animals, their personal values and cultural background that must be acknowledged and respected when exploring specific recommendations for care ("Ms. Jones suffers from chronic pain herself and frequently experiences adverse effects when she takes the medications prescribed for her. She doesn't want Fifi to experience similar adverse reactions.")

Nurses' Role as Advocates for Patient and for the Caregiver

Hospice care requires a veterinary nurse to go beyond medical skills and deliver supportive psychosocial care, understand family dynamics, and offer a nonjudgmental approach toward personal belief systems. Additional training in these areas is highly desirable.

Both animal patients and human caregivers need advocacy when they are powerless, helpless, vulnerable, or unable to communicate clearly, all of which are frequently encountered in both animals at the end of life and their caregivers. The veterinary nurse strives to see the patient as a unique sentient being with individual needs and preferences, and to understand the caregiver as a unique human being. Communication skills such as use of open-ended questions, reflective listening, expression of empathy, and attention to nonverbal cues are critical in achieving caregiver understanding. The nurse as advocate then uses this understanding to

intervene on the patient's and caregiver's behalf, taking on the role of communicator and translator of information and feelings. Veterinary nurses also help caregivers understand what the doctor said during the consultation, and help caregivers understand their own feelings in the situation (Hebert et al. 2011). Veterinary nurses must be willing and able to engage in difficult dialogs with people who are highly attached to animals who are seriously ill and may be at the end of their life. When appropriate, they may suggest or encourage caregivers to consider additional sources of support that may be available in their community, especially in the areas of spiritual support, bereavement counseling, complimentary modalities, and respite care. A proficient veterinary hospice nurse is familiar with specific resources within the community that caregivers can be confidently referred to when specific skills are needed (Adams 2013).

Nurses' Role as Educators

The veterinary nursing staff can be trained to provide information on a wide range of topics, including techniques for medicating animals, observation of animal behavior, activities of daily living, symptom recognition, and death and dying (Shanan 2015).

Like veterinary nurses' medical role, their role as educators involves all phases of the HPC process, starting at the initial contact between caregiver, animal, and the hospice team, through planning and delivery of care, patients' assessments, and participation in end-of-life decision-making. During the hospice intake interview, history taking is followed by the education portion of the interview. This includes providing answers to questions clients may have (whether conveyed explicitly by the client or not) and ensuring clients understand what has been discussed in the visit (Cornell and Kopcha 2007).

Veterinary nurses teach caregivers the necessary level of skill in performing many animal care tasks. Those include administration of oral, rectal, and injectable medications; attention to the details of medication delivery is critical to ensure the appropriate delivery of prescribed medications, food, and supplements. Other animal care tasks include bathing, setting up clean comfortable bedding, using slings and boots, recognizing subtle behavioral signs of pain, expressing flaccid bladders, and turning recumbent animals. Veterinary nurses must also be adept at teaching caregivers practical aspects of animal behavior and handling. Any task that is unfamiliar, awkward, or uncomfortable for the caregiver must be practiced until competency is demonstrated. Having the opportunity to initially perform the task once or several times in the presence of a supportive veterinary nurse frequently convinces anxious, insecure caregivers that they can perform the task (Shanan 2015). It is important to educate caregivers how to assess hydration by evaluating the moistness of the mucus membranes (gums), as well as demonstrating the skin-pinch method. Subcutaneous (SC) fluid injection techniques should be taught as a supportive and palliative treatment when dehydration is suspected (Villalobos 2011b).

Awareness of Signs of Pain

One of veterinary nurses' primary responsibilities in HPC is to increase caregivers' awareness of the strong connection between pain and the animal's QOL. Educating caregivers to recognize the sometimes-subtle manifestations of pain in their animal's behavior is a primary responsibility of the veterinary nurse (Shanan 2015). Repeatedly reinforcing the message and pointing out the behaviors when they occur is critical to achieving client adherence and is an important part of the veterinary hospice nurse's role. It is *not* veterinary nurses' responsibility, and it is not appropriate for nurses to offer their opinion on if and when euthanasia should be considered.

Hygiene and Safety

Caregivers need guidance in safely handling wounds on their pets, whether those wounds are infected or not.

It is important for the veterinary healthcare team to take the time to educate pet owners and their families in the basics of universal precautions and good hygiene practices as pets enter palliative and hospice care. Universal precautions are infection control guidelines designed to protect people from diseases spread by blood and certain body fluids. It is best to assume that all blood and body fluids are infectious for blood-borne diseases (Downing et al. 2011). Universal precautions are straightforward and easy to implement. For instance, when cleaning up blood, urine, stool, vomit, or wound secretions, the following steps should be taken:

- put on disposable gloves
- wipe up blood or body fluids with absorbent paper towels
- place contaminated paper towels in a plastic garbage bag
- clean and rinse area with whatever disinfectant is typically used
- remove gloves and place into garbage bag
- secure bag with tie
- dispose of plastic garbage bag
- wash hands
- use a mask when cleaning up inhaled irritants
- keep young children safe from any urine, stool, or vomit contamination

Sharps containers should be provided to the caregiver if injections are part of the daily care. Owners should be supplied with a snap-on fabric muzzle fitted to the pet in case the pet becomes painful but needs to be handled or moved. Any humans in the household who are immune compromised (e.g. chemotherapy, human immunodeficiency virus/acquired immune deficiency syndrome, rheumatoid arthritis) or pregnant should be excused from handling the pet's waste if possible (Downing et al. 2011).

Death and Dying

Caring for animals facing imminent death is guided by the same principles that guide caring for all hospice patients: maximizing patient physical and emotional comfort so the death experience is as peaceful, dignified, pain free, and loving as possible; and supporting the animal's caregivers so they experience peace and confidence in their own conduct and decision-making when facing the imminent death of their loved one. Emotional support, guidance, and education are provided by the hospice team to maximize caregiver's sense of having made the right choices and to minimize guilt, internal conflict, and complicated grief.

The choice between euthanasia and allowing the animal to experience a hospice-supported natural death can be difficult for highly attached caregivers, and depends on their life experiences, culture, and beliefs. It is imperative that both euthanasia and natural death be discussed as soon as possible once a "caregiver-hospice provider relationship" has been established. A discussion about euthanasia should take place with those caregivers who are planning on a natural death of their pet; likewise, the option of natural death should be discussed with caregivers planning on euthanasia.

When discussing options for how the animal's life will end, veterinary nurses must skillfully and sensitively provide an appropriate degree of detail regarding possible or probable outcomes, to minimize fear or prejudice (Lagoni et al. 1994). Any attempt – intentional or unintentional, conscious, or unconscious – to impose personal beliefs on a caregiver facing this difficult decision carries the risk of making his or her experience more painful than necessary.

When educating families in preparation for a hospice-supported natural death, a variety of likely and less likely scenarios during the last hours (and sometimes days) of the animal's life should be discussed. Protocols can be provided to ensure dying animals and their families are given the environment and the skilled care they need. Recognizing and treating pain is of utmost importance. However, veterinary hospice nurses must be familiar with natural death and skilled in helping caregivers understand that what *they experience* when the patient is actively dying may be very different from the *patient's experience*.

Educating clients about the euthanasia procedure itself and encouraging them to ask questions is an important and sensitive task. Information should be provided about the drugs that will be administered and by which route, and how long it will take for sedation and death, respectively, to occur.

Caregivers should be informed that the animal's eyes may not close at death, that agonal breathing or vocalization may occur, and that bladder and bowel control may be lost. Client handouts with community resources such as pet loss help lines, pet loss groups, and online support should be made available (Jones 2014). This can be done as early as during the first hospice meeting. It is best practice to provide families with available resources prior to the passing of the pet, as anticipatory grief can be as debilitating as the actual loss.

Conclusion

Veterinary technician nurses play an integral role in the care of HPC patients. In their medical role, veterinary HPC nurses provide professional care for seriously ill animals and support for their owners. They are trained to provide a high standard of nursing care based on a sound knowledge of the patient's condition and her or his individual needs. Veterinary nurses enable patients to achieve the best possible QOL, whatever their condition (QAA 2019). In their roles as advocates and educators, veterinary HPC nurses utilize the knowledge, understanding, and sensitivity required for communicating with the patient's emotionally vulnerable caregivers. Veterinary nurses can offer guidance and empower caregivers to make the difficult decisions they face, and must be emotionally accessible and present when most needed by caregivers. The nurse must intervene on the patient's and caregiver's behalf, taking on the role of communicator and translator of information and feelings.

References

Adams, V.H. (2013) A look at a veterinary hospice team. Proceedings 85th Annual Western Veterinary Conference. Las Vegas, NV.

American Animal Hospital Association/ American Association of Feline Practitioners (AAHA/AAFP) (2015) Pain management guidelines for dogs and cats. *J. Feline Med. Surg.*, 17, 251–72

American Association of Feline Practitioners (AAFP) (2010) Veterinary hospice care for cats. *J. Feline Med. Surg.*, 12, 728–730.

American Veterinary Medical Association (AVMA) (2015) *The Human-Animal Interaction and Human-Animal Bond.* Available at: http://www.avma.org/KB/ Policies/Pages/The-Human-Animal-Bond. aspx (accessed April 2022).

American Veterinary Medical Association (AVMA) (2016) *Guidelines for Veterinary End-of-life Care.* Available at: https://www. avma.org/resources-tools/avma-policies/ veterinary-end-life-care (accessed April 2022).

Calvo, G. (2012a) Rehabilitation nursing goals. *Proceedings WSAVA/FECAVA/BSAVA World Congress*, BSAVA 2012, Birmingham, UK.

Calvo, G. (2012b) Neurological conditions case studies. *Proceedings WSAVA/FECAVA/BSAVA World Congress*, BSAVA 2012, Birmingham, UK.

Cornell, C.C. and Kopcha, M. (2007) Client- veterinarian communication: skills for client centered dialogue and shared decision making. *Vet. Clin. North Am. Small Anim. Pract.*, 37, 37–47.

Davis, H., Jensen, T., Johnson, A., et al. (2013) 2013 AAHA/AAFP fluid therapy guidelines for dogs and cats. *J. Am. Anim. Hosp. Assoc.*, 49, 149–159.

Downing, R. (2011) Pain management for veterinary palliative care and hospice patients. *Vet. Clin. North Am. Small Anim. Pract.*, 41, 531–550.

Downing, R. and Gaynor, J.S. (2015) Therapeutic goals. Handbook of Veterinary Pain Management, 3 (eds James S. Gaynor and William W. Muir III). Elsevier: St. Louis, MO, p. 438.

Downing, R., Adams, V.H., and McClenaghan, A.P. (2011) Comfort, hygiene, and safety in veterinary palliative care and hospice. *Vet. Clin. North Am. Small Anim. Pract.*, 41, 619–634.

Drum, M., Werbe, B., McLucas, K., and Millis, D. (2014) Nursing care of the rehabilitation patient. Canine Rehabilitation and Physical Therapy, 2 (eds D. Millis and D. Levine). Elsevier/Saunders: Philadelphia, PA, p. 277.

Fox, S.M. (2014) Physical rehabilitation in the management of musculoskeletal disease. In: Pain Management in Small Animal Medicine. CRC Press: Boca Raton, FL, p. 250.

Gaynor, J.S. and Muir, W.W. (2015) Handbook of Veterinary Pain Management, 3. St. Louis, MO: Elsevier/Mosby.

Goggs, R., Humm, K., and Hughes, D. (2008) Fluid therapy in small animals 1. Principles and patient assessment. *In Pract.*, 30, 16–19.

Goldberg, M.E. (2010) The fourth vital sign in all creatures great and small, *NAVTA J.* 2010, 31–54.

Goldberg, M.E. and Shaffran, N. (2015) Pain Management for Veterinary Technicians and Nurses. Wiley and Sons, Ames, IA.

Hebert, K., Moore, H., and Rooney, J. (2011) The nurse advocate in end-of-life care. *Ochsner J.*, 11, 325–329.

Hoskins, J. (2004) The oral cavity and dental disease, Geriatrics and Gerontology of the Dog and Cat, 2. Saunders/Elsevier, St. Louis, MO, p. 154.

Humm, K., Goggs, R., and Hughes, D. (2008) Fluid therapy in small animals 2. Crystalloid solutions. *In Pract.*, 30, 85–91.

Jones, K. (2014) Pain management in hospice and palliative care. Pain Management in Veterinary Practice, 1 (eds C.M. Egger, L. Love, and T. Doherty). Wiley: Ames, IA, pp. 431–436.

Jucan, A.C. and Saunders, R.H. (2015) Maintaining oral health in palliative care patients. *Ann. Long-Term Care Clin. Care Aging*, 23, 15–20.

Kata, C., Rowland, S., and Goldberg, M.E. (2015) Pain recognition in companion species, horses, and livestock. In: Pain Management for Veterinary Technicians and Nurses, 1 (eds M.E. Goldberg and N. Shaffran). Wiley: Ames, IA, p. 16.

Lagoni, L., Butler, C., and Hetts, S. (1994) The Human-Animal Bond and Grief. W.B. Saunders: Philadelphia, PA.

Landsberg, G.M. and DePorter, T. (2011) Clinical signs and management of anxiety, sleeplessness, and cognitive dysfunction in the senior pet. *Vet. Clin. North Am. Small Anim. Pract.*, 41, 565–590.

Marrelli, T.M. (2005) Hospice and Palliative Care Handbook. Elsevier Mosby: St. Louis, MO, pp. 80, 81, 358, 382.

McKune, C.M., Murrell, J.C., Nolan, A.M., et al. (2015) Nociception and pain. In: Veterinary Anesthesia and Analgesia, 5 (eds K.A. Grimm, L.A. Lamont, W.J. Tranquilli, et al.). Wiley: Ames, IA, pp. 584–585.

McMillan, F. (2005) Stress, distress, and emotion: distinctions and implications for mental wellbeing. In: Mental Health and Well-Being in Animals (ed. F. McMillian). Wiley: Ames, IA, pp. 93–111.

Millis, D.L., Drum, M., and Levine, D. (2014) Therapeutic exercises: early limb use exercises. In: Canine Rehabilitation and Physical Therapy, 2 (eds D. Millis and D. Levine). Elsevier/Saunders: Philadelphia, PA, p. 496.

Mitchell, K.D. (2010) Enteral feeding in dogs and cats: Indications, principles and techniques. Proceedings CVC in Kansas City, KS.

Ogunkorode A. (2019) Chapter 3: Global perspectives on palliative care: Nigerian context, In: Hospice Palliative Home Care and Bereavement Support: Nursing Interventions and Supportive Care, editors: Lorraine Holtslander, Shelley Peacock, Jill Bally, Springer Nature Switzerland AG, Cham, Switzerland, p. 42

Olby, N. (2010) Patients with neurological disorders. In: BSAVA Manual of Canine and Feline Rehabilitation, Supportive and Palliative Care (eds S. Lindley and P. Watson). BSAVA Publications: Gloucester, UK, p. 169.

Quality Assurance Agency (QAA) (2019) Subject Benchmark Statement – Veterinary Nursing. Quality Assurance Agency for Higher Education. Available at www.qaa.ac.uk/docs/qaa/subject-benchmark-statements/subject-benchmark-statement-veterinary-nursing.pdf?sfvrsn=def3c881_6 (accessed April 2022).

Reid J, Nolan AM, Hughes JML, Lascelles D, Pawson P, and Scott EM. (2007), Development of the short-form Glasgow composite measure pain scale (CMPS-SF) and derivation of an analgesic intervention score, *Anim. Welfare*, 16(S), 97–104.

Reid, J., Scott, E.M., Calvo, G., and Nolan, A.M. (2017) Definitive Glasgow acute pain scale for cats: validation and intervention level. *Vet. Rec.*, 180, 449.

Senior Care Guidelines Task Force (2005) AAHA senior care guidelines for dogs and cats. *J. Am. Anim. Hosp. Assoc.*, 41, 81–91.

Shaffran, N. and Grubb, T. (2010) Pain management. In: McCurnin's Clinical Textbook for Veterinary Technicians, 7 (eds J.M. Bassert and D.M. McCurnin). Saunders/Elsevier, St. Louis, MO, p. 859.

Shanan, A. (2015) Pain management for end of life care. In: Pain Management for Veterinary Technicians and Nurses, 1 (eds M.E. Goldberg and N. Shaffran). Wiley: Ames, IA, pp. 331–339.

Shanan, A. et al. (2016) 2016 AAHA/IAAPC end of life care guidelines for dogs and cats. Available at: https://www.aaha.org/globalassets/02-guidelines/end-of-life-care/2016_aaha_iaahpc_eolc_guidelines.pdf (accessed April 2022)

Shearer, T.S. (2011) Managing mobility challenges in palliative and hospice care patients. *Vet. Clin. North Am. Small Anim. Pract.*, 41, 609–617.

Starr, L. (2013) Rehabilitation for geriatric patients. In: Canine Sports Medicine and Rehabilitation (eds C.M. Zink and J. Van Dyke). Wiley: Ames, IA, pp. 362–366.

Todd-Jenkins, K. and Bentz, A.I. (2013) Geriatric and hospice care: supporting the aged and dying patient. In: McCurnin's Clinical Textbook for Veterinary Technicians, 8 (J.M. Bassert and J. Thomas). Saunders/Elsevier: St. Louis, MO, 1358.

Villalobos, A.E. (2011a) Quality-of-life assessment techniques for veterinarians. *Vet. Clin. North Am. Small Anim. Pract.*, 41, 519–529.

Villalobos, A.E. (2011b) Assessment and treatment of nonpain conditions in life-limiting disease. *Vet. Clin. North Am. Small Anim. Pract.*, 41, 551–563.

World Health Organization (2022) *WHO Definition of Palliative Care*. Available at: http://www.who.int/cancer/palliative/definition/en (accessed April 2022).

Wrigley, H. and Taylor, E.J. (2012) Oral care for hospice patients with severe trismus. *Clin. J. Oncol. Nurs.*, 16, 113–114.

Further Reading

Adams, V.H. (2011) Meet the faces of hospice: the team, the patients. Proceedings 17th International Veterinary Emergency and Critical Care Society, San Antonio, TX.

Foster, S.C. (2007) The definition and classification of dry eye disease: report of the definition and classification Subcommittee of the International dry eye Workshop (2007). *Ocul. Surf.*, 5, 75–92.

Gelatt, K.N. (2014) Nasolacrimal and lacrimal apparatus. The Merck Veterinary Manual. Available at: https://www.merckvetmanual.com/eye-diseases-and-disorders/ophthalmology/nasolacrimal-and-lacrimal-apparatus (Accessed: October 2022).

Hancock, C.G., McMillan, F.D., and Ellenbogen, T.R. (2004) Owner services and hospice care. In: Geriatrics and Gerontology of the Dog and Cat, 2 (ed J.D. Hoskins). Saunders: St. Louis, MO, pp. 5–17.

Lewis, A., Wallace, J., Deutsch, A., and King, P. (2015) Improving the oral health of frail and functionally dependent elderly. *Aust. Dent. J.*, 60,(1 Suppl), 95–105.

Marcellin-Little, D.J. and Levine, D. (2014) Devices for ambulation assistance in companion animals. In: Canine Rehabilitation and Physical Therapy, 2 (eds D. Millis and D. Levine). Elsevier/Saunders: Philadelphia, PA, p. 496.

Rawlings, C.A. (1993). Percutaneous placement of a midcervical esophagostomy tube: new technique and representative cases. *J. Am. Anim. Hosp. Assoc.*, 29, 526–530.

Wanamaker, B.P. and Massey, K.L. (2015) General pharmacology. In: Applied Pharmacology for Veterinary Technicians, 5. (eds B.P. Wanamaker and K.L. Massey). Saunders/Elsevier: St. Louis, MO, pp. 6–8.

23

Comfort Care During Active Dying

Gail Pope and Amir Shanan, DVM

Natural Death and Euthanasia

When an emotional attachment exists between the animal and a human caregiver, the decision whether the animal's life should end by euthanasia or natural death is made by the caregiver (used in this text interchangeably with the terms pet owner or pet parent) in collaboration with the hospice team (veterinarian, veterinary nurses and technicians, and others).

Animal hospice and palliative care shares many of its clinical, philosophical, and ethical principles and objectives with human hospice and palliative care. Animal hospice and palliative care is unique, however, in that euthanasia is a legal and widely practiced intervention aimed at relieving an animal's suffering by ending life peacefully and humanely when other efforts to alleviate suffering have failed or cannot be pursued. Under such circumstances, euthanasia is recognized as an acceptable option, consistent with animal hospice principles.

The choice between euthanasia and allowing the animal to experience a hospice-supported natural death can be a difficult one and depends on the caregiver's life experiences, culture, and beliefs. It is imperative that both euthanasia and natural death be discussed as soon as possible once a "caregiver/hospice provider relationship" has been established.

A discussion about euthanasia should take place with those caregivers who are planning a natural death for their pet; likewise, the option of natural death should be discussed with caregivers planning on euthanasia.

Animal hospice team members must present all options carefully and provide detail as to the possible or probable outcomes. Options should be described sensitively, however, and with an appropriate degree of detail to minimize fear or prejudice (Lagoni et al. 1994). Any attempt – intentional or unintentional, conscious, or unconscious – by the hospice team to impose personal beliefs on a caregiver facing this difficult decision carries the risk of making his or her experience more painful than necessary. Even attempts to sway caregivers toward the hospice provider's personal preferences is unethical (see Chapter 7 in this book for more on ethical decision-making).

Many veterinarians have been taught that euthanasia is the kindest, most humane thing to do for animals that are believed to be near the end of life. This school of thought is anchored in several assumptions: that animals have no concepts of past and future, nor concepts of life and death, and therefore have no individual preferences regarding whether their lives should continue or be terminated; that if animals had such concepts and preferences, they would have no way to communicate those

Hospice and Palliative Care for Companion Animals: Principles and Practice, Second Edition.
Edited by Amir Shanan, Jessica Pierce, and Tamara Shearer.
© 2023 John Wiley & Sons, Inc. Published 2023 by John Wiley & Sons, Inc.
Companion website: www.wiley.com/go/shanan/palliative

to humans; that even if they were able to communicate their preferences to humans, their judgment regarding what is best for themselves is inferior to humans' judgment of what is best for them; lastly, that terminating life is an acceptable and desirable way to protect animals not only from ongoing suffering, but also from anticipated future suffering. The idea that "we don't want animals to suffer" serves as a rationalization for choosing euthanasia when an animal is uncomfortable but NOT suffering "yet." It is also a rationalization for caregivers and veterinarians who prefer to avoid the burden associated with providing patient-centered, end-of-life care.

As discussed in detail in Chapter 4, "Quality of life in the animal hospice and palliative care patient," recent scientific research strongly indicates that many mammalian species have the capabilities to feel and think. Considering these findings, it is reasonable to assume that animals also have the capability to exhibit behaviors reflective of whether or not they would like to continue living when experiencing discomfort, disability and/or distress. An assumption consistent with current knowledge would be that some animals would prefer to be euthanized, some would prefer to take the risk of additional discomfort hoping to continue life in their familiar surroundings with their loved one/s (as many humans do), and some animals wouldn't have a preference. The reader is encouraged to review Chapter 4 for an in-depth discussion about the relationships between pain, suffering, quality of life, and animals' individual preferences and will to live, as they apply to making end of life decisions for animals.

Findings from human hospice repeatedly show higher patient QOL and satisfaction with care in hospice compared to non-hospice medical care at the end of life (Steele et al. 2005; Bretscher et al. 1999; Wright et al. 2010). Some studies show increased longevity in hospice compared to non-hospice medical care (Temel et al. 2010). A significant number of human hospice patients (5–15%) are "discharged live"

for a variety of reasons (Teno et al. 2014). The majority (79%) of hospice live discharges occurred because the patients' condition had stabilized or improved to the extent that they no longer met hospice eligibility criteria (Kutner et al. 2004). This is a significant group of patients who fare better than their physicians' prognosis.

Those numbers (5–15%) might be suggestive of the numbers of animals who are euthanized based on inaccurate assumptions. In the course of our clinical work, the authors have come across many animals that had met their owner's or veterinarian's criteria for euthanasia before presentation for hospice care. Once in hospice care, their condition stabilized with good palliation, and they regained acceptable quality of life – some of them for months and even years (Shanan unpublished data; Pope unpublished data).

Misconceptions about hospice care and lack of knowledge about its benefits are barriers that prevent both human and animal patients and their attached, loving caregivers from enjoying the best possible care at the end of life. This includes pervasive lack of knowledge about the realities of death and dying without euthanasia.

This chapter describes the processes of dying without euthanasia, and the means of caring for patients dying a hospice-supported natural death without euthanasia. We will summarize the physiologic changes that occur as patients are dying; then describe some approaches to the management of associated symptoms; and lastly, discuss care at the time of death. Euthanasia is discussed in detail in the next chapter, "Euthanasia in Animal End-of-Life Care." The reader is encouraged to refer to the Glossary section of the IAAHPC Guidelines (IAAHPC 2017) for the authors' definitions of natural death and euthanasia. The emotional burden of caregiving experienced by animal hospice patients' human caregivers is covered in Chapters 25 and 26 in this book. Coping with loss, grief, and bereavement after the loss of a pet is a topic that has been covered by many excellent books and articles in the past several decades.

Goals of Caring for the Dying Patient

Caring for animals facing imminent death is guided by the same principles that guide caring for all hospice patients: maximizing patient physical and emotional comfort is the highest priority, with the primary goal being a death experience that is as peaceful, dignified, pain-free, and loving as possible.

A secondary but equally important goal is to support the animal's caregivers, so they experience peace and confidence in their own conduct and decision-making when facing the imminent death of their loved one. Emotional support, guidance, and education are provided to maximize the caregiver's sense of having made the right choices, and to minimize guilt, internal conflict, emotional trauma, and complicated grief.

Advance Preparation and Education of Caregivers and Hospice Team

Family caregivers, hospice service providers, and volunteers need as much advance preparation and education as possible for the hospice team to accomplish end-of-life care goals. Preparedness is particularly important when the patient is at home, because when death is imminent it is frequently preferable that patients remain with caregivers they know, rather than be transferred to a medical facility. When the home care team is well prepared, unnecessary admission for hospital care during the last hours of life can be avoided.

Clinical competence, willingness to educate, and calm, empathetic reassurance are critical to helping patients and families in the last hours of an animal's life. Team members who are inexperienced in any area will need specific training. Everyone who participates must be knowledgeable about:

- The patient's health status
- The goals for care as defined by the animal's primary caregiver in collaboration with the hospice veterinarian
- The projected time course for the patient's dying process as well as its unpredictability
- The clinical and behavioral changes associated with different types of active dying that may affect the individual patient
- The options for managing the clinical signs and syndromes associated with the dying process

When the patient is admitted to hospice care early enough, this information will have been deliberated during the hospice team's regular interdisciplinary meetings (see Chapter 3 in this book) and documented in the patient's medical record, providing an effective, detailed, and convenient source of information for the entire team's preparation.

All parties involved must plan for a variety of likely and less likely scenarios during the last hours (and sometimes days) of the animal's life. Protocols must be in place to ensure dying animals and their families are provided with the environment and the skilled care they need. Recognizing and treating pain is of utmost importance. However, members of the animal hospice and palliative care team must understand and be skilled in helping caregivers understand that *their experience* when witnessing the patient actively dying may be very different from the *patient's experience*.

Barbara Karnes, renowned end of life nurse and educator, stated: "There is a misconception that dying is painful and therefore pain medicine/narcotics should be used routinely in the last days to weeks of life. Dying does not cause pain; disease causes pain. Not all diseases create pain, so we need to look at a person's disease history to determine if we are witnessing actual physical pain, flu-like discomfort, or our own fears as we watch the labor of dying." This knowledge can be profoundly reassuring to both caregivers and hospice team members.

Written materials can provide additional support to caregivers when experts are not present. When caregivers are educated and prepared for the experience of witnessing and supporting an animal's dying process, they experience a sense of final gift giving and good parenting. If unprepared and unsupported, caregivers unnecessarily spend energy worrying; and if things do not go as hoped for, they may feel frustration, fear, or guilt long after the death. (See Chapter 25 "Caregivers' Emotional Burden" in this book for additional information). It is important to recognize the changes in behavior, appearance, and physiological function that are commonly a part of the dying process and are not to be feared as a medical failure.

The role of animal hospice team members shares some elements with that of birthing midwives. Birth and death are both moments of great vulnerability; and some of the preparation that is encouraged for birth is also valuable in preparation for death. Through this preparation and deeper understanding of the dying process, it is possible for pain to exist yet be lessened by tenderness, love, and compassion (Hayhurst 2010).

Distraction, relaxation, and social support are known to help humans suffering chronic pain (Roditi and Robinson 2011). Those are meant to be used in conjunction with pharmaceutical and physical therapies to manage pain. Similarly, when death is a long and laborious process, gentle touching, massaging, encouragement to relax and let go, gentle talking and singing, and cradling all may be greatly comforting as adjuncts to medical pain management efforts. The hospice team members in attendance should strive to practice inner stillness and be peacefully present, putting aside personal pains or sorrows. Animal hospice is a sacred service requiring a great deal of work and love.

The last days are a time most precious for caregivers to spend with their beloved animal.

Every effort should be made to focus at this time on any manifestations of peace, love, joy, celebration, and awareness of the past, present, and future of the relationship that will continue – though in a very different form.

Desirable Environment of Care

The environment in which care for imminently dying patients is provided should be conducive to privacy and intimacy and allow family and friends access to the dying beloved animal around the clock without disturbing others. During the last hours (and sometimes days) of their lives, all patients require skilled care around the clock, under the direct or indirect supervision of a licensed veterinarian. All members of the hospice team must be available to lend support if requested. This level of care can be provided in any setting if providers, caregivers, and others are appropriately prepared and supported throughout the process.

Preparedness is particularly important when the patient is at home to avoid unnecessary transfer to another facility when death is imminent. Preparation of the home or hospital environment should include:

- Providing necessary medications, equipment, and hygiene supplies
- Careful adjustment of the room temperature to keep the animal more comfortable
- Promoting relaxation and minimizing stress with environmental enrichment, augmented by using canine or feline appeasing pheromones, (Kim et al. 2010) flower essences, and essential oils (diffused into the room air when possible)
- Avoiding noise outside and inside the room and, when available, playing soft music. Music designed by psychoacoustic experts has been shown to minimize anxiety and lower heart rate (Wells et al. 2002; Boone and Quelch 2003).
- Avoiding any unnecessary disturbances to the patient and family

Animal hospice providers are expected to set high standards in designing the environment of care for imminently dying patients and serve as role models to all other animal care providers in this regard. As qualified animal hospice services are slowly becoming more widely available, it will be the responsibility of all veterinary practices to offer clients the option of referral to such a service for the animal's end-of-life care if they cannot provide that care themselves.

Prognostication

Although we often sense that the death of an animal patient will come in a matter of minutes, hours, days, or weeks, death is not possible to predict. Some human and animal patients are said to appear to be waiting for someone to visit or for a particular event to take place, and then die soon afterward. Others experience unexplained improvements and live longer than expected.

When faced with the inevitability of the death of a beloved pet, most caregivers want "to do the right thing." Often, however, they find themselves preoccupied with how to accomplish that objective and therefore highly value any prognostic information. To that end, providers should give caregivers a general idea of the disease's trajectory and how long the patient might live, but caregivers must always be advised about the inherent variability and unpredictability of the dying process – when it will start, what progression it will follow, and when it will end. An effective tool for helping caregivers cope with this unpredictability is the concept of preparing for multiple possible "scenarios." We cannot predict which of these scenarios they will be faced with or when; but whatever happens, and whenever it happens – it *will* be a "scenario" they have prepared for.

The discussion below provides information to help providers and caregivers prepare for the dying process.

Changes During Early and Late Stages of Active Dying

Available Information

Public and scientific discourse about the details of what an animal is experiencing during active dying, especially in the final phase of active dying, has suffered from lack of direct empirical data. Obtaining information about the internal experience of nonverbal patients during a once in a lifetime event for which no follow up observations are available has proven to be an insurmountable challenge to the scientific methods of investigation available to date.

Rapidly accumulating scientific evidence suggests that many mammalian species are capable of sensations, feelings, and emotions that have much in common with those of humans. The reader is encouraged to review Chapter 4 "Quality of Life in the Animal Hospice and Palliative Care Patient" for additional information. While proof may be difficult to achieve, the evidence available suggests that inferring from human experience what animals may experience can be quite informative and can complement information gathered by observing animals' behavior. The authors of this chapter have found the use of carefully assessed evidence about human patients' experience helpful in their clinical work caring for animals in the last hours of life.

Changes During Early Stages of Active Dying

Physical Changes

As animals approach the time of death, food and water intake habits change; what worked only a few weeks or days ago may not work today. It is well documented in human hospice that as patients get close to the end of life their desire to eat declines, often to the point of having no interest in eating at all. As appetite decreases and food becomes less appealing, we should become creative in seeking ways to tempt the palate; however, we must also be watchful for the time when eating has become a detriment to the patient. An increased desire for water, or no water intake at all, may be seen in the same patient in random succession.

The changes in eating and drinking habits may be due to fatigue or weakness, occult pain, or due to a variety of metabolic imbalances as the body's homeostatic mechanisms begin to fail. Metabolic imbalances can lead to dehydration and to digestive disorders and resultant nausea, vomiting, diarrhea, or constipation.

It is a common and widespread fear that an animal that stops eating will "starve to death." Human hospice patients, however, clearly verbalize that they have lost the desire for food and that *not* eating, at that point in time, is more comfortable for them than eating (McCann et al. 1994). One of the authors (Pope), who took her mother through hospice care for seven months, can well attest to how her mother lost the desire for food, and how difficult it was *not* to keep trying to tempt her to eat a little more. Human patients' reports are supported by studies showing that lack of food has the benefit of increasing production of endorphins in the brain, promoting comfort and restfulness and providing some endogenous pain relief (Reid and Pantilat 2012). Ganzini has argued that the effects of artificial nutrition and hydration (ANH) are "counterpalliative" for patients during the early stages of dying (Ganzini 2006). Water consumption habits also change and become much less predictable.

Generalized muscle weakness and loss of muscle mass progress and may result in decreased mobility and inability to maintain urinary and fecal continence. Changes in respiration may be observed, such as increased or decreased respiratory rate, panting, or open-mouthed breathing.

These changes alter the animal's appearance. Decreased food intake results in weight loss, which may lead to severe emaciation and postural changes due to weakness and discomfort. Decreased food and water intake may result in the animal's coat taking on an increasingly dull and greasy appearance. This may be compounded by the lack of grooming due to pain, weakness, fatigue, or depression. These changes are often disturbing to caregivers if they are not well prepared to recognize them as common in all species at the end of life. It's important to advise caregivers that changes in the animal's appearance do not cause significant additional discomfort for the patient.

Behavioral Changes

Some of the behavioral changes at the end of life are a progression of those typically observed as animals age. Other changes in behavior reflect the central nervous system's response to the primary disease, terminal loss of homeostasis, or the presence of chronic pain. Energy levels are often decreased, and animals may tire easily after a few steps. They may prefer interaction for short periods only or none at all. Irritability, restlessness, and vocalizing at strange times may occur. Grooming activities decrease or disappear completely. Withdrawal from relationships may be seen gradually or abruptly, as evidenced by the animal preferring to be left alone, seeking solitude, refusing to be touched or held, and/or not sleeping with the caregiver as he or she has done regularly in the past. Cats may sit in the litter box for extended periods. Cats and dogs can be seen hanging their head over a water bowl without drinking for extended periods of time. Other animals in the family often start keeping a distance from the dying. Conversely, the other animals may stay closer than usual, possibly expressing a desire to offer comfort or reassurance. At the author's (Pope) animal hospice and sanctuary, for example, animals find themselves surrounded in love by cats, dogs, and humans throughout their final stages of life.

Indications of Pain

In imminently dying patients, the possibility of pain must be considered when physiologic changes are noticed (e.g. increases in pulse rate and respiratory rate), and when any of the behaviors of pain are present, discussed extensively in Chapter 5 in this book, "Recognizing Distress," and elsewhere (e.g. Gaynor and Muir 2015, and others). In humans, grimacing and continuous facial tension are used as a measure of pain intensity (Prkachin 1992). In dogs and cats, furrowed eyebrows, squinted eyes, and a fixed glare have been described as changes in facial expression that may be indicative of pain. Holden et al. (2014) studied differences between facial expressions of painful and pain-free cats and found that those included areas of the orbit (eyes), ears, and mouth. These distinguishing features are similar to features reported to be significant in facial pain expressions of mice and rats, which included orbital tightening, nose/cheek flattening, ear changes, and whisker changes (Langford et al. 2010; Sotocinal et al. 2011). References cited at the end of Chapter 5 will help readers recognize pain in rats, mice, cats, horses, and rabbits. Assessment of pain experience during the dying process is complicated by neurological changes that may include confusion, drowsiness, agitation, and departure from the patient's normal personality. These changes make the diagnosis of pain difficult in both human and animal patients. The restlessness, agitation, moaning, and groaning that accompany terminal delirium in humans can be difficult to distinguish from pain. Detailed descriptions of terminal delirium in animals are not available, but it is likely that it occurs sometimes and may be incorrectly interpreted as pain.

Vocalization, panting, and other abnormal respiratory patterns, salivation, irritability, submissive as well as aggressive behavior, loss of appetite, over grooming, and self-mutilation may all be triggered and/or accentuated by pain (Wiese 2015). Pain is a common manifestation of some of the most common terminal medical conditions in companion animals (many types of cancer, osteoarthritic conditions) and is therefore frequently encountered in animal hospice patients. However, the dying process itself does not cause pain; disease causes pain, and not *all* diseases create pain. *A thorough acquaintance with the patient's disease history is crucial in determining if he or she is experiencing actual physical pain!* A therapeutic trial with one or more pain management modalities is in the animal's best interest if pain is suspected, even if it cannot be definitively confirmed. It is in the patient's best interests to have pain over treated rather than undertreated.

Changes During Late Stages of Active Dying

There are several signs that may indicate when an animal is close to or just hours from death. Such observable changes may include:

Behavior, Sleeping Pattern, Responsiveness

Animals who are approaching the end of their lives may experience periods of restlessness, alternating with times of peaceful sleep. They may experience drowsiness and loss of consciousness, partial or complete, interspersed with periods of alertness. In what seems like a resurgence of life, a momentary return to more normal behavior may be seen such as lucid communication and a desire for water or food. Further withdrawal from those present around the animal and a decrease in responsiveness to other stimuli may be observed.

It is not unusual to see animals lying peacefully and making eye contact with those around them, intermittently exhibiting restlessness, and sometimes crying out softly, which may or may not stop when they are given attention and comforted.

Respiration

Changes in a dying patient's breathing pattern are common and may be indicative of significant neurologic compromise. Lichter and Hunt (1990) assessed the incidence of pain, dyspnea, moist breathing, nausea and vomiting, confusion, restlessness, jerking and twitching, difficulty swallowing, incontinence and retention of urine, sweating, moaning and groaning, and loss of consciousness in 200 human patients and concluded that "many of these features can be attributed to organic brain disease consequent to metabolic disorder associated with multi-organ failure."

Breaths may become very shallow and frequent with a diminishing tidal volume. Periods of apnea and/or Cheyne–Stokes pattern respirations (an irregular pattern of rapid breaths followed by variable periods of time of no breathing at all) may develop. Periods of panting may also be observed. Accessory respiratory muscle use may become prominent. A few (or many) last reflex breaths may signal death. Dyspnea and coughing may be seen as pulmonary congestion sets in, often secondary to cardiac function failure. Fluid that accumulates in the airways may cause "rales" and "rattles" sounds, but those are not as commonly heard in animals as in humans. These breathing sounds, referred to as "death rattle," are often distressing to caregivers but are not an indication of pain or suffering (Wildiers and Menten 2002).

Eyes, Mucus Membranes, Jaw, and Extremities
The eyes generally become glazed with dilated pupils and a distant and fixed gaze. The jaw may remain slightly open. Slow, repetitive jaw motion, as if to indicate an unpleasant taste, may be seen. With the decrease in peripheral circulation, the lips and gums become pale gray, bluish, or white, and cooler to the touch, as do the distal limbs, paws, ears, and tail.

Muscle Twitching, Stretching, and the Agonal Position
Involuntary muscle twitching may occur in any part of the body, before and/or after death. When death is imminent the head may lift and tilt in a backward motion, while the front legs stretch out and forward – often seen in humans just before death. However, caregivers should be prepared for the fact that this action may

take place several times before death finally occurs, and the process can take anywhere from minutes to days.

Odor
A distinctive odor may suddenly become noticeable that is sometimes referred to as "the smell of death." It is not always present and may be related to the kidneys no longer functioning properly. Another distinctive smell could be that of a decaying cancerous mass. The "smell of death" is caused by the presence of putrescine and cadaverine, which are foul-smelling diamine compounds produced by protein hydrolysis during tissue putrefaction in living and dead animals. Putrescine and cadaverine were first described in 1885 by the Berlin physician Ludwig Brieger (1849–1919).

Summary
Signs and changes that may be seen at the end of life are summarized in Table 23.1.

NOTE: Dying is unique to each individual in regard to presentation and timing, so it is not likely that all of the changes listed below will be presented in the dying process of any single patient.

At the Time of Death

Death has been defined as an irreversible condition in which an organism is incapable of carrying on functions of life; a cessation or termination of all biological functions that sustain a living organism. Regardless of the cause of death, the journey to death, and its timing and presentation are personal and unique to each individual. What happens to one, may not be experienced or happen to another (Yaxley 2015). As eloquently articulated by Yaxley, the physiological details explaining why and how each individual journey is so unique are complex and therefore not easy to elucidate. Empirical research is difficult and knowledge about many aspects of death and

Table 23.1 Signs and changes that may be seen at the end of life.

Early phase of active dying From a few weeks to a few days	Final phase of active dying From approx. a few days – to minutes
Neurologic, behavioral, and emotional changes	
Withdrawal from social interaction, confusion, focus changing	Departure from normal personality, blank stare, glazed eyes with dilated pupils
Increased sleep, lethargy, exhaustion	Drowsiness, loss of consciousness, comatose, other worldly
Restlessness, increased agitation, disorientation, inability to be made comfortable	Severe agitation, terminal delirium
Cats lying by water bowl or in litter box	Loss of sensation in the extremities
Fly catcher's syndrome	Hallucinations
Digestive system	
Thirst diminishing or increasing decreased food intake or pica	Anorexia, cessation of all oral intake (not taking food or water by mouth)
Gradual onset of dysphagia (difficulty swallowing)	Inability to swallow, gulping
Constipation, diarrhea, fecal incontinence	Constipation, diarrhea, fecal incontinence
Musculoskeletal system	
Muscle weakness	Muscle spasms, twitching, myoclonus. Slow repetitive jaw motions
Progressive muscle mass loss, emaciation	End stage emaciation
Integumentary system	
Decreasing skin turgor	Skin turgor extremely decreased; skin stretched tight
Wound healing prolonged or absent	Wounds discharges ceasing; may appear to be healing
Urinary system	
Polyuria, dysuria	Oliguria, anuria
Abnormal urine color (dark, concentrated, or colorless)	Urine may appear thicker and darker
Urinary incontinence intermittently.	Urinary incontinence
Circulatory, cardiovascular, and respiratory system	
Dehydration, progressive	Dehydration, severe
Pulmonary and/or peripheral edema	Circulatory failure
Decreased and/or variable respiratory rate, panting	Decreased and/or variable respiratory rate
Dyspnea, flaring of nares and/or cheeks on exhalation, abdominal retractions	Cheyne–Stokes, agonal, open mouth breathing, or only gentle rising and falling of abdomen
Coughing	Accumulation of respiratory secretions ("death rattle")
Hypertension, hypotension, fluctuations in blood pressure	Hypotension, often profound
Brachycardia, tachycardia, arrhythmias	Brachycardia, tachycardia, arrhythmias
Pallor and/or cyanosis of mucous membranes and skin	Pallor and/or cyanosis, severe
Peripheral hypothermia, mild (extremities feel noticeably cooler)	Peripheral hypothermia, severe
Other	
Noticeable odor	Odor intensifies

the dying process remains anecdotal or descriptive alone. With nearly a quarter of the twenty-first century behind us, death is still a mystery.

Often at the time of death, the hind legs may be seen "kicking" and then stretching right out, followed by the front legs also stretching forward and then downwards toward the torso. The neck may extend up and back, bladder and/or bowels may empty, and mild spasms of retching can occur at the moment of death. This can sometimes come as an unexpected event for a person who is holding the animal close and saying final goodbyes. Respiration, heartbeat, and brain electrical activity cease, and all muscles go flaccid.

The Different Types of Active Death

The authors' experience has led us to forming the following categories:

1) *The Slow and Detached.* There is mostly peace and calm, sometimes for days on end as the animal slips back and forth between worlds and between degrees of unconsciousness. The last, almost imperceptible breath slips away quietly with grace and tenderness, and the animal's facial expression at the time of death is relaxed.

2) *The Slow and Engaged.* In one author's opinion (Pope), the best kind of natural dying process. Here there is contact and communication all the way to the very end. This is very precious and a time when the caregiver can hold the animal's paws, gaze into their eyes, and talk of many things. Some animals will remain in eye and finger contact as they draw their last breath. For this author, this is an extremely reassuring, comforting, and beautiful experience.

3) *The Fast Track.* The animal seems set to live a while longer, but then suddenly it experiences physical changes that lead to death in a matter of seconds or a few minutes.

4) *The Restless and Frustrating.* Referred to in human hospice as "The difficult road to

Table 23.2 "Two roads" to death.

"Usual" road	"Difficult" road
Normal	Normal
	Restless
Sleepy	Confused
	Tremulous
Lethargic	Hallucinating
	Delirious
Obtunded	Myoclonic jerks
	Seizures
Semicomatose	
Comatose	
Death	

Source: Adapted from: Freemon, F.R. "Delirium and organic psychosis." In: *Organic mental disease.* Jamaica, NY: SP Medical and Scientific Books; 1981: 81–94.

death" (See Table 23.2) Fainsinger et al. (2000) found the prevalence of difficult neurologic symptoms (delirium) requiring sedation at the end of life to be approximately 6% (9 out of 150) in a population of hospice and palliative care patients. The study's authors note that this figure is relatively low compared to others reported in the literature. They attribute the low rate to improved symptom management that has resulted in fewer distressing symptoms at the end of life. However, they advise caution in comparing results of different palliative care groups and in different cultures. Less than 1% of this type of death was experienced at BrightHaven Animal Hospice (Pope unpublished data).

Impeccable management of the patient's symptoms may significantly affect the type of death he or she will experience. Hospice teams should strive to ensure timely and effective monitoring processes are in place for patients going through hospice-supported natural death. Peaceful passings are more likely to be witnessed in practices that focus on proactive pain and symptom management. Difficult deaths are more difficult to prevent in critical care facilities seeing many patients in acute crises, whether due to trauma or decompensating. In those cases, caregivers and medical teams may have very little time to decide between initiation of curative attempts, palliative/supportive care, or euthanasia.

Managing Clinical Signs During Active Dying

Unpredictable and sometimes rapid changes in hydration, mentation, respiratory function, and pain levels, as well as unexpectedly long periods with little change, may be encountered during the last hours of life. Caregivers' ability to cope may also change unpredictably. For both patient and caregivers' needs to be managed competently, it is essential to understand the specific needs of the patient and caregivers in each scenario, know what actions will produce optimal results, and have in place the information, equipment, and support staff needed to deliver the needed services. It is also important to alleviate fear for all participants by ensuring they understand those symptoms that are common during the dying process and don't necessarily indicate the dying patient is suffering.

The patient's condition and the caregivers' ability to cope must be reassessed frequently, and the plan of care promptly modified. One such plan modification might be a decision by the animal's caregiver to request that the animal be euthanized. Caregivers and animal hospice providers are encouraged to research experienced euthanasia providers in their community so that should the need arise for euthanasia, especially in an emergency, they will know who to contact.

Management of Pain

Pain is a part of all life. In the process of evolution, mammals and other creatures developed the capacity to experience pain from the moment they begin their physical existence and throughout life. Terminal illness and dying are no exception. Yet equating the dying process with extreme suffering may be mostly a manifestation of our own fear of the unknown. Contrary to this common fear, there is no evidence to suggest that pain suddenly increases or appears during active dying (Emanuel et al. 2005).

Managing pain is an essential component of all animal hospice and palliative care, including imminently dying patients. The possibility of pain must be considered when physiologic changes are noticed (e.g. increases in pulse rate and respiratory rate), and when any of the behaviors of pain are present. Treatment of pain in the imminently dying patient follows general multimodal pain management principles (Gaynor and Muir 2015; AAHA 2015; AAHA 2016), with opioid agents serving as the foundation of effective analgesia for severe pain. Other medications that may improve comfort include neuropathic pain blockers, adjunctive analgesic agents, NSAIDS, or corticosteroids.

Analgesic medications should be administered in "breakthrough" doses, titrated to manage expressions suggestive of continuous pain. Dying patients experience altered neurologic function as well as diminished hepatic metabolism and renal perfusion. Under these circumstances effective doses of all drugs may be difficult to predict. Routine dosing or continuous infusions of most medications, including all analgesics, may increase the risk of agitation, confusion, and seizures. Therefore, close monitoring and frequent evaluations are essential for desirable outcomes. Use of doses above or below the recommended dosing range may be needed. Many patients benefit from gradually lowering doses of all drugs when they are at the end of life.

Many physical modalities can help manage pain with a low risk of side effects. For example, cryotherapy is good to treat local inflammation. Heat therapy and various massage techniques (TTouch, acupressure, *Tui-na*, Healing Touch, etc.) can relax muscle spasms and help control pain. Laser and pulsed electromagnetic field (PEMF) therapy are noninvasive and can relieve pain. Classical veterinary homeopathy, acupuncture, and animal Reiki can be effective in pain relief and, at the same time, can manage other sources of discomfort, like nausea, agitation, labored breathing, and congestion. Cannabis has proven to offer pain and anxiety relief during the dying process. Hemp, which is a strain of *Cannabis sativa*, offers all the medical benefits of cannabis without the "high-inducing" capacity of THC. Whole-plant, hemp-derived CBD oil is often easier to administer in the later stages of dying and is equally as efficacious. It absorbs quickly through the gums and must be dosed cautiously because a small amount might go a long way.

Management of Anxiety and Agitation

Neurological changes associated with the dying process in animals are poorly understood. These changes are the result of compromised blood circulation to the brain and other organs, as well as multiple biochemical imbalances at the end of life. Neurological changes include confusion, drowsiness, loss of consciousness, agitation, muscle twitching or spasming, and departure from normal personality. The changes in neurologic function can be frequent and unpredictable.

Treatment of these changes may therefore be challenging, especially in semi-conscious patients. In the treatment of imminently dying humans, combinations of opioids and benzodiazepines are frequently used because of their synergistic anxiolytic effect. This drug combination is much less predictable in canine and feline patients. Both opioids and benzodiazepines can cause paradoxical agitation and/or dysphoria in both felines and canines. Canines' rapid metabolism of benzodiazepines must also be taken into consideration. Haloperidol is a neuroleptic agent commonly used in humans to alleviate agitation. There is little clinical experience in using this drug in animals.

Landberg et al. list 1–4 mg per dog b.i.d. as a standard dose, and note that doses in the range of 0.05–0.5 mg/kg^{-1} q12–24 have been reported for dogs (Landberg et al. 2013, p. 420). Acepromazine is a low-potency neuroleptic frequently used in veterinary medicine. Its efficacy in treating agitation is unpredictable, and its possible adverse effects include hypotension, cardiac arrhythmias, and paradoxical aggression. Trazodone is a serotonin antagonist and reuptake inhibitor (SARI) class antidepressant that may be used as an adjunct in management of anxiety in dogs. Landberg et al. list 2–3 mg/kg^{-1} up to q8 h as a standard dose, and note that doses up to 10 mg/kg^{-1} up to q8 h (300 mg per dose maximum) have been reported (Landberg et al. 2013, p. 420).

Canine and feline appeasing pheromones, as well as aromatherapy, may be used as adjunctive therapy to manage anxiety. Orally administered natural therapies for anxiety include l-theanine, Harmonease (Veterinary Products Laboratory) melatonin, and α-casozepine (Landberg et al. 2013, p. 228).

Holistic modalities may also prove helpful in addressing anxiety and/or agitation, even severe. Some examples include classical veterinary homeopathy, animal Reiki, and the compassionate touch of traditional Chinese medicine, including acupuncture, acupressure, *Tui-Na*, craniosacral therapy, and *Jin Shin Jyutsu*.

Fatigue and Weakness

Weakness and fatigue often increase as the patient approaches the time of death. It is not uncommon that the patient is unable to move around or even raise his or her head (Twycross and Lichter 1998). Joints may become uncomfortable if they are not moved (Fulton and Else 1998). As the patient approaches death, providing adequate cushioning on the bed will lessen the need for uncomfortable turning. The reader can find additional information in Chapter 22 "Nursing Care for Seriously Ill Animals" in this book.

Loss of Ability to Swallow

Weakness and decreased neurologic function frequently combine to impair the patient's ability to swallow. Decreased ability to swallow may cause some involuntary retching, which does not appear to be distressing to the animal. As the gag reflex and reflexive clearing of the oropharynx decline, secretions from the tracheobronchial tree accumulate. These conditions may become more prominent as the patient loses consciousness. Buildup of saliva and oropharyngeal secretions may lead to gurgling, crackling, or rattling sounds with each breath, (Nuland 1995) called by some the "death rattle." This term, however, is frequently disconcerting to families and caregivers. This phenomenon is not encountered as frequently in dying animals as in humans. Once the patient is unable to swallow, any form of oral intake must be ceased due to the risk of aspiration. Scopolamine or Glycopyrrolate will effectively reduce the production of saliva and other secretions and can be administered subcutaneously (Storey 1998; Hughes et al. 1996) to minimize or eliminate the gurgling and crackling sounds and may be used prophylactically in the unconscious dying patient. However, this treatment is primarily for the benefit of caregivers present, and its use in the conscious patient may lead to unacceptable drying of oral and pharyngeal mucosa. If excessive fluid accumulates in the back of the throat and upper airways, it may be at least partially cleared by repositioning of the patient or postural drainage.

Respiration

Families and professional caregivers frequently find changes in breathing patterns to be one of the most distressing signs of impending death. Many fear that the patient will experience a sense of suffocation. However, *unresponsive (unconscious, comatose) patients do not experience breathlessness or suffocating* (Emanuel et al. 2005).

Supplemental oxygen may not be beneficial and may prolong the dying process. Low doses of opioids or benzodiazepines are appropriate to manage perception of breathlessness when suspected in conscious animals. There is no evidence that initiation of opioid treatment or increases in dosing of opioids or sedatives is associated with precipitation of death. In fact, the evidence suggests the opposite (Sykes and Thorns 2003).

During agonal breathing at end of life, the caregiver may gently slide a hand under the animal's head and neck for support, or cradle him/her in their arms so that the head, although lightly supported, is free to lean back. Slight elevation of the animal's head or turning them on their side may help. Most importantly, however, caregivers should realize this does not require medical intervention, but a calm, comforting, and supportive attitude.

One of the authors (Pope) has found classical veterinary homeopathy especially useful during the dying period if respiratory distress is present.

Cardiac Dysfunction and Renal Failure

As cardiac output and intravascular volume decrease at the end-of-life, there will be evidence of diminished peripheral blood perfusion. Tachycardia, hypotension, peripheral cooling, and cyanosis are expected.

Urine output falls as perfusion of the kidneys diminishes. Oliguria or anuria is not uncommon. Parenteral fluids will not reverse this circulatory shut down (Mount 1996).

Diminished Skin Vitality

Decreased blood perfusion of peripheral tissues is a common consequence of dehydration and low blood pressure. When the patient is too weak to move, there is continuous pressure on some areas of skin, particularly over bony prominences, which over time can cause skin necrosis manifesting as painful ulcers (Walker 1998). Turning the patient from side to side every

1–1.5 hours and protecting areas of bony prominence are recommended to minimize the risk of pressure ulcer formation. A draw sheet can assist caregivers to turn the patient and minimize her or his pain. A pressure-reducing surface (e.g. air mattress or airbed) can be used if turning is too distressing to the patient. As the patient approaches death, however, the need for turning lessens as the risk of skin breakdown becomes less important. Intermittent massage before and after turning, particularly to areas of contact, can both be comforting and reduce the risk of skin breakdown. Massaging areas of non-blanching erythema or actual skin breakdown should be avoided.

Mucosal and Conjunctival Care

Dryness of the mouth (and other mucosal surfaces) is an uncomfortable sensation and can be minimized with meticulous oral, nasal, and conjunctival hygiene (Lethen 1993). The oral mucosa can be moistened and cleaned frequently, every 15–30 minutes. The lips and anterior nasal mucosa can be coated hourly with a thin layer of petroleum jelly to reduce evaporation. Products that are perfumed or contain lemon and glycerin are to be avoided, as these can be both desiccating and irritating.

If eyelids are not closed, eyes can be moistened to avoid painful dry eyes. Ophthalmic lubricating gel may be applied every three to four hours. Artificial tears, physiologic saline solution, or one of the many holistic ophthalmic solutions can be applied every 15–30 minutes.

Incontinence

Fatigue and loss of sphincter control in the last hours of life may lead to incontinence of urine and/or stool. Both can be very distressing to patients and family members, particularly if they are not prepared for the fact that these problems may arise. If they occur, attention needs to be paid to cleaning and skin care. A urinary catheter may be beneficial but is not necessary if urine flow is minimal and can be managed with absorbent pads or surfaces.

Clipping fur away from the perianal area and wrapping the tail can make cleaning easier. Simple diapering can help contain messes but requires frequent changes. If diarrhea is considerable and relentless, or sphincter muscles are weakened, a rectal catheter (also called rectal tube) may benefit patients, protecting the perineal area from frequent or constant contact with loose feces. Use of the rectal catheter carries a risk of serious complications, including rectal perforation. It should be closely monitored and removed as soon as feasible.

Administration of Medications, Fluids, and Food

As discussed above, decline in homeostatic mechanisms near the time of death results in changes in patients' desire for food and water and changes in their hydration status. These changes are frequently challenging to caregivers and hospice providers alike, in that providing nutrition and hydration are considered the foundation of competent patient care and symbolically demonstrate love and dedication to caring for the sick. Similarly, administering medications is also considered foundational to competent patient care and demonstrating our concern for the patient's well-being and comfort.

It is a common and widespread fear that an animal that stops eating will "starve to death." Human hospice patients, however, clearly verbalize that they have lost the desire for food and that *not* eating, at that point in time, is more comfortable for them than eating (McCann et al. 1994). One of the authors (Pope), who took her mother through hospice care for seven months, can well attest to how her mother lost the desire for food, and how difficult it was *not* to keep trying to tempt her to eat a little more. Tube feeding has been shown in repeated studies to result in discomfort more often than in the intended added comfort from improved nutritional status. For many terminal patients, loss of appetite and thirst parallels the dying body's inability to utilize nutrients. Biochemical and metabolic changes decrease appetite, decrease awareness, and have other salutary effects on symptoms (Brody et al. 2011). Ganzini has argued that, under these circumstances, the effects of ANH are "counterpalliative" (Ganzini 2006).

Human patients' reports are supported by studies showing that lack of food has the benefit of increasing production of endorphins in the brain, promoting comfort and restfulness and providing some endogenous pain relief (Reid and Pantilat 2012). Water consumption habits also change and become much less predictable.

Contrary to the common sentiments described above, in most cases food and fluids given orally or parenterally to the terminally ill do not increase patients' quality of life, and may increase discomfort and suffering (McClave and Chang 2003). The balance between the benefits and burdens of medications becomes less predictable near death as well, in the absence of competent homeostatic mechanisms. Below are some guidelines for managing these clinical challenges in patients near the time of death.

Administration of Fluids

Maintaining a level of hydration for all physiological processes to function optimally is a critical homeostatic mechanism, honed by evolution and essential for life. It is a complex mechanism integrating brain, kidney, digestive, vascular, and endocrine organ function. When illness impairs any of these, dehydration or overhydration may develop, causing discomfort, weakness, and potentially further impairing organ function. Vigilantly tending to the patient's fluid intake is therefore critical to caring for the ill. If an animal is unable to drink unassisted, it is important to offer water via syringe or by increasing the water content of the animal's food. In one of the authors' (Pope) experience, animals seem to develop a preference for dirty water – according to one school of thought, to seek precious minerals – so adding minerals to drinking water may help improve their desire to drink. Research to

definitively confirm and possibly explain this phenomenon is lacking. A bowl of pure water and another containing water with trace minerals, colloidal silver, liquid oxygen, or flower essences added may be offered to the pet. Many animals prefer to drink from a running water source, so a fountain near to their bed may be welcomed in the early stages of dying.

When oral fluid intake is impossible or too distressing for the patient, fluids can be administered parenterally in a variety of routes. The subcutaneous route is particularly suitable for home care of patients who are not in an acute clinical crisis, and it is common for patients to show clinical and emotional improvement in response. At the end of life, however, the balance between optimal hydration and overhydration may be difficult to maintain. Symptoms such as swelling, bloating, choking, coughing, nausea, vomiting, or difficulty breathing may ensue, especially when the animal's cardiovascular function is impaired. Peripheral edema may be evident when fluids administered subcutaneously are no longer being absorbed into circulation; when this happens, fluid pockets are seen around the neck or shoulders, or fluid may follow gravitational pull and migrate down to the axillae or distal limbs, manifesting as a distinct or diffuse tissue swelling. In this event, fluid therapy should be discontinued to prevent any further discomfort to the patient from overhydration.

Furthermore, it has been documented in human hospice patients that at the end of life, dehydration is often associated with added patient comfort, rather than discomfort. Dehydration, as with lack of food, has been shown to be associated with an increase in the release of endorphins in the brain, biochemicals that provide some relief from pain and anxiety and thus enhance patients' mental status.

Dehydration does cause thirst and dry mouth, which are uncomfortable for the patient. These can be alleviated by simple, noninvasive measures such as giving small amounts of fluids or ice chips by mouth and by lubricating the lips (McCann et al. 1994).

One must keep in mind that "last-minute turn-arounds" do occur in animals appearing close to the end of life, warranting the utmost caution in making the decision to discontinue fluid therapy altogether. Instead, gradually decreasing the amounts of fluids administered is recommended while monitoring the animal closely.

Administration of Food

It is very important to continue to offer food, remain open and receptive to patient preferences, and try creative ways to encourage food intake. As the patient's eating habits change, what worked only a few weeks or days ago may not be acceptable. Caregivers may need to offer different types of food, smaller quantities, or different textures. Muscle or organ meats, as well as supplements such as liver powder sprinkled on the food, may stimulate the appetite. Adding canned food, dried chicken, Bonita flakes, nutritional yeast, or a few pieces of kibble may also stimulate appetite. Other options may include adding an egg yolk or baby food to the regular diet, or serving them alone. Raw or cooked meats can be pureed, and food can be offered by syringe, finger, spoon, or small flat plate or saucer. Food can be offered at different temperatures, too, even if the pet might not have shown any such preference in the past.

Caregivers must also be prepared for the possibility that their pet may stop eating completely or, conversely, may continue eating right up until the day of his/her death. Offering food or water by syringe should be discontinued if the patient retches or gags frequently, to avoid aspiration into the airways and lungs. Not eating is a common event in the dying process, and it is important to take cues from the animal to determine when feeding attempts should cease altogether. Food and water could continue to be offered every few hours but taken away and never forced if the pet turns away.

Studies in human patients demonstrate that parenteral or enteral feeding of patients near death neither improves symptom control nor lengthens life (Ahronheim and Gasner 1990; Finucane et al. 1999; McCann et al. 1994; American College of Physicians 1989). Anorexia may be helpful as the resulting ketosis can lead to a sense of well-being and diminish discomfort (Winter 2000).

Human beings express love for one another through the act of feeding and sharing meals. Decisions to start, withhold, or discontinue ANH are often motivated by the unfounded belief that the administering of ANH is an act of nurturing. ANH is a medical treatment, with intended beneficial effects as well as potential adverse effects and complications. When ANH is more likely to be burdensome than helpful, it should be avoided or discontinued.

Nurturing can be expressed in more helpful ways, such as gentle presence, touch, talking with the person (regardless of his/her ability to respond, as it is known that the last sense to leave is hearing), keeping the person's lips and mouth moist, gently massaging the skin using lubricants, praying with the person, or playing their favorite music selections. These alternative ways of nurturing can be very powerful and moving for both the person (or animal) with the life-threatening illness and his/her loved one (Arenella 2014).

Administration of Medications

As the animal approaches death, the need for each medication should be reassessed and the number of medications given minimized, leaving only those needed to manage the presence of clinical signs such as pain, breathlessness, nausea, excess secretions, terminal delirium, and seizures.

Administering medications orally to end of life patients can be difficult and often traumatic for both patients and caregivers. The least invasive route of administration should be chosen: the buccal, nasal, rectal, or subcutaneous routes of administration should be used whenever possible. The intravenous route is convenient if a catheter is already in place and is tolerated by the patient. The oral and the intramuscular routes of administering medications should be used only if no other options are available (Emanuel et al. 2005).

Potential long-term adverse effects such as liver failure and drug addiction are of minimal relevance; conversely, adverse effects that negatively impact patient comfort within hours require immediate reassessment of the treatment plan. Sedation is a common adverse effect of many analgesic agents, especially in higher doses. Prioritizing the gain in patient comfort versus the loss of conscious awareness at the end of life is medically challenging and can be ethically agonizing for both caregivers and animal hospice professionals.

If the animal becomes less cooperative about medications being administered, it is prudent to reassess and more aggressively treat for pain, nausea, and other symptoms that may not be well controlled. All conventional and complementary symptoms management techniques should be considered. Classical veterinary homeopathy can be effective and is particularly advantageous due to the ease of giving remedies.

If such efforts fail, however, it is likely that the animal is expressing a preference for further medical treatment to be withheld. When this happens, honoring the patient's wishes should be the highest priority. Caregivers may have a better sense that treatment is not *desired* by the animal than the hospice team members. Teamwork in which caregivers and all providers collaborate in making this important clinical decision for the animal is most likely to ensure success in keeping the dying animal comfortable.

Summary

This chapter is intended to provide both knowledge and support to those accompanying an animal on the journey to transition. We have endeavored to summarize the physiologic changes that occur as patients are dying, as well as to describe some approaches to the management of associated symptoms. We have also discussed care at the time of death with special emphasis on the symptoms or signs that may be seen during the process.

To conclude, here are some supportive tips:

- Self-care is very important for the caregiver.
- Hospice-supported, natural dying requires a team and integrative approach.
- Approaching death can be very peaceful. The unpleasant things sometimes associated with death generally occur as a part of living before the dying process begins and can be treated accordingly.
- Intuition is your ally – listen to it.
- The power of love and being present is amazing!
- Fear is natural.
- Dying is a very complex natural process involving many different physiological pathways and various organ systems, all leading to the eventual cessation of all biological activity.
- Death itself is a process.
- Death is not a failed medical event.
- It is important to learn about and embrace death as a natural, inevitable part of the circle of life.

References

Ahronheim, J.C. and Gasner, M.R. (1990) The sloganism of starvation. *Lancet*, 335: 278–279.

American Animal Hospital Association (AAHA/IAAHPC) (2016) End-of-life care guidelines for cats and dogs. Veterinary Practice Guidelines. Available at: https://www.aaha.org/globalassets/02-guidelines/end-of-life-care/

2016_aaha_iaahpc_eolc_guidelines.pdf (Accessed: May 21, 2022).

American Animal Hospital Association/American Association of Feline Practitioners (AAHA/AAFP) (2015) AAHA/AAFP 2015 pain management guidelines for cats and dogs. Veterinary Practice Guidelines. Available at:

https://www.aaha.org/globalassets/ 02-guidelines/pain-management/2015_aaha_ aafp_pain_management_guidelines_for_dogs_ and_cats.pdf (Accessed: May 21, 2022).

American College of Physicians. (1989) Parenteral nutrition in patients receiving cancer chemotherapy. *Ann. Int. Med.*, 110: 734–735.

Arenella, C. (2014) Artificial nutrition and hydration at the end of life: beneficial or harmful? American Hospice Foundation. Available at: http://americanhospice.org/ caregiving/artificial-nutrition-and-hydration- at-the-end-of-life-beneficial-or-harmful (Accessed May 21, 2022).

Boone, A and Quelch, V. (2003) Effects of harp music therapy on canine patients in the veterinary hospital setting. *Harp Ther. J.*, 8: 1, 4–5, 15.

Bretscher, M., Rummans, T., Sloan, J. et al. (1999) Quality of life in hospice patients. a pilot study. *Psychosomatics*, 40: 309–313.

Brody, H., Hermer, L.D., Scott, L.D. et al. (2011) Artificial nutrition and hydration: the evolution of ethics, evidence, and policy. *J. Gen. Intern. Med.*, 26: 1053–1058.

Emanuel, L.L., Ferris, F.D., von Gunten, C.F. et al. (2005) Module 6: last hours of living. In: Education for physicians on end-of-life care –oncology. Chicago: The EPEC Project. Available at: http://www.ipcrc.net/epco/ EPEC-O%20M06%20Dying/EPEC-O% 20M06%20Dying%20PH.pdf (Accessed: May 21, 2022).

Fainsinger, R.L., De Moissac, D., Mancini, I. et al. (2000) Sedation for delirium and other symptoms in terminally ill patients in Edmonton. *J. Palliat. Care*, 16: 5–10.

Finucane, T.E., Christmas, C., and Travis, K. (1999) Tube feeding in patients with advanced dementia: a review of the evidence. *J. Am. Med. Assoc.*, 282: 1365–1370.

Fulton, C.L. and Else, R. (1998) Physiotherapy. In: Oxford Textbook of Palliative Medicine. (eds. D. Doyle, G.W.C. Hanks, and N. MacDonald) 2nd edn. Oxford: Oxford University Press; 821–822.

Ganzini, L. (2006) Artificial nutrition and hydration at the end of life: ethics and evidence. *Palliat. Support Care*, 4: 135–143.

Gaynor, J.S. and Muir, W.W. (2015) Handbook of Veterinary Pain Management. 3edn. St. Louis, MO: Elsevier.

Hayhurst, W. (2010) Coming for to Carry Me Home: Guidelines for Living and Dying Consciously. Esher Surrey, UK: Venus Group Publishing Ltd.

Holden, E., Calvo, G., Collins, M. et al. (2014) Evaluation of facial expression in acute pain in cats, *J. Small Anim. Pract.*, 55: 615–62.

Hughes, A.C., Wilcock, A., and Corcoran, R. (1996) Management of 'death rattle.' *J. Pain Symptom Manag.*, 12: 271–272.

International Association of Animal Hospice and Palliative Care (IAAHPC). (2017) *Animal Hospice and Palliative Care Guidelines*. Available at: https://iaahpc.org/ wp-content/uploads/2020/10/IAAHPC- AHPC-GUIDELINESpdf.pdf (Accessed: 5/21/22).

Kim, Y.M., Lee, J.K., Abdel-aty, A.M. et al. (2010) Efficacy of dog-appeasing pheromone (DAP) for ameliorating separation-related behavioral signs in hospitalized dogs, *Can. Vet. J.*, 51: 380.

Kutner, J.S., Meyer, S.A., Beaty, B.L. et al. (2004) Outcomes and characteristics of patients discharged alive from hospice. *J. Am. Geriatr. Soc.*; 52: 1337–1342.

Lagoni, L., Butler, C., and Hetts, S. (1994) The Human-Animal Bond and Grief. Philadelphia, PA: W.B. Saunders Company.

Landberg, G., Hunthausen, W., and Ackerman, L. (2013) Behavior Problems of the Cat & Dog. 3 edn. Elsevier.

Langford, D.J., Bailey, A.L., Chanda, M.L. et al. (2010) Coding of facial expressions of pain in the laboratory mouse. *Nat. Methods*, 7: 447–449.

Lethen, W. (1993) Mouth and skin problems. In: The Management of Terminal Malignant Disease. (eds. C. Saunders and N. Sykes) 3 edn. Boston: Edward Arnold Publishing, pp

139–142 *Coeditor Dame Cicely Saunders, OM, DBE, FRCP (St Christopher's Hospice, London) is often regarded as the founder of the modern hospice movement.*

Lichter, I. and Hunt. E. (1990) The last 48 hours of life. *J. Palliat. Care*, 6: 7–15.

McCann, R.M., Hall, W.J., and Groth-Juncker, A. (1994) Comfort care for terminally ill patients: the appropriate use of nutrition and hydration. *J. Am. Med. Assoc.*, 272: 1263–1266.

McClave, S.A. and Chang, W.K. (2003) Complications of enteral access. *Gastrointest. Endosc.*, 58: 739–751.

Mount, B.M. (1996) Care of dying patients and their families. In: Textbook of Medicine. (eds. J.C. Bennett and F.C. Plum) 20 edn. Philadelphia, PA: W.B. Saunders Company, 6–9.

Nuland, S. (1995) How We Die. New York: Vintage Books.

Prkachin, K.M. (1992) The consistency of facial expressions of pain: a comparison across modalities. *Pain*, 51: 297–306.

Reid, T. and Pantilat, S. (2012) When should enteral feeding by percutaneous tube be used in patients with cancer and in patients with non-cancer related conditions. In: Evidence-Based Practice of Palliative Medicine. (eds. N.E. Goldstein and R.S. Morrison). Elsevier Health Sciences, 166.

Roditi, D. and Robinson, M.E. (2011) The role of psychological interventions in the management of patients with chronic pain. *Psychol. Res. Behav. Manag.*, 4: 41–49.

Sotocinal, S.G., Sorge, R.E., Zaloum, A. ct al., (2011) The rat grimace scale: a partially automated method for quantifying pain in the laboratory rat via facial expressions. *Mol. Pain*, 7: 55–126.

Steele, L.L., Mills, B., Hardin, S.R. et al. (2005) Quality of life of hospice patients: patient and provider perceptions. *Am. J. Hosp. Palliat. Care*, 22: 95–110.

Storey, P. (1998) Symptom control in dying. In: Principles and Practice of Supportive Oncology Updates. (eds. A. Berger, R.K. Portenoy, and D. Weissman). Philadelphia, PA: Lippincott-Raven Publishers, 741–748.

Sykes, N. and Thorns, A. (2003) Sedative use in the last week of life and the implications for end-of-life decision making. *Arch. Intern. Med.*, 163: 341–344.

Temel, J.S., Greer, J.A., Muzikansky, A. et al. (2010) Early palliative care for patients with metastatic non-small-cell lung cancer. *N. Engl. J. Med.* 363: 733–742.

Teno, J.M., Plotzke, M., Gozalo, P. et al. (2014) A national study of live discharges from hospice. *J. Palliat. Med.*, *17*(10), 1121–1127.

Twycross, R. and Lichter, I. (1998) The terminal phase. In: Oxford Textbook of Palliative Medicine. (eds. D. Doyle, G.W.C. Hanks, and N. MacDonald) 2 edn. Oxford: Oxford University Press, 977–992.

Walker, P. (1998) The pathophysiology and management of pressure ulcers. In: Topics in Palliative Care. (eds. R.K. Portenoy and E. Bruera) 3 edn. New York: Oxford University Press, 253–270.

Wells, D.L., Graham, L., and Hepper, P.G. (2002) The influence of auditory stimulation on the behaviour of dogs housed in a rescue shelter. *Anim. Welfare*, 11: 385–393.

Wiese, A.J., Assessing pain. (2015) In: Handbook of Veterinary Pain Management. (eds. J.S. Gaynor and W.W. Muir). 3 edn. St. Louis: Elsevier, 67–68.

Wildiers, H. and Menten, J., (2002) Death rattle prevalence, prevention and treatment. *J. Pain Symptom Manage.*, 23: 310–317.

Winter, S,M. (2000) Terminal nutrition: framing the debate for the withdrawal of nutritional support in terminally ill patients. *Am. J. Med.* 109: 723–726.

Wright, A.A., Keating, N.L., Balboni, T.A. et al. (2010). Place of death: correlations with quality of life of patients with cancer and predictors of bereaved caregivers' mental health. *J. Clin. Oncol.*, *28*(29): 4457–4464.

Yaxley P. (2015) Pathophysiology of death. Proceedings for the IAAHPC Annual Conference, San Diego, CA, October 1–4.

24

Euthanasia in Animal End-of-Life Care

Kathleen Cooney, DVM, CHPV, DACAW

Decision-Making for the Animal Hospice Patient

It is expected that caregivers will question the right time to euthanize an animal, including to determine if it is necessary at all. "Is he suffering? Am I being selfish and keeping him around just for me? Do they ever die in their sleep so I don't have to make a decision for euthanasia?" These are commonly heard questions in veterinary medicine. To hope for a peaceful natural passing is almost universal. In fact, within this author's former mobile animal hospice service, the staff found that over 90% of caregivers mention the desire for natural death. Some families want a planned euthanasia in animal hospice, but many are willing to see how far quality medical support can take them and will decide for or against euthanasia based on perceived suffering. Ultimately, the decision to euthanize is a leap of faith that comes with the belief nothing else can be done to maintain comfort; when death will be a welcomed release for everyone, including the patient. The best practitioners can do is help caregivers comprehend how an animal's condition changes over time and how to recognize signs of true suffering that might lead to a decision to humanely terminate life.

Animal euthanasia has been around for generations. In our society, it is virtually impossible to find someone who doesn't know euthanasia is performed on animals. It is ingrained in us to "let them go" when it is evident that a significant level of suffering is present. However, those caregivers choosing animal hospice are looking for the means to maintain quality of life, and perhaps delay euthanasia longer than would be possible without palliative support. They are actively choosing life, even when euthanasia offers a quicker ending. In human healthcare, it is well documented that hospice care at the end of life often extends survival time, so much so that some terminally ill patients are discharged from hospice altogether. The same is proving true in animal hospice, even though published cases of success are rare. Advocating for euthanasia too soon in the illness not only denies potential quality time for the animal, but also may harbor lingering doubts for the family for years to come. Due to advances in modern veterinary medicine, euthanasia is no longer the only means to palliate pain and distress brought on by symptoms of disease(s). We have better ways to minimize suffering and maintain considerable quality of life for our companion animals, and euthanasia remains an option when necessary.

In animal hospice, it is beneficial to openly discuss euthanasia early in the journey so everyone is clear on options and expectations.

The topic can be brought up during the caregivers' first hospice assessment. With open communication, families will readily share their hopes for care and opinions for or against euthanasia. We often learn about pertinent psychosocial concerns and what factors are fueling decision-making. Finances, previous experiences with death, physical limitations, and more can play a role. It's helpful to listen closely to concerns and then outline all options for death. Here is an example of the options for death presented to caregivers during an end-of-life assessment.

1) hospice-supported natural death (also referred to as palliated death)
2) natural death, but open to euthanasia
3) planned euthanasia

Presenting options opens the door for honest dialogue, especially when euthanasia remains more advocated for than a natural passing. Caregivers feel understood and supported. With so many unknowns in hospice, asking how the family hopes to see death achieved gives them a unique sense of control and can help minimize guilt (August et al. 2017).

What is perceived as suffering varies greatly from one person to the next, but most believe that if an animal is experiencing irremediable suffering, and when all hope of a return to "normal" life is gone, the choice to euthanize becomes acceptable. It's worth mentioning that returning to a "normal" life is not always attainable and that a "new normal" filled with unique joys can be fulfilling. If euthanasia is chosen, it is chosen for all the right reasons such as intractable pain, severe breathing difficulty, uncontrollable seizures, and/or debilitating anxiety. If a family chooses a planned euthanasia, the care leading up to it should still be considered hospice care. The goal of a natural death is ideal for some, but for many it is simply not an option (whether philosophically, practically, or both). With medical support, a natural death can be a viable option and euthanasia avoided altogether. In the family's home or comfort room, as pictured in Figure 24.1, is a wonderful place to gather.

Advance Preparation and Education of the Professional Team

Opportunities to learn about euthanasia best practices is increasing in veterinary medicine. Books, articles, and research detailing modern approaches are being produced thanks in large part to those in the animal hospice field. Many

Figure 24.1 Ideal settings for euthanasia provide comfort and reduce anxiety.

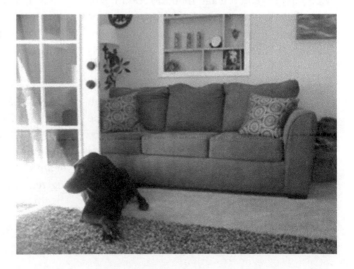

professionals in the animal welfare industry also focus great time and resources to generate useful, highly practical information. While euthanasia education in veterinary and technician colleges remains underserved, it is increasing by those who wish to see euthanasia skills improve (Dickinson 2021). Until more recently, it was assumed that if a veterinarian or technician knew how to give an intravenous injection, they knew how to euthanize an animal. With animals in the role of family members, it has become clear that all personnel performing euthanasia need to be highly skilled in the art of ending life, including communication and problem-solving. The Companion Animal Euthanasia Training Academy (CAETA), who offers a certificate program in advanced euthanasia protocols, refers to the new attention given the procedure as "the good death revolution" (Cooney 2019). Many things can go wrong, and because it is so important to have animals achieve a peaceful passing, education and training should increase the odds of success.

Understanding euthanasia begins with the fundamentals of death itself. Each living being's awareness and manifestation of death changes will be unique. That said, the physiology of death follows a general pattern in which, ideally, unconsciousness presents before awareness of cardiac arrest. Unconsciousness is followed by cessation of breathing and then the cessation of a heartbeat. In this way, feelings of pain, anxiety, or discomfort are minimized. Through unconsciousness, the animal is unaware of what is happening during physiologic death.

This is ultimately the goal of assisted death too. Humane euthanasia, according to the American Veterinary Medical Association (AVMA), is the act of bringing about as pain-free and stress-free a death as possible (Leary et al 2020). The word euthanasia is from the Greek language combining the words eu (good) + thanatos (death). With the implementation of proper techniques and preparation, a good death can be readily achieved.

The euthanasia agents used in most animal hospice cases are those commonly used in all veterinary hospitals to facilitate death and they are given via injection. The most common pharmaceutical agent is pentobarbital, a barbiturate anesthetic previously used in veterinary medicine to induce anesthesia before surgery. These days, pentobarbital is used almost exclusively as the gold-standard, injectable drug for euthanasia. Pentobarbital combination products include the addition of agents like phenytoin sodium. Euthanasia solutions in the US are manufactured by a variety of companies and typically come colored with a dye to distinguish them from other liquid substances. Other countries may use different lethal agents, include a colored dye or not, and offer pentobarbital with assorted concentrations.

Pentobarbital works on the brain to first induce unconsciousness, then cause a cessation of breathing, followed by cardiac death, all in usually less than one minute when the drug is given intravenously. It can be administered to conscious animals orally, intravenously, or into the abdomen via intraperitoneal injections (IP). Any other route requires patient unconsciousness, which is achievable through the administration of pre-euthanasia anesthetics.

In animal hospice, patients are often very weak or severely compromised. Knowing the various euthanasia techniques and when to use them will make for a smoother experience for all. While veterinarians are usually the ones performing the procedure, all hospice team members can and should learn about it. In some states, non-veterinarians are allowed to euthanize animals under direct or indirect veterinary supervision. (For a summary of state laws, see the AVMA's webpage, available at: www.avma.org/sites/default/files/2019-12/Euthanasia-Chart.pdf). A collective understanding of the entire experience, not just the techniques themselves, should elevate the team's ability to support both patient and caregiver. A procedural meeting is a great way to begin to prepare everyone for best practices (Box 24.1).

During the procedural meeting, team members can be introduced to resources providing

---

Box 24.1 Animal hospice team meeting agenda: The euthanasia experience.

Required attendance: the entire team
 Suggested time frame: two to three hours Topics:
  Reasons for euthanasia
  Family preparations
  Staff preparations
  Animal comfort
  Drugs utilized
  Reactions: expected and unexpected
  Body respect and aftercare options
  Memorializing
  Emotional support: family and team

Box 24.2 The 14 essential components of companion animal euthanasia.

G = Grief support materials provided
O = Outline caregiver and pet preferences
O = Offer privacy before and after death
D = Deliver proper technique
E = Establish rapport
U = Use pre-euthanasia sedation or anesthesia
T = Thorough, complete consent
H = Helpful and compassionate personnel
A = Adequate time
N = Narrate the process
A = Avoid pain and anxiety
S = Safe space to gather
I = Inclusion of loved ones
A = Assistance with body care

Source: Cooney (2019).

---

additional training. The books *In-home Pet Euthanasia Techniques* (Cooney 2011), *Veterinary Euthanasia Techniques* (Callan et al. 2012), and *Small Animal Euthanasia* (Marchitelli 2020) are among the few books written entirely about euthanasia. *Blue Juice*, by sociologist Patricia Morris, takes a philosophical and historical look at the act of taking life in the veterinary industry (Morris 2012). Technical manuals have been published by the Humane Society of the United States (*Euthanasia Training Manual*) and by the American Humane Association (*Euthanasia by Injection*) (Rhoades 2002; Fakkema 2008). The International Association for Animal Hospice and Palliative Care (IAAHPC) commonly offers euthanasia-focused tracks at their annual conference, and CAETA provides a certificate program plus countless learning modules in what they refer to as the "art of gentle death." Every animal hospice team should also have a copy of the AVMA's *Guidelines for the Euthanasia of Animals* accessible at all times. These guidelines are free and readily available through the AVMA website. Box 24.2 provides an outline of euthanasia best practices for teams to adhere to.

Lastly, the hospice team including euthanasia practitioner can physically and mentally prepare for a euthanasia. In an effort to reduce or prevent compassion fatigue brought on by primary or secondary traumatic stress, team members can practice self-regulation to calm nerves and relax the body. In addition, taking time to establish rapport with caregivers and patients before euthanasia has the potential to release the hormone oxytocin in the body to further set the stage for trust and tranquility.

Advance Preparation and Education of Caregivers and Family

Once the decision to euthanize has been made, caregivers will need to prepare and decide on what is important when saying goodbye. These preparations are specific to each family and will reflect different factors such as time of day, where the animal is most comfortable, and who wants to be present. A family may have ideas about how they want euthanasia to occur, but if they don't, they may ask for guidance.

There are four main factors to consider: who, where, when, and how. In the hospital setting, these factors are usually less flexible, but options certainly still exist. Except in crisis situations when the animal may have been brought to an emergency veterinary facility or when veterinary staff cannot offer home care, natural death and euthanasia will occur in the home setting. Home euthanasia is commonly chosen for those caregivers hoping to say goodbye in a more private setting, where animals can remain more comfortable with loved ones gathered close and for easier home burial logistics. Hospital euthanasia is typically chosen due to the strong bond between veterinarian/staff and the family, the presence of support staff, and convenience of the location.

There are simple, creative ways to achieve a more peaceful and fear-free environment for families that choose to bring their pet to a hospital for euthanasia. For dogs that can ambulate, it is paramount to provide nonslip flooring to prevent falls. Other ways to transform an exam room into a more comfortable space is by utilizing soft lighting and turning off overhead fluorescents. It has been documented that the utilization of canine and feline pheromone diffusers and soothing music can reduce anxiety, thus making for a more peaceful experience. Also the temperature of the room should be adjusted to suit the comfort of the pet. Provide warmth for patients that are shivering and lower the temperature for pets that are panting. For improved comfort; candles, wind chimes and a water fountain feature can also modify the room into a more serene retreat. The creation of a quiet outdoor space or garden can offer an additional location for a hospital euthanasia.

To insure the pet owner has ample time with their pet before and after the euthanasia, it is important to proactively schedule during the quiet times of the day (if possible, before or after routine appointments are completed). Various codes can be used in a multi-doctor practice to inform others that euthanasia is in progress and they should be mindfully quiet to respect the family. Examples include the placement of a special flag on a door, turning on a special light, or playing specific music. Lastly, all hospital staff should be trained in how to provide considerate aftercare of the pet's body.

When the family has decided on what is important to them, and what they believe to be important to their beloved animal, the hospice team can help them realize their requests. As shown in Box 24.3, discussing these themes is a good way to begin. If any of the requests cannot be met by the animal hospice team, hopefully suitable alternatives can be found.

Once the decision to euthanize is made, team members should describe the process in detail to help prepare those present. The euthanasia procedure itself is no time for surprises. This being said, there is such a thing as too much detail. In this author's experience, caregivers do not usually want to know specifics on why the veterinarian or nurse is choosing one technique over another or how the drugs work on the body. They will mostly want to know what is being done to keep their animal safe and comfortable.

Before the appointment during advanced preparation, the caregiver considerations outlined in Box 24.3 can be reviewed. During the appointment, payment is handled first (if not already done beforehand), as well as signing of euthanasia consent forms and body care requests and sharing grief support literature. Information is provided about the use of pre-euthanasia sedation or anesthesia and everyone who wants to be present is gathered. When the animal is sleeping or otherwise ready for euthanasia, the family is gently informed and preparations are made accordingly. Before death occurs, those present should be reasonably prepared for what death itself will look like. It helps them to accept any physical changes like open eyes, reflexive breathing, body stretches, or emptying of the bowels, as normal and simply part of the process. This should be minimized so as not to cause unnecessary worry.

Box 24.3   Caregiver considerations before euthanasia.

1) Who: Immediate family members
   Extended family members and friends
   Their household pets
   Primary hospice veterinarian or routine care veterinarian
   Other hospice team members, including those for spiritual support
   Cemetery or crematory staff to help with body care
2) Where: Inside the home
   Outside the home
   Local part or community area
   Clinic or hospital
   Specialty pet euthanasia care center
3) When: Day or night
   Weekday or weekend
   On a day of significance to the caregiver(s)
   Before, during, or after a crisis event if one presents
   In accordance with any event that brings unmanageable suffering
4) How: Simple and straightforward
   Ceremonial with possible music, readings, candles, etc.
   Use of pre-euthanasia sedation or anesthesia (often preset by the team regardless)
   Euthanasia method determined by patient signalment, veterinarian preferences
   Length of appointment catered to everyone's needs

As with so many things in life, predicting the exact time and manner of death is impossible. Nevertheless, euthanasia offers us some control over such things. Yet even a planned euthanasia still requires a conversation about the unanticipated, such as what to do if the animal declines in health unexpectedly before everyone is ready. Advance preparation and education of the caregiver(s) includes the provision of emergency drugs to administer in times of crisis. These emergency drugs aim to induce sleep and minimize suffering until animal hospice personnel arrive at the home or the animal can be transported to a veterinary facility. These medicines can be given before euthanasia with the understanding that, once given, the person performing the euthanasia will be able to do so within an hour or two. Caregivers who keep these emergency drugs in their home should be instructed on how to safely store and administer them if and when

necessary. Ideally these drugs will give the animal the relief it needs and allow the veterinary staff to perform the euthanasia procedure they are most comfortable with. If these emergency drugs are never used, the caregiver will need to properly dispose of them in accordance with state and federal drug disposal laws.

Euthanasia Setting: Desirable Environment of Care

In this author's opinion, the most important component of any euthanasia is compassion. A close second is skill, and third is trust. Compassion and the bond between caregiver and pet remain front and center, always. The environment where the bond is honored can be shaped to hold special touches that keep the space inviting, calm, and safe. Whether in the home or hospital, loved ones are welcome and time allowed for meaningful goodbyes.

Caregivers benefit when given space to share their needs, hopes, and fears around euthanasia. A desirable environment includes the chance to openly communicate about their feelings. This deepens the understanding between caregiver and hospice team and helps everyone align. Euthanasia is a procedure with no "do-overs" and as such, requires trust and honesty between all parties from the start.

Euthanasia settings in hospice are often the home environment. Family, friends, children, and other pets are regularly present. It is common to gather in various rooms of the home or outdoors; wherever the patient is content and loved ones can openly mourn. Caregivers desire to have some control over how their pet's final moments will be, regardless of where the procedure ultimately takes place. Some need a little; some need a lot. The veterinary team's role is to be a guide during euthanasia, a shepherd or chaperone.

Useful tips to create safe space, home or hospital:

- Understand the needs of the pet owner before entering
- Move slowly with soft body posture
- Learn everyone's name
- Take deep breaths throughout the appointment
- Include natural elements – trees, flowers, water
- Provide time to hear stories
- Perform a technically strong euthanasia

Euthanasia Techniques and Criteria

When deciding upon a euthanasia technique, veterinary staff must choose one that is appropriate for the situation and take all factors into consideration. The method of euthanasia chosen will depend on many things:

1) practitioner's comfort with the technique
2) supplies available
3) the presence of onlookers
4) the type of euthanasia solution and the amount available
5) the use of sedation or anesthesia
6) the signalment and physical condition of the animal
7) the need for a postmortem exam

Every technique should be checked against the AVMA's criteria for euthanasia (Box 24.4). Not every one of these 14 criteria can always be met, but they should at least be considered as the technique is chosen. Caregiver(s) will not need to know exactly why a particular method is chosen over another; however, generalizations may be made for those seeking to know details.

The use of pre-euthanasia sedation or anesthesia to induce unconsciousness is commonplace in modern euthanasia best practices. The benefits of sedation for the animal and involved personnel generally are accepted as greatly

---

Box 24.4   AVMA Euthanasia Criteria.

1) Ability to induce loss of consciousness and death without pain or anxiety
2) Time required to induce loss of consciousness
3) Reliability
4) Safety of personnel
5) Irreversibility
6) Compatibility with requirement and purpose
7) Documented emotional effect on observers and operators
8) Compatibility with use of tissue, examination
9) Drug availability and human abuse potential
10) Compatibility with species and health status
11) Ability to maintain equipment in working order
12) Safety for predators/scavengers should the body be consumed
13) Legal requirements
14) Environmental impacts of the method or carcass disposition

Source: Adapted from AVMA Euthanasia Guidelines 2020.

outweighing any potential negative effects (Robertson 2020). Providing sleep before death has proven useful to reduce pain, anxiety, and stress for the patient in their final moments of life. Unconsciousness brought on by the administration of anesthetics is required for intraorgan injections, when sedation may not be enough to prevent pain. Common sedatives include benzodiazepines (e.g. midazolam), opioids (e.g. butorphanol), α2 agonists (e.g. dexmedetomidine), and phenothiazines (e.g. acepromazine). Common anesthetics include dissociatives (e.g. ketamine), hypnotics (e.g. propofol), neurosteroids (e.g. alfaxalone), and anesthetic gases (e.g. isoflurane) (Cooney 2021). This author advocates for sedation or anesthesia be provided to the patient via subcutaneous or intramuscular injection before necessary restraint for all euthanasia methods. This approach is widely used within animal hospice as a whole and aligns well with the mission of gentle death.

With any of these techniques, veterinary personnel should take their time and be consistent. If the first chosen technique is not going to work, readily moving on to another should help ensure things continue smoothly for those present and the animal. The author encourages veterinary personnel to learn as much about different techniques as possible, even for those species rarely seen. Poorly performed euthanasias, defined as dysthanasia by CAETA, complicates the mourning process. With proper education and training in euthanasia, the incidence of bad euthanasia should decrease, which is essential for everyone involved. Listed here are brief descriptions of common techniques for the euthanasia of companion animals, such as dogs and cats, using pentobarbital solution.

Intravenous Injection

Pros
 Fast and effective
 Standard dosing of solution
 Sedation not required but recommended

Cons
 Venous access necessary
 Blood pressure concerns
 Requires moderate skill

In order to perform an intravenous (IV) injection, one needs to find a vein to work with. The accessory cephalic and cephalic veins in the front leg and the medial and lateral saphenous veins in the back leg are easy to see and feel. The dorsal pedal vein near the tarsus is also a popular choice. The practitioner chooses the one that is most appropriate under the circumstances.

Intravenous injections using a barbiturate like pentobarbital require dosing of 85 mg/kg^{-1} of body weight (Leary et al. 2020). If the euthanasia solution is extremely thick, it can be diluted with saline to ease its movement through the needle and/or catheter. If the plan is to insert the euthanasia syringe with needle directly into the patient's vein, it is prudent to draw back and check for blood. To be safe, one should draw back at least once during venous administration to make sure that the needle is still placed correctly. Indwelling IV catheters are the best way to guarantee the euthanasia solution remains in the vein during injection.

Euthanasia solution is injected slowly and steadily during IV injections (Figure 24.2). When all of the solution has been injected into the vein, the needle can be removed. Pressure is briefly applied to the site to stop any bleeding. An IV catheter can be flushed with saline to ensure it is cleared of the euthanasia solution. When performing an IV injection, it is important to remember that death occurs very quickly, the effects of the injection typically noticeable within approximately 30 seconds. A slower rate of administration in sedated patients can reduce active signs of death (Cooney 2021). Once death has occurred, the injection site may be wiped to clean the area.

Intracardiac Injection

Pros
 Fast and effective
 Eliminates venous pressure concerns
 Provides a large surface area to inject

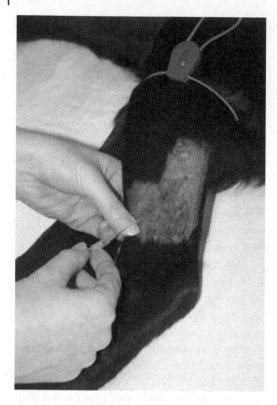

Figure 24.2 Demonstration of intravenous injection in a dog.

Cons

    Perception as gruesome

    Requires advanced skill

    Requires unconsciousness

The intracardiac (IC) injection is a useful technique for many reasons, the primary being the avoidance of veins with poor blood pressure, a common occurrence in hospice patients. The easiest way to give an IC injection is to have the animal laying in lateral recumbency on either their right or left side. This author prefers to have the patient lying on his or her right side because the heart is easier to auscult from the left and the left ventricle is usually the largest available chamber to inject. The heart in most dogs and cats will reside from the 2nd or 3rd intercostal space (ICS) to the 5th or 6th ICS and from the sternum to about two-thirds of the way up the thorax (Pasquini and Spurgeon 1992). Other species have variable

heart locations, so it is important to know the anatomy before attempting to inject. Often, the heart is located more cranial and ventral than expected.

When auscultating the heart, the provider needs to pinpoint the point of maximum intensity (PMI). On the left side of the chest, this will likely be the point of the aortic valve located in the 4th ICS at the level of the shoulder. On the right side, the right aortic valve will be the loudest and is also in the 4th ICS at the level of the olecranon/elbow. The olecranon is located near the 5th ICS so there will be little heart caudal to this point. A stethoscope or hand is used to locate the PMI on the chest wall. Then, the lower antebrachium is grasped and the elbow pressed up the chest wall to simulate where it would normally be if the animal were standing. A good place to insert the needle is just a bit cranial to the point of the elbow. Combining the location of the PMI with this landmark should help to safely locate the heart (Figure 24.3).

The patient must be fully unconscious and should not react to the injection in any way. Pre-euthanasia anesthesia is required to prevent patient pain and distress. This remains true for any intraorgan injection.

When injecting into the heart, it is essential to draw back blood to ensure proper needle placement into a chamber. This requires a little extra room in the syringe, so a larger syringe is needed than is necessary to hold the euthanasia solution alone. For example, if giving 6 ml of solution, a 12-ml syringe will provide enough room for the solution and for blood to be aspirated before the injection begins. This is also helpful if fluid such as a pulmonary effusion is accidentally drawn up in the syringe. Similarly, if the tip of the syringe is within an airway, the practitioner will draw back air. A little extra space in the syringe is helpful to overcome the added volume. The AVMA Euthanasia Guidelines recommend 85 mg/kg^{-1} of pentobarbital solution, just like IV injections. This is a minimum requirement and one may always give more to a patient if needed.

Figure 24.3 Anatomical location of the intracardiac injection in a dog.

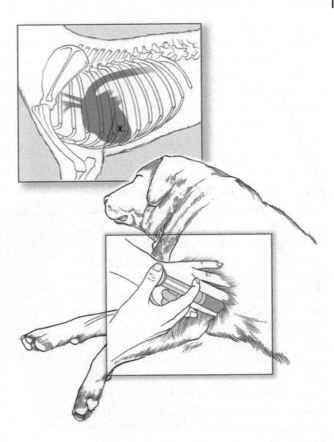

When performing an intracardiac injection in larger animals, it is necessary to use a long needle. Smaller animals may only require a short 1-inch needle. Larger dogs often require a 2-inch needle or longer. The needle can be attached directly to a syringe or to a short extension line (Cooney 2021). When preparing to enter the chest wall, the needle should be kept perpendicular to the body. Angling the needle will increase the amount of tissue through which the needle needs to travel before reaching the heart. If a rib is encountered during penetration of the chest wall, the injection can be started over or the needle tip gently "walked off" the rib edge.

When the needle is believed to be in the heart, the plunger is drawn back. If negative pressure is encountered, the needle tip is within something solid (e.g. the myocardium, a tumor, etc.). The needle is then pushed farther or angled slightly different and the plunger

drawn back again. When there is rush of blood into the syringe, the euthanasia solution is administered. Time to death is rapid, usually less than one minute when properly performed.

Intraperitoneal Injection

Pros
    Easy to perform
    Works well in smaller companion animals
    Sedation not required but recommended
Cons
    Longer time to absorb
    More solution needed
    Risk of injecting organs if still conscious

An IP means the euthanasia solution is given into the peritoneal space (the abdomen). The solution must therefore miss neighboring organs or the administration will be considered intraorgan and without sedation is considered painful (Wadham 1997, Laferriere and

Pang 2020). Even though pre-sedation is not required for this technique, this author's preference is to always give it.

The typical area for injection is low on the right lateral abdomen just caudal to the umbilicus. This region should be more amenable to injection with reduced organ presence. The needle should be inserted at an angle slightly toward the head and the syringe plunger pulled to aspirate for negative pressure or air. If no blood or fluid is seen in the syringe, the practitioner can proceed to inject. Because the euthanasia solution is moving into the bloodstream through absorption across abdominal organ membranes and serosa linings, it may take longer to achieve cardiac death. Three times the IV dose is required for this technique (Leary et al. 2020). If the patient is not pre-sedated and is still conscious after 15–20 minutes, more solution is administered, especially with the caregiver present. IPs will typically cause death within 15–30 minutes. This technique takes longer than most, which can be challenging for anyone expecting a rapid death. However, this added time provides opportunity for storytelling and sharing of memories common in animal hospice work. When necessary, the abdomen can be massaged to help the solution absorb.

Intrahepatic Injection

Pros

    Simple technique

    Provides a large surface area to inject

Cons

    Requires unconsciousness

    More solution needed

The liver is large, highly vascular, and is usually easy to palpate. Veterinarians choose intrahepatic (IH) injections over IP injections because of the improved uptake of the euthanasia solution. The liver is highly vascular and should speed the drug's uptake to the brain. When an IV injection is not viable, an IH injection can be a great alternative. Like IC injections, IH injections need to be done under anesthesia or a state of unconsciousness (Figure 24.4).

It is necessary to choose a needle length that is sufficient for reaching the liver. With small animals, a 1-in. needle should be adequate, but in larger animals, a 1.5-inch or 2-inch needle may be necessary. The AVMA recommends 170 mg/kg^{-1} of euthanasia solution. The expected time to death using the IH method is under two minutes. If the liver is missed, death may not occur as rapidly. Administering a second dose should shorten time to death.

To inject the liver, the needle is placed in the notch on either side of the xyphoid process and aimed cranially, up under the last rib of the laterally recumbent animal (Callan et al. 2012). Some pressure can be applied inward with the syringe or with a free hand to allow the needle to move deeper. There is no need to draw back and check for blood. IH injections work well from either the left or right side. At the start of

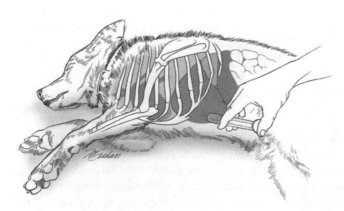

Figure 24.4 Anatomical placement of an intrahepatic injection.

the injection, it is prudent to inject a tiny amount of pentobarbital solution to ensure no patient response before infusing the total volume. If the patient is not fully unconscious, they may react in pain. Time can then be provided to allow for deeper sleep before the total volume is administered. The same is true for all other intraorgan injections.

Intrarenal Injections

Pros

    Well suited to cats and small mammals

    Fast and effective

Cons

    Requires unconsciousness

    Requires moderate skill

This method is a great choice when venous access is difficult or when preparing a catheter site is too obtrusive. As with IH injections, the kidneys will speed the rate of absorption over standard IP injections. As with cardiac and hepatic injections, anesthesia is required. This technique has gained popularity in felines and other small mammals. Canines tend to have significant musculature along the back, which can make kidney injections more difficult, however thin body conditioning may make it possible.

The goal with an intrarenal (IR) injection is to locate a kidney, then hold it in position for the injection of euthanasia solution. When choosing which kidney to inject, the practitioner selects the one that can be easily isolated from surrounding abdominal tissue. If the patient is in renal failure, the kidneys may be smaller, have a nodular feeling, or be difficult to locate but the technique may still be used.

Once the patient is unconscious, the caregiver can hold them on their lap or the patient can be gently placed on any soft surface. The practitioner then gently runs their hands along the abdomen to find the kidney and feel for any abdominal muscle tensing. If the patient tenses, they are not unconscious enough for the renal injection, and more anesthetic must be administered until no response is noted.

When ready to inject, the practitioner uses one hand to push the kidney upward, from the patient's (lower) downside, into the other hand to hold the kidney firmly in place, raising it up parallel with the spine (Figure 24.5). The kidney is best held in this manner throughout the entire injection. If the kidney is accidentally released mid-injection, the practitioner can attempt to finish the injection by directing the needle toward the kidney deep in the abdomen. If the kidney cannot be found, the syringe is gently advanced toward the liver and the injection completed.

IR euthanasia requires more solution than an intravenous (IV) injection would. The standard injection amount is three times the IV dose, or 255 mg/kg^{-1} (Leary et al 2020). This recommended amount is anecdotal based on reported practitioner successes, and further study may indicate less can be used. While less solution may effectively facilitate death, more solution is beneficial in case the needle must be redirected to locate the target.

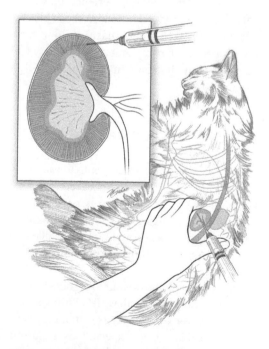

Figure 24.5 Anatomical placement of an intrarenal injection.

Upon injection, the practitioner should feel the kidney swell. This is a good indication that the needle is positioned properly within the renal cortex. The rest of the solution can then be injected. If certain that the needle is positioned correctly and the kidney does not swell, the needle might be inadvertently placed into the renal pelvis, which will slow uptake into the vasculature. Kidney swelling does not guarantee immediate death, but it does increase the success rate. It is common for patients to stop breathing before the injection is complete. As with IH injections, it is good practice to let the caregiver know ahead of time that their animal may pass immediately or within just a few minutes.

Following any of these techniques, personnel will listen to the heart to confirm death. When achieved, those present should be informed that death has occurred and when possible, private time offered. The body can remain with the family as long as they wish or the hospice team can help expedite body care, such as cremation or burial. The important thing is that the entire experience flows at a pace suitable to loved ones and those providing the care. When euthanasia is done well, loved ones will be very grateful and likely feel safe choosing it again in the future if the need arises.

Variability and Unpredictability

Those who've performed euthanasia long enough have likely experienced variable responses to drugs and protocols, or the misfortune of a challenging procedure. Euthanasia like any medical act can be unpredictable and complex. As animal hospice providers, our mission is to provide a gentle death, which is exactly what caregivers want too. There is nothing inherently wrong with variety during euthanasia, however consistency is better, especially when caregivers have expectations regarding how things should proceed. Many have gone through the procedure before with other pets. Hospice team members also benefit when the appointment progresses in a stable, secure manner. Unpredictability is most likely to occur when using different drugs, when working with novel species or breeds, and when faced with a challenging patient condition, e.g. aggression, breathing difficulty, seizures.

Dysthanasia is a term used to define a bad euthanasia experience, the opposite of a good death. As of 2021, the word is still being shaped by what caregivers and veterinary professionals believe equals a bad death. When it occurs in practice, there remains the opportunity to address it and mitigate negative emotions as a result. By recognizing a dysthanasia has happened, the animal hospice team and/or euthanasia practitioner sets a clear resolution plan in place.

A dysthanasia case example with resolution plan: The hospice team has decided what equals a quality euthanasia appointment. They have put protocols in place to deliver a safe and meaningful euthanasia for the patient, and a gentle experience for the caregiver and their team. During the appointment, however, things go awry, the technique of choice doesn't work, and the euthanasia becomes an unpleasant, drawn-out ordeal for all involved. The caregiver is visibly upset, and the team is shaken. According to the established protocols, the appointment is labeled a dysthanasia, and the next step is to adequately address what happened, first with a team debriefing to discuss what went wrong and troubleshoot solutions to prevent future occurrences, and then of equal importance, reaching out to the caregiver with empathy and a discussion about what happened.

Talking about a dysthanasia will never be easy, but connecting with caregivers afterward, to answer questions and belay fears of the unknown, is always necessary. According to CAETA who fields dysthanasia calls from pet owners around the United States, the number one concern is pain during death. Gently and compassionately reviewing the facts helps put things in perspective and calms fears. Lead the conversation with, for example: "Yesterday did not go as we all expected. While some things are beyond our control, I want to thank you for your patience with the process, and for allowing me [and my team] to move forward in the best way possible. What questions can I answer for you?"

Professionally, animal hospice teams must forgive themselves, learn from the experience, and use the dysthanasia as a legacy for improvement. Some hospitals, especially those with a large euthanasia appointment volume, hold rounds focused on euthanasia, or at least include successes and challenges each time they meet. Dysthanasia begs to be talked about,

not only to address the technical issues, but also to provide space for team members to share their experiences.

Embracing the three C's:

- Provide *Compassion*. Things may go wrong but maintain the desire to love and serve.
- Portray *Confidence*. This increases trust in the team's ability to handle the situation.
- Maintain *Control*. The euthanasia is completed, or the decision is made to postpone until issues can be resolved.

References

August, K., Cooney, K., Hendrix, L., et al. (2017) Animal Hospice and Palliative Care Guidelines. International Association for Animal Hospice and Palliative Care (IAAHPC). Available at: https://iaahpc.org/wp-content/uploads/2020/10/IAAHPC-AHPC-GUIDELINESpdf.pdf (Accessed: July 6, 2021).

Callan, R., Chappell, J., Connally, B. et al. (2012) Veterinary Euthanasia Techniques: A Practical Guide. Ames, IA: Wiley Blackwell.

Cooney, K. (2011) In-Home Animal Euthanasia Techniques: The Veterinarian's Guide to Helping Families and their Pets Say Goodbye in the Comfort of Home. Amazon Press.

Cooney, K. (2019) The 'Good Death Revolution' – companion animal euthanasia in the modern age. Veterinary Practice News. Available at: https://www.veterinarypracticenews.com/good-death-revolution-companion-animal-euthanasia-modern-age (Accessed: August 3, 2021).

Cooney, K. (2021) Euthanasia protocols. Clinician's Brief. Available at: https://www.cliniciansbrief.com/article/euthanasia-protocols (Accessed: August 15, 2021).

Dickinson, G.E., Cooney, K., and Hoffmann, H. (2021) Euthanasia education in veterinary schools in the United States. *J Vet Med Educ.*, 48(6): 706–709. https://doi.org/10.3138/jvme-2020-0050

Fakkema, D. (2008) Euthanasia by Injection – Training Guide. American Humane Association.

Leary, S., Underwood, W., Anthony, R. et al. (2020) AVMA Guidelines for the Euthanasia of Animals. American Veterinary Medical Association (AVMA). Accessed August 31, 2021. https://www.avma.org/sites/default/files/2020-02/Guidelines-on-Euthanasia-2020.pdf

Laferriere, C.A. and Pang, D.S. (2020) Review of intraperitoneal injection of sodium pentobarbital as a method of euthanasia in laboratory rodents. *J. Am. Assoc. Lab. Anim. Sci.*, 59(3): 254–263.

Marchitelli, B.(2020) Euthanasia in Veterinary Medicine. Small Animal Euthanasia; Updates on Clinical Practice. Elsevier.

Morris, P. (2012) Blue Juice. Philadelphia: Temple University Press.

Pasquini, C. and Spurgeon, T. (1992) Anatomy of Domestic Animals, 5. Pilot Point: Sudz Publishing.

Rhoades, R. (2002) Euthanasia Training Manual. Washington, D.C.: Humane Society of the United States.

Robertson, S. (2020) Pharmacologic Methods: An Update on Optimal Presedation and Euthanasia Solution Administration. *Vet. Clin. N. Am. -Small Anim. Pract.*, 50(3):525–543.

Wadham, J, Townsend P, Morton D. (1997) Intraperitoneal injection of sodium pentobarbitone as a method of euthanasia for rodents. *ANZCCART News* 1997; 10(4):8

Part III

Caregiver Needs: Providing Support

25

Caregivers' Emotional Burden: Understanding, Acknowledging, and Addressing Caregivers' Emotional Burden

Amir Shanan, DVM

Efforts to assess caregivers' burdens and resources are made only in rare instances in the veterinary healthcare system. Referral to skilled animal palliative care practitioners early in the course of animals' illness enhances the physical and emotional wellbeing of both the animal patient and her human caregivers. This increases the referring veterinary practices client satisfaction and retention.

In her new book, *Just Like Family: How Companion Animals Joined the Household* (Laurent-Simpson 2021), sociologist Andrea Laurent-Simpson asserts the American family structure is changing to include nonhuman species. "American pet owners are transforming the cultural definition of family," Laurent-Simpson says. "Dogs and cats are treated like children, siblings, grandchildren." The American Veterinary Medical Association found that "85% of dog owners and 76% of cat owners think of their pets as family. The same is true for 57% of the owners of pet birds and 47% of the owners of pet horses." (AVMA 2018) With seventy percent of U.S. households owning a pet (APPA 2022), this means that between one third and one half of the US total population think of their pets as family.

It should come as no surprise, then, that caregiving at the animal's end of life is a significant event in the lives of many people. This was documented by research over 20 years ago

(Adams et al. 2000; Lagoni et al. 1994) With the profound significance of animals in humans' lives and the deep emotional connections recognized, there is growing awareness that as animals near the end of their lives, these animals' human primary caregivers face increased responsibilities and experience significant emotional turmoil. The author's observations during 28 years of clinical veterinary end-of-life care practice support the idea that what pet caregivers experience shares important features with the experience of caregivers of seriously ill/dying human patients. This is supported by a study (Britton et al. 2018) comparing burden and positive aspects of caregiving in owners of a seriously ill companion animal and caregivers of a family member with dementia. The study showed both differences and similarities between the two groups. Its findings suggest that both groups show comparable experiences of fearing the future, guilt, and financial strain; and that in both groups experiencing positive aspects of caregiving was associated with a lower burden.

The experience of caregiving for seriously ill companion animals and its impact on the caregiver's mental health has been studied in recent years (See Chapter 26 in this volume). Mental health considerations relevant to caregiving for seriously ill and dying human patients, however, have been studied for nearly

Hospice and Palliative Care for Companion Animals: Principles and Practice, Second Edition.
Edited by Amir Shanan, Jessica Pierce, and Tamara Shearer.
© 2023 John Wiley & Sons, Inc. Published 2023 by John Wiley & Sons, Inc.
Companion website: www.wiley.com/go/shanan/palliative

half a century. This chapter highlights issues described in the human caregiver burden literature, which in the author's experience, are relevant to caregiving for animals at the end of life. The reader will therefore find throughout the chapter extrapolations to caregiving for animals from references written about caregiving for human patients. Those extrapolations are supported by the many thousands of hours the author has spent listening to and providing support for caregivers of animals nearing the end of life.

Caregiving Experience

Caregiving requires outlays of time, money, and physical work provided to loved ones for no financial compensation. Thus, it is a financially thankless and often lonely experience. According to *Caregiving in the United States 2020* (AARP and National Alliance for Caregiving 2020), an estimated 53 million adults (more than 20% of the US population) are caregivers, having provided care to an adult or child with special needs at some time in the past 12 months. Of those, nearly 70% use no paid help for their caregiving, and 33% (more than 17 millions) provide care alone, with no paid or unpaid help. The percentages of caregivers providing care with no paid help and/or alone are certainly higher among caregivers of seriously ill companion animals.

Caregivers of dying patients face complex and multifaceted responsibilities (Stewart et al. 1999). Family caregivers' role in the patients' day-to-day life varies, depending on the physical and mental condition of the dying patient and on the caregivers' physical, emotional, and financial resources. The caregiver's most immediate task may be about the physical aspects of care: helping a loved one eat, stay clean, or even breathe – whether that loved one is a person or an animal. In addition, caregivers perform the emotional tasks of sharing love and compassion, reflecting on the relationship and remembering good times.

Caregivers are expected to assess and report information regarding the patient's pain, including the source, nature, and amount of pain. They must identify and report side effects of the patient's therapy as well as new symptoms experienced by the patient. Caregivers make day-to-day decisions that determine a patient's comfort, such as which medication to administer, when to give it, and at what dosage. These decisions may be complex and even overwhelming, especially when the patient is unable to assist in carrying them out. Caregivers are asked to keep records, and fill and refill prescriptions – responsibilities that presuppose such skills as the ability to follow medical instructions and the ability to anticipate the need for refills ahead of time (Glajchen 2003, 2004).

Caregivers of seriously and/or terminally ill patients have specific needs that include having the time to say goodbye, being present when the patient died, and being able to talk with staff after the patient's death about events surrounding the terminal illness. Caregivers may need a place to safely discuss their fears (Hinds and Kelly 2010). An important need of many caregivers is for medical care to meet the patients' needs: in a qualitative study to identify aspects of patient and family quality of life, families indicated that the patient's needs were more important than theirs (Wadhwa et al. 2013). Lagoni et al. (1994) list the needs of caregivers with emotional bonds to their seriously ill companion animals in Box 25.1.

Among the challenges that caregivers of hospice and palliative care patients universally face, uncertainty looms large. Caregiver's lives are less secure or predictable than they once were because changes in the patient's condition is rarely predictable. Caregivers make important decisions, the consequences of which are rarely known with certainty. Concerns that treatments will not work or cause unpleasant side effects, resulting in discomfort for the patient, are reality based and distressing. Making plans for life after the loss is difficult because the loss will change

<table>
<tr><td>

Box 25.1 Caregivers' emotional needs related to the bond with their companion animal.

- trust
- personalized and focused attention
- information
- acknowledgement of the human–animal bond
- confidence in veterinary team's ability to identify and respond to sensitive issues
- validation of intuition, observations, and perceptions regarding the pet's health
- communication skills that sooth anxiety and fear
- a feeling of partnership during decision-making and treatment procedures
- direct honest communication
- access to veterinarian/Approachable and available staff
- referrals to specialists and related experts
- commitment to identify and work through differences
- skilled support during crises, pet loss, and emotionally vulnerable times
- empathy

Source: Adapted from Lagoni et al. (2001).

</td></tr>
</table>

aregivers' lives in some yet unknown ways. It may impact relationships, interfere with caregivers' ability to function normally, and may have long lasting ramifications

Uncertainty leads to feeling vulnerable along with a myriad of other reactions that often include anxiety, anger, sadness, or fear. These reactions may interrupt sleep or interfere with caregivers' ability to concentrate or participate in activities they previously enjoyed. Coping with uncertainty is an important part of caregivers' efforts to stay emotionally healthy.

Uncertainty is often distressing when caregivers face making difficult decisions about their loved ones' end-of-life care, while they themselves are experiencing the intense emotions of anticipatory or acute grief. Pet caregivers have power to influence the comfort and suffering and life and death of a beloved animal, who has wishes and preferences but can't verbally express them, requiring caregivers to be skilled at interpreting animal behavior. The uncertainty about what the patient really wants is emotionally challenging and can be overwhelming, and fear of making decisions that are inconsistent with "what the animal wants" is a common source of caregiver distress.

The decisions made about the animal's end of life care can greatly influence the caregivers' subsequent process of adjusting to and reconciling the loss. Caregivers commonly feel a huge burden when making decisions about whether or not the animal's death will be assisted by euthanasia, and if so when. The uncertainty about what the patient really wants is complicated by uncertainty about the consequences of each of the available choices. Adding to this pressure can be financial and time considerations, and resultant guilt that can be paralyzing if pending decisions are perceived by the caregiver as "wrong" or "selfish."

At the time of death or euthanasia, caregivers face many decisions about the details of the transition process. Some of the decisions that pet caregivers have to make at the time of impending death or euthanasia are listed in Box 25.2.

Wadhwa et al. (2013) evaluated the quality of life and mental health of caregivers of human cancer patients who were at an advanced (but not terminal) stage of the illness and were not receiving hospice or other palliative care. The study showed that caregivers experienced substantial emotional distress. Caregivers' *overall quality of life* was shown to be significantly impacted by patients' *physical* health: caregiving demands and challenges increased exponentially when the patient's condition progressed and his or her needs increased. Caregivers' *mental health*, specifically, was more directly impacted by patients' *emotional* well-being: the more the patient is suffering emotionally, the more his or her

---

Box 25.2 Decisions that have to be made at the time of an animal's death.

- Who will be with the patient at the time of death?
- How long will the caregiver stay with the deceased animal before the body is removed?
- When, how, and who covers or wraps the body?
- Will a ritual be performed (such as reciting a prayer)?
- Where will the body be transported? By whom?
- Will the body be cremated or buried?
- If cremated, how will the cremains be handled?
- If buried, where, how, and when?
- How can the life that ended best be memorialized and honored?

Source: Adapted from Shanan (2011).

---

family caregivers do. Wadhwa et al. (2013) describe factors that influence the end-of-life caregiving experience as caregiver, patient, and care-related.

- Patient factors include the type and stage of disease process as well as personality traits and coping style.
- Care-related factors include location, duration, intensity, and cost of care, as well as the availability of caregiver support.
- Caregiver factors include physical and mental health, living arrangements, financial resources, and the quality of the relationship between caregiver and patient.

All of those considerations apply to caregivers of animal patients. In addition, "reading" animals' state of emotional well-being requires caregivers to be skilled at interpreting animal behavior. As mentioned above, the risk of misjudging what the animal is experiencing and making "wrong" choices – resulting in less than optimal care for the animal – is

another potential source of future regret and guilt for caregivers.

Family members of seriously ill human patients experience as much emotional distress, or more, than the patient does (Gilliland and Fleming 1998; and others). This distress results from both the caregiver responsibilities and from witnessing the patient's suffering (Ferrell et al. 1991). Schumacher et al. (2000) found that family members of terminally ill humans may need as much or more support as the patient because they are facing an imminent loss, experiencing anticipatory grief, attempting to provide emotional and tangible support to the patient, empathizing with the ill patient, feeling guilt, and worrying about being left behind. Wadhwa et al. (2013) conclude that early palliative care interventions at the patient level are likely to benefit caregivers as well. For example, without the benefit of effective support, many caregivers gravitate to assuming the worst when asking themselves: "Is my animal suffering?" The commonly held myth that "animals hide pain" serves to further reinforce caregivers' overly pessimistic outlook because it casts doubt over accepting the animal's displays of positive emotions at face value: in effect, the animal is saying, "Hey guys, I'm doing ok," to which the caregivers respond, in their thoughts, "C'mon, we know you're suffering." Believing the animal is suffering more than she actually does places an unnecessary and significant burden on caregivers. Referral to palliative and hospice care early in the disease process can minimize this unnecessary burden.

On the positive side, the caregiving experience can offer meaningful psychological rewards and satisfaction as well. One study found that levels of distress were reduced when positive feelings outweighed the negative feelings of caregiving (Kinney et al. 1995). Another study demonstrated that home-based palliative caregiving resulted in life enriching experiences for many caregivers, including opportunities for reciprocity, finding meaning in the situation, and spending time with the patient (Stajduhar 2003). Still another study found that caregivers had an overall sense of having accomplished something difficult and extremely valuable; as a result, positive bereavement outcomes were found to predominate over negative reactions in home-based family caregiver situations (Koop and Strang 2003).

The author routinely shares with his clients the following statement: "Caregiving is a noble undertaking. Parts of it are deeply meaningful and there are happy moments. You are committed to caring for your animal out of love, dedication, and the desire to 'do the right thing.' Parts of caregiving can be very stressful and/or painful for you. Please know that, from my team's point of view, what you're doing is equally valuable and challenging; supporting you is as important to us as providing comfort for your animal."

The Mental Health Impact of Caregiving

Caregiving responsibilities near the end of an animal's life have a significant impact and may be experienced as a burden on personal resources of time, physical energy, and finances, as well as an emotional and spiritual burden that can be exhausting (Carmack 1985).

Animal caregiving is a highly individual experience. People in caregiving roles may experience feeling depressed, anxious, burdened, resentful, guilty, devastated, traumatized, or suicidal. They may also experience feeling enlightened, relieved, refreshed, or blessed (Mader 2013; McAdam and Puntillo 2009; Pochard et al. 2001). Many caregivers of animal patients at the end of life are ill-prepared for the demands of this role and as a result experience profound psychological strain. Hence, the caregiving experience frequently and significantly affects the mental health of caregivers with strong emotional and psychological attachments to an animal at the end of the animal's life.

Studies conducted by Adrian and Stitt (2017) found that 63% of the 343 pet owners who participated reported that they had experienced "slight, some, marked or complete" functional impairment at the time of their animal's death. Of the pet owners evaluated, significant psychological distress in the form of complicated grief (CG) resulting from pet loss was present in 3.4%, and 5.7% met the criteria for posttraumatic stress disorder (PTSD). CG is characterized as a maladaptive coping mechanism persisting for at least six months or more after the traumatic loss of a loved one. Half of the pet owners experiencing CG in this study had lost their pet 15 months or longer prior to the study, indicating the emotional suffering by some of those affected is prolonged. PTSD is an anxiety-based reaction to a traumatic stressor either witnessed or experienced (DSM-IV-TR 2000). As measured by the PTSD checklist questionnaire (Weathers et al. 1994), 12.61% of this study population reported feeling moderately disturbed by memories/thoughts of their pet's death; 10.03% suddenly felt as if they were reliving the experience; 14.70% felt very upset when reminded of their loss; 16.05% reported avoidance around thinking or talking about the experience; 10.06% had trouble falling asleep; and 12.39% reported being super-alert following the demise of their animal.

While 3.4% and 5.7% may not sound like high figures, they represent a significant mental health risk for millions of people. These findings suggest that early referral to animal hospice and palliative care, if it can indeed mitigate pet loss related psychological distress, may be tremendously beneficial both to individual pet caregivers and to mental health in our society at large. It is the duty of animal hospice and palliative care providers to respect and support caregivers' relevant emotional needs and desires, as well as beliefs, spirituality, religion, and cultural identities (See also Chapter 27).

Wallston et al. (1987) described the following issues as significantly influencing caregivers' psychological well-being in the context of end of life care for human patients. Those issues are pertinent for animal caregiving as well:

Emotional Distress. Caregivers' emotional well-being is under assault by feelings that are commonly triggered by the reality of the [*animal's*] impending loss – often referred as *anticipatory grief.* This term is used to describe a situational emotional constellation of depression, uncertainty, anxiety, fear, and worry. A struggle to find meaning in the [*animal's*] illness or death is commonly experienced and contributes to caregivers' emotional and spiritual distress. Uncertainty, unmet needs, and financial concerns further exacerbate caregivers' emotional distress.

Dignity/Esteem. Positive self-esteem is an important component of psychological well-being. Caregivers' self-esteem is profoundly influenced by their sense of competence in caregiving, which is in turn influenced by the patient's level of comfort; hospice, and palliative care's focus on patient comfort directly reflects recognition of the impact of successful symptom management on patient and caregiver self-esteem. Caregiver self-esteem is also influenced by a sense that one's [*animal*] loved one had the opportunity to die a dignified death. A dignified death is characterized as one in which the care given:

- honors the dying patient's by respecting his or her preferences
- protects the one who is dying from abject suffering; and
- conveys that dignity resides in the patient (not their physical attributes)
  (The Institute of Medicine, Committee on Care at the End of Life 1997).

For animal caregivers, the dignity of a dying patient could also refer to issues of presentation, i.e. soiling, offensive odor, emaciated appearance, or the presence of nonhealing wounds. These may be secondary concerns to the dying animal but can

negatively influence caregivers' sense of competence and hence their self-esteem.

Sense of Control, Autonomy. Dying is a critical time when both patients and families may feel they have few opportunities for choice and control. Thus, the degree to which caregivers feel they were presented with and understood various options, and felt in control of the choices, is important. Control can also be defined in terms of control over the entire process of dying, a perception that the animal was able to "die on her or his own terms," on the one hand, or that the caregiver had the desired control over the animal's dying by scheduling euthanasia, on the other. Caregivers' sense of control is enhanced when their preferences are honored regarding the approach to care and the degree of use of medical treatments. This is referred to as "self-determined life closure" by the National Hospice and Palliative Care Organization. Supporting self-determination by the patient and family is an important objective of hospice care.

Resilience. Resilience has been defined as the ability to maintain emotional equilibrium under stressful circumstances. Resilience depends the individual's physiologic and psychological reserve – one's unused capacity available to be called upon in a time of stress or crisis.

Supporting Caregivers' Emotional Needs

A serious effort to assess caregivers' resources, including patient management skills and coping skills, is made only in rare instances in the veterinary health care system, and caregivers receive little or no support. The hospice team's presence offers a unique opportunity to help as caregivers prepare for the loss, at the time a pet dies and immediately afterwards. Caregivers are likely to be in vulnerable emotional states during this journey. They may be overwhelmed, in a state of shock, crying, or feeling numb.

They may also be surprised, confused, or embarrassed by their own emotions.

The goal in supporting someone who is experiencing pet caregiving burden is to help them work though the myriad of reactions described above and to determine what will best help them cope with the challenging reality. Emotional support can enhance caregivers' morale and self-esteem, improve coping ability, increase sense of control, and reduce anxiety and depression.

Hospice team members can draw from their understanding of the tasks and processes of caregiving to help caregivers maintain a balance as they oscillate between coping with today's challenges, reminiscing the past, and preparing for the impending loss. Remembering the past may be associated with a sense of loss even while the animal is still alive – a loss of what the relationship was like before the animal's illness, injury, or aging.

Animal hospice team members who are not mental health professionals can support caregivers emotionally by building effective helping relationships, described in detail in Chapter 8 "Supporting Relationships: Providers' Nonmedical Roles" in this book. In a helping relationship, support can be offered by communicating empathy verbally and/or nonverbally. Empathy can be shown verbally by acknowledging, validating, and normalizing what caregivers are feeling. Nonverbally, empathy can be expressed by body posture, facial expressions, and eye contact with caregivers. Nonverbally communicating respect for caregivers' feelings is extremely important, often more so than words. It can be done with few words or in silence.

The animal hospice team can support caregivers as they make difficult decisions. It is essential to *listen* to what is most important to a family under the circumstances – what their concerns are, how they want to spend their time as options become limited, and what kinds of trade-offs they are willing to make – *before* offering information and advice. The information offered must include multiple options for caregivers to choose from. The information about each option must be balanced and sufficient for caregivers to form their own opinion on that option. The objective of discussing options is to help families find the best way to achieve what they want to accomplish. This gives families some control over the process leading to the inevitable loss – control that in turn promotes healthy grieving and emotional growth.

This is especially true of the decisions made at the time of impending death or euthanasia. It is common for caregivers in acute grief to struggle even when decisions have been made in advance, because they feel insecure, guilty, anxious, or confused. Hospice team members can remind caregivers of the decisions that they have to make or have already made. That can be best accomplished by asking guiding questions in a quiet, patient manner. Closely watching caregivers' emotional state helps choose the most appropriate time to offer such guidance. Hospice team members can also help caregivers make decisions by gently providing factual information and answering questions. Reducing the degree of uncertainty inherent to the end-of-life situation can help to offset some of the intensity of caregivers' emotions. *Encouraging caregivers to trust themselves is paramount.* Caregivers' ideas should be supported, but any risks involved pointed out. Reminding caregivers to remain flexible – a challenging task for many – can be helpful.

An important goal for the hospice and palliative care (HPC) team members is to help caregivers realize that making *perfect decisions* is rarely possible. Making the *best possible decisions* is an attainable goal and therefore a better one to focus on. Validating that they did their best for a beloved animal, with the information available at the time, helps caregivers cope and forgive themselves if haunted later on by questioning their decisions. This can be especially important if some of the outcomes of those decisions were different than they had expected.

When emotions are freely expressed, the process of positive emotional growth related to the loss experience is facilitated. It is *not* helpful to try to distract caregivers or tell them what they should be doing, thinking, or feeling. Additionally, it is essential not to attempt to talk them out of their feelings, even if they are in great emotional pain (Lagoni et al. 1994). Clinical experience shows that, when the expression of an emotional experience is restricted in some way, processing and restoration of balance are impeded. Openly expressing guilt or anger is healthier than clamming up. Telling a caregiver "you have no reason to blame yourself (or someone else)" rarely helps. A support person should encourage the expression of feelings because blocking them may paradoxically reinforce the negative or painful feelings. It may be helpful, however, to point out to the caregiver that the *feeling* of guilt (for example) is real, but it is most likely a reflection of the uncertainty common to end-of-life caregiving and *rarely a reflection of a reality of caregiving failure.*

Glajchen (2004) describes interventions developed to support human cancer patients' caregivers that apply well to animal HPC caregivers. Glajchen describes the following types of interventions to promote caregivers' physical and emotional well-being:

Educational interventions are intended to increase caregivers' knowledge.

Education is an effective tool for helping cancer patients and their families understand the disease process, pain, other symptoms, and treatment options (Glajchen et al. 1995). Information about the disease trajectory, the anticipated course, and the range of emotions experienced by families helps normalize caregivers' experience, enhances sense of control, and helps decrease anxiety. Due to the wide range of tasks that need to be mastered at different points in the patient's illness, caregivers' information needs change over time. Wong et al. found caregivers' most important information and education needs included management of pain; management of weakness/ fatigue; and the types of home care services available to facilitate patient care (Wong et al. 2002).

In the area of pain management, caregivers need to understand pharmacologic issues and medication instructions. Specifically, caregivers need instruction about which medications to use for pain relief, when to give the medication, how to assess the efficacy of pain control, how to monitor for and how to manage side effects, and how to identify negative results or ineffectiveness. Caregivers have been shown to benefit from education in nonpharmacologic strategies for reducing pain, such as massage, use of lotions and ointments, and use of heat and cold compresses. Caregivers have responded favorably to education in distraction and relaxation techniques, as such skills promote caregiver confidence and reduce helplessness. Similarly, skills in positioning with pillows, mobilizing the patient, and assisting with ambulation in an effort to promote pain relief can be taught (Ferrell et al. 1991).

Problem solving and skill building interventions are intended to increase caregivers' confidence. Throughout the caregiving process, caregivers assume a variety of new and complex roles and frequently lack the requisite resources or skills to undertake these roles. Nine core caregiving processes that have recently been identified are listed in Box 25.3:

Mastery of each of these skills can be daunting for caregivers; therefore, interventions designed to help caregivers master these skills should be employed.

The COPE problem-solving model was developed to maximize caregivers' effectiveness, sense of efficacy, and satisfaction (Houts et al. 1996). The acronym stands for Creativity, Optimism, Planning, and Expert information. Caregivers are encouraged to develop creative solutions to challenging situations. The model addresses the emotional aspect of problem-solving, combining optimism with realism, teaches caregivers the rationales for what they do and helps caregivers develop specific plans to meet their individual situations.

Box 25.3   Nine core caregiving processes.
1) Monitoring (ensuring changes in the patient's condition have been noted)
2) Interpreting (making sense of what is observed)
3) Making decisions (selecting a course of action)
4) Taking action (carrying out decisions and instructions)
5) Providing hands-on care (carrying out nursing and medical procedures)
6) Making adjustments (progressively refining caregiver's actions)
7) Accessing resources (obtaining what is needed)
8) Working with the patient (providing illness related care in a way that is sensitive to the preferences of both patient and caregiver)
9) Negotiating the healthcare system (ensuring patient's needs are adequately met)
Source: Adapted from Schumacher et al. (2000).

Box 25.4   Goals of counseling interventions.
• Feeling less overwhelmed and more in control
• Exploring the meaning of the illness, disability, or loss experience
• Managing difficult feelings, such as depression and anxiety
• Communicating effectively with the health care team
• Addressing relationship issues and financial concerns that are causing distress
• Exploring options and getting feedback about important decisions
• Talking about concerns about the future
• Understanding and adjusting to changes
Source: Adapted from Amer. Soc. Clin. Oncology (2015).

Effective skills training programs combine guidance, support, and nursing home visits(Ferrell et al. 1991). Nurse-led transition coaching programs prepare caregivers for the next level of care, teach communication skills, and follow patients to the home, providing continuity of care through a single point of contact (Naylor 2006). Such programs are very applicable to, and needed in, providing support to caregivers of pets at the end of life. When caregivers are more skilled in providing care, they are more confident and engaged in the end-of-life experience, which facilitates an easier adjustment to their loss.

Counseling interventions are designed to help people respond to challenges and the associated emotions in healthy ways. Grief therapy may be needed when challenges interrupt the bereaved person's ability to work through the pain of the grief and to adjust in a healthy and timely manner to the loss (Worden 2009).

Counselors cannot always solve problems, but they provide a safe environment for caregivers to talk about their concerns. Counseling is most needed when caregivers experience distress that is long lasting and/or interferes with the ability to carry out daily activities, but may be helpful even if the level of distress is less severe. A wide range of goals can be addressed through counseling, listed in Box 25.4.

The Role of a Licensed Mental Health Professional

Utilizing the skills of a licensed mental health professional in an appropriate and timely way is an ethical responsibility of animal hospice providers to their clients.

In 2002, Dr. Elizabeth Strand coined the term "veterinary social work" and began a program at the University of Tennessee School of Social Work that offers specialty certification in that field. The Veterinary Social Worker's primary roles are to provide emotional support to clients and staff, short term interventions, and psychoeducational programs. Taking specific online classes, a one week in-person component at the University of Tennessee, and completing an internship, in addition to a master's degree in social work (MSW), are required to become a Certified Veterinary Social Worker (CVSW). As of 2020, approximately 200 social workers have completed CVSW certification programs.

However, there are no identified or accepted standards and qualifications for licensed mental health professionals who desire to work in providing support and consultations for people involved in end-of-life care for animals. Examples of when to consider contacting a mental health professional are listed in Box 25.5.

Box 25.5   Consider contacting a mental health professional when a caregiver...

- Is unclear about his or her own needs, gives mixed messages, is unable to define or express what they want for themselves and for their animal; yet expresses anxiety, concern, worry, fear, and/or upset about the animal's care plans and end-of-life decisions.
- Has pervasive feelings of confusion about the animal's health and/or about decisions that need to be made.
- Is "stuck," unable to adjust to changes; is unable to accept the seriousness of an animal's health condition; expresses not being ready to say goodbye.
- Does not follow through with agreed upon care plans.
- Genuinely cares about their beloved animal yet inhibits the animal hospice team's effectiveness by repeatedly exhibiting disruptive behavior, e.g. being angry, inebriated, or chronically canceling appointments.
- Shows emotional instability. (If unsure, consult with the MH professional on your animal hospice team.)
- Expresses or hints or says that they are feeling misunderstood by their family and friends.
- Hints at wanting "another opinion" regarding understanding and coping with their feelings or emotions.
- Wants guidance on how to include, or talk with, child family members about death (may hide a deeper concern of the parent or responsible adult).
- Asks you to lie to a child or to anyone in the family.

- Expresses having chronic or overwhelming thoughts or feelings of guilt, regret, or remorse.
- Shares stories about traumatic life experiences they say are being recalled or remembered resulting from caring for or by being around their dying animal.
- A person in the animal's home hospice environment shows interest in being close to the animal patient and/or in being involved in discussions about care plans, yet appears to be ignored or dismissed by a more dominant caregiver.
- Multiple caregivers consider themselves as having primary decision-making rights and are locked in disagreement about matters relevant to care plans.
- Hints about, jokes about, or simply says that when his or her animal dies, he or she will no longer have a reason to live. A caregiver may or may not use direct language like "killing myself" or "wanting to commit suicide." Any hint or forthright comment indicating the possibility of suicidal intent or ideation must be taken seriously as an urgent emergency. If an animal hospice provider has any doubt about what actions to take to protect the well-being of the caregiver, an immediate consultation with a licensed mental health professional is warranted. For urgent situations contact your area's mobile crisis unit or call 9-1-1. Wait with the caregiver until qualified assistance arrives.

Source: Adapted from IAAHPC Animal Hospice and Palliative Care Guidelines (2017).

Qualified Mental Health Professionals

Mental health professionals must complete specialized training and pass a state examination before becoming a licensed counselor. Therefore, the use of clinically trained, licensed mental health professionals is recommended to ensure that a minimum level of education and skill has been met and that legal and ethical care is being provided. (Mader 2013) Types of licensed mental health and counseling professionals are listed in Box 25.6. The emerging field of animal hospice and palliative care would benefit greatly from participation of clinically trained, licensed mental health professionals in AHPC teams. Research to further develop strategies that can be most helpful in grief counseling and support for people involved in end-of-life care for animals is urgently needed. Some counselors, social workers, or pastoral counselors practice without being licensed. It's advisable to seek licensed mental health professionals.

Establishing a business relationship with a licensed mental health professional as an independent contractor offers potential benefits such as ease of referral and transition of care and familiarity with hospice team approaches and procedures. Before establishing the relationship, AHPC providers are encouraged to check state laws regarding this type of business relationship. Using a clinically trained, licensed mental health professional protects the referring animal hospice provider as well as the caregivers referred to them (Mader 2013). The ideal candidates to consider are professionals with expertise in treating loss (grief and bereavement), crisis and trauma, families,

---

Box 25.6   Types of licensed mental health and counseling professionals.

Psychiatrists. These are medical doctors who specialize in the diagnosis and treatment of mental disorders. In addition to providing counseling, psychiatrists can prescribe medications to treat mental disorders and emotional problems.

Psychologists. These professionals have a master's or doctoral degree and advanced training in diagnosing and treating mental disorders. They are qualified to do psychotherapy, teaching, and research, but in most states they cannot prescribe medication.

Clinical social workers. These professionals have a master's degree and are qualified to counsel people with emotional concerns but also specialize in finding ways to adapt the environment to the client's needs. This may include coordination of care, finding resources in the community, or function as a case worker or manager.

Psychiatric clinical nurse specialists. These professionals, also called psychiatric nurse practitioners, are registered nurses who have at least a master's degree in psychiatric mental health nursing. They specialize in treating mental disorders, and they are trained to conduct counseling.

Marriage and family therapists (MFT). MFTs are mental health specialists with at least a Master's level of training who specialize psychotherapy and counseling with couples and families.

Licensed professional counselors. These professionals, also called licensed mental health counselors, have at least a master's degree in counseling and advanced skills in individual, family, and group counseling.

Licensed pastoral counselors. These professionals have at least a master's degree in ministry or divinity and specialized training in counseling. Licensed pastoral counselors conduct counseling within the context of religion and spirituality.

Source: Adapted from Amer Soc Clin Oncology (2019).

and suicidology. It is imperative to inquire about the candidates' *personal* feelings toward euthanasia, palliative care, animal hospice, and hospice-supported natural death for animals.

In addition to the diverse clinical training of mental health and counseling professionals, different types of counseling are available. Caregivers' should be encouraged to search for the type of counseling that best fits their specific needs, personal preferences, and financial resources. The options include the following:

Individual counseling. This provides a one-on-one interaction with a counselor to talk about troubling circumstances, thoughts, and feelings. The counselor will listen attentively, express caring concern, ask questions, and offer feedback.

Couples or family counseling. When meeting with a couple or with multiple family members, a counselor listens objectively to all participants and helps identify how specific thoughts and behaviors may be contributing to conflict. Family members learn new ways to support one another during stressful times.

Group counseling. A group of individuals with similar concerns may meet together with a counselor who leads the discussion and provides support and guidance. Individuals learn from both the counselor's insights and the perspectives of the other members of the group.

Support groups. Social support can be helpful to people who are stressed, struggling with grief, and feeling alone. Caregivers who feel supported by family and friends fare better psychologically than those without such personal resources. The company of others with similar experiences may lessen feelings of social isolation and not being understood. Proficiently led support groups can serve this need, especially for caregivers who do not have the benefit of a supportive family or community, by promoting information exchange and informal networking. Support

groups are available specifically for people coping with an impending death, or have experienced the loss of their beloved pets. Such groups are commonly listed with local humane societies, pet burial, and crematory businesses, local or state veterinary associations, and even some (human) hospice bereavement programs (Stroebe et al. 2008).

Support is also available from books and on the Internet through various pet loss-related websites (search term "pet loss"); some pet loss websites hold virtual candlelight ceremonies and offer supportive online "chat rooms." Proper research into the group providing this support is encouraged.

Summary

The role of a family caregiver for a seriously ill family member – human or animal – is challenging and is often both emotionally exhausting and rewarding. Hospice teams in human healthcare include bereavement counselors, chaplains, and licensed mental health professionals available to address patients' and caregivers' emotional needs. Animal hospice and palliative care teams should strive to include emotional and spiritual support professionals as well. Developing close relationships with counseling and mental health professionals in the community as the first-in-line resource for consultations and referrals for particularly vulnerable caregivers is a good first step toward realizing this goal (Mader 2013).

The social, psychological, emotional, and spiritual impact of caregiving for an animal nearing the end of life should be identified and supported by the entire hospice team. Recognizing the psychological vulnerability among caregivers throughout the trajectory of the animal's illness is essential in implementing specific interventions to promote coping, alleviate anxiety, and encourage problem solving.

References

AARP and National Alliance for Caregiving (2020) Caregiving in the United States 2020. Washington, D.C.: AARP.

Adams, C.L., Bonnett, B.N., and Meek, A.H. (2000) Predictors of owner response to companion animal death in 177 clients from 14 practices in Ontario. *J. Am. Vet. Med. Assoc.*, *217*(9): 1303–1309.

Adrian, J.A. and Stitt, A. (2017) Pet loss, complicated grief, and post-traumatic stress disorder in Hawaii, *Anthrozoös*, 30: 123–133.

American Pet Products Association (APPA). (2022) 2021-2022 APPA National Pet Owners Survey. Available at: https://www.american petproducts.org/pubs_survey.asp (Accessed: November 15, 2022).

American Psychiatric Association. (2000). Diagnostic and Statistical Manual of Mental Disorders. (DSM-IV-TR). Arlington, VA: American Psychiatric Association.

American Veterinary Medical Association (AVMA) (2018) Pet ownership stable, veterinary care variable. Available at: https://www.avma.org/javma-news/2019-01-15/pet-ownership-stable-veterinary-care-variable (Accessed: April 17, 2022).

Britton, K., Galioto, R., Tremont, G. et al. (2018) Caregiving for a companion animal compared to a family member: burden and positive experiences in caregivers. *Front Vet Sci.*, 5: 325.

Carmack, B.J. (1985) The effects on family members and functioning after the death of a pet. *Marriage Fam. Rev.*, 8(3–4): 149–161.

Ferrell, B.R., Rhiner, M., Cohen, M.Z. et al. (1991) Pain as a metaphor for illness, I: impact of cancer pain on family caregivers. *Oncol. Nurs. Forum*, 18: 1303–1309.

Gilliland, G. and Fleming, S. (1998). A comparison of spousal anticipatory grief and conventional grief. *Death Studies*, 22: 541–569.

Glajchen, M. (2003) Caregiver burden and pain control. In: Cancer Pain. (eds. R. Portenoy and E. Bruera) New York: Cambridge University Press.

Glajchen, M. (2004) The emerging role and needs of family caregivers in cancer care. *J. Support Oncol.*, 2: 145–155.

Glajchen, M., Blum, D., and Calder, K. (1995) Cancer pain management and the role of social work: barriers and interventions. *Health Soc. Work*, 20: 200–206.

Hinds, P.S. and Kelly, K.P. (2010) Helping parents make and survive end of life decisions for their seriously ill child. *Nurs. Clin. North Am.*, 45: 465–474

Houts, P.S., Nezu, A.M., Nezu, C.M. et al. (1996) The prepared caregiver: a problem-solving approach to family caregiver education. *Patient Educ. Couns.*, 27: 63–73.

Institute of Medicine, Committee on Care at the End of Life. (1997) Field MJ, Cassel CK, Editors: *Approaching Death: Improving Care at the End of Life.*

International Association of Animal Hospice and Palliative Care (IAAHPC). (2017) *Animal Hospice and Palliative Care Guidelines.* Available at: https://iaahpc.org/wp-content/uploads/2020/10/IAAHPC-AHPC-GUIDELINESpdf.pdf (Accessed: 5/21/22).

Kinney, J.M., Stephens, M.A., Ranks, M.M. et al. (1995) Stresses and satisfactions of family caregivers to older stroke patients. *J. Appl. Gerontol.*, 14: 3–21.

Koop, P.M. and Strang, V.R. (2003) The bereavement experience following home-based family caregiving for persons with advanced cancer. *Clin. Nurs. Res.*, 12: 127–144.

Lagoni, L., Butler, C., and Hetts, S. (1994) The Human-Animal Bond and Grief. Philadelphia, PA: W.B. Saunders Company.

Lagoni, L., Morehead, D., Brannan, J. et al. (2001) Guidelines for Bond-Centered Practice, Fort Collins, CO: Argus Institute, Colorado State University.

Laurent-Simpson, A. (2021) Just Like Family: How Companion Animals Joined the Household. New York: New York University Press.

Mader, B. (2013) Palliative care, animal hospice, and mental health care. Proceedings for the Third Annual IAAHPC Conference, Denver CO.

McAdam, J.L. and Puntillo, K. (2009) Symptoms experienced by family members of patients in intensive care units. *Am. J. Crit. Care*, *18*(3): 200–210.

Naylor, M. (2006) Transitional care: a critical dimension of the home healthcare quality agenda. *J. Health Care Qual.*, 28: 20–28.

Pochard, F., Azoulay, E., Chevret, S. et al. (2001). Symptoms of anxiety and depression in family members of intensive care unit patients: ethical hypothesis regarding decision making capacity. *Crit. Care Med.*, 29: 1893–1897.

Schumacher, K.L., Stewart, B.J., Archbold, P.G. et al. (2000) Family caregiving skill: development of the concept. *Res. Nurs. Health*, 23: 191–203.

Shanan, A. (2011) A veterinarian role in helping pet owners with decision making. *Vet. Clin. North Am.*, 41: 644

Stajduhar, K. (2003) Examining the perspectives of family members involved in the delivery of palliative care at home. *J. Palliat. Care*, 19: 27–35.

Stewart, A.L., Teno, J., Patrick, D.L. et al. (1999) The concept of quality of life of dying persons in the context of health care. *J. Pain Symptom Manage.* 2: 93–108.

Stroebe, M., Hansson, R., Schut, H. et al. (2008). Handbook of Bereavement Research and Practice Advances in Theory and Intervention. Washington, D.C.: American Psychological Association.

Wadhwa, D., Burman, D., Swami, N. et al. (2013) Quality of life and mental health in caregivers of outpatients with advanced cancer. *Psycho-Oncology*, 22: 403–410.

Wallston, K.A., Wallston, B.S., Smith S. et al. (1987) Perceived control and health. *Curr. Psychol. Res. Rev.*, 6: 5–25.

Weathers, F.W., Litz, B.T., Huska, J.A. et al. (1994) PTSD Checklist--Civilian Version PCL-C for DSM-IV. Boston: National Center for PTSD--Behavioral Science Division.

Wong, R.K.S., Franssen, E., Szumacher, E. et al. (2002) What do patients living with advanced cancer and their carers want to know? – a needs assessment. *Support. Care Cancer*, 10: 408–415.

Worden, J.W. (2009) Grief Counseling and Grief Therapy a Handbook for the Mental Health Practitioner. 4 edn. New York: Springer Publishing Company.

26

Caregiver Burden in the Companion Animal Owner

Mary Beth Spitznagel, PhD and Mark D. Carlson, DVM

Humans providing care for a companion animal with protracted, serious illness frequently experience "caregiver burden," a term used to describe strain from the challenges of caregiving. Because extended caregiving is often experienced in animal hospice and palliative care (AHPC) contexts, it is important to understand what caregiver burden is, how it affects everyone in the AHPC setting, how to recognize it, and how to appropriately respond to such burden.

What Is Caregiver Burden?

Caregiver burden is distress or strain experienced in response to providing care for a loved one who is ill (Zarit et al. 1980). Burden includes the response to objective challenges and caregiving responsibilities such as having less time for oneself or the physical demands of caregiving, as well as subjective experiences including guilt, anger, or frustration (Hébert et al. 2000). Although caregiving can be highly rewarding, with many individuals reporting positive aspects of caregiving (e.g. feeling needed or useful, experiencing an enhanced appreciation of life; Tarlow et al. 2004), it also carries risk for adverse physical and emotional conditions, social repercussions, and financial

strain for the caregiver (Paradise et al. 2014). More than four decades of caregiver burden research in the human medicine literature position us well to understand burden in the companion AHPC setting. Research points to both similarities and differences in the caregiving experience for a human family member versus a companion animal (Britton et al. 2018), providing rationale for the study of companion animal caregiving within its own distinct context.

A Word About Research Data, the Terminology Used, and this Article's Audience

The research data reviewed here come from a variety of samples. Some work has been done with hospice/palliative clients, while other work has been done with social media pet caregiver groups or veterinary hospitals (both general and specialty referral). To further complicate matters, because AHPC is not a regulated field, veterinarians serving the clients sampled for the research vary greatly in their skill sets, caseload, and in their interpretation of the core mission of AHPC.

In veterinary practice, the humans providing care for their companion animals are generally referred to as "pet owners" and/or "veterinary

Hospice and Palliative Care for Companion Animals: Principles and Practice, Second Edition.
Edited by Amir Shanan, Jessica Pierce, and Tamara Shearer.
© 2023 John Wiley & Sons, Inc. Published 2023 by John Wiley & Sons, Inc.
Companion website: www.wiley.com/go/shanan/palliative

clients." In AHPC, they are referred to as "animal caregivers." Individuals working in AHPC providing care for animals and/or humans are referred to as "hospice team members" and/or "service providers."

Since the data reviewed in this article reflect a sample of people who identified themselves as "pet owners" and/or "veterinary clients," they are mostly referred to in the article using those terms, used interchangeably with "animal caregiver." The terms "pet," "animal" and "companion animal" are also used interchangeably.

The audience for this book is broad and diverse. It is primarily aimed at veterinarians, veterinary team members, and others working as members of an AHPC team. However, the audience also includes social workers and other mental health professionals; individuals providing care for companion animals independently (massage therapists, alternative medicine providers, pet sitters and others); animal chaplains; those interested in human–animal interactions; those interested in how animals are treated by humans; bioethicists; and pet caregivers preparing for the end of a beloved animal companion's life or reflecting on their struggles in the past.

Caregiver Burden Is Present in Owners of Seriously Ill Companion Animals

In an early qualitative study exploring caregiving for an ill companion animal, Christiansen and colleagues (Christiansen et al. 2013) conducted interviews with 12 owners of elderly or ill dogs. This work identified concerns consistent with caregiver burden, including greater care needs for the animal, strain from meeting needs related to work and finances, negative effects on social life, and emotional distress. More recent quantitative work (Spitznagel et al. 2017, 2019a) demonstrated that caregiver burden is greater in owners of a seriously ill cat or dog, compared to those with a healthy companion animal. Notably, both quantitative studies found that the average level of caregiver burden in owners of a seriously ill companion

animal was above a threshold considered clinically meaningful in human caregiving samples. While not all owners of a seriously ill companion animal will suffer clinically elevated levels of distress, it is important to recognize that many do experience burden in this context.

How Caregiver Burden Differs from Other Client Experiences in this Context

Because companion animal caregiver burden has received relatively little attention until recent years, Spitznagel and Carlson (2019) noted that burden is sometimes confused with other owner experiences that have seen greater focus in in the veterinary medicine literature, namely grief and quality of life. As reviewed in that work, differentiation of these issues is important, as recognizing each within the appropriate context may foster more effective communication between the veterinarian and client.

Whereas burden is strain due to the challenges of caregiving, grief is a response to loss (Prigerson et al. 2009), or an expected loss in the case of anticipatory grief (Reynolds and Botha 2006). Owner anticipatory grief and caregiver burden may both be present in the owner during hospice and palliative care, but they differ in etiology and emotional experience (Spitznagel and Carlson 2019). Quality of life, in contrast, is not context-specific, but a general assessment of satisfaction with one's life across various domains (WHO 1999). Recent factor analytic work examining measures assessing caregiver burden, anticipatory grief, and quality of life in owners of a seriously ill or elderly cat or dog showed that these constructs are conceptually distinct from one another (Spitznagel et al. 2021a). However, these experiences can sometimes overlap within an individual. Specifically, cluster analysis of these measures demonstrated four separate owner profiles, summarized in Figure 26.1.

In this work, some owners exhibited a "Distressed" presentation, with pervasive

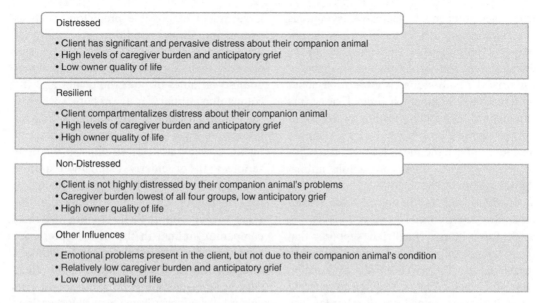

> **Distressed**
> • Client has significant and pervasive distress about their companion animal
> • High levels of caregiver burden and anticipatory grief
> • Low owner quality of life
>
> **Resilient**
> • Client compartmentalizes distress about their companion animal
> • High levels of caregiver burden and anticipatory grief
> • High owner quality of life
>
> **Non-Distressed**
> • Client is not highly distressed by their companion animal's problems
> • Caregiver burden lowest of all four groups, low anticipatory grief
> • High owner quality of life
>
> **Other Influences**
> • Emotional problems present in the client, but not due to their companion animal's condition
> • Relatively low caregiver burden and anticipatory grief
> • Low owner quality of life

Figure 26.1 Profiles of owners of a seriously ill or elderly companion animal. *Source:* Mary Beth Spitznagel, PhD.

distress about the companion animal. Others showed a "Resilient" presentation, defined by compartmentalization of their distress about the companion animal. A third, "Non-Distressed" presentation also emerged, in which owners were relatively unaffected by their companion animal's problems. A final group of owners showed distress due to "Other Influences," with clear emotional difficulty that was not closely linked to the companion animal's condition.

While problems in domains of caregiver burden, anticipatory grief, and quality of life occurred simultaneously for some individuals (e.g. Distressed owners showed high caregiver burden, high anticipatory grief, and low quality of life), this was not the case for all owners (e.g. Resilient owners showed high caregiver burden and high anticipatory grief, but good quality of life). Each group exhibited distinguishing features that may benefit from communication strategies tailored to the prevailing issues. These will be discussed in greater detail later in this chapter.

How Does Caregiver Burden Affect the Veterinary Client?

Emotional distress does not exist in a vacuum. When caregiver burden is present in the veterinary client, it has the potential to impact the client's well-being, and also that individual's decisions about their companion animal.

Impact of Caregiver Burden on the Client

Research robustly demonstrates that compared to those with a healthy companion animal, owners of a seriously ill companion animal report significantly greater problems on measures of stress, anxiety, and depression (Spitznagel et al. 2017, 2019a). Indeed, average levels of depressive symptoms endorsed by research participants with a seriously ill companion animal from both studies (one of which drew a sample from social media, the other from a general veterinary hospital) met a threshold for clinical significance – if an individual presented for a psychological evaluation with the number of depressive symptoms observed, on average, in the owners of a seriously ill animal, that individual might be diagnosed with a formal depressive disorder. Importantly, both studies showed that about half of the ill companion animal caregivers experienced clinically meaningful levels of burden, defined as greater than 1.5 standard deviations above the mean level of burden for owners of a healthy companion animal (Spitznagel and Carlson 2019).

The cross sectional design of these studies precludes determination of directionality, but work from human medicine supports that these relationships are not simply driven by individuals with psychosocial dysfunction who are experiencing caregiving as burdensome. Rather, prolonged caregiver burden may actually to lead to depression (Epstein-Lubow et al. 2008). It is thus possible that presence of caregiver burden in owners of a companion animal with serious illness could be causal in development of several negative psychosocial outcomes.

Impact of Caregiver Burden on the Patient

The links between caregiving and distress in the companion animal owner warrant consideration of whether burden in the owner affects decision-making for the animal. A recent study investigated how owner distress impacts consideration of euthanasia for an elderly or ill companion animal (Spitznagel et al. 2020). First, a measure was developed to assess the steps that have been taken toward a decision to euthanize, with items asking about experiences associated with these steps. For example, has the owner had thoughts about euthanasia? Have they had discussions with family or a veterinarian about euthanizing the companion animal? Has an actual euthanasia appointment been scheduled? The total of this "consideration of euthanasia" measure was strongly correlated with actual euthanasia of the pet within the following 30 days (r = 0.70). Consideration of euthanasia was then examined in the context of a

large model of possible predictors, such as companion animal condition (e.g. quality of life), owner psychosocial factors (e.g. caregiver burden, anticipatory grief), and demographic variables of both the owner and the companion animal (e.g. age of both, species of the animal, income of the owner). Caregiver burden emerged as the strongest predictor of owner consideration of euthanasia for their seriously ill or elderly companion animal after controlling for the animal's quality of life. The owner who is experiencing high levels of burden is more likely to euthanize their companion animal in the near future, even after removing the influence of the animal's quality of life from that relationship. Findings suggest it is possible that presence of caregiver burden contributes to earlier decisions to euthanize.

Taken together, research suggests that when caregiver burden is present in the owner of a seriously ill companion animal, it may have significant repercussions for both the owner and the animal. As such, it is worthwhile to consider what actions might be taken to reduce burden for the client.

Research-Based Suggestions for Interacting with the Burdened Owner

Recommendations for working with clients who are experiencing caregiver burden can be made on the basis of research examining predictors of this burden. Some of these have been covered in past work (Spitznagel and Carlson 2019) and will be briefly summarized and updated here. An important caveat for all recommendations provided is that best practices for alleviating caregiver burden in the veterinary client are still a work in progress.

Understand the Owner's Perspective

Recognize, acknowledge, and validate burden when you see it. Clients in distress may be comforted knowing that companion animal caregiving is stressful for many owners (Spitznagel et al. 2017, 2019a). Watch for telltale signs of burden, including a client who is exhibiting stress and anger, talking about feelings of overwhelm or loss of control, or expressing uncertainty or guilt (Zarit et al. 1980). When these signs are present in a hospice or palliative care context, they may indicate burden. Let caregivers know you recognize their burden by expressing empathy, verbally and/or nonverbally. Communicate that they are not alone, and direct them toward education on the topic, such as www.petcaregiverburden.com.

Understand and acknowledge the benefits of caregiving. Companion animal caregivers report greater positive aspects of caregiving than those providing care for human family members (Britton et al. 2018). Caregivers may experience many benefits, such as feeling needed, useful, and appreciated, or more positive toward life. Understanding and asking about the presence of these benefits may allow the caregiver to reframe their burden in a manner that reminds them WHY they are making the sacrifices they are making. This may also help with client connection, rapport, and trust.

Collaborate on the Care Approach

Get on the same page. It is essential that the client's expectations for what hospice or palliative care can accomplish are realistic. Higher levels of burden are observed when interventions are perceived by the owner as ineffective (Shaevitz et al. 2020). If an owner expects improvement from a treatment that is being used with the goal of enhancing the animal's comfort, the owner's perception of poor treatment efficacy could contribute to burden. Being clear about what constitutes "success" of any treatment is essential.

Collaborate on the care plan. Greater burden is present when the client's daily routine has to be altered or the client perceives the care plan as difficult to follow (Shaevitz et al. 2020; Spitznagel et al. 2019a). Collaborative decision-making is a joint intellectual effort, useful for moving clients closer to addressing their pets' medical issues within the context of a complex life (O'Grady and Jadad 2010). Collaborative decision-making is a supportive environment, helping clients gain confidence in their problem-solving ability and increasing their sense of control over their situation. Working together with the client to develop a clear and concrete plan, with consideration of the client's typical routine (Spitznagel and Carlson 2019) and "wiggle" room to change the plan if necessary, reinforces the sense of client–veterinary team partnership and promotes optimal decision-making.

Help with problem-solving. Caregiver burden is predicted by a client's sense of control or mastery of a situation (Spitznagel et al. 2018). Anticipate the likely problems (e.g. food refusal) and make sure the client has access to a list of possible solutions (i.e. lists of common fixes to try). Encourage the client to use small, sequential actions (i.e. "scientific method") to test out different strategies as they manage the challenges that arise (Spitznagel and Carlson 2019).

Lighten the Load

Minimize medications/treatments. Some research has suggested that greater quantity of medications is closely related to caregiver burden (Shaevitz et al. 2020). Fewer overall treatments predict lower burden, even after controlling for disease severity (Spitznagel et al. 2020). Reducing the number of treatments or medications when possible may be of benefit.

Praise good solutions. The owner's sense of mastery or efficacy is predictive of caregiver burden (Spitznagel et al. 2018). Feelings of competence in managing a difficult situation may be boosted by simple praise or encouragement, which may help reduce burden for that owner (Tremont et al. 2005). Increase owners' sense of mastery by recognizing and praising small steps toward successfully solving caregiving problems.

One Size Does Not Fit All: Toward Individualized Client Interactions

Studies examining caregiver burden in companion animal owners are largely based on average levels of burden detected within samples of owners. It is important to be mindful that individual differences will exist across owners, and that the experience of each owner may not be fully captured by group averages. The cluster analytic work undertaken to understand common profiles of clients caring for an elderly or seriously ill companion animal (Spitznagel et al. 2021a) begins to address the diversity of experiences in these owners, showing that some owners exhibit a "Distressed" presentation, some are "Resilient," others appear "Non-Distressed," and still others ("Other Influences") experience significant turmoil for reasons other than their companion animal's condition.

Greater understanding of how owner profiles interact with patient presentations, how to identify an individual aligning with a specific profile, and knowledge of recommended approaches for connecting with individuals of each profile may be useful for most effectively helping clients. Considerations for interacting with clients of each profile are described below and summarized briefly in Figure 26.2.

Interacting with the Distressed Client

The Distressed client is experiencing not only elevated burden, high levels of anticipatory grief, and low quality of life, but also shows clinically meaningful symptoms of depression and stress. These owners describe their companion animal's quality of life as poor and may be strongly considering euthanasia, having taken several steps toward this decision. Because Distressed clients have high levels of caregiver burden, which has been linked to a greater need for communication from the veterinary clinic (Spitznagel et al. 2019a), they may come across as being needy, demanding, or dependent. The high levels of depressive symptoms and stress in this group could result in a greater likelihood of complaint or lashing

---

Distressed: Pervasive turmoil while navigating end-of-life issues

- *Owner:* Elevated symptoms of depression and stress
- *Companion animal:* Quality of life is low; Owner is likely considering euthanasia
- *How to identify:* Owner might seem needy or prone to complaint; Interactions may be emotionally challenging for your team
- *Approaches to consider:* Understand the source of their behavior; Be prepared to take extra time; Set appropriate boundaries

Resilient: End-of-life issues not impacting other life domains

- *Owner:* Compartmentalized distress about companion animal; Significant stress and depression absent
- *Companion animal:* Quality of life is low; Owner is likely considering euthanasia
- *How to identify:* "Keeping it together" while caring for their pet; May have high communication needs due to caregiver burden
- *Approaches to consider:* Proactively ask about their concerns; Focus on active and collaborative problem-solving

Non-Distressed: Not distressed by companion animal's problems

- *Owner:* Caregiver burden and anticipatory grief are not clinically meaningful; Significant stress and depression absent; Lowest level of companion animal attachment
- *Companion animal:* More likely to have chronic presentation, relatively better quality of life
- *How to identify:* May appear to care less (lower attachment); Might exhibit greater non-adherence to treatment recommendations
- *Approaches to consider:* Provide clear rationale for specific work-up or treatment, ensuring these work within client parameters

Other Influences: Many life stressors; distress is not primarily due to companion animal

- *Owner:* Significant stress and depression; Caregiver burden and anticipatory grief are relatively low
- *Companion animal:* Relatively better quality of life; Owner not likely to be considering euthanasia
- *How to identify:* May be in obvious distress; Companion animal may be low on priority list
- *Approaches to consider:* Focus on pragmatically meeting patient needs

Figure 26.2 Considerations for veterinary clients of each profile. *Source:* Mary Beth Spitznagel, PhD.

out, as depressive symptoms can be related to expressions of anger (Koh et al. 2002). For these reasons, it may be emotionally challenging to work with Distressed clients. Recognizing that caregiving burden is the basis of some or all of their difficult behaviors, being prepared to take extra time and setting appropriate boundaries may be helpful in interacting with the Distressed client.

Interacting with the Resilient Client

Resilient owners also experience high levels of burden and anticipatory grief, but they report a better quality of life compared to the Distressed client. Interestingly, the Resilient client reports similarly low quality of life in their companion animal as the Distressed client, and they have also taken several steps toward the euthanasia decision. In contrast to the Distressed owner, however, they do not show high levels of depressive symptoms or stress. Together, findings suggest that they are better able to compartmentalize their distress about the companion animal, and it does not pervade their life. Because the Resilient owner exhibits high levels of caregiver burden, their communication needs may also be high (Spitznagel et al. 2019a). However, their distress may not be obvious, as the strain they are under is non-pervasive. For this reason, a proactive approach may be beneficial, such as asking the Resilient client, "What concerns/questions do you have?" (rather than "Do you have any concerns/questions?"). Combining a proactive approach with a focus on collaborative, active problem-solving may be of greatest benefit.

Interacting with the Non-Distressed Client

Non-Distressed owners, with high quality of life and low burden and anticipatory grief, appear to feel relatively unaffected by their companion animal's condition. They also show few depressive symptoms and low stress. The companion animal itself is more likely to have a condition that is perceived by the owner as chronic rather than terminal, which could help explain the lower levels of distress

observed in these owners; however, notably, the Non-Distressed owner's attachment to the companion animal is also the lowest of all four groups. It is thus important in working with the Non-Distressed client to be aware of issues that could be related to lower attachment, including the potential for nonadherence to the care plan. Because the companion animal's illness is more likely to be chronic in this situation, ensuring that communications include clear rationale regarding recommendations is important, as well as understanding and working within the parameters (e.g. economic, lifestyle) of the Non-Distressed client.

Interacting with the "Other Influences" Client

Lastly, owners experiencing distress related to other influences experience relatively low levels of caregiver burden and anticipatory grief, but also report low quality of life and high levels of depressive symptoms and stress. Factors beyond the companion animal's condition appear to drive their emotional turmoil. Although this client may be observably distressed, the care of their companion animal might not be a high priority. If this is the case, meeting care needs for the animal in the most practical manner possible may be useful.

Being knowledgeable about caregiver burden and how it interacts with other client experiences in the context of hospice and palliative care can help providers of hospice and palliative care avoid a "one-size-fits-all" approach. Adjusting communication strategies may, in turn, facilitate understanding of the client's perspective and optimize communication between the AHPC team and clients who are experiencing distress.

More than Compassion Fatigue: When Client Burden Transfers to the Clinician

Reading about profiles of caregivers of a seriously ill or elderly companion animal might bring various clients to mind, and perhaps even a visceral response when thinking about emotionally challenging interactions or non-adherent clients. Recent research suggests that caregiver burden in the owner of an animal with serious illness can underlie stressful encounters with providers, effectively transferring the owner's burden to veterinary personnel (Spitznagel et al. 2021b). This "burden transfer" is in turn related to stress and burnout for individuals working in the field (Spitznagel et al. 2019b).

The Burden Transfer DANCE

Factor analytic work has demonstrated five domains of veterinarian-client interactions, referred to in combination as the "Burden Transfer DANCE;" these interactions are correlated with caregiver burden in the veterinary client and predict stress and burnout for veterinarians (Spitznagel et al. 2019b). DANCE is an acronym for the five specific domains of client behaviors or interactions: **D**aily Hassles (e.g. clients requesting impossible predictions, having difficulty making decisions, following others' advice about the companion animal health care needs, shopping around to compare costs), **A**ffect (e.g. clients requiring euthanasia counseling, demonstrating anxiety or sadness), **N**on-Adherent/ Inconsiderate (e.g. clients declining recommended workup or treatment, not showing for appointments), **C**onfrontation (e.g. clients blaming, refusing to pay for services, making a complaint), and **E**xcess Communication (e.g. overly frequent phone calls or email contact). Both the frequency of these client interactions and the clinician's individual reaction to them (how bothered they felt by the situation), predict the experience of stress and burnout for the clinician.

DANCE interactions might serve as a mechanism for commonly discussed sources of occupational distress in veterinary medicine like moral stress (Moses et al. 2018) and compassion fatigue (Cohen 2007). For example, a client who is experiencing burden related to financial strain might refuse a recommendation

or request euthanasia for a treatable problem (a behavior fitting into the "Nonadherence" DANCE category). The burden of the client may transfer to the veterinarian with an outcome of moral stress, if the ethical conflict of being unable to help an otherwise treatable animal is upsetting. Another example would be interacting with a tearful client who is experiencing caregiver burden due to uncertainty about the future for their seriously ill companion animal (a behavior fitting into the "Affect" DANCE category). Over time, interactions of this nature may lead to client burden transferring to the veterinarian in the form of compassion fatigue. Beyond moral stress and compassion fatigue, the veterinary provider's reaction to other DANCE interactions, including Daily Hassles, Confrontations, and Excess Communication may lead to additional negative outcomes related to stress and burnout in the field.

Importantly, research suggests that it is not only the frequency of these DANCE interactions, but also the clinician's reaction to them (Spitznagel et al. 2019b) that may lead to stress and burnout. The notion of burden transfer suggests that negative occupational outcomes in veterinary medicine might be reduced through: (i) Reducing caregiver burden and, in turn, client DANCE behaviors; and (ii) Reducing reactivity to these DANCE situations in veterinary personnel. Approaches and techniques helpful in reducing clients' caregiver burden are described in detail in Chapter 25 in this volume. Veterinarians perform important nonmedical helping roles in their interactions with clients facing pet loss, described eloquently by Lagoni et al. (1994) as supporting, educating, guiding, and facilitating. In the hospice and palliative care setting, veterinarians interact multiple times a day with clients facing pet loss. Educating, supporting, guiding, and facilitating with AHPC clients is most effectively performed by an interdisciplinary team (IDT). See Chapter 3 in this volume for additional information about the important role of the IDT in hospice and palliative work.

As interdisciplinary AHPC teams become more commonplace in the future, it is possible that veterinarians' share of facing DANCE behaviors and experiencing burden transfer will decrease.

Research is still needed to determine if reducing clients' caregiver burden will lead to significant changes in their DANCE behaviors. For this reason, it is important to consider how we might reduce the reactivity of those working in veterinary medicine. This reactivity to challenging client encounters is a potentially modifiable risk factor for occupational stress in the field. Pilot work (Spitznagel et al. 2021b) examining a skills-based educational intervention tailored to reducing reactivity from stressful veterinary client interactions has shown high rates of acceptability and use by participants, as well as significant reductions in burden transfer. Reductions in raw scores of stress and burnout were also observed; although these were not significant in the small pilot trial, raw data changes from before to after the intervention were promising. This work overall suggests it may be possible to improve occupational distress for the veterinary healthcare team by targeting burden transfer.

Because the hospice and palliative care setting necessitates interaction with owners who may be experiencing caregiver burden, it is important that those working in this setting recognize the potential for burden transfer. Tailoring communications with the burdened client might help reduce the client's caregiver burden and, in turn, reduce the likelihood of client DANCE behaviors resulting in burden transfer. Concurrently, veterinarians and AHPC team members are likely to benefit from increased awareness of their own reactions to difficult client behaviors, and from developing skills for effectively managing difficult client interactions.

Conclusions

Recognizing and addressing pet caregiver burden is a central goal for individuals working in AHPC. Caregiver burden experienced by AHPC clients potentially impacts the client's well-being, often to a degree that meets the symptom threshold for a formal depressive disorder. Caregiver burden may impact the care that clients provide their companion animal, including an increased risk of making the decision to euthanize earlier. Many research-based recommendations have been made for working with and potentially reducing burden in the client, but it is important to recognize that clients will differ in regard to the experience of caregiver burden. Many will experience significant and pervasive distress while providing care for their seriously ill companion animal, but others appear less affected, perhaps due to greater compartmentalization or lower levels of attachment to the animal. Watching for burden and personalizing communication strategies may facilitate connection between the veterinary and/or AHPC team and the client. Being aware that caregiver burden in the client may transfer to veterinary personnel through difficult client interactions, and taking stock of one's own reaction to these situations, may be helpful in reducing occupational distress for individuals working in AHPC and in veterinary medicine.

References

Britton, K., Galioto, R., Tremont, G. *et al.* (2018) Caregiving for a companion animal compared to a family member: Burden and positive experiences in caregivers. *Front. Vet. Sci.*, 5: 325.

Christiansen, S.B., Kristensen A., Sandoe, P. *et al.* (2013) Looking after chronically ill dogs: impact on the caregiver's life. *Anthrozoös*, 26: 519–533.

Cohen, S.P. (2007) Compassion fatigue and the veterinary health team. *Vet. Clin. North Am. Small Anim. Pract.*, 37: 123–134.

Epstein-Lubow, G., Davis, J.D., Miller, I.W. *et al.* (2008) Persisting burden predicts depressive symptoms in dementia caregivers. *J. Geriatr. Psychiatry Neurol.*, 21: 198–203.

Hébert, R., Bravo, G., and Préville, M. (2000) Reliability, validity and reference values of the Zarit Burden Interview for assessing informal caregivers of community-dwelling older persons with dementia. *Can. J. Aging*, 19: 494–507.

Koh, K.B., Kim, C.H., and Park, J.K. (2002) Predominance of anger in depressive disorders compared with anxiety disorders and somatoform disorders. *J. Clin. Psychiatry*, 63: 486–492.

Lagoni L, Butler C, and Hetts S. (1994) The Human-Animal Bond and Grief. Philadelphia, PA: W.B. Saunders Company.

Moses, L., Malowney, M.J., Boyd, J.W. (2018) Ethical conflict and moral distress in veterinary practice: a survey of north American veterinarians. *J. Vet. Intern. Med.*, 32: 2115–2122.

O'Grady, L. and Jadad, A. (2010) Shifting from shared to collaborative decision making: a change in thinking and doing. *J. Participat. Med.*, 2: e13

Paradise, M., McCade, D., Hickie, I.B., *et al.* (2014) Caregiver burden in mild cognitive impairment. *Aging Ment. Health*, 19: 72–78.

Prigerson, H.G., Horowitz, M.J., Jacobs, S.C., *et al.* (2009) Prolonged grief disorder: psychometric validation of criteria proposed for DSM-V and ICD-11. *PLoS Med.*, 6: e1000121

Reynolds, L. and Botha, D. (2006) Anticipatory grief: its nature, impact, and reasons for contradictory findings. *Couns. Psychother. Health*, 2: 15–26.

Shaevitz. M., Tullius, J., Callah, R.T., *et al.* (2020) Early caregiver burden in owners of pets with suspected cancer: relationship to owner psychosocial outcomes, communication behavior, and treatment factors. *J. Vet. Intern. Med.*, 34 (6): 2636–2644.

Spitznagel, M.B. and Carlson, M.D. (2019) Caregiver burden and veterinary client well-being. *Vet. Clin. North Am. Small Anim. Pract.*, 49: 431–444.

Spitznagel, M.B., Jacobson, D.M., Cox, M.D., *et al.* (2017) Caregiver burden in owners of a sick companion animal: a cross-sectional observational study. *Vet. Rec.*, 181 (12): 321.

Spitznagel, M.B., Jacobson, D.M., Cox, M.D., *et al.* (2018) Predicting caregiver burden in general veterinary clients: contribution of companion animal clinical signs and problem behaviors. *Vet. J.*, 236: 23–30.

Spitznagel, M.B., Cox, M.D., Jacobson, D.M., *et al.* (2019a) Assessment of caregiver burden and associations with psychosocial function, veterinary service use, and factors related to treatment plan adherence among owners of dogs and cats. *J. Am. Vet. Med. Assoc.*, 254: 124–132.

Spitznagel, M.B., Ben-Porath, Y., Rishniw, M., *et al.* (2019b) Development and validation of a Burden Transfer Inventory measure for predicting veterinarian stress related to client behavior. *J. Am. Vet. Med. Assoc.*, 254: 133–144.

Spitznagel, M.B., Marchitelli, B., Gardner, M., *et al.* (2020) Euthanasia from the veterinary client's perspective: psychosocial contributors to euthanasia decision-making. *Vet. Clin. North Am. Small Anim. Pract.*, 50: 591–605, https://doi.org/10.1016/j.cvsm.2019.12.008.

Spitznagel, M.B., Anderson, J.R., Marchitelli, B., *et al.* (2021a) Owner quality of life, caregiver burden, and anticipatory grief: how they differ and why it matters. *Vet. Rec.* 188 (9): 74.

Spitznagel, M.B., Updegraff, A.S.G., Twohig, M.P., *et al.* (2021b) Reducing occupational distress in veterinary medicine personnel with acceptance and commitment training: a pilot study. *NZ Vet. J.*, 70 (6): 319–325.

Tarlow, B.J., Wisniewski, S.R., Belle, S.H., *et al.* (2004) Positive aspects of caregiving: contributions of the REACH project to the development of new measures for Alzheimer's caregiving. *Res. Aging*, 26: 429–453.

Tremont, G., Davis, J.D., Spitznagel M.B. (2005) Understanding and managing caregiver burden in cerebrovascular disease. In: Vascular Dementia: Cerebrovascular Mechanisms and Clinical Management. (ed. R.H. Paul, R. Cohen, B.R. Ott et al.). Totowa, NJ: Humana. p. 305–321.

World Heath Organization (WHO). (1999) Annotated Bibliography of the WHO Quality of Life Assessment Instrument–WHOQOL. Geneva, Switzerland: WHO.

Zarit, S.H., Reever, K.E., and Bach-Peterson, J. (1980) Relatives of the impaired elderly: correlates of feelings of burden. *Gerontologist*, 20: 649–655.

27

Addressing Spiritual Needs of Caregivers

Carol Rowehl, LVT, MAR, STM

Adjunct Chaplain at The Hospital of the University of Pennsylvania, Philadelphia, PA

Whether providing human or animal hospice care, it is important to address the spiritual needs of the caregiver. Galek et al. analyzed the empirical and theoretical literature that explored the spiritual concerns and needs of patients in a human hospital and discerned the following overarching themes of spiritual needs: "belonging, meaning, hope, the sacred, morality, beauty, resolution, and a deeper acceptance of dying" (Galek et al. 2005). The most important spiritual needs identified among human patients with cancer and their families were "being positive, loving others, finding meaning, and relating to God" (Taylor 2006). The spiritual needs of veterinary clients and caregivers of patients in animal hospice may be similar to those seen in human patients and their loved ones. Ignoring spiritual needs may lead to spiritual distress, which "can have a detrimental effect on physical and mental health" (Anandarajah and Hight 2001).

Spirituality has historically been "an integral part of the mission and practice" of human healthcare institutions and providers (Puchalski and Ferrell 2010). It "is an important, multidimensional aspect of the human experience that is difficult to fully understand" or scientifically measure, yet evidence-based studies show it has a beneficial role in the practice of human medicine (Anandarajah and Hight 2001). Cultural, religious, and spiritual practices and rituals tend to provide solace and meaning to people. The term "cultural," as used here, refers to a "set of beliefs, values, and practices arising out of the primarily secular community with which a particular individual identifies" (Mann 2006). The Standards of Practice for Professional Chaplains (Association of Professional Chaplains 2015b) defines "religion" as "an organized system of beliefs, practices, rituals, and symbols designed (i) to facilitate closeness to the sacred or transcendent (God, higher power or ultimate truth/reality) and (ii) foster an understanding of one's relationship and responsibility to others in living together in a community" (Koenig et al. 2001), and "spirituality" as "the way individuals seek and express meaning and purpose, and the way they experience their connectedness to the moment, to self, to others, to nature, and to the significant or sacred" (Puchalski et al. 2009). Even those who self-identify as atheist, agnostic, or nonbeliever have a relationship with the transcendent through their choice to reject it. Many atheists describe themselves as spiritual (Sulmasy 2006). Spiritual support should be available to all individuals, including those who do not self-identify as spiritual or religious.

Hospice and Palliative Care for Companion Animals: Principles and Practice, Second Edition.
Edited by Amir Shanan, Jessica Pierce, and Tamara Shearer.
© 2023 John Wiley & Sons, Inc. Published 2023 by John Wiley & Sons, Inc.
Companion website: www.wiley.com/go/shanan/palliative

Spiritual Needs of Caregivers

A study on spiritual needs, conducted in a human hospital setting, found that the families of patients are more likely to be involved in a search for meaning than the patients themselves. As they wait and hope for the best, they worry about and fear the worst (VandeCreek and Smith 1992). Families who prayed and used other religious activities to help them cope with stress while a loved one was having a surgical procedure were reported to benefit more from their religious coping practices than from nonreligious forms of support (Jankowski et al. 2011). Spirituality has been shown to help people cope with a serious illness, as well as adapt to the death of a loved one (Wall et al. 2007).

The more people consider companion animals to be a member of the family, the more the veterinarian-client-patient relationship becomes like the pediatrician-parent–child relationship (Shaw et al. 2004). The quality of provider-client communication has been shown to play a significant role in the strength of the provider-client bond, directly impacting the loyalty of the client to a veterinarian and, ultimately, the care the animal receives (Lue et al. 2008). The ability and willingness of a veterinary professional to discuss spiritual matters with clients is essential to good communication. Addressing spiritual matters with clients could improve provider-client communication, strengthen the provider-client bond, and increase client loyalty. In addition, there could be a positive effect on the client's ability to cope with their companion animal's terminal illness, the quality of life of the client and animal, client-provider and client-staff relationships, client compliance with prescribed treatment for the animal, and possibly the overall course of the animal companion's illness, as has been shown in human healthcare (Koenig 2013).

Families tend to appreciate healthcare practitioners inquiring about and integrating the spirituality of the family into decisions around illness and end of life (Robinson et al. 2006). A study done with human inpatients at the University of Chicago Medical Center showed that satisfaction with care was significantly greater for those who had discussions about their religious or spiritual concerns while in the hospital, including those who initially did not want to discuss such concerns (Williams et al. 2011). Once medical issues have been addressed, patients tend to be receptive to healthcare practitioners inquiring about or discussing their spiritual concerns (MacLean et al. 2003). Veterinary clients may also be receptive to veterinary professionals addressing spiritual matters once the medical issues of their animal companion are addressed.

An Australian study found that veterinary clients were influenced by their religious beliefs when making decisions regarding the euthanasia of their animal companion, as well as how they conceptualized and dealt with their grief. The religions represented by the participants in the study were Christian, Baha'i, Buddhist, Sikh, Spiritualist, Wiccan, Pagan, Universal, atheist, agnostic, and "none." Not all who self-identified as religious believed in some form of afterlife for their animal companion, whereas some who self-identified as nonreligious did. Participants deeply appreciated when their veterinarian was sensitive to their feelings and grief, showed respect for their animal, appreciated their animal's individuality, or reached out after the death of their animal companion. Providing clients with clear information about their animal's health situation and giving them sufficient time to make decisions about treatment options, euthanasia, and aftercare of their animal companion's body gave them an enhanced sense of control or helped them find meaning in the animal's illness and subsequent death (Davis et al. 2003).

Spiritual Distress

Spiritual distress tends to occur when the things that bring meaning, hope, love, peace, comfort, strength, connection in (Anandarajah and Hight 2001), and purpose to one's life are compromised; when one is unable to find a source of spiritual strength to cope with a difficult or traumatic situation (Wintz 2013); or when one's beliefs are in conflict with the events occurring in their life (Anandarajah and Hight 2001). They may appear anxious, angry, or depressed; have trouble sleeping; question or express anger at God or a higher power; express regret; feel "a sense of emptiness or loss of direction" (Healthcare Chaplaincy 2012); or question the fairness of life or life choices made. Spiritual issues, such as "hopelessness, despair, guilt, shame, anger, and abandonment by God," tend to arise, leading people to feel alienated from themselves, others, God, or their ultimate source of meaning, and provoking deep suffering (Puchalski and Ferrell 2010). People anticipating the loss of an animal companion may experience feelings of guilt or failure, or "bargain with God for the restored health of their animal." They may question their beliefs, or feel abandoned or betrayed by God, and need a source of spiritual strength when an animal companion dies (Lagoni et al. 1994).

Acting as the surrogate decision maker for a child or family member unable to make decisions regarding their own medical care places someone under considerable psychological stress and uncertainty. Since the veterinary client (caregiver) always has to act as the surrogate decision maker for their animal companion, they tend to experience stress when faced with making complex healthcare decisions on the animal companion's behalf.

The understanding and approach to decision-making regarding the treatment and care of a child with an illness, disability, or in end-of-life care tends to be affected and influenced by the spiritual perspectives of the parents and the spiritual resources they turn to for help (Robinson et al. 2006). Whether justified or not, parents who believe they are directly or indirectly responsible for their child's illness or condition may feel guilty, helpless, hopeless, angry, or frustrated. They may hold in their emotions or redirect their anger and frustration at others, including the medical staff. Others may think God is angry at them or punishing them for a past transgression. They might be angry at, feel betrayed by, or have lost faith in God if they believe God allowed, caused, or failed to prevent the child's illness or death (Fosarelli 2006).

Caring for an animal companion with a chronic or terminal illness may require a large time and financial commitment from the caregiver, yet the same social services or support systems available to people caring for a chronically or terminally ill human family member are not currently available to the person caring for an animal. The caregiver could become socially isolated. Employers may not grant a leave of absence, and they may have to leave their job to provide hospice care for their animal. If self-employed, they may be unable to run their business while caring for their animal. If they have limited financial resources, they may be faced with the difficult choice between the health or life of their animal and their financial well-being, which could lead to spiritual distress.

Veterinary clients may experience heightened emotions when their animal companion is undergoing a medical or health crisis, causing stress to ripple through the personnel of the entire veterinary practice (Figley and Roop 2006). In addition, people working in veterinary practices bond and form relationships with the clients and animal patients, which could span the entire lifetime of the animal. They share in the joys and sorrows of the client and grieve when the animal dies or the relationship with the client and animal ends. Since animals have a relatively short life span in comparison, veterinary personnel will experience many losses, their own as well as their client's, over the course of their career. The cumulative effect of these losses, as well as repeated exposure to the pain and suffering of clients and animals, are among the sources of compassion fatigue in veterinary settings that need to be counterbalanced with good self-care, including identifying and addressing one's spiritual needs. Addressing emotional and spiritual needs will help to counteract burn out and compassion fatigue (Ayl 2013).

Taking a Spiritual History

When faced with death, one is compelled to confront what gives one ultimate meaning, which may lead to reflection on "the universal values of love, justice, peace, and acceptance" (Puchalski 2006). During this time, people often turn to spiritual resources for comfort or help or question their beliefs and values or the purpose and meaning of life (Mann 2006). Spiritual care "involves compassion, presence, listening, and the encouragement of realistic hope," and may not always involve a discussion of God or religion (Anandarajah and Hight 2001). Therefore, it "can and should be performed to a greater or lesser degree by all healthcare professionals" (Handzo 2012). Someone may be struggling with spiritual issues if they talk about searching for meaning, feeling a sense of isolation or hopelessness instead of connection or hope, or fearing the unknown (Anandarajah and Hight 2001).

Within the human healthcare setting, physicians are encouraged to take a spiritual history on family members of patients. A spiritual history helps identify those who "may be experiencing a high level of religious or spiritual distress or a possible spiritual crisis" (Jankowski et al. 2011) and provides an awareness of, and respect for, the cultural, religious, and spiritual concerns and resources (Mann 2006) of the caregiver, as well as what

they may need to help them cope with the impending death of their loved one. Animal hospice providers could conduct a spiritual history on caregivers and their families by listening to and learning about their beliefs, and asking open-ended questions. Doing so could help providers identify possible spiritual needs or issues, as well as recognize when someone is experiencing spiritual distress. As a guide, if the caregiver is wearing religious jewelry, clothing, or has a religious or spiritual text in the home, the provider could ask direct questions about their spiritual beliefs, such as, "Do you have spiritual beliefs or practices that help you cope with stress?" and "Will your beliefs influence the end of life care decisions you make for your animal companion?" (adapted from Puchalski 2006).

To learn more about the caregiver's social and emotional support systems, the provider could ask questions such as, "Are you a member of a cultural, spiritual, or religious community? Is this of support to you, and how? Is there a group of people you really love or who are important to you?" (Puchalski 2006) and "Do you have friends or family nearby to help you?" (Mann 2006).

To remain within ethical and professional boundaries, veterinary professionals are advised to let the caregiver direct any discussion on spiritual concerns. They should conduct themselves in a respectful manner, without imposing their own beliefs, and honor the privacy of the caregiver and their family. The following guidelines from human healthcare could be applied to the animal hospice setting (adapted from Puchalski 2006):

- Spiritual histories are caregiver centered.
- Professional chaplains are recognized as the experts for spiritual care.
- Proselytizing is unacceptable and unethical.
- Caregivers should not be coerced to address spiritual issues.
- If more in-depth spiritual counseling is needed, it should be under the direction of a

professional chaplain or other appropriate spiritual leader or counselor.

It is important to recognize that veterinarians and other animal hospice providers should not initiate prayer, unless the hospice chaplain or other spiritual leader is unavailable, and the caregiver requests it. If the caregiver wants to pray, the veterinarian/animal hospice provider can stand by in silence. The caregiver has called the hospice provider at a vulnerable time in their life and likely views the provider as a person of authority. The provider should take care to not abuse that authority (adapted from Puchalski 2006).

Veterinary professionals may be uncomfortable, reluctant, or resistant to adding spiritual support to their practice, especially if they are not spiritual or religious themselves. However, as investors in the human-animal bond, veterinary professionals also take care of the people who are bonded with the animal patient. In human healthcare, the spiritual needs of the patient and their family should determine whether a physician takes a spiritual history, not the physician's spiritual or religious beliefs, or how comfortable they are talking to patients about spirituality and religion (Koenig 2013). The same could be said about the spiritual needs of veterinary clients and staff. To help them explore their own spirituality and connect with their clients, veterinary professionals could ask themselves the following questions:

- What gives meaning in my life?
- What beliefs and values are most important in guiding my life?
- What does religion mean to me?
- What does spirituality mean to me?
- How would a life-threatening illness change the way I find meaning, values, or beliefs in life?
- What spiritual resources do I bring to my work? What connections have I made between spirituality and my life experiences of suffering, grief, losses, and such? (Bryson 2004)

When to Call in the Experts (and Who Are the Experts?)

In the human healthcare setting, chaplains are considered the primary experts in spiritual care. In this context, the title "chaplain" refers to a professional, board-certified chaplain who has met all of the requirements of the Common Standards for Professional Chaplaincy (Association of Professional Chaplains 2004b) and the Common Code of Ethics for professional chaplains, which "prohibits proselytizing or imposing one's own beliefs and practices" on a person in their care (Association of Professional Chaplains 2004a). A chaplain certified through the Board of Chaplaincy Certification, Inc. (BCCI), an affiliate of the Association of Professional Chaplains (APC), assures the chaplain has met established national standards for professional competence. Board certified chaplains practice evidence-based care, which includes ongoing evaluation of new practices, and, when appropriate, contribute to or conduct research. The requirements to apply for board certification include a bachelor's degree, theological graduate education, four units (1600 hours) of Clinical Pastoral Education (CPE), ordination or other similar standing in, and current endorsement by, the ecclesial body or faith group the chaplain represents, a minimum of 2000 hours of work experience as a chaplain, and demonstration of 29 professional chaplain competencies (Board of Chaplaincy Certification, Inc. 2015a).

Board certified chaplains with three years of experience in human hospice and palliative care can apply for specialty certification in hospice and palliative care, designated BCC-HPCC (board certified chaplain-hospice/palliative care certified). The competencies and requirements for BCC-HPCC specialty certification are based on the guidelines for chaplains from the National Consensus Project for Quality Palliative Care, which published clinical guidelines for all disciplines serving in human hospice and palliative care (National Consensus Project for Quality Palliative Care 2013). These guidelines are recognized as the professional norm for hospice and palliative care chaplains practicing in the United States (Board of Chaplaincy Certification, Inc. 2015b). Currently, a specialty certification for Board Certified Chaplains serving in a veterinary or animal hospice setting does not exist. However, BCC-HPCC chaplains are considered to be competent in all hospice and palliative care settings, which could also apply to animal hospice and palliative care.

Many human hospitals and hospices employ chaplains as fully integrated and vital members of the interdisciplinary healthcare team. Chaplains assess and address the spiritual and existential needs of patients, family, and staff. They come from many different faith traditions and provide spiritual support to all, not just those who identify as religious or spiritual. Chaplains are clinically trained to integrate theology and the behavioral sciences (Koenig 2013) to help people find their own sources of spiritual strength and resilience in the face of illness or death "regardless of religion or beliefs" (Handzo 2012).

The most important intervention chaplains provide is listening to and offering a safe and sacred space for individuals to share their "emotions freely without judgment or advice." They are present to others in an attentive, compassionate, and non-anxious way, which helps the other "find the things that bring them strength, comfort and renewal." Since the chaplain is seen as a neutral member of the healthcare team who does not diagnose, treat, or provide direct care to the patient, individuals tend to be more comfortable sharing their concerns with them (McClung et al. 2006). Chaplains are especially helpful when difficult decisions are being made and end of life discussions are taking place between physicians, medical staff, patients, and the patient's family.

Although chaplains are not widely used within veterinary medicine at this time, they could be of great benefit to families and hospice professionals and hopefully will begin to be integrated into interdisciplinary care teams. If the animal hospice provider is not comfortable with conducting a spiritual history, or does not have time to complete one, the chaplain could conduct it. When the spiritual history indicates the caregiver is struggling with spiritual issues or experiencing spiritual distress, the chaplain conducts a spiritual assessment, "an extensive, in-depth, ongoing process of actively listening to a [person's] story as it unfolds in a relationship." Spiritual assessments help determine the degree to which someone "may be experiencing issues with purpose and meaning, loss of self control, or spiritual pain and suffering" (Jankowski et al. 2011). Due to their complex nature, spiritual assessments should only be done by board certified chaplains because they have the special clinical training necessary to perform them (Puchalski and Ferrell 2010). The chaplain formulates a spiritual care plan from the spiritual assessment. It is appropriate for the chaplain to complete a spiritual assessment even when the caregiver does not identify with, or express an interest in, religion (Association of Professional Chaplains 2015b).

As a member of the animal hospice team, the chaplain could be contacted before the initial consultation with the caregiver of the animal patient (client) and accompany the provider and team on that first visit. In addition to conducting spiritual histories and assessments, chaplains serving in an animal hospice practice could:

- help the caregiver create an advance directive (Pierce 2012) if one was not prepared when the animal patient was healthy. In human hospitals, chaplains assist patients and families with the preparation of advanced directives. Veterinary chaplains could do the same for clients on behalf of their animal companion.
- encourage the caregiver to fully discuss all treatment options with the hospice provider, as well as ask for information about the

euthanasia procedure, hospice-supported natural death, and active dying process.

- provide emotional and spiritual support before the hospice provider arrives and remain as long as needed after the provider or hospice team leaves.
- sit with the client while the animal patient is receiving care.
- when the caregiver requests, and if practical, sit with the animal patient during treatment procedures.
- provide spiritual support to the caregiver, caregiver's family, provider, and animal hospice staff throughout the continuum of care.
- provide a supportive presence when difficult decisions need to be made.
- help the client explore the decision-making process leading to the authorization for euthanasia.
- help the client work through *all* their feelings before arriving at a decision to choose euthanasia or hospice-supported natural death.
- if other family members are involved in the decision on when to euthanize, facilitate discussion to ensure that everyone's feelings are taken into account.
- provide a supportive presence before, during, and after euthanasia procedure or the death of the animal patient.
- remain with a client after the animal's death for as long as needed so the staff can leave and move on to next appointment or task.
- be available to the hospice team members to help them debrief, as well as help them manage their potential for compassion fatigue.
- perform rituals and memorial services for the client and staff.
- communicate with, refer to, interact with, and be a liaison to religious leaders in the local community.
- refer the caregiver or a team member to a mental health professional or other services in the community when necessary.

It needs to be emphasized that the caregiver is always free to reject chaplaincy care at any time and be offered chaplaincy care if they change their minds at a later point in time. The chaplain should respect their choice without offense, question, or judgment.

Spiritual Questions Unique to Veterinary Practice and Hospice and Palliative Care

People anticipating the death of their animal companion may wonder about or question whether their animal has a soul or an afterlife. If what they were taught regarding the soul and afterlife of animals conflicts with what they have come to believe, or if a religious authority or others close to them do not agree with their belief, they might experience considerable anxiety or spiritual distress. For example, many pet caregivers wonder whether animals go to heaven. A chaplain would be the spiritual care expert best able to help clients struggling with this issue, as they are open and available to listen to the client's beliefs and concerns without imposing their own beliefs. Although grounded in the religious or faith tradition they represent, chaplains are available to meet others wherever they are on the religious or spiritual spectrum, help them answer their own questions, and come to their own conclusions based on their own beliefs and traditions, and find solace and peace. In comparison, religious leaders or authorities may avoid, dismiss, treat insensitively, ridicule, or feel unable to address this issue because of their beliefs or the beliefs, traditions, expectations, or policies of their ecclesial body or faith tradition.

Similar to their counterparts in human hospice, animal hospice providers and team members provide palliative care to terminally ill and dying patients, provide comfort and support to the patient's family, frequently experience the death of a beloved patient – the accumulative effect of grief upon grief, and may need or benefit from professional spiritual care. Unlike human hospice and palliative care, euthanasia is an available therapeutic option in veterinary medicine. Considered to be "one of life's most painful yet loving and unselfish acts" (Ayl 2013), euthanasia can raise ethical or moral questions around the intentional killing of an animal (Pierce 2012) and cause euthanasia-related stress, known as the "Caring-Killing Paradox," which affects the emotional well-being of veterinary professionals and staff (Ayl 2013). When a long and intensive period of hospice care ends in a decision to euthanize, veterinary clients may also experience euthanasia-related stress, especially if they believe they are killing or causing the death of their animal companion. Chaplains are trained and experienced in addressing the spiritual and emotional needs of those caring for the terminally ill and dying, helping them debrief and manage their potential for compassion fatigue or burnout (Koenig 2013), which could be applied to euthanasia-related stress in the veterinary and animal hospice setting.

Including a Chaplain on the Interdisciplinary Veterinary/Hospice Team

Since assumptions and misconceptions about the role of the chaplain exist in human healthcare, veterinary professionals may also have doubts about adding a paid staff chaplain to the veterinary or animal hospice team. Like many of their medical counterparts, they may not be aware that chaplains have extensive specialized training that integrates behavioral science with theological and ministerial skills (Cahners 2009) and, therefore, assume that a referral to clergy in the local community will adequately meet the spiritual needs of their clients and staff. A white paper about providing support to people in the veterinary setting, created by an ad-hoc committee of the American Animal Hospital Association (AAHA), suggests that veterinary professionals partner with religious leaders in the local community who are "sensitive to the human-animal bond,"

empathic to the loss of an animal, and "know how to comfort people regarding death and the afterlife" to provide spiritual care to clients and staff (American Animal Hospital Association 2012). However, community clergy may not have time to visit their own congregants who are hospitalized to "perform religious rituals, pray, or provide in-depth spiritual counsel," especially if they serve in a large or aging congregation (Koenig 2013). If community clergy do not have the time to visit their own hospitalized congregants, it is unlikely that they will have time to provide spiritual care to a congregant with a sick or recently deceased animal companion. Since "approximately one-third of Americans ... have not attended a religious service in the past six months" (Koenig 2013), veterinary clients may not belong to a community of faith or have a trusted spiritual leader to contact in times of spiritual need. The spiritual needs of those who are "spiritual, but not religious," atheist, or agnostic also need to be considered, and are not mentioned in the white paper.

In addition, religious leaders sensitive to the human-animal bond may be difficult to find. In our culture, grief over the loss of an animal companion tends to be minimized, discounted, or belittled, denying the griever the important ritual of telling the story of "what happened" (Rosell 2005) and causing their grief to be disenfranchised, "not socially sanctioned, openly acknowledged, or publicly shared" (Doka and Davidson 1998). Many organized religions do not offer help, comfort (Netting et al. 1984), or solace to those mourning the loss of an animal (Sife 2014). When asked to conduct a "religious ceremony or ritual normally associated with human death," religious leaders need to use their professional judgment and will decline if they are obligated to follow the particular beliefs and norms of their religious tradition (Netting et al. 1984). Clients belonging to a faith community rarely contact their religious leader when an animal companion dies, as they would when a human family member dies. They may be afraid their religious leader will ridicule them or not support them in their grief (Netting et al. 1984). They may think asking for spiritual support during the illness or following the death of an animal will be an imposition on the religious leader. When the caregiver's religious tradition or leader is not available or supportive, chaplains could provide spiritual support, and create and preside over a funeral service for a beloved animal (Rosell 2005). Chaplains are more available, flexible, and qualified than community clergy to provide spiritual care in veterinary and animal hospice settings.

In human healthcare, chaplains have been shown to be one of the most cost-effective resources to facilitate communication and increase family and staff satisfaction (BCC 2015a). Chaplaincy care is provided as a non-billable service. Chaplains are employed by the hospital or hospice as paid staff members. The hospital or hospice might have adjunct (volunteer) chaplains in addition to the paid staff chaplains. Adjunct chaplains typically are local clergy members from various faiths and denominations who have completed one or more units of CPE at an Association of Clinical Pastoral Education (ACPE) accredited CPE center. The ACPE is "a multicultural, multifaith organization devoted to providing education and improving the quality of ministry and pastoral care offered by spiritual caregivers of all faiths" (The Association for Clinical Pastoral Education 2016a), and is considered to be "the standard-setting, accrediting, certifying, resource agency in the field of clinical pastoral education (CPE)" (McGee 1990). Like the American Veterinary Medical Association Council on Education (AVMA COE), the ACPE is nationally recognized as an accrediting agency by the U.S. Secretary of Education through the U.S. Department of Education (The Association for Clinical Pastoral Education 2016a). Hospitals and hospices that are accredited CPE centers have at least one ACPE certified supervisor to train and supervise CPE students (residents, interns, and externs). CPE residencies are paid positions,

whereas interns and externs serve as volunteers. A listing of CPE centers accredited by the ACPE can be found on their website (The Association for Clinical Pastoral Education 2016b). Clinical training completed in ACPE accredited CPE centers could be applied to the veterinary and animal hospice setting.

Veterinary practices and hospices are not currently used as clinical placements for CPE students. An increase in the awareness of and demand for trained and competent chaplains in veterinary settings could result in veterinary teaching hospitals, larger veterinary practices, and veterinary emergency and specialty clinics employing a ACPE certified supervisor, adjusting the CPE curricula to the veterinary or animal hospice context, and seeking ACPE accreditation as CPE centers, providing clinical placements and training for "veterinary chaplains." Evidence-based chaplaincy research exploring the benefits of, developing standards of practice for, and continuously improving the quality of chaplaincy care in the veterinary setting could be conducted at these larger facilities.

The physical presence of a chaplain is tantamount to effective chaplaincy care. A chaplain available on-site, or as a member of the animal hospice team, would be available and ready to respond to any emergent situation. Ideally, a veterinary clinic or animal hospice organization would employ and pay the salary of at least one professional chaplain who would provide spiritual care to clients and staff, as well as supervise other staff and adjunct chaplains. If a veterinary practice or animal hospice is located near an ACPE accredited CPE center, CPE students at that center might be interested in serving as volunteer chaplains. Veterinary clinics or animal hospice organizations with an insufficient volume of clients to sustain full and part-time staff chaplains could have on-call chaplains on scheduled days and hours, available if and when the clinic or animal hospice needs them. Veterinary clinics or animal hospice organizations lacking the funds to pay for a full-, part-time, or on-call chaplain could fund these services through individual donations to a special fund created by the veterinary clinic, religious organization of the chaplain, or a nonprofit organization formed to provide chaplains in veterinary and animal hospice settings. Funding could also be pursued through grants written to pet food manufacturers, veterinary associations, pharmaceutical and animal health industries, and other animal-related companies and organizations.

"Veterinary chaplaincy" is an emerging field, and it may be difficult for a veterinarian to find a chaplain. Veterinary and animal hospice practices or organizations wanting to employ a staff chaplain could submit a job posting on the website of the Association of Professional Chaplains (Association of Professional Chaplains 2015a).

There are nonprofit corporations and organizations that offer spiritual care and support services to the employees and families of small and large businesses at a reasonable cost. Marketplace Chaplains, founded in 1984, has over 1800 chaplains serving in the United States (nationwide: mchapusa.com), Canada (mcares.ca), Mexico (mchapmx.com), the United Kingdom, and Puerto Rico. They have placed chaplains to serve the clients, family, and staff of animal hospitals and veterinary emergency and specialty centers. Their chaplain teams consist of two trained, experienced, and diverse professional chaplains, who make rounds on a weekly basis to develop relationships and provide individual spiritual care and support to veterinary staff and clients who choose to engage with a chaplain. The chaplain team is available to employees on a 24/7 basis and includes crisis care. Confidential, face to face care is available off-site, on-site, and remotely via their app, "MyChap." There are no limits imposed on the amount of time or frequency for an individual to meet with a chaplain. Practices choosing to have a "chaplain" on their interdisciplinary team can opt to contract with "Marketplace Care Partners," where the same chaplains serve under the title, "Care Partner."

Workforce Chaplains (www.workforce chaplains.com) offers on-site spiritual and emotional support to small and large businesses located primarily within the state of Indiana, as well as remote care nationwide. Their chaplain teams consist of six trained, experienced, and diverse professional chaplains to provide a listening ear, and spiritual care and support that is nondenominational and confidential and follows the Common Code of Ethics for professional chaplains (Association of Professional Chaplains 2004a). Interacting with a chaplain is optional. The frequency of in-site care is flexible and can be provided on an as-needed, once-a-week, or once-a-month basis.

TeleChaplaincy is a cost-effective, remote service offered primarily to medical institutions via telehealth by The Health Care Chaplaincy Network (HCCN). Professional chaplains deliver spiritual and emotional support to the staff, overnight inpatients, outpatients, and family caregivers of a medical institution when a professional chaplain is not available on-site. One of the three models of chaplaincy care offered, "Talk to the Chaplain Live," provides on-call chaplains to serve remotely throughout a specified period of time. This service can be customized to meet the needs of a veterinary or animal hospice practice. To inquire about how chaplaincy care can be provided to clients and staff in your veterinary or animal hospice practice or set up a contract with HCCN for TeleChaplaincy service, see the contact information listed under "Resources" in this chapter.

Veterinary or animal hospice practices in rural areas unable to find a chaplain locally could interview local clergy, such as priests, pastors, rabbis, imams, or clergy with one or more units of CPE training, to find those who are animal-friendly and willing, able, and available to provide this service. Clergy who are retired or currently not serving a congregation would be more likely to have the time to provide spiritual care in the veterinary and animal hospice setting. Some clients might prefer spiritual care provided by clergy from their own religious tradition. For rural, mobile, and small veterinary practices, "Chat with a Chaplain" may be a good option. Provided by the HCCN through their "Chaplains On Hand" website (chaplainsonhand.org), this service is free to anyone wanting or needing to connect with a professional chaplain (by email, phone or video call) to listen and offer spiritual care and support.

As opposed to the professional model of chaplaincy care, there are websites where ordination or certification as a chaplain can be purchased by someone with minimal to no qualifications, education, or training. These web-based institutions offer education, training and/or certification to become an animal chaplain through online or correspondence courses, submitted essays or papers, or by simply submitting an online application and fee. The institutional requirements for training and credentialing animal chaplains are quite variable, and the online institutions that educate, train, and certify them lack program, ecclesial, and professional oversight, and are not postsecondary institutions or programs accredited by the U.S. Department of Education. In addition, animal chaplains may be ordained and/or certified by the same institution that trained them, instead of by an independent body. These animal chaplains, therefore, may not be held accountable to an ecclesial body or faith group, professional chaplain association, accrediting agency, professional standards, or code of ethics, unlike professional, board certified chaplains.

Currently, veterinary or animal hospice chaplaincy is not recognized as a specialty by professional chaplaincy or religious organizations. In addition, the AAHA does not address meeting the cultural, spiritual, and religious needs of veterinary clients and staff as a standard of quality care required for AAHA accreditation, and the American Veterinary Medical Association (AVMA) mentions spiritual care only in the context of self-care for managing burn out and compassion fatigue in veterinary professionals (American Veterinary Medical Association 2015a,b,c,d) and in a caption for one particular veterinary social worker

(Larkin 2015). There is no organization collecting statistics on the number of chaplains employed by, or serving in, veterinary or animal hospice settings, as well as how many are paid or volunteer, staff, or on-call, what kind of education or chaplaincy training they have, and what, if any, credentials they have to practice as a chaplain. Anecdotally, there are religious leaders and chaplains interested in and serving as chaplains in veterinary settings. The increased emphasis on client care in veterinary medicine could lead to a greater awareness of the importance of spirituality for caregivers, providers, and staff. Evidence-based research on the spiritual needs and spiritual care of veterinary clients and staff may give a better picture of the state of veterinary chaplaincy, and lead to provision of on-site spiritual care in veterinary and animal hospice settings (Dobbs 2015).

Resources

Marketplace Chaplains
Website: mchapusa.com
Address: 2001 W. Plano Parkway, Suite 3200, Plano, TX 75075

Marketplace Care Partners at MAU (in partnership with Marketplace Chaplains since 2013)
Website: www.mau.com/carepartners
MAU Workforce Solutions (www.mau.com)

Marketplace Care Canada
Website: https://mcares.ca
Address: 10060 Jasper Avenue, Tower 1, Suite 2020, Edmonton, AB T5J 3R8
Mailing Address: PO Box 2262, Beaverlodge, AB, T0H 0C0

Marketplace Chaplains Mexico (Capellanes Marketplace de México)
http://mchapmx.com
Address: Calle Nieve No. 344, Col. Satélite, Querétaro, Oro., CP, 76110, Mexico

Workforce Chaplains
Website: www.workforcechaplains.com
Address: P.O. Box 517, Brownsburg, IN 46112

TeleChaplaincy (for inquiries, contact the person below, not the person listed on their website)
Health Care Chaplaincy Network (HCCN)
Contact: Jose Hernandez, Chief Operating Officer
Website: healthcarechaplaincy.org/telechaplaincy
Address: 505 Eighth Avenue, Suite 900, New York, NY 10018

Chat with a Chaplain – Chaplains On Hand
Health Care Chaplaincy Network (HCCN)
Website: http://chaplainsonhand.org
Address: 505 Eighth Avenue, Suite 900, New York, NY 10018

Association of Professional Chaplains (APC)
Website: www.professionalchaplains.org
Address: 2800 W. Higgins, Suite 295, Hoffman Estates, IL 60169

Board of Chaplaincy Certification, Inc. (BCC), an affiliate of APC
Website: https://bcci.professionalchaplains.org
Address: 2800 W. Higgins, Suite 295, Hoffman Estates, IL 60169

Association of Clinical Pastoral Education (ACPE)
Website: acpe.edu
Address: 55 Ivan Allen Jr. Boulevard, Suite 835, Atlanta, GA 30308

References

American Animal Hospital Association (AAHA). (2012) *Human support in veterinary settings*. AVMA. Available at: http://vetsocialwork.utk.edu/wp-content/uploads/2018/01/HumanSupport-Document_Final.pdf (Accessed:21 October 2022).

American Veterinary Medical Association (AVMA). (2015a) *Model program for wellness*. AVMA. Available at: https://www.avma.org/resources-tools/wellbeing/model-program-wellness (Accessed: 21 October 2022).

American Veterinary Medical Association (AVMA). (2015b) *Self care for veterinarians*. AVMA. Available at: https://www.avma.org/resources-tools/wellbeing/self-care-veterinarians (Accessed: 21 October 2022).

American Veterinary Medical Association (AVMA). (2015c) *Work and compassion fatigue*. AVMA. Available at: https://www.avma.org/resources-tools/wellbeing/work-and-compassion-fatigue(Accessed: 21 October 2022).

American Veterinary Medical Association (AVMA). (2015d) For human needs, some veterinary clinics are turning to a professional. Available at: https://www.avma.org/javma-news/2016-01-01/human-needs-some-veterinary-clinics-are-turning-professional (Accessed: 15 October 2022).

Anandarajah, G. and Hight, E. (2001) Spirituality and medical practice: using HOPE questions as a practical tool for spiritual assessment. *Am. Fam. Physician*, 63: 81–89.

Association for Clinical Pastoral Education, Inc (ACPE). (2016a) *About ACPE*. ACPE. Available at: https://acpe.edu/about-acpe (Accessed: 22 October 2022).

Association for Clinical Pastoral Education, Inc (ACPE). (2016b) *Accredited CPE Centers*. ACPE. Available at: https://profile.acpe.edu/accreditedcpedirectory (Accessed: 22 October 2022).

Association of Professional Chaplains (APC). (2004a) *Common Code of Ethics for Chaplains, Pastoral Counselors, Pastoral Educators and Students*. APC. Available at: http://www.professionalchaplains.org/files/professional_standards/common_standards/common_code_ethics.pdf (Accessed: 7 Nov 2004).

Association of Professional Chaplains (APC). (2004b) *Common Standards for Professional Chaplaincy.* APC. Available at: http://www.professionalchaplains.org/files/professional_standards/common_standards/common_standards_professional_chaplaincy.pdf (Accessed: 7 Nov 2004).

Association of Professional Chaplains (APC). (2015a) *Post a Job.* APC. Available at: http://www.professionalchaplains.org/content.asp?admin=Y&pl=217&sl=78&contentid=218 (Accessed: 22 Jan 2016).

Association of Professional Chaplains (APC). (2015b) *Standards of Practice for Professional Chaplains.* APC. Available at: http://www.professionalchaplains.org/Files/professional_standards/standards_of_practice/Standards_of_Practice_for_Professional_Chaplains_102215.pdf (Accessed: 22 Jan 2016).

Ayl, K. (2013) When Helping Hurts: Compassion Fatigue in the Veterinary Profession AAHA Press, Lakewood, CO.

Board of Chaplaincy Certification, Inc (BCC). (2015a) *Advocating for Professional Chaplaincy: The Benefits of Board Certification.* BCC. Available at: http://033012b.membershipsoftware.org/Files/benefits_of_bcc.pdf (Accessed: 22 Jan 2016).

Board of Chaplaincy Certification, Inc (BCC). (2015b) *Hospice and Palliative Care Specialty Certification.* BCC. Available at: https://bcci.professionalchaplains.org/content.asp?pl=42&contentid=45 (Accessed: 22 Jan 2016).

Bryson, K.A. (2004) Spirituality, meaning, and transcendence. *Palliat. Support. Care*, 2: 321–328.

Cahners, N. (2009) What does a hospital chaplain do again? Trying to explain the meaning of making meaning in the work of medical ethics. In: *Medical Ethics in Health Care Chaplaincy.* (eds. W. Moczynski, H. Haker, and K. Bentele), pp. 317–329. Berlin: LIT Verlag.

Davis, H., Irwin, P., Richardson, M. *et al.* (2003) When a pet dies: religious issues, euthanasia and strategies for coping with bereavement. *Anthrozoös*, 16: 57–74.

Dobbs, K. (2015) Professional Chaplaincy in Veterinary Medicine. *Veterinary Team Brief.* July, 51–53, Available at: https://files.brief.vet/migration/article/23986/sf_professional-chaplaincy-in-veterinary-medicine-23986-article.pdf (Accessed: 21 October 2022).

Doka, K.J. and Davidson, J.D. (eds.) (1998) *Living with Grief: Who we Are, how we Grieve.* New York: Routledge Taylor & Francis Group.

Figley, C. and Roop, R. (2006) Compassion Fatigue in the Animal-Care Community Washington, D.C.: Humane Society Press.

Fosarelli, P. (2006) The spiritual issues faced by children and adolescents at the end of life. In: *A Time for Listening and Caring: Spirituality and the Care of the Chronically Ill and Dying.* (ed C. M. Puchalski), pp. 83–100. New York: Oxford University Press.

Galek, K., Flannelly, K.J., Vane, A. *et al.* (2005) Assessing a Patient's spiritual needs: a comprehensive instrument. *Holist. Nurs. Pract.*, 19: 62–69.

Handzo, G. (2012) The process of spiritual/pastoral care: a general theory for providing spiritual/pastoral care using palliative care as a paradigm. In: *Professional Spiritual & Pastoral Care: A Practical Clergy and Chaplain's Handbook.* (ed. S. B. Roberts), pp. 21–41. Woodstock, VT: SkyLights Path Publishing.

HealthCare Chaplaincy. (2012) Chaplaincy Care Volunteer Training Manual. New York: HealthCare Chaplaincy.

Jankowski, K.R., Handzo, G.F., and Flannelly, K.J. (2011) Testing the efficacy of chaplaincy care. *J. Health Care Chaplain.*, 17: 100–125.

Koenig, H.G. (2013) Spirituality in Patient Care 3. West Conshohocken, PA: Templeton Press.

Koenig, H.G., King, D.E., and Benner Carson, V. *et al.* (2001) Handbook of Religion and Health. New York: Oxford University.

Lagoni, L., Butler, C., and Hetts, S. (1994) The Human-Animal Bond and Grief. Philadelphia, PA: W.B. Saunders Company.

Larkin, M. (2015) For human needs, some veterinary clinics are turning to a professional.

JAVMAnews. Available: https://www.avma. org/News/JAVMANews/Pages/160101a.aspx (Accessed:16 Dec 2015).

Lue, T., Pantenburg, D.P., and Crawford, P.M. (2008) Impact of the owner-pet and client-veterinarian bond on care that pets receive. *J. Am. Vet. Med. Assoc.*, 232: 531–540.

MacLean, C.D., Susi, B., Phifer, N. *et al.* (2003) Patient preference for physician discussion and practice of spirituality. *J. Gen. Intern. Med.*, 18: 38–43.

Mann, S. (2006) On sacred ground – the role of chaplains in the care of the dying: a partnership between the religious community and the healthcare community. In: *A Time for Listening and Caring: Spirituality and the Care of the Chronically Ill and Dying.* (ed C. M. Puchalski), pp. 115–128. New York: Oxford University Press.

McClung, E., Grossoehme, D.H., and Jacobson, A.F. (2006) Collaborating with chaplains to meet spiritual needs. *Med. Surg. Nurs.*; 15: 147–156.

McGee, L.L. (1990) Certification. In: *Dictionary of Pastoral Care and Counseling.* (ed R.J. Hunter), p. 135. Nashville: Abingdon Press.

National Consensus Project for Quality Palliative Care (2013) *Clinical Practice Guidelines for Quality Palliative Care.* 3rd edition. Pittsburgh, PA: National Consensus Project for Quality Palliative Care. Available at: https://www. nationalcoalitionhpc.org/ncp/ (Accessed: 22 October 2022).

Netting, F.E., Netting, K.A., Wilson, C.C. *et al.* (1984) Pastors, parishioners, and pets. *Pastoral Psychol.*, 33: 126–135.

Pierce, J. (2012) The Last Walk: Reflections on our Pets at the Ends of their Lives. Chicago: University of Chicago Press.

Puchalski, C. (2006) Spiritual Care: Practical Tools. In: *A Time for Listening and Caring: Spirituality and the Care of the Chronically Ill and Dying.* (ed. C. M. Puchalski), pp. 229–251. New York: Oxford University Press.

Puchalski, C. and Ferrell, B. (2010) Making Health Care Whole: Integrating Spirituality into Patient Care, West Conshohocken, PA: Templeton Press.

Puchalski, C., Ferrell, B., Virani, R. *et al.* (2009) Improving the quality of spiritual care as a dimension of palliative care: the report of the Consensus Conference. *J. Palliat. Med.*, 12: 885–904.

Robinson, M., Thiel, M.M., Backus, M.M. *et al.* (2006) Matters of spirituality at the end of life in the pediatric intensive care unit. *Pediatrics*, 118: 719–729.

Rosell, T. D. (2005) Grieving the loss of a companion animal: pastoral perspective and personal narrative regarding one Sort of disenfranchised grief. *Rev. Expositor*, 102: 47–63.

Shaw, J.R., Adams, C.L., and Bonnett, B.N. (2004) What can veterinarians learn from studies of physician-patient communication about veterinarian-client-patient communication? *J. Am. Vet. Med. Assoc*, 224: 676–684.

Sife, W. (2014) The Loss of a Pet: A Guide to Coping with the Grieving Process when a Pet Dies 4, Nashville, TN: Howell Book House.

Sulmasy, D. (2006) The healthcare professional as person: the spirituality of providing care at the end of life. In: *A Time for Listening and Caring: Spirituality and the Care of the Chronically Ill and Dying.* (ed. C. M. Puchalski), pp. 101–114. New York: Oxford University Press.

Taylor, E.J. (2006) Prevalence and associated factors of spiritual needs among patients with cancer and family caregivers. *Oncol. Nurs. Forum*, 33: 729–735.

VandeCreek, L. and Smith, D. (1992) Measuring the spiritual needs of hospital patients and their families. *J. Pastoral Care*, 46: 46–52.

Wall, R., Engelberg, R. A., Gries, C. J. *et al.* (2007) Spiritual care of families in the intensive care unit. *Crit. Care Med.*, 35: 1084–1090.

Williams, J.A., Meltzer, D., Arora, V. *et al.* (2011) Attention to inpatients' religious and spiritual concerns: predictors and association with patient satisfaction. *J. Gen. Intern. Med.*, 26: 1265–1271.

Wintz, S. (2013) Caregivers for the ill need care, too. The Huffington Post. Available at: http:// www.huffingtonpost.com/the-rev-sue-wintz/ spirituality-and-caregiving_b_4086329. html?utm_hp_ref=gps-for-the-soul&ir=GPS%20 for%20the%20Soul (Accessed: 14 Oct 2013).

28

Factors Contributing to the Decision to Euthanize Pet Dogs and Cats

Nathaniel Cook, DVM, CVA, CVFT, CTPEP and Beth Marchitelli, DVM, MS

Introduction

The factors that contribute to a decision to euthanize a pet dog or cat are complex and multifactorial. Literature on euthanasia decision-making factors (also called triggers) for pet dogs and cats has grown significantly over the last decade, with studies examining both patient factors and pet owner factors. (Mallery et al. 1999; Nogueira Borden et al. 2010; Reynolds et al. 2010; Gates et al. 2017; Niessen et al. 2017; Testoni et al. 2017; Bussolari et al. 2018; Bennett and Cook 2019; Marchitelli et al. 2020; Persson et al. 2020; Spitznagel et al. 2020; Pegram et al. 2021; Spitznagel et al. 2021) Understanding these factors is critically important to the success of both the pet's healthcare providers in making recommendations and the pet's owner in implementing care.

Patient factors can be divided into two categories. The first patient category is the presence of symptoms or clinical signs that negatively affect quality of life, which may or may not be associated with a known disease process. The second patient category is the diagnosis of a specific disease, which often comes with a set of expected symptoms, consequences, potential treatment options, medical prognosis, and disease trajectory. Pet owner factors, which are often referred to in the hospice literature as "psychosocial," involve the interplay of the needs, abilities, and beliefs of the owner in relation to their pet. These categories of patient factors and pet owner factors, though not mutually exclusive, present unique challenges to the human–animal bond and often require different responses from veterinary hospice professionals as they try to provide the best help and care for animals and their human families. This chapter will highlight and discuss these three major categories that, whether independently or collectively, often trigger a decision to euthanize.

Pet Factors: Symptoms and Clinical Signs that Affect Quality of Life

Pet owners, particularly those with an aged animal, often find it very difficult to ascertain what exactly is responsible for their pet's declining health and quality of life. Pet owners can and do observe changes in their pet and notice symptoms of illness, but they are often unable to describe these symptoms to the veterinary team in a medically meaningful way, nor do they understand what these symptoms might mean in terms of a diagnosis or prognosis. In many cases, changes and symptoms develop insidiously and incrementally over a

Hospice and Palliative Care for Companion Animals: Principles and Practice, Second Edition.
Edited by Amir Shanan, Jessica Pierce, and Tamara Shearer.
© 2023 John Wiley & Sons, Inc. Published 2023 by John Wiley & Sons, Inc.
Companion website: www.wiley.com/go/shanan/palliative

relatively long time period, leaving pet owners uncertain about when the change or symptom began or how it developed. When symptoms first occur, they may be sporadic or mild, and are often attributed to general age-related changes as opposed to disease symptoms or progression. The observations of pet owners, of course, are often also complicated by a pet's instinct and ability to compensate for or mask symptoms of illness or discomfort. It is tempting to assume that obtaining a specific diagnosis will fully explain all changes and symptoms a pet is displaying, but unfortunately this is also often not the case. The diagnostic process can itself be problematic. Chasing down a diagnosis can be time consuming, expensive, and sometimes even invasive or life threatening for the animal patient. Further complexities of understanding occur in cases where pets have a number of comorbidities or where symptoms cannot be directly linked to any known diagnosis and may be more representative of general age-related decline than a specific illness.

While diagnosis of a specific disease may be required to offer the gold standard of a cure, obtaining a diagnosis cannot be the only means of providing therapies for symptom management. There are numerous cases where a specific diagnosis will not be pursued or will remain beyond reach. Likewise, even if there is a specific diagnosis, in many cases there is no cure or no targeted therapy for the disease diagnosed. For example, a pet owner may state that if their pet were younger, they would pursue a full diagnosis and, after diagnosis, an aggressive or potentially curative treatment plan. A decision not to pursue a diagnosis is not necessarily a decision for euthanasia, and therefore, whether there is a definitive diagnosis or not, treatment for symptom management is still needed in order to improve or maintain the pet's comfort and quality of life. The symptoms that a pet may experience over the course of a diagnosed illness may be more predictable, and so a diagnosis is valuable, but it is also certainly possible to manage symptoms as they develop,

and to use the combination of symptoms encountered to better understand a pet's overall condition and prognosis.

In this section, we will describe some of the most common symptoms associated with decreased quality of life in dogs and cats. Again, the cause of these symptoms may be unknown, due to age-related decline, or due to a specific disease or combination of disease processes. Although any one of these symptoms could be a trigger for euthanasia, it is also often true that the interaction of multiple symptoms can compound the effect on a pet's quality of life. Therefore, all of these symptoms should be carefully considered in a quality-of-life evaluation, and if applicable investigated for treatment potential. While the cause and surrounding circumstances do not necessarily change the symptom itself, context often does change how a given symptom affects an animal and how the pet owner perceives this effect. For example, general age-related decline may compound the challenges of predicting or understanding a disease trajectory, and the unknown can be incredibly stressful to pet owners. On the other hand, for middle-aged and younger pets experiencing symptoms associated with the diagnosis of a severe or terminal disease, the retained vibrancy of other bodily systems and physiologic processes can confound the ability to ascertain when suffering has become intolerable. No matter the cause or surrounding circumstances, understanding, identifying, discussing, and implementing treatment for symptoms is possible without the burden of making a diagnosis or potentially even without knowing a pet's full medical history.

Appetite and Weight Loss

Appetite

It is well established that dysrexia, defined as a disruption or distortion of normal appetite and food intake, is a common trigger for euthanasia in pets. Any major change of appetite or food intake can be problematic, whether increased or decreased. Hyporexia (reduced appetite/food intake) and anorexia (no appetite/food intake) are generally more problematic though, and so more likely to require intervention or trigger a decision for euthanasia in pets. Appetite and food intake are important beyond the basic needs for energy and nutrients, and so there are a number of both physical and emotional consequences (to the pet and pet owner) of reduced or lack of appetite. Some of the important consequences to a pet of reduced appetite include an inability to meet nutritional requirements, unwillingness to eat a specific or therapeutic diet necessary for disease management, unwillingness to take oral medications (which are generally given in food or treats), and unwillingness to eat a diet that an owner can afford. It is important to also point out that appetite, understood as psychological interest in and desire to ingest food, cannot be directly observed but rather is inferred based on actual food intake (Johnson and Freeman 2017). This can be confusing for pet owners because pets will often seem interested in eating (sniffing, eagerly approaching the food bowl) only to walk away without ingesting food.

As dogs and cats age, food preferences and volume of food intake often change. This can be due to many processes, some benign and some related to underlying disease. Examples of benign processes include reduced energy requirement due to a less active lifestyle or simply preferring a different type of food, but still eating normally otherwise. Pet owners will often describe pets as becoming more "picky or finicky," if a dog begins to prefer canned food over dry food or if a cat is ingesting only the liquid portion of canned food. Pet owners will also often attribute a change in their pet's food intake to difficulty in finding the right food. Pet owners will assert that their pet will not eat consistently because their pet gets bored easily, and their pet frequently changes preferences in terms of the form, texture, or flavor of food.

As appetite wanes further, pets often will refuse dog and cat food entirely. These pets may still be willing to eat treat foods or "human food," with the scope of these new food preferences generally becoming narrower and narrower over time. A pet's reduced appetite or refusal of food can be particularly emotionally unsettling for pet owners, because offering food is one of the ways we show our pets that we love and care about them – and we know that they have to eat in order to feel good and go on living. Refusal of food coupled with an inability to give needed oral medications can cause great anxiety and distress to pet owners because they know it will mean they are not able to manage their pet's health conditions. Not surprisingly, the same feelings of anxiety and distress have been described for human caregivers of human family members in hospice and palliative care (Namasivayam-MacDonald and Shune 2018; Tana et al. 2019).

When looking at appetite differences based on age, pets who are younger (i.e. juvenile or adult versus senior or geriatric) may continue to be more physiologically driven to eat as compared to older pets. There are likely many factors that contribute to appetite changes in older animals, some related to diagnosable disease processes and some not. In addition, younger pets are likely to have fewer comorbidities and visual cues of illness/malaise, meaning that they appear "healthy" in certain domains despite failing in others. For example, younger pets will most likely have a healthier appearance with supple skin, a shiny coat, clear eyes, decent oral health, and acute perceptual abilities (specifically vision and hearing). They often also have better reserves in terms of muscle mass, strength, and flexibility, and may show greater interest in eating and playing. This can complicate assessing the decline in quality of life and can therefore make end-of-life decision-making particularly burdensome.

The reality is that in many cases a change in appetite is a sign of a degenerative aging process such as reduced smell or taste or an underlying health condition or disease process. Unless the cause of a reduced appetite can be addressed effectively, the reduction in appetite will generally progress, with worsening effects on a pet's health over time. Reduced appetite is so common because it is a consequence of numerous diseases and degenerative processes. Because of this, symptomatic therapy for reduced appetite can be complicated. For example, if the cause of a reduced appetite and/or changes in food preferences is due to oral pain from dental disease, appetite could potentially be restored with appropriate dental therapies. On the other hand, chronic nausea caused by conditions such as pancreatitis, organ failure, or cancer may all cause reduced appetite, and symptomatic treatment with an anti-nausea drug may help in all of these cases even without therapy targeted at the specific disease process. In addition, the cause of waning appetite in older pets may have no readily identifiable cause or successful treatment intervention. Therefore, while it can be helpful to have a specific diagnosis, offering symptomatic treatment for causes of reduced appetite is nearly always appropriate.

Paradoxically, pets may also continue to eat normally, and in some cases voraciously (i.e. polyphagia), even when quality of life is poor, which can also cause confusion and consternation for pet owners trying to assess quality of life. In a pilot study by Marchitelli conducted from 2018–2019, 36 of 126 dogs (29%) were reported to have a normal appetite at the time of euthanasia. In contrast, only 2 of 50 cats (4%) were reported to have a normal appetite at the time of euthanasia. Species differences between dogs and cats may come into play here as cats generally appear to be more susceptible to disruptions in appetite when ill (Marchitelli et al. 2020). This difference between dogs and cats is likely multifactorial including difficulty in meeting preferences for form, texture, and flavor when offering human food to cats, the ease of consumption of human food by dogs, differences in the prevalence of disease processes between the species, and other physiologic differences between the two species.

Weight Loss

Weight loss, which can be a direct or indirect trigger for euthanasia, is included under the heading of appetite here, but can exist independently in the face of normal to increased appetite. Although we may assume that weight loss is always related to "decreased" food intake, a number of disease states cause weight loss through altered metabolism and undesirable changes in body composition such as fat redistribution in endocrine disorders and cachexia with neoplasia and organ failure. Medication side effects, such as those seen with long-term corticosteroid use, can have similar effects. Therefore, weight loss and obvious changes in physical appearance due to changes in body conformation can occur in the face of an increased, normal, or poor appetite. Sarcopenia, meaning a decrease in muscle mass that is age-related is a well-defined phenomenon, but the exact mechanism is not well understood, and it is very difficult to prevent (Pagano et al. 2015; Lorke et al. 2017). Common ways that weight loss may indirectly contribute to a decision for euthanasia include general weakness, decreased mobility, and changes in appearance. Pet owners are not necessarily equipped to understand the different causes and consequences of weight loss, but they do see and feel the ways that weight loss can negatively affect their pet's quality of life and their ability to effectively care for their pet. The visual and tactile observation by pet owners of weight loss/decreased muscle mass can influence euthanasia decision-making.

Elimination Disorders

Changes in a pet's elimination habits can be especially difficult to manage. While these issues do not always cause physical or emotional distress or frustration to pets or pet owners, in some cases they do. Pet owners will ascribe feelings such as a loss of dignity, embarrassment, or shame to pets who urinate and defecate in the house and/or on themselves. Poor hygiene, understood as the inability to keep clean after urinating/defecating, is listed on several quality to life assessment scales, illustrating its importance in end-of-life decision-making (Villalobos 2011; Ohio State University Veterinary Medical Center 2019). Broadly, end of life elimination disorders can be broken down into three groups:

- Conditions that cause abnormal urination or defecation, but where there is no house soiling.
- House soiling, where the location of urination or defecation becomes problematic and there may or may not be other abnormalities of urination and defection, but the cause is not incontinence.
- Incontinence (which often includes house soiling) where there is a loss of function, neurological or otherwise, causing lack of control over normal elimination.

In many cases, changes in elimination are multifactorial and may be either intermittent or inconsistent and so there can be great difficulty and frustration in identifying potential causes and solutions.

- **Inappropriate or Abnormal Urination/ Defecation without House Soiling**

Conditions causing changes in elimination but without house soiling or incontinence are generally easier for a pet owner to tolerate but are not necessarily easier on a pet. Common examples could include chronic diarrhea due to inflammatory bowel disease of gastrointestinal lymphosarcoma, polyuria/polydipsia due to hyperadrenocorticism or chronic kidney disease, and constipation due to megacolon. All of these conditions can cause significant discomfort to pets but may only present minor issues to pet owners. For pets, there can be significant pain or discomfort associated with diarrhea, excessive thirst/urination, and constipation, all of which may or may not be recognized by their owner. Typically, these conditions trigger a decision to euthanize when they impact other quality-of-life factors

such as decreased appetite, weight loss, or weakness.

- **Inappropriate or Abnormal Urination/ Defecation with House Soiling**

It can be particularly distressing to pet owners when dogs and cats who have previously been well trained to eliminate outdoors or in a litter box begin to urinate and/or defecate indoors or out of the litter box. There are both physical and emotional tolls on the pet and the pet owner as a result of house soiling. For the pet, these issues may necessitate the need for additional cleaning or bathing (which they may or may not like), can be emotionally taxing, and can be a sign of an underlying disease process causing pain or discomfort. Common medical conditions that lead to house soiling are gastrointestinal disorders, conditions causing polyuria/polydipsia, lower urinary tract disease, cancer, pain (arthritic or otherwise), and cognitive dysfunction syndrome. For pet owners, these visual cues of their pet's illness along with the need for constant cleaning and potential damage or destruction of property, can be exhausting.

In older dogs, particularly large breed dogs with hind-limb pain and/or weakness, inappropriate defecation is common and often precedes or occurs independently from inappropriate urination. Owners will describe these dogs as walking while defecating or defecating while lying down without awareness that they are doing so, sometimes just after having gone outside. These dogs generally have normal anal tone and are not truly incontinent, but are defecating inappropriately due to difficulty posturing, a lack of sensory feedback, decreased anal sphincter control, cognitive decline, or a combination of these. For similar reasons, older cats frequently defecate in close proximity to, but not quite inside, the litter box. Dogs and cats with poor ambulation and/or proprioceptive deficits may also fall into their feces, increasing the demands of nursing care. Solutions such as diapers, bellybands, and/or urinary pads, additional litter boxes, and so forth, can be helpful, but are not always implemented or well-accepted by pet owners. Inappropriate urination in cats, often caused by lower urinary tract disease, is almost always intolerable for pet owners in the long-term and once behavioral and medical solutions have been exhausted, almost always results in euthanasia or abandonment (Carney and Sadek 2014).

- **Incontinence**

Incontinence is more commonly diagnosed in dogs than in cats, and there are numerous causes of incontinence, some primary and some secondary. Unfortunately, depending on the cause, treatment and management strategies can be very different, and therefore symptomatic therapy is often not straightforward. Two important confounding factors in trying to address incontinence are first that pet owners frequently describe all conditions causing abnormal elimination as incontinence and second that pet owners often do not recognize incontinence as being present unless it is severe and constant. As an example, pet owners often assume that urinary incontinence in older female dogs is part and parcel of natural aging and in some cases may be unaware that this is a treatable condition. While it is true that urinary incontinence is diagnosed more frequently in older spayed female dogs due to the absence of estrogen, it should not be considered normal and left untreated. Like most chronic health conditions, there are consequences of uncontrolled or refractory urinary incontinence, the most notable of which is urinary tract infection. Ongoing hygiene issues associated with incontinence generally lead to both physical and emotional strain on the bond between pet and pet owner. No matter the underlying cause, when incontinence is difficult to manage or cannot be managed, it can contribute to euthanasia decision-making.

Impaired Mobility

Impaired mobility is one of the most frequently reported triggers for euthanasia, especially for dogs (Marchitelli et al. 2020). Degenerative joint disease such as osteoarthritis is likely the most common cause of gradual mobility impairment, but many other causes and contributing comorbidities are also possible. Mobility changes can be acute or gradual, but in the context of age-related decline, it is common that a slowly progressive condition culminates with the pet's inability to walk and even stand. The degree to which impaired mobility impinges on quality of life can depend on a number of interrelated factors. Some of these include the pet's previous mobility and activity level, the pet's acceptance of their mobility status, the owner's ability to assist their pet with mobility, environmental factors (such as stairs and flooring), and the presence of comorbidities. Because impaired mobility is directly associated with the sequelae of not being able to accomplish activities of daily living (ADLs) in a normal way, other problems typically result such as unreliable eating and drinking habits, elimination disorders such as house soiling, injuries due to falling, and also injuries to pet owners from trying to assist their pet with mobility. Pet owners will often go to great lengths to help pets with their mobility, but in many cases providing this help can be physically and emotionally exhausting and can also be quite costly.

- **Progressive Worsening versus Acute Loss of Mobility**

Chronic and progressive impaired mobility can be a trigger for euthanasia. Impaired mobility can present as a gradual decline with the eventual inability to stand unassisted. More subtle and chronic signs of mobility impairment reported by pet owners can be mistaken for changes in behavior or preference as opposed to being attributed to impaired mobility. For example, pet owners may assume a pet who was able to jump up on furniture or counters to get to favorite places is no longer doing so out of preference rather than due to lack of ability. Pet owners commonly report changes such as unsteadiness/incoordination, difficulty standing up or sitting down gracefully, slipping on flooring, tiring more easily, and losing interest in activities such as going for a walk.

Acute worsening or complete loss of mobility/ambulation (with or without prior significant mobility issues) is also a frequent trigger for euthanasia and in some cases can be harder for pets and pet owners than incremental mobility changes. The acute inability to stand and/or walk can result from a variety of causes such as intracranial disease, peripheral vestibular disease, hemodynamic/bleeding events, thromboembolic events, spinal cord compression (e.g. due to Intervertebral Disc Disease (IVDD), neoplasia, etc.), and generalized weakness due to metabolic disease. Acute loss of mobility is particularly likely to be a euthanasia trigger for owners of large and giant breed dogs, where helping a "down dog" accomplish critical daily activities may simply be beyond the physical capacities of most people. Owners may be able to assist small/medium breed dogs and cats with mobility more easily. However, it may be harder to identify mobility impairment in smaller pets due to the ease with which they can be assisted. The level of challenge posed by loss of mobility is dependent on both the pet owner's ability to provide help and the pet's ability to accept help.

● **Neurological Deficits and Weakness**

Mobility impairment due to neurological deficits may or may not carry with it the component of pain that is typically present with musculoskeletal conditions such as arthritis. Whether pain is present or not, neurological disease can compound the effects of musculoskeletal causes of mobility impairment, resulting in worsening mobility. Neurological deficits typically manifest as symptoms of weakness and/or ataxia (including the very common finding of hindlimb proprioceptive deficits in older dogs). The exact etiology of neurological deficits is often undiagnosed because a diagnosis could be risky and/or costly if it involves anesthesia and advanced imaging. Conditions such as spondylosis deformans, chronic intervertebral disc disease,

degenerative myelopathy, and undifferentiated degenerative neurological conditions are common in geriatric dogs and cats. Neurological causes of mobility impairment are particularly frustrating because they are generally very difficult to manage and are relentlessly progressive. This is also reported in human medicine in the geriatric population and may contribute to falls and instability (Goble et al. 2009; Jahn et al. 2019).

Impaired mobility can serve as a trigger for euthanasia as a result of the physical constraints described above. Impaired mobility also affects the human–animal bond as pets and pet owners may no longer be able to enjoy extended walks or exuberant play time together. Although less strenuous activities can be substituted, the relationship can nevertheless be impacted.

Sensory and Cognitive Decline

Symptoms of sensory and cognitive decline can have an insidious onset and waxing and waning progression. Most upsetting to both pets and pet owners, cognitive and sensory decline can drastically change the way a pet is able to interact with their living environment including their human family. A significant divide between human and animal often develops when restrictions have to be put into place for protection of the pet (gates, enclosures) and interactions are no longer the same or even pleasant due to behavior changes. This divide is frequently a trigger for euthanasia as the human–animal bond is damaged or broken.

● **Sensory Decline**

Sensory decline, defined as impairment, changes in, or complete loss of the special senses of touch, vision, hearing, smell, and taste, can negatively impact quality of life as well as the relationship of the pet with their owner. These senses help our pets interact with us and the world around them, and so it only follows that any change could be problematic. For example, a pet with a nasal or oral tumor is likely to have impairment or loss of smell and/

or taste, which could compound issues with loss of appetite, making it difficult for their owner to get them to eat. In many cases, sensory decline is gradual and includes a level of compensation particularly in older pets. In all cases sensory decline exacerbates and contributes to underlying quality-of-life issues. This is best mitigated when the pet's environment is consistent. For example, a pet who is blind often navigates very well in their own home, but if furniture is rearranged or if they are moved to a new environment, they may have great difficulty and are at risk of potential injury if encountering hazards such as stairs. Further changes in the relationship between pet owners and pets can occur as a result of sensory decline. For example, pet owners may no longer be greeted at the door when they return home because their pet cannot hear their car approaching. There are also some examples of how impairment of the senses could be potentially beneficial, such as hearing loss in a dog with noise phobias, but these examples are far less common than those where sensory decline is detrimental.

- **Cognitive Decline**

Cognitive decline can be difficult or impossible to differentiate from sensory decline, but the two often coexist and compound the effects of each other. Cognitive decline can present as undesirable behavioral changes such as loss of pleasure in activities, changes in attachment style, anxiety, insomnia or disrupted sleep/wake cycles, vocalization, restlessness, or pacing, and in some cases aggression (Dewey et al. 2019, Landsberg et al. 2010, 2011, 2012). Cognitive decline may lead to a diagnosis of Cognitive Dysfunction Syndrome, but at present this is a diagnosis based on behavioral changes versus identifiable structural changes in the brain. It is often difficult to ascertain the cause or driving factors of behavioral changes, especially when related to cognitive decline (Černá et al. 2020, Gunn-Moore 2011, Ozawa et al. 2019).

In many cases these changes in behavior will negatively alter the way that pets interact with their owners over time. Behavior changes can broadly be grouped into those resulting from a reduced stimulation level or a heightened stimulation level. Examples of a reduced stimulation level include disinterest in activities once enjoyed, hiding, no longer engaging with other pets or human family members, and loss of learning or difficulty with new learning. Examples of a heightened stimulation level include anxiety, increased attachment, disrupted sleep/wake cycles causing insomnia, vocalization, restlessness/pacing, and aggression. Initially, a pet owner might love the experience of a once relatively independent pet following them everywhere but over time this can become exhausting or disruptive. Insomnia, often including vocalization, pacing, or needing extra attention at night, can be particularly destructive to the human–animal bond because it will also result in alterations in the pet owner's sleep quality and duration. Loss of sleep and the exhaustion that results for pet owners cannot be underestimated in contributing to euthanasia decision-making. Anxiety can be the driving factor for many behavioral changes in animals and is often treatable, particularly if pain is well managed.

Dyspnea and Respiratory Compromise

Dyspnea, defined here as difficult, troubled, or labored breathing, is one of the most common symptoms encountered in palliative and hospice care and is often considered to be the most problematic symptom in terms of quality of life. All major quality-of-life monitoring scales include dyspnea as a parameter. In fact, both Bennett and Cook and Gates et al. reported dyspnea as a contributing factor for a decision to euthanize for approximately 10% of all dog and cat patients (Gates et al. 2017; Bennett and Cook 2019). Three major challenges in managing dyspnea are that there is no standard or single therapy that will always be effective, there are numerous reasons why dyspnea occurs, and there is often an acute onset and rapid progression with dyspnea, so it is often a true emergency. The condition of dyspnea in human palliative and hospice care patients has recently been reviewed in a two-part series by Kamal et al. to highlight the complexities of diagnosis and management to maintain comfort. (Kamal et al. 2011, 2012) Their findings are relevant to caring for veterinary palliative and hospice patients.

Perception of Pain

Although there is agreement that pain is an unpleasant and often even intolerable experience, it remains that pet owners and veterinary healthcare professionals alike struggle to diagnose, monitor, and treat pain in pets. There are three main reasons for this: (i) pets are often experts at masking expressions of pain, (ii) consensus on how to identify and evaluate pain in pets has been historically lacking and, (iii) treating pain often requires multiple treatment modalities and frequent adjustments over time. Several types of pain scale are now available that can help in identifying pain, but these are generally much more suited to veterinarians than to pet owners. Over the past couple of decades, despite a much stronger push from pet owners, attention from veterinary healthcare providers, and innovations from within the pet care industry at large, pain often still remains undiagnosed and poorly managed.

Pet owners are frequently concerned about pain for their pets, but in published studies, pain has rarely been reported as a symptom triggering euthanasia (Gates et al. 2017; Bennett and Cook 2019). On the other hand, despite adequate pain management on exam with a veterinarian, pet owners may insist that their pet is in pain and thus make the decision to euthanize. This puzzling phenomenon may have two explanations. First, significant discomfort and morbidity can be present without pain but may appear as pain to a pet owner. Second, any perception of pain or discomfort can cause emotional distress to the pet owner, and therefore increase the pet caregiver burden (Spitznagel et al. 2018).

Pet Factors: Severe Illness Diagnosis

In recent years, there has been increased attention in the literature to how veterinary decisions are made in the face of diagnosis of a serious or terminal illness. There are some interesting distinctions when comparing this data focused on illness diagnosis to the data focused on symptoms. First, there is the time of diagnosis, where there may or may not be severe symptoms that prompted the diagnosis. For example, incidental diagnosis of a splenic mass prior to rupture and hemoabdomen is a very different experience for a pet and pet owner than emergency diagnosis with all of the complications and urgency of hemoabdomen. That being said, in the face of a severe and/or terminal diagnosis, some pet owners will elect euthanasia immediately, or before there is progression of the illness. Otherwise, once treatment interventions are instituted, decisions will generally be more heavily weighted based on symptoms and quality of life than the actual diagnosis itself. In veterinary medicine, as in human medicine, there are certain health conditions that spark strong emotions at the time of diagnosis, and just the diagnosis can be hard to overcome in terms of considering treatment interventions. Here we will review recent literature pertaining to three such diagnosis: cancer, congestive heart failure (CHF), and diabetes mellitus (DM).

Cancer

Cancer is a common diagnosis in older pets, but at the same time there is tremendous variability in terms of body systems affected, treatment interventions available, and prognosis after diagnosis. Just speaking the word "cancer" though, can be distressing to pet owners, largely because cancer is serious and often fatal. Therefore, it is critical that veterinary healthcare providers are well versed in how pet owners respond to a cancer diagnosis for their pet, and how to help the pet and pet owner achieve the best treatment outcomes possible. In a 2010 study, Bowles et al. looked at pet owner perceptions of interventions with the chemotherapeutic drug carboplatin as well as other palliative treatments for dogs and cats (Bowles et al. 2010). Missing from this study was a group receiving palliative therapies without chemotherapy as well as a full description of how additional palliative care therapies were provided. Even still, there is the very interesting finding that while only 43% of pet owners reported that they would treat their pet with chemotherapy prior to a cancer diagnosis, after instituting treatment, 89% reported that they did not regret the decision for chemotherapy. This is in the face of 57% of the pets experiencing side effects related to chemotherapy.

An older but still very timely study by Slater et al. looked at pet owner satisfaction with cancer treatments for cats (Slater et al. 1996). In this study, cats were treated with a broader group of therapies, including surgery, chemotherapy, and radiation. Cat owners were interviewed soon after diagnosis as well as six months after diagnosis. At the initial interview, Slater et al. found that cat owners expressed satisfaction with their decision to euthanize at the time of diagnosis if at that time their cat was displaying symptoms of diminished capacity or inability to groom, eat, and play. For those cats where treatment intervention(s) were chosen, a number of factors contributed to cat owner satisfaction at the six-month interview. Most notable of these were if their cat was still living, if caregivers had fully understood the treatment's appointment schedule, components, and cost, if they understood the potential side effects/complications of treatment, and their perception of their cat's quality of life. Likewise, there was a finding of a strong negative effect on satisfaction if a cat owner felt that there was a communication breakdown surrounding their expectations for their pet's life span/prognosis or the cost of treatment. Probably most notable, though, was the finding that cat owners expressed the value and benefit of their veterinarian directly discussing the emotional strain of caregiving. While there was no group receiving only palliative care, and palliative care in relation to other treatment interventions was not the topic of this study, it is clear that these cat owners wanted and appreciated a more complete care program that also addressed their needs as caregivers.

Organ Failure: Congestive Heart Failure

A diagnosis of CHF is always serious, but there is significant variation in recommended treatments and prognosis based on the specifics of the diagnosis. Similar to a cancer diagnosis, the severity of presentation, presence of comorbidities, and potential emotional baggage associated with a diagnosis of CHF will all come into play. In fact, it is very common that a previous pet or human family member or friend will have suffered with CHF, especially since heart disease is so common.

In 1999, Mallery et al. published a prospective study of dogs diagnosed with CHF who were euthanized over an approximately two-year time period (Mallery et al. 1999). After euthanasia, the dog's owners were interviewed to discuss what symptoms their dog had experienced, perceptions about their dog's quality of life, and what were the most important factors influencing the decision for euthanasia. Mallery et al. found that more than 70% of dogs were reported to have experienced hyporexia or anorexia, weight loss, weakness, dyspnea, coughing, and exercise intolerance, but that for pet owners, anorexia and weakness were named as the most concerning of these symptoms. As triggers for a decision to euthanize, pet owners listed recurrence of decompensation of CHF, a generally poor perception of quality of life, and discussion with the veterinarian in which the animal was given a poor prognosis.

Another study looking at CHF in dogs from Oyama et al. in 2008 looked more specifically at the relative importance of quality of life versus quantity of life to pet owners of dogs who were still living but had been diagnosed with CHF (Oyama et al. 2008). In general, pet owners conveyed the importance of being able to detect if their pet was suffering, and whether their pet was able to continue normal interactions with the family. In terms of willingness to trade survival time for quality time, 86% of pet owners agreed that they would do so, and 52% stated that they would be willing to trade up to 6 months of survival time for quality time. Oyama et al. found a correlation between pet owners being more willing to trade survival time for quality of life if the dog was being treated for respiratory issues or fainting episodes on an outpatient basis versus in an emergency hospital. This study also found that dog owners of younger dogs experiencing fainting episodes were more willing to trade survival time for quality of life. While there may be a number of unreported factors at play in these decisions, this study does highlight the importance of quality of life to pet owners of dogs diagnosed with CHF, and also the importance of discussion of survival versus quality of life with pet owners.

Endocrine Disorders: Diabetes Mellitus

A third serious illness that is relatively common, but still complex and often dreaded by veterinary healthcare professionals and pet owners alike, is DM. DM carries similar baggage as cancer and CHF, in that pet owners understand that it is a serious illness that can be very difficult to manage or even terminal. In addition, they often have experiences with other pets or humans who have been diagnosed with this disease. Another unique feature of the treatment for DM is that most pets will require insulin therapy for good management, which has schedule demands, the need to give injections, and associated costs that are already more than many pet owners can handle. In 2017, Niessen et al. published the results of a worldwide study termed the "Big Pet Diabetes Survey," whose aim was to better understand the frequency and triggers for euthanasia of pets diagnosed with DM (Niessen et al. 2017). Perhaps not surprising to

veterinarians, pet owners elected euthanasia at the time of diagnosis of DM for about 10% of pets, and within a year of diagnosis another 10% of pets were euthanized. What may be more surprising though, is that when veterinarian respondents were asked whether they would treat their own cat or dog with insulin injections if diagnosed with DM, only 93.2% responded that they would "certainly" treat their cat, and only 95.3% said that they would "certainly" treat their dog. Again, these findings highlight the gravity of a diagnosis of DM.

While specific details of how pet owners make these decisions is not completely clear from this study as it was based on surveys completed by veterinarians, not pet owners, there are still a number of important findings. First, veterinarians listed presence of concurrent disease (45%), cost of treatment (44%), pet age (37%), issues with disease management (35%), overall quality of life and pet welfare (35%), and impact to a pet owner's lifestyle (32%) all as being important as triggers for euthanasia. A correlation was also found between pets treated in rural or mixed practices being more likely to be euthanized at time of diagnosis or within one year of diagnosis versus pets who were treated at referral or specialty hospitals. While it is not possible to fully understand all of the complexities of these pet owner decisions from these data alone, it is again clear that numerous pet and pet owner factors came into play in these decisions.

Pet Owner Factors: Psychosocial Factors of Caregiving

The effect of pet caregiver burden on pet owners has been brought to light in recent years by the work of Dr. Marybeth Spitznagel at Kent State University. Greater pet caregiver burden has been associated with euthanasia decision-making (Spitznagel et al. 2020). Specific clinical signs and problem behaviors have also been identified as contributing to pet caregiver burden (Spitznagel et al. 2018). The concept of frailty, which is well established in human geriatric medicine, has not been well defined or studied in veterinary medicine. A recent paper by Banzato et al. established a frailty index for dogs and correlated this measure with mortality (Banzato et al. 2019). Such measures along with evidence-based studies on the impact of age-related deterioration on quality of life will be of great value in contributing to our understanding euthanasia decision-making. In addition, psychosocial factors such as previous experiences with pet death/euthanasia, financial constraints, employment variables (working from home or outside the home), and pet owner social/psychological support all contribute to euthanasia decision- making. An exhaustive discussion of such factors is beyond the scope of this chapter, but each deserves to be mentioned here. (See Chapter 25 in this volume for an in-depth discussion of factores related to a pet caregiver's emotional burden.)

Conclusion

Our pets are living longer lives, partly due to advances in veterinary healthcare and partly due to pet owners seeking more comprehensive care for their pets and having increased awareness of the many options for treating and supporting dying animals. Still, the role of euthanasia within this complex realm of veterinary medicine – especially what factors drive caregivers and veterinary professionals to seek out and/or continue palliative and hospice care or to choose euthanasia – has remained underexplored. The paucity of scientific literature and relative inquiry on the subject has made it harder for veterinarians, other members of a veterinary hospice and palliative care team, and the general public to support pet owners who are faced with decision-making about the timing and appropriateness of euthanasia.

Now, with increasing attention to factors or triggers that may lead caregivers to choose euthanasia, the veterinary hospice provider is better equipped to offer guidance. Based on available research, three major groups of contributing factors can be identified: (i) pet-based factors related to symptoms or clinical signs that affect or appear to affect quality of life, (ii) pet-based factors related to serious disease diagnosis, and (iii) pet-owner factors, also called psychosocial factors. We know based on recent publications that each of these groups of factors will apply differently for each pet and their family, but that also, through applying this knowledge in the format of focused hospice and palliative care, we have the potential to further improve the care offered to both pet patients and their families.

References

Banzato, T., Franzo, G., Di Maggio, R. et al. (2019) A frailty index based on clinical data to quantify mortality risk in dogs. *Sci. Rep.*, 9 (1): 16749. https://doi.org/10.1038/s41598-019-52585-9. PMID: 31727920; PMCID: PMC6856105.

Bennett, C. and Cook, N. (2019) Palliative Care Services at Home: viewpoint from a multidoctor practice. *Vet. Clin. North Am. Small Anim. Pract.*, 49 (3): 529–551. https://doi.org/10.1016/j.cvsm.2019.01.018. Epub 2019 Mar 5. PMID: 30846375.

Bowles, D.B., Robson, M.C., Galloway, P.E. et al. (2010) Owner's perception of carboplatin in conjunction with other palliative treatments for cancer therapy. *J. Small Anim. Pract.*, 51 (2):104–12. https://doi.org/10.1111/j.1748-5827.2009.00891.x. Epub 2010 Jan 11.

Bussolari, C.J., Habarth, J., Katz, R. et al. (2018) The euthanasia decision-making process: A qualitative exploration of bereaved companion animal owners. *Bereavement Care*, 37 (3): 101–108. https://doi.org/10.1080/02682621.2018.1542571

Carney, H.C. and Sadek, T.P. (2014) How to save the house-soiling cat from abandonment or euthanasia. *J. Feline. Med. Surg.*, 16 (7): 545–545. DOI: https://doi.org/10.1177/1098612X14539085. PMID: 24966279.

Černá, P., Gardiner, H., Sordo, L. et al. (2020) Potential Causes of Increased Vocalisation in Elderly Cats with Cognitive Dysfunction Syndrome as Assessed by Their Owners. *Animals*, 10 (6): 1092. https://doi.org/10.3390/ani10061092.

Dewey, C.W., Davies, E.S., Xie H. et al. (2019) Canine Cognitive Dysfunction. *Vet. Clin. North Am. Small Anim. Pract.*, 49 (3): 477–499. DOI: https://doi.org/10.1016/j.cvsm.2019.01.013. Epub 2019 Mar 5. PMID: 30846383.

Gates, M., Hinds, H. and Dale, A. (2017) Preliminary description of aging cats and dogs presented to a New Zealand first-opinion veterinary clinic at end-of-life. *N Z Vet. J.*, 65 (6): 313–317. DOI: Epub 2017 Aug 9. PMID: 28747096.

Goble, D.J., Coxon, J.P., Wenderoth, N. et al. (2009) Proprioceptive sensibility in the elderly: degeneration, functional consequences and plastic-adaptive processes. *Neurosci. Biobehav. Rev.*, 33 (3): 271–8. https://doi.org/10.1016/j.neubiorev.2008.08.012. Epub 2008 Aug 26. PMID: 18793668.

Gunn-Moore, D.A. (2011) Cognitive dysfunction in cats: clinical assessment and management. *Top. Companion Anim. Med.*, 26 (1): 17–24. https://doi.org/10.1053/j.tcam.2011.01.005. PMID: 21435622.

Jahn, K., Freiberger, E., Eskofier, B.M. et al. (2019) Balance and mobility in geriatric patients: assessment and treatment of neurological aspects. *Z. Gerontol. Geriatr.*, 52 (4): 316–323. English. https://doi.org/10.1007/s00391-019-01561-z. Epub 2019 Jun 3. PMID: 31161336.

Johnson, L.N. and Freeman, L.M. (2017) Recognizing, describing, and managing reduced food intake in dogs and cats. *J. Am. Vet. Med. Assoc.*, 251 (11): 1260–1266. https://doi.org/10.2460/javma.251.11.1260. PMID: 29154711.

Kamal, A.H., Maguire, J.M., Wheeler, J.L. et al. (2011) Dyspnea review for the palliative care professional: assessment, burdens, and etiologies. *J. Palliat. Med.*, 14 (10): 1167–1172. https://doi.org/10.1089/jpm.2011.0109.

Kamal, A.H., Maguire, J.M., Wheeler, J.L. et al. (2012) Dyspnea review for the palliative care professional: treatment goals and therapeutic options. *J. Palliat. Med.*, 15 (1): 106–114. https://doi.org/10.1089/jpm.2011.0110.

Landsberg, G.M., Denenberg, S., and Araujo, J.A. (2010) Cognitive dysfunction in cats: a syndrome we used to dismiss as 'old age'. *J. Feline. Med. Surg.*, 12 (11): 837–848. DOI: https://doi.org/10.1016/j.jfms.2010.09.004. PMID: 20974401.

Landsberg, G.M., Deporter, T., and Araujo, J.A. (2011) Clinical signs and management of anxiety, sleeplessness, and cognitive dysfunction in the senior pet. *Vet. Clin. North Am. Small Anim. Pract.*, 41 (3): 565–590. https://doi.org/10.1016/j.cvsm.2011.03.017. PMID: 21601747.

Landsberg, G.M., Nichol, J., and Araujo, J.A. (2012) Cognitive dysfunction syndrome: a disease of canine and feline brain aging. *Vet. Clin. North Am. Small Anim. Pract.*, 42 (4): 749–768. https://doi.org/10.1016/j.cvsm.2012.04.003. Epub 2012 May 17. PMID: 22720812.

Lorke, M., Willen, M., Lucas, K. et al. (2017). Comparative kinematic gait analysis in young and old Beagle dogs. *J. Vet. Sci.*, *18* (4): 521–530. https://doi.org/10.4142/jvs.2017.18.4.521 PMID: 28385001; PMCID: PMC5746446.

Mallery, K.F., Freeman, L.M., Harpster, N.K. et al. (1999) Factors contributing to the decision for euthanasia of dogs with congestive heart failure. *J. Am. Vet. Med. Assoc.*, 214 (8): 1201–1204. PMID: 10212683.

Marchitelli, B., Shearer, T., and Cook, N. (2020) Factors contributing to the decision to euthanize: diagnosis, clinical signs, and triggers. *Vet. Clin. North Am. Small Anim. Pract.*, 50 (3): 573–589. https://doi.org/10.1016/j.cvsm.2019.12.007. Epub 2020 Mar 2. PMID: 32139081.

Namasivayam-MacDonald, A. M. and Shune, S. E. (2018) The burden of dysphagia on family caregivers of the elderly: A systematic review. *Geriatrics (Basel, Switzerland)*, *3* (2): 30. https://doi.org/10.3390/geriatrics3020030 PMID: 31011068; PMCID: PMC6319247.

Niessen, S.J.M., Hazuchova, K., Powney, S.L. et al. (2017) The big pet diabetes survey: Perceived frequency and triggers for euthanasia. *Vet. Sci.*, *4* (2): 27. https://doi.org/10.3390/vetsci4020027 PMID: 29056686; PMCID: PMC5606606.

Nogueira Borden, L.J., Adams, C.L., Bonnett, B.N. et al. (2010) Use of the measure of patient-centered communication to analyze euthanasia discussions in companion animal practice. *J. Am. Vet. Med. Assoc.*, *237* (11): 1275–1287. https://doi.org/10.2460/javma.237.11.1275 PMID: 21118013.

Ohio State University Veterinary Medical Center. (2019) How will I know? Assessing quality of life and making difficult decisions for your pet. The Ohio State University Veterinary Medical Center Honoring the Bond Program. https://vet.osu.edu/vmc/sites/default/files/files/companion/HTB/Difficult%20Decisions%20brocure-web%20layout%20%282019%29%20digital.pdf (Accessed: June 19, 2021).

Oyama, M.A., Rush, J.E., O'Sullivan, M.L. et al. (2008) Perceptions and priorities of owners of dogs with heart disease regarding quality versus quantity of life for their pets. *J. Am. Vet. Med. Assoc.*, 233 (1): 104–108. https://doi.org/10.2460/javma.233.1.104

Ozawa, M., Inoue, M., Uchida, K., et al. (2019) Physical signs of canine cognitive dysfunction. *J. Vet. Med. Sci.*, *81* (12): 1829–1834. https://doi.org/10.1292/jvms.19-0458. Epub 2019 Nov 1. PMID: 31685716; PMCID: PMC6943310.

Pagano, T.B., Wojcik, S., Costagliola, A. et al. (2015) Age related skeletal muscle atrophy and upregulation of autophagy in dogs. *Vet. J. (London, England : 1997)*, *206* (1): 54–60. https://doi.org/10.1016/j.tvjl.2015.07.005 Epub 2015 Jul 6. PMID: 26257260.

Pegram, C., Gray, C., Packer, R. et al. (2021) Proportion and risk factors for death by euthanasia in dogs in the UK. *Sci. Rep.*, *11* (1): 9145. https://doi.org/10.1038/s41598-021-88342-0 PMID: 33947877; PMCID: PMC8096845.

Persson, K., Selter, F., Neitzke, G. et al. (2020) Philosophy of a 'good death' in small animals and consequences for euthanasia in animal law and veterinary practice. *Animals (Basel)*, *10* (1): 124. https://doi.org/10.3390/ani10010124. PMID: 31940971; PMCID: PMC7022873.

Reynolds, C.A., Oyama, M.A., Rush, J.E. et al. (2010) Perceptions of quality of life and priorities of owners of cats with heart disease: Quality of life in cats. *J. Vet. Intern. Med.*, *24* (6): 1421–1426. https://doi.org/10.1111/j.1939-1676.2010.0583.x Epub 2010 Aug 24. PMID: 20738770.

Slater, M.R., Barton, C.L., Rogers, K.S. et al. (1996) Factors affecting treatment decisions and satisfaction of owners of cats with cancer. *J. Am. Vet. Med. Assoc.*, *208* (8): 1248–1252. PMID: 8635966.

Spitznagel, M.B., Jacobson, D.M., Cox, M.D. et al. (2018) Predicting caregiver burden in general veterinary clients: Contribution of companion animal clinical signs and problem behaviors. *Vet. J. (London, England : 1997)*, *236*: 23–30. https://doi.org/10.1016/j.tvjl.2018.04.007. Epub 2018 Apr 13. PMID: 29871745.

Spitznagel, M.B., Marchitelli, B., Gardner, M., et al. (2020) Euthanasia from the veterinary client's perspective: Psychosocial contributors to euthanasia decision making. *Vet. Clin. North Am. Small Anim. Prac.*, *50* (3): 591–605. https://doi.org/10.1016/j.cvsm.2019.12.008. Epub 2020 Feb 27. PMID: 32115280.

Spitznagel, M.B., Anderson, J.R., Marchitelli, B. et al. (2021) Owner quality of life, caregiver burden and anticipatory grief: How they differ, why it matters. *Vet. Rec.*, *188* (9): e74. https://doi.org/10.1002/vetr.74. Epub 2021 Feb 2. PMID: 33960467.

Tana, C., Lauretani, F., Ticinesi, A. et al. (2019) Impact of nutritional status on caregiver burden of elderly outpatients. A cross-sectional study. *Nutrients*, *11* (2): 281. https://doi.org/10.3390/nu11020281.

Testoni, I., De Cataldo, L., Ronconi, L. et al. (2017) Pet loss and representations of death, attachment, depression, and euthanasia. *Anthrozoös*, *30* (1): 135–148. https://doi.org/10.1080/08927936.2017.1270599.

Villalobos A. E. (2011) Quality-of-life assessment techniques for veterinarians. *Vet. Clin. North Am. Small Anim. Prac.*, *41* (3): 519–529. https://doi.org/10.1016/j.cvsm.2011.03.013. PMID: 21601744.

29

Supporting Other Needs

Shea Cox, DVM, CHPV, CVPP and Mary Ellen Goldberg, CVT, LVT, SRA-retired, CCRVN, CVPP VTS-lab animal-retired, VTS-Physical Rehabilitation-retired, VTS-anesthesia/ analgesia-Honorary

Family caregiving toward the end-of-life entails considerable emotional, social, financial, and physical costs for caregivers, all of which need to be addressed in the hospice relationship.

Caring for the Caregiver: Addressing Emotional and Physical Needs

Caregivers tend to be overlooked and are often referred to as the "hidden patients" (Kristjanson and Aoun 2004). Caregivers are defined in animal hospice and palliative care as the animal's owner, and/or any others involved directly in the animal's daily care and decision-making surrounding the animal and its health care. The term "caregiving family" may be used to designate multiple people assuming responsibilities of ownership and care.

Evidence suggests that a solid support system can improve caregiver psychological outcomes (Aoun et al. 2015), and caregivers who are able to embrace, learn, and develop effective coping skills are far better equipped to care for themselves as well as the pet who is in hospice. Coping refers to the mental and behavioral changes that people exert to manage stressful burdens or circumstances Caregivers' emotional and spiritual needs have been addressed in Chapters 24 and 25. This chapter will address caregivers' burdens in the realms of time management, financial planning, and physical labor as related to caring for their seriously ill pet.

Coping strategies that can be recommended to any caregiver are (Baran et al. 2009):

- take it slow;
- seek education and training;
- acknowledge feelings;
- vent when necessary and appropriate;
- seek help from others who are supportive;
- be confident in your judgment and abilities.

Ultimately, caregivers need to keep in mind their personal quality of life. Important questions they need to address, to help them assess their quality of life and identify where they may need help, include (Argus Institute in Conditions and Illness, Senior Pets 2020):

- How much of my time will go toward taking care of my pet?
- How much time do I have to devote to caregiving?

Hospice and Palliative Care for Companion Animals: Principles and Practice, Second Edition.
Edited by Amir Shanan, Jessica Pierce, and Tamara Shearer.
© 2023 John Wiley & Sons, Inc. Published 2023 by John Wiley & Sons, Inc.
Companion website: www.wiley.com/go/shanan/palliative

- What cost will I incur in taking care of my pet? What other financial responsibilities do I have?
- What other responsibilities do I have in my life (job, parenting)? Who else do I need to consider (partner, children, and other pets)?
- Who can help me?
- What other stresses and obligations do I have in my life right now?

Maintaining Self-Care

Engaging in self-care activities will improve the welfare of all caregivers involved and, in turn, the pet receiving hospice care. Caregivers often become so focused on caring for the pet that they can begin to neglect their own emotional, physical, and spiritual health. Caregiver demands on the body, mind, and emotions can easily begin to overwhelm, leading to fatigue and ultimately to burnout. Therefore, it is an important objective for the hospice team to help caregivers make a personal commitment to practicing self-care, and to attend to their own healthcare needs. Health is much more than the absence of disease. It is a positive quality, emphasizing physical, social, intellectual, emotional, and spiritual well-being. The key aspects of basic self-care that can be addressed include nutrition, rest, exercise, and relaxation.

Maintain Personal Nutrition and Sleep

Optimum nutrition, providing all nutrients in both kind and amount, is the cornerstone of good health and the cutting edge of prevention. The foods caregivers eat, and the nutrients these foods provide, are important continuing environmental factors influencing caregivers' functional abilities and health.

Caregivers find themselves fatigued at different times during their caregiving experience due to sleep disturbances and extended responsibilities. Pet caregivers who are tired can have trouble paying attention and staying focused.

Other consequences of fatigue include reduced motivation, irritability, memory lapses, impaired communication, diminished reaction time, slowed information processing and judgment, and loss of empathy. Making a conscious effort to minimize sleep loss and maintain good sleep habits such as following a daily routine and making the sleep area comfortable can help caregivers stay fresh and avoid fatigue.

Engage in Exercise

Regular physical activity plays an important role in improving and maintaining one's health. Although many people are aware of the benefits of regular activity, many do not meet the recommended guidelines. Long-term physical activity adherence may be strengthened by promotion of the individual's basic psychological need satisfaction. Adherence is most likely to occur when the value of participation becomes internalized over time as a component of the physically active self. (For more on exercise and self-care see Costello et al. 2011.)

Make Time for Relaxation

"Burnout" has been defined as a persistent, negative, task-related state of mind in "normal" individuals. Burnout is primarily characterized by exhaustion and accompanied by distress, a sense of reduced effectiveness, decreased motivation, and the development of dysfunctional attitudes and behaviors. This psychological condition develops gradually but may remain unnoticed for a long time by the individual involved.

Additionally, burnout is a work outcome, defined by prolonged occupational stress in an individual that presents as emotional exhaustion, depersonalization, and diminished personal accomplishment (Maslach and Jackson 1981). Nurses and those providing daily care experience high levels of burnout syndrome (Buckley et al. 2020).

Relaxation interventions that aim to induce a state of mental or bodily calmness, or both, to counteract the agitation caused by stress, are extremely helpful. This can be achieved by being a passive recipient of a massage or by actively performing various exercises. Thus, focus is directed toward a specific relaxing activity and away from the unpleasant thoughts and feelings associated with stress.

Sometimes, in order to continue, *one must step back and refuel*. Caregivers need to take breaks, daily, and weekly. Activities that may be restorative include massage, being out in nature, listening to music or comedy, watching movies, dining out, being with family, spending time with little children, seeing beauty at an art museum or shopping at a mall, taking up a new hobby or activity, and being creative. Discovering what energizes the individual caregiver and maintaining balance is important. Acknowledging how the circle of life continues and how we are all a part of it can provide needed relief from spiritual stress. Caregivers who need more time away can consider enlisting the services of a pet sitter or respite care provider who is qualified to care for their pet in their absence. (For more on the role of relaxation in self-care see Ruotsalainen et al. 2015.)

Time Considerations of Hospice Care

Each pet owner has his or her own personal lifestyle, tolerance, and time considerations. Caring for an aging, chronic or terminally ill pet takes dedicated time, which can in turn affect physical health and the ability to function at one's best. Discovering, respecting, and honoring the amount of time one can healthily give to another helps maintain emotional and physical health balance, allowing caregivers to do more for their pets.

Managing Time Commitments of Care

Steps to managing time are:

1) *Make a list of the tasks that need to be accomplished.* A list of tasks, from the mundane to the critical, helps to get a handle on what needs to get done.

2) *Balance the effort.* Work daily on small portions of tasks that will be due by the end of the week, starting with the most important tasks first.
3) *Focus on the most productive time of day.* Some people work better in the morning, and some are more focused in the evening.
4) *Manage time in increments.* Statistics have proven that 45 minutes of work followed by a 10-minute rest is best for the average individual.
5) *Take breaks.* Those help to clear the mind, refresh, and refocus.
6) *Keep track of progress.* Cross things off the list as they are completed.
7) *Reassess the list.* Rewrite and prioritize the list on a regular basis.
8) *Leave time for fun.* While there are times when it is necessary to power through a long list of tasks, it's important to take time to let loose.
9) *Sleep for 7–8 hours every night.* Getting the proper amount of sleep helps to stay alert and energetic, able to think clearly, and function at a high level.

Tips for Balancing Caregiving with Ongoing Responsibilities

When in a caregiving role, an individual might feel that it's impossible to give her full commitment to both work and personal responsibilities. But there are steps to take to make life more manageable:

- Get organized using scheduling programs and tools to manage time more effectively.
- Talk honestly with your boss about your situation and be assertive about what you can and can't handle.
- Reach out to colleagues for support and try to help them with their own responsibilities when you have extra time.

Understanding the Physical Labor of Care

Hospice care requires an active and physical commitment from all caregivers, especially from the pet parent who becomes the primary caregiver, ensuring that their pet's life continues, and ends, as comfortably as it can. If an owner decides that hospice care is the right course, they will become their pet's primary nurse, which can often take a considerable physical toll, especially with larger pets who can't walk or eliminate independently. Proper education with regards to the physical aspects of care is an important consideration, and the need to care for one's own body while caring for another cannot be emphasized enough.

Utilizing Proper Body Mechanics During Delivery of Care

Ergonomics is the study of body mechanics. Caregiver education into body mechanics is an effective intervention for increasing knowledge and promoting correct lifting techniques (Holmes et al. 2008). Some of the most common injuries for which caregivers are at risk are severe musculoskeletal strains. Many injuries can be avoided by the conscious use of proper body mechanics when performing physical labor. Body mechanics is the utilization of correct muscles to complete a task safely and efficiently, without undue strain on any muscle or joint (Lockette 2013).

Principles of good body mechanics (drawn from Hughey 2007)
1) Maintain a stable center of gravity. The line of gravity should pass vertically through the base of support.
   - Keep the center of gravity low.
   - Keep the back straight.
   - Bend at the knees and hips.
   - Keep the object being lifted close to the body.
2) Maintain a wide base of support. This provides maximum stability while lifting.
   - Keep the feet apart.
   - Place one foot slightly ahead of the other.
   - Flex the knees to absorb jolts.
   - Turn with your feet.
3) Maintain proper body alignment.
   - Tuck in the buttocks.
   - Pull the abdomen in and up.

- Keep the back flat.
- Keep the head up.
- Keep the chin in.
- Keep the weight forward and supported on the outside of your feet.

Techniques of body mechanics (Hughey 2007)
1) Lifting:
   - Use the stronger leg muscles for lifting.
   - Bend at the knees and hips; keep the back straight.
   - Lift straight upward, in one smooth motion.
2) Reaching:
   - Stand directly in front of and close to the object.
   - Avoid twisting or stretching.
   - Use a stool or ladder for high objects.
   - Maintain a good balance and a firm base of support.
   - Before moving the object, be sure that it is not too large or too heavy.
3) Pivoting:
   - Place one foot slightly ahead of the other.
   - Turn both feet at the same time, pivoting on the heel of one foot and the toe of the other.
   - Maintain a good center of gravity while holding or carrying the object.
4) Avoid stooping:
   - Squat, bending at the hips and knees.
   - Avoid bending at the waist.
   - Use your leg muscles to return to an upright position.

General considerations for performing physical tasks (Hughey 2007)
- It is easier to pull, push, or roll an object than it is to lift it.
- Movements should be smooth and coordinated rather than jerky.
- Less energy or force is required to keep an object moving than it is to start and stop it.
- Use the arm and leg muscles as much as possible, the back muscles as little as possible.
- Keep the work as close as possible to your body. It puts less of a strain on your back, legs, and arms.

- Rock backward or forward on your feet to use your body weight as a pushing or pulling force.
- Keep the work at a comfortable height to avoid excessive bending at the waist.
- Keep your body in good physical condition to reduce the chance of injury.

Reasons for the use of proper body mechanics (Hughey 2007). Use proper body mechanics in order to avoid the following:

- Excessive fatigue.
- Muscle strains or tears.
- Skeletal injuries.
- Injury to the patient.
- Injury to others assisting in getting the task completed.

Environmental Considerations of Hospice Care

Caregivers should rely on veterinary nurses and other hospice team members to advise them on equipment and methods for maintaining cleanliness around the animal, to ensure that the animal is on comfortable bedding appropriate for his or her condition, and to institute measures to protect the animal from self-injury. The veterinary nurse can help caregivers select and install assistive devices in the home environment such as ramps, gates, and enhanced floor traction.

Assessment of the Physical Space

Making the pet's living space safe and comfortable takes a significant burden off of the caregivers' long list of concerns. It is only through direct observation, careful open-ended questioning, and active listening that the caregiver and hospice team members can work together to make the pet's living space as comfortable as possible.

Most often the veterinary technician nurse, with or without the veterinarian, can make a house call to advise the caregiver about modifications that can be made to the home for the pet's comfort.

Household and Environmental Modifications

Comfort-driven home modifications are limited only by what the caregiver and veterinary hospice team can envision. The following list is a good foundation from which to begin:

- Cover slick floors (hardwood, tile, sheet vinyl) with nonskid surfaces (rubber backed/area rugs, permanent carpet, thin foam flooring like that found in gyms and weight rooms).
- Provide nonskid additions to the stairs, especially at the top and bottom of the stairs.
- Use secure baby gates to block entrance to stairways (top and bottom) for pets who should negotiate stairs only with supervision.
- Provide an appropriate sleeping surface based on the pet's individual needs. Some dogs prefer orthopedic foam beds. Some dogs prefer a plusher surface. Move outdoor dogs indoors. Some cats like beds built like tents to facilitate hiding.
- Provide a ramp for entry into and exit from the family vehicle for dogs.
- Consider a ramp for short clusters of steps such as those leading into or out of the home.
- Consider step stairs to allow pets to climb onto a couch or into a bed more easily.
- Raise food and water dishes to between shoulder and elbow height for animals that are still ambulatory (including cats).
- Provide absorbent pads and fleece under pets with continence issues to wick moisture away from the body.
- Provide absorbent pet diapers for ongoing incontinence.
- Provide and facilitate using carts (also called wheelchairs) to maximize mobility for those pets still capable of using them. Look for a cart that is lightweight, custom-fit, and easy-on/easy-off.

Financial Considerations of Hospice Care

Veterinary hospice care can be an expensive undertaking. While costs may decrease with the amount of duties the caretaker can accept, there are still built-in costs of care that will remain a part of the hospice plan.

The veterinarian and the rest of the hospice care team should develop a method for ensuring transparency and accord between the client's needs and the anticipated cost of services. Eric Clough created a list of questions a client might consider when requesting hospice care to gain a realistic view of what to expect and whether the veterinary care team can match the client's needs to the available finances (Clough 1998).

- Do I accept that this is a dying animal, and no more efforts will be made to cure his or her illness?
- Have I discussed with my veterinarian my pet's medications and their effects?
- Do I have enough time in my schedule to spend the necessary hours looking after my pet?
- Does my family realize what home hospice care will entail?
- Can I cover the projected costs of hospice care?
- Are there sufficient veterinary staff personnel to support me and my family throughout my pet's course of disease?
- Will someone be available 24 hours a day if my pet's condition changes?
- What is the expected outcome, how might death occur, and what arrangements will I make following my pet's death?

Cost of Medications

Costs for pet medications have increased with the level of sophistication and general increases in costs of health care, and this expense needs to be factored into the hospice plan (Carrns 2012). Prescriptions can be dispensed by the veterinarian, written and filled at a local pharmacy, or ordered online.

Cost of Diagnostics

Oftentimes, blood and urine tests are recommended during the course of hospice care to evaluate response to treatment and ensure that the treatments being provided are not causing harm (such as with the use of nonsteroidal anti-inflammatory drugs or chemotherapy agents). Although more extensive tests are often declined in lieu of comfort care, they are sometimes indicated by the veterinarian or requested by the client. These can include radiographs, advanced imaging, or more specialized blood tests that carry a higher cost. Be sure to discuss any diagnostics that may be anticipated during the course of treatment so that costs can be properly accounted and prepared for.

Cost of Other Healthcare Providers

Discussions should be held with the pet owner regarding the cost of additional professional services outside of the hospice and palliative care core team. Examples include veterinary acupuncturists, pain management specialists, pet massage therapists, rehabilitation practitioners, alternative medicine specialists, and pet nutritionists.

Cost of Environmental Modifications

The cost of environmental modifications needs to be considered when evaluating the total cost of hospice care. These modifications can include, but are certainly not limited to, the cost of pet beds, ramps, gates, mobility devices, wheelchairs, and hygiene care needs. Prices can vary widely between suppliers, and investing the time researching prices may result in considerable savings.

Cost of End-of-Life Care

Hospice care ends when a pet dies naturally or when a family has elected humane euthanasia. With end of life comes additional expenses, and these anticipated costs should be discussed with families *prior* to the death of the pet. The total cost of end-of-life care will depend on many factors, including:

- the type of euthanasia service used, such as bringing a pet to a clinic setting versus having a veterinarian come to the home for euthanasia;
- the geographical location of the pet and family, such as a rural versus urban setting;
- the timing of the euthanasia, such as on weekends, evening, or holidays;
- the aftercare option chosen by the family, such as burial and private, semiprivate, or communal cremation;
- the choice of urn or memorialization options by the family.

Helping to Defer Costs of Hospice Care

Pet Health Insurance

Pet health insurance has grown more popular since it was first introduced in the United States three decades ago. However, its use is still not widespread. About 1.4 million pets in the United States and Canada were covered by a plan at the end of 2014, according to the North American Pet Health Insurance Association, a trade group. That's less than 1% of about 174 million pet cats and dogs (Walker 2016). Many pet insurance companies cover, in some part, the cost of hospice care, and it is recommended that pet owners contact their provider to obtain full details of what is covered under their policy, and what documentation is required to fulfill the reimbursement of insurance claims.

Equipment Rental, Recycling, and Reduced Cost Programs

Some businesses provide equipment rentals, recycling, and reduced cost programs, such as Eddie's Wheels, a company that makes wheelchairs for pets. Owners of deceased pets can also resell their pet's wheelchair through Eddie's Wheels' website, allowing a new owner to purchase at a substantially lower cost (eddieswheels.com). Donations of equipment are often made to healthcare professionals or businesses that supply mobility aids, and in good faith, these items are donated back to families with limited financial resources. Working with pet-related businesses in your area can oftentimes lead to the creation of resources that were unknown or previously unavailable.

Creating a Memorial Fund

A potential way for hospice care providers to help defer the cost of care to families with financial limitations is to consider beginning a memorial fund. Families can donate in honor and in memory of their deceased pet and, in turn, those donations can be used to offset the cost of hospice or end of life care for another family in need. Memorial funds can be established as a 501c3 nonprofit or simply as a "good faith" program. One of the authors (Cox) has created a memorial fund, and between the donation of her time and the financial donations from families, she is able to provide complete hospice and/or end-of-life care for at least one family each month. Providing a way for families to turn loss into helping another can be very healing for them.

Creating a Donation Bank

Another way to help reduce the cost of care for owners is for healthcare providers to begin a donation bank. Oftentimes, when a pet passes, families are left with various medications, supplies, and food that they do not wish to keep. Creating a donation bank allows these needed items to go to another family and eliminates unnecessary environmental waste. The same author has been able to defray thousands of dollars in medication and supply costs to other families, while providing another means for families of deceased pets to feel that their pet is able to "make a difference" for another.

References

Aoun, S.M., Grande, G., Howting, D. *et al.* (2015) The impact of the carer support needs assessment tool (CSNAT) in community palliative care using a stepped wedge cluster trial. *PLoS One*, 7: 1–16.

Argus Institute in Conditions and Illness, Senior Pets (2020). *Considering your pets quality of life in the midst of disease.* James L. Voos Veterinary Teaching Hospital, Colorado State University. Available at: http://csu-cvmbs.colostate.edu/vth/diagnostic-and-support/argus/Pages/quality-of-life-self.aspx (Accessed: April 2015).

Baran, B.E., Allen, J.A., Rogelberg, S.G. *et al.* (2009) Euthanasia-related strain and coping strategies in animal shelter employees. *J. Am. Vet. Med. Assoc.*, 235: 83–88.

Buckley, L., Berta, W., Cleverley, K. et al. (2020) What is known about paediatric nurse burnout: a scoping review, *Hum. Resour. Health*, 18(1):9, 1–23 https://doi.org/10.1186/s12960-020-0451-8.

Carrns, A. (2012) My lesson in the high cost of drugs for pets. *The New York Times*, October 10. Available at: http://bucks.blogs.nytimes.com/2012/10/10/my-lesson-in-the-high-cost-of-drugs-for-pets/?_r=0 (Accessed: Sept. 2016).

Clough, E.A. (1998) Gentle departure: hospice care for pets. *PetLife*, Spring Special Issue.

Costello, E., Kafchinski, M., Vrazel, J. et al. (2011) Motivators, barriers, and beliefs regarding physical activity in an older adult population. *J. Geriatr. Phys. Ther.*, 34: 138–147.

Holmes, W., Lamb, P.Y., Elkind, P., et al. (2008) The effect of body mechanics education on the work performance of fruit warehouse workers. *Work*, 31: 461–471.

Hughey, M. (2007) Nursing Fundamentals I, Subcourse MD0905 Edition 100 Body Mechanics. [Based on the text of a correspondence course produced by the Academy of Health Sciences, United States Army Medical Department, San Antonio, TX.] Available at: http://brooksidepress.org/nursing_fundamentals_1/?page_id=62 (Accessed: October 2022).

Kristjanson, L. and Aoun, S. (2004) Palliative care for families: remembering the hidden patients. *Can. J. Psychiatry*, 49: 359–365.

Lockette, K. (2013) Good body mechanics for caregivers. [Adapted from: *The Pocket Physical Therapist: A Caregiver's Complete Guide for Mobility and Independence in the Home.* Langdon Street Press, 2010.] Available at: www.cdss.ca.gov/agedblinddisabled/res/VPTC2/4%20Care%20for%20the%20Caregiver/Good_Body_Mechanics_for_Caregivers.pdf (Accessed: Sept. 2016).

Maslach, C., and Jackson, S.E. (1981) The measurement of experienced burnout. *J. Organ. Behav.*, 2(2): 99–113.

Ruotsalainen, J.H., Verbeek, J.H., Marine, A. et al. (2015) Preventing occupational stress in healthcare workers. *Cochrane Database Syst. Rev.*, (4): CD002892. https://doi.org/10.1002/14651858.CD002892.pub5

Walker M. (2016) Is pet insurance worth the cost? *Consum. Rep.*, 81(5): 12–14.

Further Reading

Ackerman, N. (2015) Setting up veterinary nurse clinics. *In Pract.*, 37: 199–202.

Akerstedt, T. and Wright, K.P. Jr. (2009) Sleep loss and fatigue in shift work and shift work disorder. *Sleep Med. Clin.*, 4: 257–271.

American Veterinary Medical Association (AVMA) (2015) *Guidelines for Veterinary Hospice Care.* Available at: http://www.avma.org/KB/Policies/Pages/Guidelines-for-Veterinary-Hospice-Care.aspx (Accessed: April 2015).

Aoun, S.M., Deas, K., Toye, C., et al. (2015) Supporting family caregivers to identify their own needs in end-of-life care: qualitative findings from a stepped wedge cluster trial. *Palliat. Med.*, 29: 508–517.

Dobbs, K. (2013) Hospice: the last hope. should pet insurance companies cover hospice care for their clients? *Veterinary Practice News*. Available at: http://www. veterinarypracticenews.com/Vet-Editorial-Blog/Staff-Safari/Hospice-The-Last-Hope (Accessed: Sept. 2016).

Douglass, J.A. (2014) Overextended: fighting the fatigue of long shifts. *Nursing*, 44: 67–68.

Downing, R. (2011) Pain management for veterinary palliative care and hospice patients. *Vet. Clin. North Am. Small Anim. Pract.*, 41: 531–550.

Geiger-Brown, J. and Trinkoff, A.M. (2010) Is it time to pull the plug on 12-hour shifts? Part 3. Harm reduction strategies if keeping 12-hour shifts. *J. Nurs. Adm.*, 40: 357–359.

Keller, S.M. (2009) Effects of extended work shifts and shift work on patient safety, productivity, and employee health. *AAOHN J.*, 57: 497–502.

Krehl, W.A. (1983) The role of nutrition in maintaining health and preventing disease. *Health Values*, 7: 9–13.

Rogers, A. (2008) The effects of fatigue and sleepiness on nurse performance and patient safety. In: Patient Safety and Quality: An Evidence-Based Handbook for Nurses. (ed. R.G. Hughes). Rockville, MD: Agency for Healthcare Research and Quality, pp. 509–533.

Shanan, A. (2015) Pain management for end of life care. In Pain Management for Veterinary Technicians and Nurses, 1 (ed. M.E. Goldberg and N. Shaffran). Ames, IA: Wiley, pp. 331–339.

Shearer, T.S. (2011) Pet hospice and palliative care protocols. *Vet. Clin. North Am. Small Anim. Pract.*, 41: 507–518.

Springer, J.B., Lamborn, S.D., and Pollard, D.M. (2013) Maintaining physical activity over time: the importance of basic psychological need satisfaction in developing the physically active self. *Am. J. Health Promot.*, 27: 284–293.

Villalobos, A.E. (2011) Assessment and treatment of nonpain conditions in life limiting disease. *Vet. Clin. North Am. Small Anim. Pract.*, 41: 551–563.

Wolf, C.A., Lloyd, J.W, and Black, J.R. (2008) An examination of US consumer pet-related and veterinary service expenditures, 1980–2005. *J. Am. Vet. Med. Assoc.*, 233: 404–413.

30

Aftercare
Coleen A. Ellis, CT, CPLP

One of the most important aspects of the hospice experience is that pet parents are allowed and encouraged to find meaning in the dying process, before and after the actual death occurs. The veterinarian, or a pet loss professional, can be an integral part of the family's journey by giving them permission to honor their animal's life, to acknowledge their feelings of grief, to help them create rituals to celebrate the passing or pending passing of their companion, and to find meaningful ways to permanently memorialize a life shared. Pet parents want to know that their beloved pet was treated with the same dignity and respect shown for humans. From the care of the emotions to the actual physical care of the body, pet parents want to know they did everything for their pet and had the support and care of those around them throughout the process.

Hospice Options and Accompanying Rituals

For those families fully vested in their pet's care during life, many are likely to desire a meaningful and mindful death. However, they might not know how to verbalize their wants or needs and may need guidance in creating a fulfilling end-of-life (EOL) passage with their pet. It is imperative for a hospice provider to be fully tuned into these pet owners, whose behavior will often signify that they will want to do all they could in death as well as in life. Be proactive in conversations with the family and don't assume that because they didn't bring it up that they wouldn't want to do something more. Again, they may not know how to ask for more and may not even know what more is. The role of the pet care professional should be to give educational information and let the pet owner decide what they want to pursue.

In a recent study published in *Topics in Companion Animal Medicine*, 2043 pet owners who have made EOL decisions were surveyed on various aspects of the final experience (Cooney et al. 2021). The research found that over half of the participants wanted information about the dying process, disposition of their animal's body, and memorialization options (Table 30.1).

Whether it's pet loss or even human loss, the subject of death and loss is difficult. However, this is also the area where many misunderstandings and regret can be eliminated through clear communication about options When broached gently and in an inquisitive way, the conversation about what a "perfect ending" might look like for a family can help to uncover the perfect details of what the pet and family loved to do together, or what the family most

Hospice and Palliative Care for Companion Animals: Principles and Practice, Second Edition.
Edited by Amir Shanan, Jessica Pierce, and Tamara Shearer.
© 2023 John Wiley & Sons, Inc. Published 2023 by John Wiley & Sons, Inc.
Companion website: www.wiley.com/go/shanan/palliative

Table 30.1 Owner preference for amount of information given about specific death/dying and aftercare aspects. *Kathleen A. Cooney et al. 2021 / With permission of Elsevier.*

	I Want All the Details	I Want General Information but I Don't Need All the Small Details	I Would Prefer to Just be Told What I Need to Know
The death/dying process (euthanasia, hospice)	763 (37.8%)	943 (46.7%)	314 (15.5%)
What happens to my pet after death while still at the veterinary hospital (before being transported to cemetery or crematorium)	618 (30.6%)	770 (38.1%)	632 (31.3%)
What happens to my pet at the cemetery or crematorium	572 (28.3%)	696 (34.5%)	752 (37.2%)
Options to memorialize my pet	912 (45.1%)	687 (34.0%)	421 (20.8%)

wants to remember about their pet. Imagine, for example, the cat who loved his male owner's sock drawer, and a final memory of the euthanasia being performed there.

The discussion can involve gently asking open-ended questions of a family, such as:

- What happened the last time you euthanized a pet?
- What do you want to be different this time?
- What did you find peaceful and memorable the last time?
- How will we make the end perfect for this perfect kitty?

This questioning process will help the family and the veterinary professional create those final memories and take that EOL time from an event to loving, memorable experiences.

Grief specialist Dr. Alan Wolfelt wrote, "When in grief, we have a huge need to be understood but very little capacity to understand." Families in the final days of their pet's life are trying to process the loss of their pet and may not be thinking about memory-creating experiences. Hospice professionals, through guidance and gentle questioning, can help the family see beyond the immediate loss to create beautiful and unforgettable rituals that will remain meaningful long after the passing of their animal. This final time together is one where the statement begs to be said "Let's make this final walk together one where

when it's reflected upon six months from now, there will be no regrets, no comments of 'I wish I would've' or 'I didn't know I could do that.'" This is a time of no do-overs.

For many pet owners, rituals while their pet was living happen daily. These include routine rituals of every day, including sleeping, outside time, eating, treats, walks, and play time, as well as various special holiday rituals throughout the year. Photos with Santa, dog park outings, holiday ornaments on the tree, Halloween costumes, and bunny ears at Easter-pet parents can be found doing any or all these things in their role as a caring and loving pet owner. Therefore, performing rituals during the final days of a pet's life should be very organic and natural. Oftentimes, pet parents just need ideas and information through a gentle questioning process. They also need permission to openly express their love through rituals, however quirky these might appear from the outside. There is power in knowing that other pet parents love their pets just as much and in seeing what they do to show their love for their furry family members.

Consider some of these rituals to share with families, as they search for special events to do with their pets for the final time:

- Let the animal eat what he wants. Was it steak, French fries, pizza, or candy that intrigued them as they watched you indulge? Let them indulge.

- What brought the animal the most joy? Car rides? McDonalds? The dog park? Grandma and Grandpa's? Do these special things often in the final days.

- Guide pet parents in how to engage an elderly or sick animal in play rituals. A dog who loved to chase a ball can still get great pleasure from having a ball gently rolled several inches from her nose, just to where she can comfortably retrieve it. Help the pet parent find creative ways to keep the animal doing the things she loves to do.

- Have a "pre-morial." This is a service held before death occurs. Have friends and family members over, especially those who have animals who are friends with the aging or sick pet, for an evening of reminiscing. Allow those in attendance the opportunity to say their goodbyes and give their final kisses. This might also be a good time for those in attendance to share their sentiments and memories with the pet owner about the dying animal. These are all beautiful ways to show support to the family during this emotionally heavy time.

- Encourage pet owners to take this time to make video and audio recordings. It's heartwarming to have a pet's "voice" recorded for posterity. Furthermore, each pet parent knows their pet's barks and meows – the barks that say I'm happy, the barks that say I'm hungry, and the barks that are meant for the UPS driver. They are all just as unique as hearing another human voice!

- Make paw print projects. Every pet owner remembers the muddy paws, the paws that wipe away the tears, the paws that call themselves to our attention. Therefore, capture these paw prints to forever remember those times. From jewelry with paw prints to special garden rocks that sport a pet's paw print, these are all special pieces that will always be treasured. As a teachable moment for a child, guide them in making their own clay paw print and/or stepping stone, a piece the child will have forever as they fondly remember their childhood pet friend.

- Use technology to gather emotional support. Many pet parents, when dealing with the terminal diagnosis of a pet or with the realization that a pet's age is taking its toll, will create bucket lists for these pets. These lists are then posted on social media sites to allow others the opportunity to show their support for the pet owners as they face their devastating loss. The viral nature of these posts is amazing as this affinity group of pet parents *want* to find others who share in their love for their pet and *need* the support.

- Use technology to capture final days and moments. Suggest hiring a photographer to chronicle final days and events or to have a final "sunset photo session," capturing the tenderness of the human–animal bond. Post photos or video on social sites so that others can share in their support for the pet's family.

- Guide pet parents in the simple art of journaling about the emotions, their day, the animal's day, the fears, the questions, the desires. Journaling can help with the healthy release of emotions and can provide a record of the pet's day-to-day health, which can help shape the pet's care plan.

- Help parents help the children in the household. Things like letter writing, planting a flower, or planting a tree as a tribute to the pet are great ways to assist in getting children ready for the day that they will have to say goodbye to their friend. Give parents the permission and guidance to do these things with their children. Many parents fear the reaction their children will have to the impending death of a pet, so they shy away from a powerful teachable moment. Children are great mourners. They just need a safe venue to do what they organically know how to do and that is to be real and to be present in the now. (A great lesson for adults, wouldn't you say?) Of course children may cry; they are facing a time that will forever affect them as a person. Crying represents a healthy release of emotion. Pet care professionals can be a valuable resource for parents as they not only struggle with their own grief but search for the strength to help their child.

- Practice the art of giving. Find a charity and establish a memorial fund in honor of the pet and request donations, either monetary or practical. Of course, an organic charity of choice would be an animal shelter or rescue facility. What a wonderful way to give back in the pet's name and memory.

Emotional Support: Honoring the Journey

Whether it is guidance and support in the rituals a family might want to perform or support for the emotional journey, pet parents are looking for every ounce of strength and support they can get during the final days of their pet's life.

When the time has come for old age to take over a young body or when an animal has been given a terminal diagnosis, the family's grief journey begins with a process called "anticipatory grief." In anticipatory grief, the emotions and feelings are similar to those experienced when death occurs. It's during this time that a family will look to a pet care professional for the information needed to give the final days those quality moments that are desired.

The anticipatory grief process, much like grief experienced after a death has occurred, can be emotionally draining. Pet owners need to have their feelings of fear validated and acknowledged during this time. They want to know it's okay to be scared, to be angry, and to be distraught. The role of a pet care professional is to honor these feelings and to walk with the family for support – not lead them, not walk behind them, but walk *beside* them.

With this time of anticipatory grief, the anxiety of the final days of a pet's life are full of the fear of the unknown. Questions arise such as:

- Will I have to make a decision about euthanasia?
- If so, how will I know when the time is right?

- What does the disease progression look like?
- Will there be pain in my beloved pet?
- What will I do after he/she does die?
- What are my options for the care of the body?
- What questions do I ask about the one that will be taking care of my pet's remains?
- I don't want to regret anything but what else is there to do?
- Will I be shamed if I ask for other options because I want to explore everything?
- What does the new normal look like?
- How will I survive without him/her?

Open and transparent conversations, where the pet owner is viewed fully as a team member and participating in the pet's care, will assist in alleviating many of these fears. Families need a plan, which many times might include homework. "Homework" is a wonderful word for mourning work, which is needed for a grieving family. We feel the grief, but to make movement in our grief journey we must mourn, with mourning being the active version of grieving. Give the family homework to do during the time between medical team visits. They can be given such tasks as taking photos daily to share with the medical team, journaling about the emotional well-being of the pet and themselves, and actively seeking to maximize quality of life for the animal. Getting the family actively involved with care will help allay fears of the unknown. This is also the perfect time for them to do more than just preparing for the final day, as this is the time for some unforgettable Bucket List events. Help them create a perfect ending.

Help pet parents craft what the end will look like. What are their goals for the pending death – hospice-assisted natural death or euthanasia? And, with both options, map out for them what it will look like, how it might feel, and what they should be doing during this time of the active dying process.

Perhaps most important, give them permission throughout the entire journey to change their mind, whether about the timing of euthanasia or any other hard-stop rules that they themselves have established.

Assisting Children, Other Pets, and Family Members in Their Journey

As mentioned previously, it's important to let children be as much a part of the pet's EOL care and dying process as they wish. When a pet dies, children should have the opportunity to say their final good-byes to their friend. Help pet parents to embrace this process – even their child's tears – as a wonderful, tender moment that the family can share together.

Interestingly, children are amazing mourners. They seem to know how to mourn a loss and perform the task naturally and in a very healthy way. Watch a child when he's in a situation like this. The child will dose himself by letting in a bit of the pain briefly and then returning to play or another activity to distract himself. When he feels like it, he will let in another little bit of pain. To adults, it can appear that the child is doing well with the loss, which can sometimes mean the child is forgotten in the grief journey. However, children do hold onto the grief and need the permission and opportunity to join in the entire family's grieving and mourning rituals.

Other pets in the family also need the opportunity to see and smell their deceased friend. Educate families on how animals process information, especially when one of their own has died. They need to smell the animal and to perform their own mourning rituals. So many anecdotes have been cited where a pet was put into the car to go to the veterinary clinic for euthanasia. The family returns from that visit, obviously without the pet, and the surviving pets at home become confused, search for their pet friend, and even appear to be depressed. By giving them the opportunity to smell and see the deceased pet, they have confirmation of what has happened, and they too can begin their own kind of grieving.

There is wonderful healing for a family in slowing down after the death and giving everyone in the family the opportunity to say their goodbyes. From surviving pet friends, children, and other friends and family members, creating a visitation time much like we do for human loved ones is incredibly cathartic. When given this opportunity to spend some special quality time after a death with their beloved pet, families have found this is the perfect time for extra I love you's, I'm sorry's, a final toast, or even a funeral service.

After-Death Care Options

Understanding the final arrangement options available for a pet's body is another part of the healing process for a family. Knowing the decision they made for their pet's body was the right decision given their living situation, their religious preferences, and other unique elements surrounding this subject gives a family peace of mind. Educating a family on their various options and helping them find what's right for them, is a meaningful way to be a responsible and caring pet care professional.

In pet death care, there are four generally accepted options: taxidermy, freeze-drying, cremation, and burial. The choice among these options can be fraught with questions and concerns. The *Topics in Companion Animal Medicine* research project (Cooney et al. 2021) found that families have common concerns when it comes to their pet's final arrangements (see Table 30.2).

This research also explored what respondents consider acceptable or unacceptable in the holding and transportation of their pet's body (Table 30.3).

Many families will choose burial for their pet. Pet burials have been undergoing an evolution, with many human cemeteries now applying for zoning changes and rededication of their grounds to allow pets and people to be buried together or, at minimum, to have pet sections housed within human cemeteries. Cemeteries nationwide are being asked for permission to have their family plots now include the *entire* family, furry children included. If it's burial that

Table 30.2 Concern and views regarding after-death body care. *Kathleen A. Cooney et al. 2021 / With permission of Elsevier.*

	1 – Not Concerned at All	2	3	4	5 – Very Concerned
That my pet might be mislabeled or lost (n = 1942)	358 (18.4%)	262 (13.5%)	301 (15.5%)	439 (22.6%)	582 (30.0%)
That I won't be able to memorialize or honor my pet the way I want (n = 1950)	393 (20.2%)	300 (15.4%)	375 (19.2%)	423 (21.7%)	459 (23.5%)
The cost of my pet's after-death body care (n = 1950)	227 (11.6%)	186 (9.5%)	346 (17.7%)	545 (27.9%)	646 (33.1%)
How my pet is physically handled by other people after their death (n = 1948)	247 (12.7%)	208 (10.7%)	380 (19.5%)	461 (23.7%)	652 (33.5%)
The type of container my pet is stored in immediately after their death (before burial or cremation) (n = 1938)	360 (18.6%)	292 (15.1%)	390 (20.1%)	440 (22.7%)	456 (23.5%)
The type of container my pet is stored in permanently (n = 1930)	281 (14.6%)	209 (10.8%)	360 (18.7%)	470 (24.4%)	610 (31.6%)
Keeping my pet separate from other deceased pets immediately after their death (before burial or cremation) (n = 1927)	376 (19.5%)	278 (14.4%)	369 (19.1%)	419 (21.7%)	485 (15.2%)
Keeping my pet with the physical keepsakes they loved in life (e.g. toys, blanket) immediately after their death (n = 1945)	358 (18.4%)	241 (12.4%)	328 (16.9%)	427 (22.0%)	591 (30.4%)
Minimizing the amount of time between my pet's death and their final resting state (burial, cremation) (n = 1929)	201 (10.4%)	172 (8.9%)	351 (18.2%)	544 (28.2%)	661 (34.3%)

Table 30.3 Participants' views on acceptability of after-death body storage options (before burial or cremation). *Kathleen A. Cooney et al. 2021 / With permission of Elsevier.*

	Unacceptable	Neutral	Acceptable
Blanket/shroud	87 (4.3%)	596 (29.5%)	1334 (66.1%)
Trash bag	1290 (64.0%)	413 (20.5%)	314 (15.6%)
Designated cadaver bag	163 (8.1%)	789 (39.1%)	1065 (52.8%)
Casket	152 (7.5%)	831 (41.2%)	1034 (51.3%)

a family is looking for, here are some questions to ask of the pet cemeteries:

- What is the perpetual care aspect of the cemetery, ensuring that it will be dedicated as a pet cemetery forever?
- What are the burial requirements – casket, vault, marker?
- If a cemetery is deemed a "green cemetery," what kinds of materials are required for burial shrouds or caskets?
- Can the family be present for the burial?
- Does the cemetery allow for preplanning and prefunding burial arrangements?

While burial has traditionally been the most common choice for animals, following trends in human death care, cremation is growing far more popular. One of the main reasons for this is the increasing mobility of our society. People are not living in the same houses or even the same towns for their entire lives like they did in the past. Instead, we are a more transient society, making cremation a more practical choice because a pet's ashes can be taken with us when we go.

Veterinary professionals are nearly always the transactional agent between the family and the crematory. As such, it is imperative for veterinary professional to know the details chapter about their chosen cremation facility's standard operating procedures and business practices. With cremation, there are a variety of educational questions and information to share with a family. First and foremost, it's implied that you, the pet care professional, have fulfilled your responsibility in doing due diligence on the crematory partner being used by your clinic. It is imperative that this part of your business model has been put through the paces, ensuring that pets entrusted to this facility are being cared for correctly.

There are three ways to cremate a pet: private, partitioned, and communal. Their definitions according to the Pet Loss Professional Alliance are as follows:

Private Cremation. A cremation procedure during which only one animal's body is present in the cremation unit during the cremation process. All retrievable cremated remains should be collected from each cremation prior to placing the next animal's body in the cremation unit. Operators should not use the word "private" in the title or description of any service in which more than one animal is cremated in any part of a single cremation unit at the same time, but should use descriptions like "semiprivate," "privately partitioned."

Partitioned Cremation. A cremation procedure during which more than one pet's body is present in the cremation chamber and the cremated remains of specific pets are to be returned. By virtue of multiple pets being cremated within the same unit at the same time, active commingling of cremated remains will occur.

Communal Cremation. A cremation procedure where multiple animals are cremated together without any form of separation. These commingled cremated remains are not returned to owners.

Many veterinary professionals or caregivers have never had the cremation process properly defined. Cremation is a two-part process. The first part of the process is heating to reduce human or animal remains to bone fragments. The second part of cremation is the removal of the skeletal remains from the retort, followed by the processing that reduces bone fragments to unidentifiable dimensions, or ashes as they are commonly known.

Other terms that pet care professionals should know are:

Commingling. Mixing of cremated remains.

Active Commingling. Commingling that occurs between animals during the cremation and/or retrieval process when multiple animals are cremated together at the same time. This type of comingling can be minimized with effective partitioning, but it is impossible eliminate commingling entirely. This type of commingling cannot, by definition, occur with a private cremation.

Residual (Incidental) Commingling. This refers to unavoidable incidental commingling between cremations, which occurs despite best efforts to recover all cremains from each cremation. This will occur to varying degrees with any type of cremation. This definition is the minimal type of commingling that takes place even in cremations performed in succession, both in human cremations and private pet cremations.

As a pet care professional, finding a reputable crematory should override finding the cheapest in the market. Find a crematory business to partner with, versus one who will just function as a supplier. Family's needs and demands are changing and knowing you can stay in your area of expertise, animal medicine, and let the pet loss professionals do the elevated work will create a beautiful symbiotic level of care for a family.

The pet owner should ask these questions so that a cremation partner can provide a full disclosure of this process:

- How are the pets held before cremation?
- How are pets identified and tracked during this process?
  - Many organizations will use a metal tracking process, much like a toe-tag for a human, which will attach to the pet. This tag will follow the pet throughout the process, ensuring the safety and security of the body and cremation. There are a few companies that will also use electronic tracking, much like a shipping company. With this, providers can log in to a portal at any time and see where the pet is in the cremation progression.
- How long are the bodies held before cremation?
- When will the ashes be ready to be returned to the family?

- How will the ashes be returned?
- What else is included in the package?
- Can a pet owner visit the facility?
  - Is there an open-door policy for the cremation provider? If they will not let people visit the facility at any time, one might wonder what's being hidden, and a new crematory provider should probably be chosen. Good and reputable pet cremation providers pride themselves in having an open door and full transparency in the process. This gives the pet parent and pet care professional the peace of mind in knowing that the business is being run in a caring and ethical manner.
- Can the pet owner witness the cremation process?
- Is there an opportunity to have a viewing or ceremony at their establishment?
- Will they provide transport the pet's body from the home or clinic with the high level of care desired?
  - Many cremation providers will use a cot or a casket, not a bag, to remove pets so that families get that extended level of care and respect for the body. If a family is dedicated enough to provide hospice care for their pet, don't take them all the way to the end and then let the care in this area fail.
- What type of other services do they provide?
  - Pet loss support groups?
  - Assistance with children and other pets in grief?
  - Opportunities for a service or visitation?

There are two other options available for the final arrangements of a pet's body: taxidermy and freeze drying. Taxidermy involves the preservation of an animal's body by stuffing or by mounting the skin over mold. Freeze-drying uses extremely cold temperatures and vacuum pressure to halt decomposition by removing moisture from an animal's body. Like taxidermy, cryopreservation leaves an animal looking like they did on the day they died.

Summary

Pet parents who pursue hospice and palliative care are generally those same pet parents who desire an EOL journey that respects the individuality and dignity of their pet, during death and beyond. They want to be given guidance and support in paying tribute to the unique being who shared his or her life with them.

References

Cooney, K., Kogan, L., Brooks, S. et al. (2021) Pet Owners' expectations for pet end-of-life support and after-death body care: exploration and practical applications, *Topics in Companion Animal Medicine*, 43: 100503. https://doi.org/10.1016/j.tcam.2020.100503.

Index

Hospice and Palliative Care for Companion Animals: Principles and Practice, Second Edition.
Edited by Amir Shanan, Jessica Pierce, and Tamara Shearer.
© 2023 John Wiley & Sons, Inc. Published 2023 by John Wiley & Sons, Inc.
Companion website: www.wiley.com/go/shanan/palliative